Practical Paediatrics

Practical Paediatrics

Edited by

M. J. Robinson MD FRACP
Reader in Paediatrics, University of Melbourne

Foreword by

P. D. Phelan Bsc MD FRACP
Stevenson Professor of Paediatrics,
University of Melbourne, Chief Thoracic
Physician, Royal Children's Hospital, Melbourne

SECOND EDITION

CHURCHILL LIVINGSTONE
MELBOURNE EDINBURGH LONDON AND NEW YORK 1990

CHURCHILL LIVINGSTONE
Medical Division of Longman Group UK Limited

Distributed in Australia by Longman Cheshire Pty Limited,
Longman House, Kings Gardens, 95 Coventry Street, South
Melbourne 3205, and by associated companies, branches and
representatives throughout the world.

First edition 1986
Second edition 1990

ISBN 0-443-04053-2

British Library Cataloguing in Publication Data
Practical paediatrics 2. – 2nd ed.
  1. Children. Diseases
  I. Robinson, M. J. (Maxwell James)
  618.92

Library of Congress Cataloging in Publication Data
Practical paediatrics 2/edited by M. J. Robinson; foreword
  by P. D Phelan. – 2nd ed.
      p. cm.
    Includes bibliographical references.
    ISBN 0-443-04053-2
    1. Pediatrics. I. Robinson, M. J. (Maxwell James)
    II. Title:
  Practical paediatrics two.
    [DNLM: 1. Pediatrics. WS 100 P8953]
  RJ45.P6583 1990
  618.92–dc20
  DNLM/DLC
  for Library of Congress   89-24012

Produced by Longman Singapore Publishers (Pte.) Ltd.
Printed in Singapore

Foreword

The first edition of *Practical Paediatrics* rapidly established itself as the most popular undergraduate textbook of general paediatrics in Australia and has been extremely well received in the United Kingdom, Europe and North America. It has been widely used by medical students, resident medical officers and general practitioners.

While the book is written from an Australian perspective, it is easy to see why the first edition has proven so popular in other parts of the world. The title *Practical Paediatrics* is very appropriate because first and foremost this is a practical book for all of those responsible for the health care of children in developed societies.

Much material has been added to this volume. There are new sections on endocrinology, the special senses, emergencies in paediatrics and on intrauterine and perinatal infections. There are a number of new contributors from the various paediatric centres in Australia. Most of the major sections from the first edition have been rewritten and revised to include updated material.

The high standards of the first edition are maintained in this new edition. It covers in detail the common health problems of children and adolescents which should be known by medical students. Chapters on less common disorders put these into proper perspective and so allow this to be a very useful reference book as well. The clinical approach of the book is essential for students and general practitioners, and practical advice is given on appropriate investigations and management. The problem orientated approach of many chapters will also be found very helpful.

Undoubtedly, the second edition will continue the popularity of this book and it is to be highly recommended to undergraduate medical students as their basic text in paediatrics. It will continue to be useful to general practitioners and others involved in child health care.

Melbourne, 1989   P. D. Phelan

Preface

It is pleasing to edit a second edition of *Practical Paediatrics* just three years after the first. This book has been revised extensively and a number of chapters rewritten completely. The contents have been rearranged into what I believe is a more logical sequence. The sections on neonatology, endocrinology and infection have been enlarged and a new section entitled 'Special senses' incorporating chapters on the eye, ear, nose and throat, and the teeth has been added. Two additional chapters 'The collapsed child' and 'Disorders of connective tissue' have also been included.

Practical Paediatrics has an extra 22 contributors bringing the total number to 55. It has been a great pleasure and a privilege to work with this distinguished group of Australian paediatricians. We have almost managed to keep the size of this volume to that of the first edition, despite increasing the number of chapters by eight, and substantially increasing the number of photographs, diagrams, charts and other types of illustrations. *Practical Paediatrics* should remain as it is –

a textbook for the undergraduate student rather than a reference volume. Nonetheless, I believe that there is sufficient material in this book to both inform and stimulate the student to further enquiry. It should also be useful to doctors who treat children in general practice and to nurse educators in paediatrics.

The teaching of paediatrics in most Western universities is given over approximately 12 weeks. Reading one chapter of *Practical Paediatrics* each day will enable the student to cover this entire book during the paediatric term.

I hope that this revised version will be seen to be even more practical than the first. More emphasis has been given to management; but at the same time the commitment to social and preventive paediatrics has been continued and the problem orientated approach maintained.

Melbourne, 1990   M. J. Robinson

Acknowledgements

Preparation of the second edition of *Practical Paediatrics* has been simplified thanks to the help received from many people. I should like to personally thank Professor Peter Phelan, Stevenson Professor of Paediatrics at the University of Melbourne, for advice and encouragement in the preparation of this manuscript. Dr Lyn Gilbert, Director of Microbiology at the Royal Children's Hospital, provided invaluable criticism and advice in rewriting Chapters 29 and 31, whilst Dr Paul Lancaster, Head, National Perinatal Statistics Unit, Sydney, provided much statistical information on infant mortality which has been incorporated into Chapter 1. The Medical Illustration Department of the University of New South Wales and teaching hospitals provided the radiographs used in Chapter 52. The Department of Radiology of the Royal Children's Hospital, Melbourne, provided the many other radiographs included in the text. I thank the Director, Dr David Boldt, and his staff for help in the selection of films. The Educational Resource Centre at the Royal Children's Hospital gave freely of their time and expertise in the preparation of the many tables, diagrams and illustrations and I would particularly like to thank Ms Gabrielle Posetti, Ms Gigi Nieuwenhuis, Ms Jocelyn Bell, Ms Sue Panckridge, Ms Joanne Sullivan and Mr Cornell Papov.

It is again a pleasure to acknowledge the diligence and skills of my secretary, Ms Mary Reddan. I cannot imagine the delays that would have occurred without her willing help.

Thanks are also due to my publishers, Churchill Livingstone, and in particular, to Ms Judy Waters, Mrs Sandra Tolra, Mrs Hilly Wilson and Ms Fiona Julian.

Contributors

Robert Adler D FRACP
Professor and Director, Department of Child and
Family Psychiatry, Royal Children's Hospital,
Melbourne

Agnes Bankier MB BS FRACP(Paed)
Medical Geneticist, Royal Children's Hospital,
Melbourne

Graeme Barnes MD FRACP
Director of Gastroenterology, Royal Children's
Hospital, Melbourne

John Boulton BSc MD FRACP
Foundation Professor of Paediatrics, University of
Newcastle, New South Wales

G. K. Brown MB BS PhD(Syd)
Senior Lecturer (Human Genetics), Department of
Paediatrics, University of Melbourne, Melbourne

A. D. Bryan MB BS(Qld) FRACP
Deputy Director, Department of Child Development
and Rehabilitation, Royal Children's Hospital,
Melbourne; Consultant Paediatrician, Yooralla Society
of Victoria, Melbourne

Neil Buchanan FRACP PhD
Professor of Paediatrics, University of Sydney, Sydney

John Burke FRACP
 Nephrologist, Mater Misericordiae and Royal
Children's Hospitals, Brisbane

Allan Carmichael MD FRACP
Director of Regional Paediatric Services, Royal
Children's Hospital, Melbourne; Chairman, Victorian
Child Protection Council, Melbourne

A. C. L. Clark MD FRACP
Professor of Paediatrics, Monash University, Monash
Medical Centre, Melbourne

W. G. Cole MB BS MSc PhD
Associate Professor Department of Paediatrics,
University of Melbourne, Melbourne

Kevin J. Collins MB BS FRACP
Neurologist, Department of Neurology and
Department of Child Development and
Rehabilitation, Royal Children's Hospital, Melbourne;
Paediatric Neurologist, Monash Medical Centre,
Melbourne

John M. Court MB BS FRACP
Physician and Director, Department of Adolescent
Medicine, Royal Children's Hospital, Melbourne

David M. Danks MD FRACP
Director, Murdoch Institute for Research into Birth
Defects, Royal Children's Hospital, Melbourne;
Professor of Paediatric Research, University of
Melbourne, Melbourne

Geoffrey Davidson MD FRACP
Director, Gastroenterology Unit, Adelaide Children's
Hospital, Adelaide

Henry Ekert MD BE FRACP FRCPA
Director, Department of Clinical Haematology and
Oncology, Royal Children's Hospital, Melbourne

Peter Fergin MB BS FACD
Dermatologist, Melbourne

G. L. Gilbert FRACP FRCPA
Director of Microbiology and Infectious Diseases,
Royal Children's Hospital, Melbourne

Philip Graves MRCP FRACP DCH
Senior Lecturer, Department of Paediatrics, Monash
Medical Centre, Clayton; Consultant Paediatrician,
Office of Intellectual Disability Services, Victoria

A. A. Haan MB BS BMedSc FRACP
Medical Geneticist, Department of Genetics, Adelaide
Children's Hospital, Adelaide

Roger K. Hall MDSc(Melb) FRACDS
Director, Department of Dentistry, Royal Children's
Hospital, Melbourne; Senior Associate, Departments
of Paediatrics, Community and Preventive Dentistry

and Dental Medicine and Surgery, University of Melbourne, Melbourne

Geoffrey Harley MB BS DO FRACO
Department of Ophthalmology, Royal Children's Hospital, Melbourne

Ross Haslam MB BS FRACP
Director, Neonatal Intensive Care, The Queen Victoria Hospital, Rose Park, Adelaide

I. J. Hopkins MD FRACP
Senior Neurologist, Royal Children's Hospital, Melbourne; First Assistant, Department of Paediatrics, University of Melbourne

Cliff Hosking MD FRACP FRCPA
Clinical Immunologist, Department of Immunology, Royal Children's Hospital, Melbourne

Andrew Kemp MB BS PhD FRACP
Head, Department of Immunology, Royal Alexandra Hospital for Children, Camperdown, Sydney

Geoffrey Klug MB BS FRACS
Neurosurgeon, Royal Children's Hospital, Melbourne

Louis I. Landau MD FRACP
Professor of Child Health, University of Western Australia, Perth

Rae Matthews FRACP MRCP DCH
Clinical Haematologist, Royal Children's Hospital, Melbourne

D. A. McCredie BSc MD FRACP
Senior Physician, Royal Children's Hospital, Melbourne

Craig M. Mellis MB BS FRACP
Head, Department of Respiratory Medicine, Royal Alexandra Hospital for Children, Camperdown, Sydney

Malcolm Menelaus MD FRCS FRACS
Director, Department of Orthopaedics, Royal Children's Hospital, Melbourne

Bernard W. Neal MD FRACP Dip Ed
Senior Physician and Dean of Postgraduate Studies, Royal Children's Hospital, Melbourne

Kim Oates MD MHP FRAMA FRCP FRACP DCH
Professor of Paediatrics and Child Health, The University of Sydney; Chairman, Division of Medicine, Royal Alexandra Hospital for Children, Camperdown, Sydney

Frank Oberklaid MB BS FRACP
Director, Department of Ambulatory Paediatrics, Royal Children's Hospital, Melbourne; Senior

Associate, Department of Paediatrics, University of Melbourne, Melbourne

Anthony Olinsky MB MCh FCPSA FRACP
Director, Professorial Department of Thoracic Medicine, Royal Children's Hospital, Melbourne

Robert Ouvrier MB BS BSc(Med) FRACP
Head, Department of Neurology, Royal Alexandra Hospital for Children, Camperdown, Sydney

John Pearn MD PhD(Lond) BSc FRCP(UK) FRACP DCH
Head, Department of Child Health, University of Queensland, Brisbane

James Penfold MB BS FRACP
Senior Lecturer, Department of Paediatrics, University of Adelaide; Director, Endocrine and Diabetic Clinics, Adelaide Children's Hospital, Adelaide

P. D. Phelan BSc MD FRACP
Stevenson Professor of Paediatrics, University of Melbourne; Chief Thoracic Physician, Royal Children's Hospital, Melbourne

H. R. Powell MB BS FRACP
Director, Renal Unit, Royal Children's Hospital, Melbourne

D. M. Roberton MD FRACP
Professor of Paediatrics, University of Adelaide, Adelaide

John G. Rogers MB BS DCH FRACP
Director, Department of Genetics, Royal Children's Hospital, Melbourne; Medical Geneticist, Murdoch Institute for Research into Birth Defects; Clinical Geneticist, Queen Victoria Medical Centre, Melbourne

Andrew R. Rosenberg MB FRACP
Head, Department of Nephrology, Prince of Wales Children's Hospital, Sydney

Frank Shann MD FRACP
Director, Department of Intensive Care, Royal Children's Hospital, Melbourne

L. J. Sheffield FRACP BMedSc MSc DCH
Medical Geneticist, Royal Children's Hospital, Melbourne; Head of Genetics Clinic, Royal Women's Hospital, Melbourne; Medical Geneticist, Royal Victorian Eye and Ear Hospital; Head of Epidemiology Section, Murdoch Institute for Research into Birth Defects, Melbourne

L. K. Shield MB BS BSc FRACP
Director, Department of Neurology, Royal Children's Hospital, Melbourne

Martin Silink MD FRACP
Director, Ray Williams Institute of Paediatric
Endocrinology, Diabetes and Metabolism, Princess
Alexandra Hospital for Children, Camperdown,
Sydney

Arnold Smith MB BS FRACP
Deputy Director, Department of Gastroenterology,
Royal Children's Hospital, Melbourne

Geoffrey P. Tauro MB BS FRACP FRCPA
Director, Department of Laboratory Haematology,
Royal Children's Hospital, Melbourne

D. I. Tudehope MB BS(Monash) FRACP
Director of Neonatology, Mater Mothers Hospital,
Brisbane Clinical Reader in Neonatal Paediatrics,
Department of Child Health, University of
Queensland, Brisbane

George A. Varigos MB BS FACD
Head of Dermatology, Royal Melbourne Hospital,
Royal Children's Hospital, Melbourne

A. W. Venables MD FRACP
Emeritus Director, Department of Cardiology, Royal
Children's Hospital, Melbourne

Garry L. Warne MB BS FRACP
Director of Endocrinology and Diabetes, Royal
Children's Hospital, Melbourne

Keith Waters MB BS FRACP
Deputy Director, Department of Clinical
Haematology and Oncology, Royal Children's
Hospital, Melbourne

Robert Webb MB BS FRACS DLO(Melb)
Otolaryngologist, Royal Children's Hospital,
Melbourne

George Werther MB BS FRACP MSc(Oxon)
Department of Endocrinology and Diabetes, Royal
Children's Hospital, Melbourne

J. Wilkinson MB ChB FRCP(Lond)
Director, Department of Cardiology, Royal Children's
Hospital, Melbourne

Victor Y. H. Yu MD MSc(Oxon) FRACP, FRCP(Lond) DCH
Director of Neonatal Intensive Care, Monash Medical
Centre; Clinical Associate Professor of Paediatrics,
Monash University, Melbourne

Contents

SECTION 1
Paediatrics in the nineties

1. Child health and disease   3
   M. J. Robinson

2. Ethics in paediatrics   12
   Bernard W. Neal

SECTION 2
Genetics

3. Birth defects   19
   David M. Danks, John G. Rogers

4. Genes and chromosomes   26
   G. K. Brown

5. Molecular genetics   33
   G. K. Brown

6. Prenatal diagnosis   41
   L. J. Sheffield

7. Approach to the dysmorphic child   45
   Agnes Bankier

8. Genetic counselling   55
   John G. Rogers

SECTION 3
Clinical assessment

9. The clinical history and physical examination   61
   M. J. Robinson

10. Posture and common orthopaedic problems   69
    Malcolm Menelaus

11. Developmental screening and assessment   77
    Kim Oates

SECTION 4
Social and preventive paediatrics

12. The child and the family   85
    M. J. Robinson

13. Nutrition   90
    John Boulton

14. Immunization   99
    Cliff Hosking

15. Child trauma   103
    John Pearn

16. The child with school problems   111
    Frank Oberklaid

17. The physically disabled child   117
    A. C. L. Clark

18. The intellectually disabled child   122
    Philip Graves

19. The family in difficulty   129
    M. J. Robinson

20. Failure to thrive   140
    M. J. Robinson

21. Child abuse   145
    Allan Carmichael

SECTION 5
Allergy and immunity

22. Factors involved in resistance to infection   153
    D. M. Roberton

23. The atopic child   163
    Andrew Kemp

SECTION 6
Neonatal problems

24. Prematurity and low birthweight   173
    Victor Y. H. Yu

25. The infant with respiratory distress   181
    D. I. Tudehope

26. The jaundiced infant   192
    Ross Haslam

27. Congenital and perinatal infections 200
G. L. Gilbert

28. Inborn errors of metabolism 208
A. A. Haan

SECTION 7
Infection in childhood

29. Infectious diseases of childhood 217
M. J. Robinson, G. L. Gilbert

30. Infections of bone and joint 228
W. G. Cole

31. Meningitis and encephalitis in infancy and childhood 235
M. J. Robinson, G. L. Gilbert

32. Pyrexia of unknown origin (PUO) 244
M. J. Robinson

SECTION 8
Paediatric emergencies

33. The collapsed child 251
Frank Shann

SECTION 9
Respiratory disorders

34. The epidemiology of acute respiratory infections 261
P. D. Phelan

35. Clinical patterns of acute respiratory infections 265
P. D. Phelan

36. The child who wheezes 275
Craig M. Mellis

37. Asthma in childhood 284
Louis I. Landau

38. The child with a persistent cough 292
Anthony Olinsky

SECTION 10
Cardiac disorders

39. Heart disease in infancy and childhood 307
A. W. Venables

40. Common congenital heart lesions 320
J. Wilkinson

SECTION 11
Haematology and oncology

41. The pale child 333
M. J. Robinson

42. Iron deficiency in childhood 342
Geoffrey P. Tauro

43. Abnormal bleeding 349
Henry Ekert

44. The thalassaemias 357
Rae Matthews

45. The problem of malignancy 363
Keith Waters

SECTION 12
Disorders of the nervous system

46. Convulsions and epilepsies 375
I. J. Hopkins

47. Cerebral palsy and cerebral degeneration 385
Robert Ouvrier, Kevin J. Collins

48. Neuromuscular disease 394
L. K. Shield

49. The child with a large head 403
Geoffrey Klug

50. Neural tube defects 412
A. D. Bryan

SECTION 13
Fluid and electrolyte homeostasis. Renal disorders

51. Fluid and electrolyte physiology 421
H. R. Powell

52. Urinary tract malformations and infection 430
Andrew R. Rosenberg

53. Glomerulonephritis and related diseases Hypertension 437
John Burke

SECTION 14
Endocrinology and metabolism

54. Growth 447
James Penfold

55. Thyroid disorders in children 467
George Werther

56. The child with ambiguous genitalia 474
Garry L. Warne

57. Childhood diabetes and hypoglycaemia   480
    Martin Silink

58. Disorders of calcium metabolism and bone   488
    D. A. McCredie

SECTION 15
Problems of gastrointestinal tract and liver

59. Vomiting in infancy and childhood   497
    M. J. Robinson

60. The child with diarrhoea   505
    Graeme Barnes

61. Malabsorption   514
    Geoffrey Davidson

62. The child with abdominal pain   526
    M. J. Robinson

63. The problem of liver disease   532
    Arnold Smith

SECTION 16
Behaviour

64. Common behavioural disturbances   543
    Robert Adler

65. Major psychiatric disorders in children and
    adolescents   550
    Robert Adler

66. Adolescence   556
    John M. Court

SECTION 17
The skin

67. The neonate with a rash   565
    George A. Varigos, Peter Fergin

68. The child with a rash   567
    Peter Fergin

69. Skin lesions in systemic disease   579
    M. J. Robinson

SECTION 18
Special senses

70. The eye   591
    Geoffrey Harley

71. Ear, nose and throat problems   599
    Robert Webb

72. The teeth   610
    Roger K. Hall

SECTION 19
Disorders of connective tissue

73. Connective tissue disorders   621
    M. J. Robinson, D. M. Roberton

SECTION 20
Pharmacology

74. Drug therapy in childhood and adolescence   633
    Neil Buchanan

Index   645

Paediatrics in the nineties

1. Child health and disease

M. J. Robinson

Paediatrics has changed dramatically since the last generation when paediatricians and other child health workers were preoccupied with the management of infectious illness. Although the problem of infection has by no means been solved (witness the emergence of AIDS) the morbidity and, in particular, the mortality due to infection has been so reduced in developed societies that those concerned with the health of children are able to become involved in other areas and other issues. Examples are many, but of particular importance is the greatly reduced incidence of tuberculosis, chronic suppuration of chest, bone and ear, rheumatic fever and rheumatic heart disease and streptococcal infections of all types. Disease patterns have changed because of improved standards of living with better nutrition, less overcrowding, immunization and a better educated society. It should be noted that the incidence of all infections was falling before the advent of antibiotic and chemotherapeutic drugs, which, incorrectly, have often been given the major credit for control of infection.

In evaluating disease incidence and health status of a community, mortality and morbidity figures are used. Mortality has been the most widespread criterion, the figures being readily obtained because of compulsory reporting of death. They are of limited value in assessing the health status and heatlh needs of a community. It is the morbidity which really determines the need for and type of health services. To be reliable, morbidity statistics need to be prospective and reflect accurate diagnosis and complete case reporting. This is very difficult to achieve so it is not surprising that there have been few good morbidity data since the One Thousand Families study in Newcastle-upon-Tyne in 1947. Reliable morbidity data for acute illness in Australia are not available. The studies of Fergusson et al (1982) in New Zealand are producing very reliable morbidity data which may have relevance to other developed societies.

Definitions

The following definitions are important in collecting data on mortality.

Live births

This is defined as the complete expulsion or extraction from its mother, irrespective of the duration of pregnancy, of a product of conception, which after separation breathes or shows other evidence of life such as heart beat.

Still birth

This is a product of conception weighing at least 500 grams but if the weight is not known, a product of conception of at least 22 weeks' gestation which, after expulsion or extraction from its mother, did not breathe or show any other evidence of life such as heart beat.

Stillbirth rate

The number of stillbirths per 1000 of all births live and stillborn.

Neonatal mortality rate

The number of deaths of live born infants within 28 days of birth per 1000 live births.

Perinatal mortality rate

This is expressed as the number of perinatal deaths (neonatal deaths plus stillbirths per 1000 births live and still).

Post-neonatal mortality rate

This is expressed as the number of deaths between 28 days and 1 year per 1000 live births.

Table 1.1   Infant mortality in the States and Territories of Australia for 1984–1986

State/Territory	Neonatal death rate	Post-neonatal death rate	Infant death rate	Live born infants (1984)
NSW	5.8	3.6	9.3	81 752
VIC	5.7	3.4	9.1	60 304
QLD	5.7	3.6	9.3	7 178
SA	4.6	3.6	8.2	20 140
WA	5.7	3.8	9.5	23 138
TAS	6.8	5.2	12.0	7 128
NT	9.4	6.4	15.8	3 057
ACT	5.6	3.2	8.8	3 896
Australia	5.7	3.6	9.3	206 593

Table 1.1 lists the total number of births, the neonatal, postnatal and infant death rates, 1984–86 and the number of live born infants 1984, in the States and Territories of Australia. Of particular note is the high infant mortality in the Northern Territory, an area with a particularly high percentage of Aboriginal births (33% of total).

The infant mortality rate of Australia between 1901 and 1986 is shown in Figure 1.1. This shows a very satisfactory fall from a rate of approximately 100 per 1000 live births at the turn of the century to the current figure of 9.3. Table 1.2 lists the comparative mortality figures for a number of developed countries.

Australia is at present seventeenth on the list. Reduction in Aboriginal infant mortality would significantly improve the Australian figure. Comparative infant mortality rates for Mexico are 40, the Philippines 60, and Malawi in excess of 100. The sex ratio and age of death is shown in Table 1.3. The preponderance of male over female infant deaths is worldwide.

Aboriginal confinements in selected States and Territories of the Commonwealth of Australila are listed in Table 1.4. The infant mortality in Western Australia is 24, that in the Northern Territory 33.8 – surely a sad reflection on the continuing poor health of the Aboriginal people.

Table 1.2   International comparisons of infant mortality for 1985

Country	Infant mortality rate/1000 live births
1. Japan	5.5
2. Finland	6.3
3. Sweden	6.7
4. Switzerland	6.9
5. Hong Kong	7.5
6. Canada	7.9
7. Denmark	7.9
8. Netherlands	7.9
9. France	8
10. Norway	8.5
11. German Federal Republic	8.9
12. Ireland	8.9
13. Singapore	9.3
14. United Kingdom	9.3
15. Belgium	9.4
16. German Democratic Republic	9.6
17. AUSTRALIA	9.9
18. Spain	10.5
19. United States	10.6
20. New Zealand	10.8
21. Italy	10.9
22. Austria	11
23. Israel	12.3
24. Greece	14
25. Czechoslovakia	14

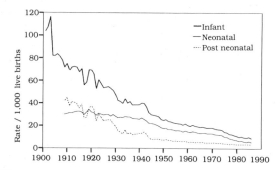

Fig. 1.1   Infant mortality rate in Australia, 1901–1986.

MORTALITY STATISTICS

It is convenient to consider 3 groups:

1. Neonatal
2. Postnatal – 28 days to 1 year
3. 1 year to 14 years

Neonatal

Figure 1.2 lists the major causes of death in the neonatal period. Hypoxia includes disorders of labour and the

Table 1.3 Sex ratio and age of death of Australia for 1981–1986

Age at death	Infant death rate/1000 live births		Sex ratio male:female
	Boys	Girls	
Less than 1 day	3.8	3	127.7:100
1–6 days	1.8	1.4	124.5:100
7–27 days	1.2	1	121:100
28–364 days	4.1	3.1	130.5:100
All ages	10.8	8.5	127.4:100

Table 1.4 Aboriginal confinements in the States and Territories of Australia for 1984

States/Territories	Confinements	Total confinements (%)
VIC	306	0.5
SA	291	1.5
WA[a]	1192	5.2
ACT	38	1.0
NT	1019	33.5

[a] Births instead of confinements.

complications of pregnancy and of the placenta. It should be noted that immaturity due to prematurity is not currently listed as a cause of death, but is a major factor in a large number of deaths in the hypoxia group. Congenital malformations and neonatal infections are not significantly associated with prematurity. Future improvements in infant mortality will undoubtedly be the result of further improvements in obstetrical and neonatal care (which is already at a very high level) and a more complete understanding of the causes of prevention of prematurity and congenital malformations.

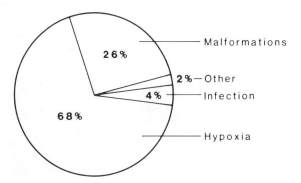

Fig. 1.2 Major causes of death in the neonatal period.

The incidence of low birthweight as a percentage of all births in the Australian State of New South Wales is shown in Figure 1.3. It should be remembered that birthweight is dependent on:

1. The duration of gestation
2. The intrauterine growth rate.

Thus low birthweight may be the result of a short gestation viz. prematurity, intrauterine growth retardation or both in combination.

Clearly there has been little change in the groups studied. Figure 1.4 demonstrates the relative importance of known factors involved in intrauterine growth retardation in a developed country.

Major postnatal causes of death between 28 days and 1 year

These are illustrated in Figure 1.5. At present the incidence of the Sudden Infant Death Syndrome (SIDS)

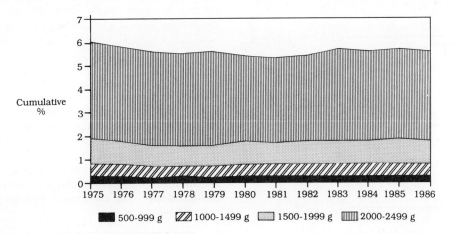

Fig. 1.3 Low birthweight incidence in New South Wales, 1975–1986.

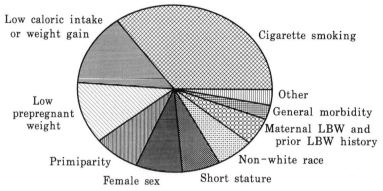

Fig. 1.4 Relative importance of established factors with direct causal impacts on intrauterine growth retardation in a developed country. Abbreviation: LBW = low birthweight (after Kramer 1987).

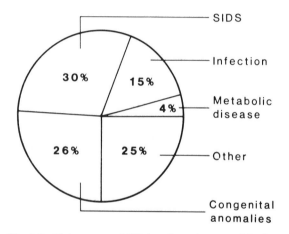

Fig. 1.5 Major postnatal (28 days–1 year) causes of death.

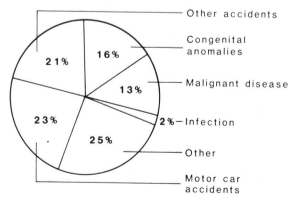

Fig. 1.6 Major causes of death between 1 and 14 years.

is 2 per 1000 live births. This rate is likely to continue until the aetiology is defined.

Causes of death between 1 and 14 years

These are listed in Figure 1.6. Accidents are by far the major cause of death after the age of 1 year. Recent legislation in respect to labelling and packaging of drugs, the manufacture of non-inflammable clothing and the fencing of swimming pools has significantly reduced mortality and morbidity due to these causes. However, the mortality from motor car accidents continues and is likely to continue until further research with proper legislation and community action is taken to prevent them (see Ch. 15).

Of some interest is the number of deaths due to asthma in childhood. A recent survey in the Australian State of Victoria has shown that the death rate of asthma has not decreased despite significant improvements in the pharmacological agents used in management.

MORBIDITY STATISTICS

As has already been mentioned, the health needs and the health programmes of the community relate to the morbidity of that community. Accurate morbidity data are not available in Australia. These are needed urgently. However certain statements in respect to acute illness can be made with reasonable confidence.

In the age group from birth to 1 year infection of one system or another is responsible for over two-thirds of the morbidity. The commonest systems involved in order of frequency are:

1. Upper respiratory tract including the middle ear

2. Lower respiratory tract
3. Skin
4. Bowel.

Other major problems in this age group involve feeding, vomiting, colic and teething. Parental anxiety and inadequacy are also common contributing factors.

In the age group 1 to 4 years infection is the basis of almost three-quarters of the presentations to a primary care facility. Again the systems most commonly involved in order of frequency are the respiratory tract, skin and bowel. Specific exanthemata are common here as is asthma.

In the age group 4 to 9 years infection is still the commonest problem accounting for almost half of initial presentations. Trauma (cuts, bruises, fractures, etc.) are now much more important as is asthma.

In the age group over 9 years infection accounts for one-third of acute presentations and asthma continues to be a major problem. Less frequent, but important problems in the child over 9 years include burns and scalds, psychological problems, blood disorders, tumours and non-febrile seizures.

An excellent five-year prospective study on childhood morbidity has been completed in New Zealand. A cohort of 1265 children were studied, 88.8% of whom were still in the study at the end of 5 years – a remarkable feat for a study of this type. The workers concluded that, by the age of 5 years, children had made an average of 18 medical consultations for morbidity and a further 4.7 for preventative health care procedures. In addition, 38% had been admitted to hospital on at least one occasion and 62% of the group had made one or more attendances at a hospital outpatient department. The following tables summarize the major groups of conditions requiring medical attention; at general practitioner level (Table 1.5), hospital outpatient clinics (Table 1.6) and the rate of hospital admissions per 1000 children (Table 1.7).

HANDICAP

In addition to acute problems, modern child care is very much concerned with the long-term management of a number of disorders associated with physical and intellectual handicap. These will be dealt with in separate chapters. Many of these disorders are genetically determined and until comparatively recently were fatal in early life. Examples include cystic fibrosis, thalassaemia major, spina bifida, phenylketonuria, haemophilia and various malignancies. An increasingly important cause of handicap is the very low birthweight baby (less than 1000 grams). With modern technology approximately

Table 1.5 Major reasons for general practitioner consultation (0–5 years)

Reason for consultation	Total consultation (%)
Respiratory illness	49.5
Skin lesions	13.3
Gastrointestinal illness	11.1
Accidents	5.1
Other disorders	20.8

Table 1.6 Major reasons for hospital outpatient attendances (0–5 years)

Reasons for attendance	Total outpatient attendance (%)
Accidents	32.2
Musculoskeletal conditions	11.4
Respiratory illness	8.8
Visual problems	8.2
Congenital heart murmur/related conditions	4.2
Genitourinary conditions	3.8
Abnormal growth	3.7
Behaviour problems	3.5
Common minor surgery	3.2
Inadequate home environment	3.0
Other conditions	18.2

Table 1.7 Major reasons for hospital admission (0–5 years)

Reason for admission	Total hospital admission (%)
Respiratory illness	21
Common minor surgery	19.5
Accidents	14.6
Inadequate home environment	8.6
Feeding management	8.5
Gastrointestinal illness	8.2
Febrile convulsions	4.3
Musculoskeletal conditions	2.9
Genitourinary conditions	2.4
Other conditions	9.8

two-thirds of these infants will survive although significant handicap will remain in up to 25% of survivors. Handicaps include cerebral palsy, mental retardation, auditory and visual problems, epilepsy – alone or in combination.

The causes of prematurity are far from established. Figure 1.7 lists the known factors believed to be important in the cause of prematurity in developed countries.

Emotional and behavioural problems

The management of behavioural and emotional problems of childhood probably accounts for at least

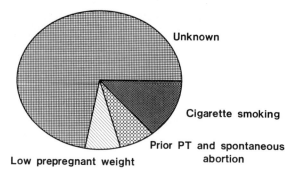

Fig. 1.7 Relative importance of established factors with direct causal impacts on prematurity (PT) in a developed country (after Kramer 1987).

10% of all paediatric consultations. These problems are encountered in all age groups. Often they present as organic, illness, e.g. abdominal pain, headache, tiredness, lethargy, etc. Some present as behaviour disturbances such as temper tantrums, sleep disturbance, feeding problems, whereas others may be more overly psychological, e.g. school phobia, depression, deliquency, anorexia nervosa and so on. Many can be managed by primary care physicians, others require paediatric consultation and a minority require the care of a child psychiatrist. There can be little doubt that the majority of these relate, at least in the first instance, to an unsatisfactory home environment with maternal depression being very significant. A great deal of paediatrics and child psychiatry is concerned with the management of the child in the context of the family.

Malignant disease

Malignant disease is assuming greater importance, as specific therapy is now available in many instances. Management is at a very sophisticated level, particularly in acute lymphatic leukaemia where cures are now common. The outlook for some solid tumours is also improving.

The care of children with chronic disease, malignancy and other handicapping conditions places heavy demands on health care systems, but these must be met.

Social factors

It is now recognized that social factors significantly modify disease and must be taken into account if total care is to be provided. Social factors include family size, financial status, physical characteristics of the home, behaviour and way of life of parents, their education, attitudes, habits, relationships and their capacity to

select and use the various types of care available. Often these factors are compounded in migrants and some other minority groups. It has been extremely difficult to measure these in scientific terms, but it is vital that they are assessed as their effects on illness are cumulative. Perhaps the best common denominator in respect to social factors is the occupational status of the father. Classification based on this was first used in 1911 by the Registrar General in the United Kingdom, when he described five classes or groups of families (Example 1.1).

Example 1.1 Classification of social class	
Occupation	**Social class**
Professional, other managerial groups, commissioned officers in the armed forces, clergy, etc.	1
Lesser managerial groups, teachers, higher clerical workers	2
Skilled artisan workers, craftsmen, etc. Some clerical workers	3
Semiskilled workers	4
Unskilled workers	5

This classification can also be related to behavioural disturbances and educational achievements of the children. Although widely used in statistical research, this grouping does not provide for unemployed persons, children without parents and families of different ethnic backgrounds and cultures. This socioeconomic classification has now been extended to involve 17 groups, each of which is thought to contain people whose social, cultural and recreational standards of behaviour are similar. Although in clinical practice such a classification would be unwieldly and impracticable it does illustrate the necessity to view illness in children against the social background.

Australian society differs from that of the United Kingdom in many respects and the above classification of social classes is not applicable. Unfortunately, data relating to social class are not available for the Australian environment; however, one good indicator is the number of years of formal education of the mother.

SUDDEN INFANT DEATH SYNDROME (SIDS)

This is the commonest cause of death in the first year of life excluding the neonatal period. It occurs in all societies with an incidence of approximately 2 per 1000 live births although this level is much lower in some Scandinavian countries. The clinical history obtained is of a previously healthy baby who is unexpectedly found dead in the cot – hence the term 'cot death'. The maximal age of incidence is between 2 and 6 months, and it is uncommon after the age of 12 months. Occasionally parents remark on a preceding mild respiratory infection, but this is usually so mild that medical attention has not been sought. Autopsy in most infants shows no significant abnormalities other than those associated with sudden death or changes of a minor respiratory infection but insufficient to explain the fatal outcome. In a few infants perceived by their parents to have been well and who are unexpectedly found dead, a disease such as myocarditis, pneumonia or epiglottitis is found at autopsy. Homicide is suspected in some SIDS.

The aetiology of SIDS remains unknown despite intensive research and it is possible that what we today label as SIDS may even include subgroups of deaths from different causes. Numerous theories of causation have been proposed, but the most convincing is that SIDS is related to a brain stem abnormality in neuroregulation of cardiorespiratory control. In support of this theory there is evidence to suggest that infants with prolonged sleep apnoea, excessive periodic breathing and other breathing abnormalities, decreased chemo-receptivity and impaired arousal to hypercardia or hypoxia are at risk to the terminal prolonged apnoeic attack which constitutes SIDS.

The incidence of SIDS is increased in infants with a history of unusual intrauterine and perinatal problems and in those who have been nursed in intensive care units. SIDS occurs more commonly in the cold weather and in families who are in poor socioeconomic circumstances. Infants of mothers who are drug addicts and subsequent siblings of an infant who has died of SIDS also appear to be at greater risk. Unfortunately, predicting SIDS in infants with these risk factors has not been successful.

In an attempt to reduce the incidence of SIDS, respiratory and cardiac monitoring has been used in infants regarded to be at risk. In the past most monitors have been simply apnoeic alarms and have often been beset by technical problems. It seems clear that when monitoring is to be used, a combination apnoea and cardiac monitor would be most appropriate. However, few would claim that monitoring for SIDS has reduced the incidence. Nonetheless, monitoring will continue to be a research tool and will often be required for groups of parents who have lost an infant with SIDS and who are extremely anxious for their next infant. Such requests would seem to be reasonable and should not be denied.

The physician has an important role to play in supporting those parents whose infant has suddenly and unexpectedly died. Parent support groups have become established in many countries both to promote research and to support the families of infants who have died in this way. It is important that parents are given the opportunity to discuss the death of their infant and to express their feelings and work through their grief. Unless this is done psychological problems within the family will be almost inevitable. It is generally accepted that having further children should be discouraged until the mourning process has been completed. This will take at least a year for most couples.

Near-miss sudden death syndrome

This is a term applied to infants who, in the opinion of parents or attendants, had experienced an episode in which death was imminent. This is usually an apnoeic attack with or without cyanosis. The infant is frequently noted to be cold. It will be appreciated that this is a subjective opinion which is not verifiable and there could be a good case for avoiding the term near-miss sudden death syndrome altogether, but it is now so firmly ingrained in the paediatric literature that it is likely to remain. Near-miss sudden death syndrome implies:

1. An alarming event
2. An immediate call for help by parents or attendants
3. Admission to hospital for observation
4. That no other cause for the emergency has been found.

This syndrome is far from rare and a wide spectrum exists. The severity may be such that recovery is rapid and complete. On the other hand, death may be immediate and mimic the sudden infant death syndrome. Most children recover completely after resuscitation, but in a few the recovery is incomplete with permanent neurological sequelae.

Most of these infants will be admitted to hospital when a variety of investigations will be performed in an attempt to define the cause for the emergency. Investigations usually performed include chest radiograph, an ECG, barium swallow, EEG, metabolic screening of blood and urine and an intense search for sepsis. Subsequently, one of a number of possible causes may be found. These include:

1. Severe and overwhelming infection
2. Severe anaemia, particularly in a preterm babe
3. Hypoglycaemia
4. Some other metabolic disturbance
5. Gastro-oesophageal reflux with aspiration
6. Impaired regulation of breathing.

In the majority of infants investigated for near-miss

SIDS no cause is found. When these infants are monitored subsequently a number will exhibit apnoeic attacks (both obstructive and mixed) compared to controls. Fortunately the great majority of these infants recover and very few die suddenly and unexpectedly.

The management of near-miss SIDS is far from easy. Parents will to some extent be reassured that no gross abnormality has been detected on investigation, but most are now very well aware of SIDS so that few will be completely reassured and relaxed. Some parents will request and receive apnoea monitors. Fortunately, however, the vast majority of these infants do not have further attacks and do not die suddenly.

DEATH, THE CHILD AND THE FAMILY

Human society from its earliest times, has evolved rituals and myths in its attempts to give meaning to death.
Raphael (1983)

Children's concepts of life and death change with time and are influenced by their families, religion and culture as well as by their own experiences. The young child tends to attribute life to everything. Later, only moving things are seen as living and finally only animals and people. Common fantasies about death relate to abandonment, going away, being punished or being attacked. Themes of death and coming alive again are common in children's play. These games are thought to represent the child's need to understand death and to control it. Usually, the adolescent has a more physiological understanding of death but fantasies of reunion with loved ones often persist into adult life. Death defying behaviour is common in adolescence.

Bereavement

The death of a person whom one loves leads to bereavement which is a natural expression of sadness at the loss. The child's response will be determined by the closeness of the relationship, the child's developmental stage and ability to understand death and the way in which remaining family members respond. Even young children may show marked distress at the death of a parent. The parent's failure to return may be interpreted as punishment or rejection. The normally concrete thinking of the young child may lead to requests to go to heaven to be with the dead parent. The surviving parent may be angry with the child's apparent lack of grief.

Seeing the dead parent and attendance at the funeral – unless there are strong cultural sanctions against such involvement in the mourning ritual – are often helpful for the child's grieving. With adequate support and understanding the child's grief will gradually abate. The early experience of parental death may leave the child more vulnerable to the effect of later separations and bereavement.

A child's death may occur suddenly as in the case with SIDS or a motor vehicle accident. In this case there is no time for family members to prepare themselves emotionally for the death. This may make the grief more intense, particularly the feelings of disbelief, guilt and anger. Because of their preoccupation with their own grief, parents may overlook the grief of surviving siblings. Some parents may try to replace the dead child by having another baby as quickly as possible. Generally it is better to advise parents to wait for a while before embarking on another pregnancy.

In many cases children die as a result of a prolonged illness. The mourning process, for parents at least, usually begins at the time of diagnosis of a potentially fatal illness. After the initial shock, many parents will seek a second opinion or they may turn to alternative medicine in search of a cure. Most will embark on treatment, pinning their hopes on a successful outcome and plunging into the depths of despair if the child's condition deteriorates. These days, more parents are electing to have their dying child at home rather than in hospital. Hospital staff have a vital role to play in supporting local doctors and community nurses as well as the family in this situation.

Also hospital staff often experience grief in response to the death of a child, especially one whom they have cared for over a period of time. This grief may lead to doubts about one's clinical skills and if not recognized to 'burn-out'.

The dying child

The terminally ill child may be aware that something is seriously wrong even at a very young age. Principally, this will be the result of separation, often painful procedures and emotional changes in key family members. Modern paediatric practice of encouraging parents to stay with their sick children can go a considerable way towards allaying anxiety and alleviating fears of abandonment.

Older children may be afraid of dying, of being left alone or of not having their pain relieved. They will often ask questions about dying or play games about going away. Honest answers to these questions are generally the best way of reducing the associated anxiety.

Adolescents facing death may become quite depressed and withdrawn or they may be very angry. Feelings of hopelessness may lead to non-compliance with treatment and to giving up at school. Anger about their aborted future may be overt and apparently irrational or it may take the form of quite serious risk taking. Many adolescents will respond well to a confiding relationship. Children and families attending clinics for seriously ill children will be acutely aware of the progress of other children. Therefore, when deaths occur there should be some opportunity for discussion if the family requests it.

REFERENCES

Fergusson D M, Beautrais A L, Horwood L J, Shannon F T 1982 The prevalence of illness in a birth cohort. New Zealand Medical Journal 95: 6–10
Kramer M S 1987 Intrauterine growth and gestational determinants. The Australian Bureau of Statistics 80(4): 502–511

Raphael B 1983 The anatomy of bereavement. Basic Books, New York

FURTHER READING

Hunt C E, Roulette M D 1987 Sudden infant death syndrome. Perspective. The Journal of Pediatrics 1105: 669–678
Simpson H, MacFadyen U M, Paton J Y 1986 'Near-miss' or 'near myth' for sudden infant death syndrome. Clinical observation on 57 infants. Australian Paediatric Journal Supplement 1: 47–51
Williams A L 1986 Scientific research into the sudden infant death syndrome. Australian Paediatric Journal Supplement 3–4

2. Ethics in paediatrics

Bernard W. Neal

THE ROLE OF ETHICS

The rest of this book deals with the things that can be done in paediatrics; this chapter deals with whether they should be done – whether it is right or wrong to do (or not to do) them.

Almost everyone would agree that there is a difference between right and wrong. In other words almost everyone holds certain moral values, whether derived from religious belief, from personal intuition or from some other source. How we think about and discuss these values is the subject matter of ethics. In a sense every decision in paediatrics has an ethical dimension. Every time advice is given it is presumably given on the basis that the doctor feels there is a duty to give it and/or some good will flow from following it. Often, this ethical dimension is not obvious since usually there is no ethical problem. However, it should not be forgotten that many everyday situations in paediatrics may have important ethical aspects. For instance, how far should the doctor go in meeting parental wishes for treatment that the doctor does not think is clinically indicated? (Antibiotics for viral infections? Sedation for troublesome behaviour? Circumcision? Tonsillectomy?)

MAJOR TOPICS

Most of the ethical debate in paediatrics of recent years has centred on a few major topics of far reaching importance. These have included:

- the management of a newborn with a severe handicap, especially spina bifida and Down syndrome
- the management of the very low birthweight infant
- organ transplantation
- medical research with children
- the rights of minors (may an adolescent girl be prescribed the contraceptive pill without her parents' knowledge?)
- the rights of the retarded (may a retarded girl be sterilized to avoid pregnancy?)

- The child's right to know – or to not know (for instance about true parentage, family history, karyotype, or AIDS antibody status)

There are no easy answers to these questions but consideration of the moral values upon which decisions may be based should at least assist us to think clearly about the problems.

BASIC MORAL VALUES

Although the basis for ethical decision making is difficult and much debated (see below) it seems likely that four basic moral obligations will be accepted by almost everybody in the moral community we inhabit: that we respect each other's autonomy, that we aim to do at least some good (beneficence), that we refrain from doing harm (non-maleficence) and that we act justly.

Autonomy

There is broad consensus that ultimately patients must decide about their own medical care, and that whilst doctors and nurses have a duty to help in decision making, they must respect the patient's autonomous decision and assist in carrying it out. This view is opposed to the extreme variety of paternalism ('doctor knows best', 'doctor's orders'). Doctors have been much attacked for allegedly extending their role as medical experts to include acting as moral experts as well. In practice, however, it must be recognized that not only medical tradition, but also the wishes of patients, and even the law itself sometimes require some degree of medical paternalism.

Informed consent

The doctrine of informed consent derives directly from the moral value of respect for the patients' autonomy. According to this doctrine the patient has the overriding right to not only give or withhold consent to medical treatment, but to be given a clear account of just what the treatment entails. Whilst most people would agree with the doctrine in principle, there is fierce debate about the details of what it means in practice, whether there should be a statute law on the subject, and if so what the law should be. The view that the patient should be told everything possible cannot be seriously entertained. However, it does seem desirable that patients (their own needs being taken into account) receive enough information to make a reasoned choice. Many doctors argue that this is what a 'reasonable doctor' does anyway, and it is what a 'reasonable patient' expects.

Other corollaries of the value of respect for autonomy are that patients have a right to be told the truth, and to have their confidentiality respected. None of these rights (informed consent, truth telling, and confidentiality) are absolute and in paediatrics there are some important reservations. Nevertheless, it must be remembered that children, in so far as they are able to exercise them, have exactly the same rights as adults. The fact that the patient is a child in no way diminishes the right, for example, to confidentiality of the personal medical record.

A good case can be made out that full autonomy is dependent upon personhood. John Locke, the 17th century British philosopher, defined a 'person' as a 'thinking intelligent being that has reason and reflection and can consider itself as itself, the same thinking thing, in different times and places'. These qualities are not already present in the newborn and may never appear in some handicapped newborns. According to this argument, it is the beginning of the life of the person, rather than of the physical organism that is crucial so far as rights are concerned. Some would argue that even the right to life itself is dependent upon personhood. Others, of course, strongly maintain that full human rights obtain from the moment of conception, or at least from some other point in time, such as the moment of birth. The view that one takes on this issue will clearly be of relevance when discussing issues such as the care of the handicapped newborn, or nursery policy in respect to the very low birthweight infant.

Whilst parents are traditionally, and rightly, given the right to make decisions on behalf of the young or incompetent child, there should be reasonable satisfaction in one's mind that the parents are making the decision that the child, if able, would make and that appears to be in the child's best interests. When, however, a child is of sufficient intelligence and maturity to make personal decisions, then that child should be permitted to do so even if still legally a minor. An important judgement in the House of Lords found that, provided certain criteria were met, it was right to prescribe contraceptives to minors without parental knowledge or consent. This, thereby, gave legal recognition to the principle that a degree of autonomy rightly belongs to a person of less than adult years and that confidentiality is an important right, even though the patient is a child.

Beneficence

It is a basic principle of ethical medical practice that the doctor aims to do some good for the patient. The community expects that the doctor will always act in the best interests of patients in general, and of his own patient in particular. Indeed, this fundamental principle is one of the distinguishing characteristics of a profession, as opposed to a mere trade.

Some qualifications of the duty of beneficence should be borne in mind: it does not override the duty of respect for autonomy (one should not do good to the patient against his/her will). And it should be remembered that doing good to the patient does not always coincide with doing what the patient wants.

The other duties listed above may also constrain to some extent the exercise of beneficence. The principle of non-maleficence requires that the potential good is not outweighed by a potential harm. For instance, it may not be acceptable to subject a child to a painful investigation if the likelihood of good flowing to the child from the investigation is remote. Finally, the principle of justice requires that the doctor in doing good to one patient is not thereby being unfair to other patients. It is not just, for example, to provide a favoured patient with access to a scarce resource ahead of others with better claims.

Non-maleficence

The phrase 'primum non nocere' (above all do no harm) has traditionally been accorded great importance in medical ethics. However, like most other aphorisms it has considerable limitations as a rule for behaviour. Despite philosophic differences in the precise meaning of the two concepts of beneficence and non-maleficence, in practice they go hand in hand, and some degree of harm to the patient must commonly be accepted if some good is to be achieved. The principle of non-maleficence should be understood as simply meaning that the prospects of harm should be carefully weighed against the prospects of good before deciding on a course of action.

An important if mundane example of the duty of non-maleficence in ordinary practice is that doctors must interview and examine children in a gentle and understanding manner, so that they are not unnecessarily hurt.

Justice

The duty of justice requires that doctors allocate the resources they control (including their own time and skill) in a fair way. It is not always easy to decide what is the fairest way to allocate a scarce resource. For instance, how does one decide which premature baby is to be given the last available incubator? Most doctors tend to make such decisions on the basis of pure medical need, but it may be argued that other factors such as welfare maximization (give to the patient who is likely to have the best outcome), or merit or social worth should be taken into account. Others have argued that once general medical suitability has been established, the decision should be made by lot. As is often the case in ethical decision making, it is easier to say what is not acceptable: the decision should not be made because of mere personal preference.

In addition to these questions of micro-allocation of resources, the principle of justice is involved also in the macro-allocation of resources. (For example, how much of the health budget should be spent on infant incubators in relation to other demands on the budget?) These are questions for governments to decide, but doctors caring for children have a duty to see that the claims of children, who cannot speak for themselves, are given due prominence.

THE BASIS OF ETHICS

The practice of medicine requires every doctor to be a participant in moral decision making; and in so far as doctors have a rational basis for their decisions, they are also ethical theorists. Therefore, it is appropriate for the doctor to have, at least in broad outline, some knowledge of the major ethical theories which have been advanced to distinguish good from bad. Two theories (or sets of theories) have predominated in modern times: utilitarianism and deontology.

Utilitarianism

John Stuart Mill proposed in the 19th century that acts are right that 'produce the greatest happiness for the greatest number'. From this basic concept has flowed an enormous amount of ethical theory. But all utilitarian theories have in common that the rightness of action is to be judged in some way by its consequences. Such thinking is familiar in medicine and the concept is the basis of cost/benefit analysis and modern methods of medical decision making. Also, utilitarianism is immediately attractive because it suggests a rational approach to the solving of ethical problems. However, a number of difficulties are commonly raised in considerations of utilitarianism. The first difficulty is in deciding just how we define a good outcome. Even if we can do this, it may be very difficult in practice to make reasonable estimates of the probability of various costs and benefits. A second objection is the assertion that to the utilitarian 'the end justifies the means'. In a particular context the question might be argued that if it is in the interest of a suffering, handicapped newborn to die, is it morally acceptable to actively terminate his life? Another aspect of utilitarian theory that gives rise to certain objections is the proposition that acts must be judged not only on their consequences to the individual but on the consequences for society as a whole. Clearly the common good is a desirable outcome, but should it be achieved by the sacrifice of an innocent individual? Further objections are that utilitarianism pays too little regard to widely held values such as personal freedom and rights.

Do children have the right to be given truthful answers to their questions, even though the answer (that there is a family history of Huntington disease, for example) is likely to have painful consequences?

Utilitarian philosophers have of course advanced arguments in rebuttal of all these objections. For instance, *rule* utilitarianism holds that it is not so much individual actions that should be judged but rather social rules or practices. For instance, the provision of expensive facilities for the care of a very low birthweight individual infant might be difficult to justify on various grounds; but the provision of such facilities as a rule in such circumstances might be to the ultimate good of society.

Deontology

In philosophic theory the four basic obligations referred to above would be included as pertaining to a deontological theory of ethics. These theories are based on the proposition that we all have moral duties, and that an act is right in so far as it is performed in accordance with our moral duty. It is not, says the deontologist, to be judged by its outcome. These theories derive from Immanuel Kant, the 18th century German philosopher, who proposed the categorical imperative – the universal principle that good behaviour demands that we all respect other people and ourselves.

Duties may be positive or negative. Negative duties are seen as being universally binding and hence we should never, for example, lie to a child, but the positive duty to tell the truth is not so strong, since we may have the option of remaining silent. Likewise there is a universal negative duty not to kill where as the positive duty to provide care may be limited. For instance, this theory would require the doctor to refrain from actively killing the child with a mortal illness, but would not require him necessarily to use every possible means to keep the child alive. The concept of duties is closely related to the concept of rights – indeed, rights and duties may be seen as two sides of the same coin. Although the concept of rights is bandied about very loosely, some difficult problems are associated with any theory of rights. For example, who has the rights in considering abortion, does one consider the fetus to have the same rights as the mother?

Also, there are many other objections that may be raised against various deontological theories. Nonetheless, like utilitarianism, deontological theories do have an immediate appeal to our ordinary moral thinking. Whilst it is true that there is never-ending debate between deontologists and utilitarians, it is likely that most doctors in practice will base their ethical decisions on elements of both sets of theories, however philosophically unsatisfactory this may be. Doctors looking after children in their concern to do what is right are likely to consider their duty to their child patients, and the rights of that child, as well as the likely consequences of their actions. The major ethical problems in paediatrics, as opposed to medicine in general, arise from the dependent status of the child, and the diminished capacity to exercise their own autonomy. The fundamental question underlies almost all ethical debates in paediatrics: who should decide for himself?

Parents

When a child is too young or too ill to make a personal decision it is usually understood that the parents make the decision. This is based on the assumption that parents are the ones most likely to know what is in their own child's best interest and to act in accordance with it. Whilst this is generally true it must be remembered that there are some problems with parents as substitute decision maker. Ideally, the substitute decision maker would make the same decision as the patient, were the patient able to make a personal decision. In the case of the retarded infant for example, there is no reason to believe that the parent is better able than anyone else to divine what the infant would wish. Similarly, parents will not necessarily be the best judges of what really is in the 'best interest' of the child. We know that some competent adults decide that it is in their best interest to continue enduring a life of suffering, whilst others do not. The great love that most parents feel for their children must always be respected, but it must also be recognized that parents may, knowingly or unknowingly, be influenced by factors other than the best interests of the child. For instance, they may be faced with a very painful 'conflict of interest' when counting the cost of the care of a handicapped child in terms of the welfare of the rest of the family.

Nurses and doctors

It is generally accepted that doctors and nurses have a clear duty to provide parents with adequate technical information on which they may base their decisions. Also, it is commonly supposed that this information will be supplied in an objective manner. However, experience shows that this is not possible, and that the moral opinion of the person providing the information is very likely to influence the manner in which the information is presented. This is not to say that the doctors and nurses should not try to be as objective as possible; however, they must realize that despite the popular criticism of 'paternalism' they will be involved to a greater or lesser degree in the ethical decision making, and many parents will expect them at least to assist in the decision making process.

Doctors must be clear that their first duty lies to their child-patient, and sometimes difficult situations arise where the carrying out of their duty brings them into conflict with the wishes of parents. An extreme example of this situation might arise if permission was refused to carry out an operation for the relief of intestinal obstruction in a newborn infant with Down syndrome. Usually, sympathetic discussion resolves such problems, but as a last resort appeal to a court of law may be necessary. Less dramatically, there are numerous everyday clinical occurrences in which the doctor's primary duty to serve the best interests of the child-patient must take precedence over the carrying out of parental wishes, such as the prescribing of antibiotics or the carrying out of operations which are not clinically indicated.

Ethics committees

Institutional Ethics Committees may also become involved, but it is impractical and undesirable for such committees to assume the role of decision maker in individual cases. They may come to fulfil a useful role as resource centres to which the doctor may turn for helpful guidance. Such committees already exist in all hospitals and institutions receiving National Health and Medical Research Council (NH & MRC) grants and in many others. So far, their role has been conferred primarily to research.

RESEARCH OF CHILDREN

The NH & MRC has set out the principles governing

research on children in its statement on Human Experimentation. The relevant section is quoted verbatim.

Scientific research is essential to advance knowledge of all aspects of childhood disease. Such research, however, may be performed only when the information sought cannot in practice be obtained by other means.

All research must be based on sound scientific concepts and must be planned and conducted in such a fashion as will reasonably ensure that definite conclusions will be reached. Some programmes may offer direct benefit to the individual child, while others may have a broader community purpose. In appropriate circumstances both may be ethical.

In all centres undertaking research in children, the following special responsibilities of the institutional ethics committee are emphasized:

(i)   protecting the rights and welfare of children involved in research procedures;
(ii) determining the acceptability of the risk/benefit relationship of any research study conducted;
(iii) ensuring that informed consent from parents/guardian and where appropriate the child, is obtained in a manner appropriate to the study;
(iv) encouraging the performance of necessary and appropriate research;
(v)   preventing unscientific or unethical research.

Consent to research should be obtained from:

(i)   the parents/guardian in all but exceptional circumstances (e.g. emergencies); and
(ii) the child where he or she is of sufficient maturity and intelligence to make this practicable.

In this context 'consent' means consent following a full and clear explanation of the research planned, its objectives and any risks involved.

Risks of research may be considered in terms of:

(i)   therapeutic research (where the procedure may be of some benefit to the child). In determining whether there is an acceptable relationship between potential benefit and the risk involved, it is essential to weigh the risk of the proposed research against customary therapeutic measures and the natural hazards of the disease or condition.
(ii) non-therapeutic research (where the procedure is of no direct benefit to the child). The risk to the child should be so minimal as to be little more than the risks run in everyday life. Risks of research in this context include the risk of causing physical disturbance, discomfort, anxiety, pain or psychological disturbance to the child or the parents rather than the risk o serious harm, which would be unacceptable.

Advances in medicine generally and in paediatrics in particular are occurring at a very rapid rate. This applies especially in the fields of molecular biology, transplantation, virology, immunology and in vitro fertilization to name but a few. The research involved and the implications of research to treatment will have very significant ethical considerations. It is most important that the community and the medical profession are prepared to face the ethical issues that these scientific advances will pose and at the appropriate time. There must not be undue delay between scientific advances in medicine and relevant ethical considerations.

FURTHER READING

Brody H 1981 Ethical decisions in medicine. Little, Brown and Co, Boston

Gorovitz S, Jameton A L, Macklin R et al 1976 Moral practices in medicine. Prentice-Hall, Englewood Cliffs, New Jersey

Nicholson Richard H 1986 Medical research for children. Oxford University Press, Oxford

Genetics

3. Birth defects

David M. Danks, John G. Rogers

Terminology

Birth defect is generally preferred to congenital malformation, a term which became devalued by imprecise usage. Birth defect is used to describe any abnormality, structural or functional, identified at any age, provided that the condition began before birth. Anencephaly is obviously a birth defect, but so also are phenylketonuria (PKU), cystic fibrosis, muscular dystrophy and Huntington disease.

Malformation is retained to describe structural defects considered due to a fault in embryonic development. *Deformation* has been introduced to describe structural abnormalities imposed upon the developed fetus, especially those due to external physical forces in the uterus. Dysmorphic is an ugly, but useful word, used to indicate that a child's appearance departs from normal in ways which are considered, by the observer, to be significant. It has replaced the unfortunate colloquial phrase 'funny-looking kid' (FLK).

CAUSES OF BIRTH DEFECTS

Birth defects may have genetic or non-genetic causes. Among the genetic causes, gross derangements of gene dosage, as seen in chromosomal trisomies, generally cause multiple abnormalities, both physical and functional (e.g. trisomy 21 – Down syndrome). Single gene defects may result in functional disturbances (as in phenylketonuria) or physical defects (as in Meckel's syndrome – polycystic kidneys, exomphalos and encephalocele).

Non-genetic causes may come from the intrauterine environment (as in physical deformations imposed by a septate uterus), from maternal factors (as in the mother with untreated phenylketonuria), from maternal nutritional habits or toxin ingestion (as in the fetal alcohol syndrome) or from the wider environment, as that term is more often used (as in methyl mercury pollution of water supplies).

PHYSICAL ABNORMALITIES AND SYNDROMES

Physical abnormalities may involve single body parts (e.g. abnormalities of one hand) or organ system (e.g. ventricular septal defect) or may involve multiple organs and parts of the body.

Progress towards understanding of the more complex structural abnormalities begins with classification of arrays of defects as syndromes. At present over 1200 syndromes are defined and named. Once a syndrome is defined the search for a cause can begin. Syndromes may be sporadic in occurrence, may cluster in families or may cluster in time and space.

Familial occurrence indicates generally a major genetic contribution to the cause, but may indicate a recurring maternal influence (e.g. mental retardation and heart defects in children of women with untreated PKU, or fetal alcohol syndrome in children of a chronic alcoholic woman). A simple Mendelian pattern in families suggests a defect in a single gene.

Clustering in time and space implies an environmental factor such as a viral infection or a nutritional or toxic chemical influence. Only a very few environmental causes are firmly established.

Major chromosomal alterations generally occur sporadically, clustering neither in families nor in time and space. Trisomy for whole chromosomes (21, 18, 13), deletions of parts of chromosomes and partial trisomies (duplications of chromosome segments) are recognized by chromosomal banding techniques. Even with the best techniques lesions involving chromosome segments smaller than about 100–200 genes remain invisible. Smaller invisible lesions of autosomes may still cause mental retardation and physical defects, explaining some of the sporadically occurring syndromes which have no explanation at present and also some of the 'private' sets of malformations unique to single patients.

Other defects occurring sporadically may be the result of new single gene mutations – lethal dominant mutations can be recognized only if an occasional patient lives to reproduce and pass the condition on to half of the children or when both of identical twins are affected.

Parental age influences the frequency of some sporadically occurring conditions. Most chromosomal trisomies occur more often among the offspring of older women. Precise risk figures are known for trisomy 21 (Down syndrome) and the limited information available about other autosomal trisomies follows a similar pattern. The risk of trisomy 21 increases from less than 1 in 1000 in the mid-twenties to 1 in 200 at 37, 1 in 100 at 40 and 1 in 40 at 45 years. It is generally agreed that paternal age has no significant effect on this risk, nor does the number of previous pregnancies. The chances of new single gene mutation does increase with advancing paternal age, which is, therefore, associated with sporadic cases of dominantly inherited conditions.

Correct identification of a syndrome allows the paediatrician to use accumulated knowledge of the condition in treating the patient, advising the parents about the child's prognosis, and predicting the chances of recurrence of the condition in future pregnancies.

The task of remembering more than 1200 syndromes is very difficult indeed and various computerized aids have been developed t complement the many textbooks describing syndromes. Most doctors are familiar with only a few of these syndromes and referral to a clinical geneticist is generally indicated in any child with multiple physical defects, or with one major defect plus more minor dysmorphic features. Referral is particularly important and urgent when a baby with multiple defects seems likely to die in the neonatal period. Some doctors feel anxious and insecure, or even personally affronted after delivering a seriously abnormal baby and may react by trying to protect the parents and baby from 'needless tests'. However, tests in life, and autopsy, may be essential to diagnose the condition present and allow accurate counselling about future pregnancies.

FUNCTIONAL DEFECTS

Disturbances of cellular function, which are present from birth, are now generally regarded as birth defects even when symptoms and abnormal physical signs develop only months or years after birth. Phenylketonuria and many degenerative brain diseases fall into this category. In many instances the natural history is one of progressive damage to the target organs, but treatment may be able to prevent this.

Inevitably, most of the diseases classified as functional birth defects are genetically determined, because only then can one know that the cause was present before birth. A disorder like vaginal adenocarcinoma in a girl exposed to diethyl stilboestrol in utero would rank as a rare example of a non-genetic disorder in this class.

Some of these defects involve proteins which serve constructional roles in the body. Genetic defects in the structure of quantity of collagen can cause a range of defects of bone and skin, including osteogenesis imperfecta, the Ehlers-Danlos syndrome and the Marfan syndrome. Red cell disorders like spherocytosis and elliptocytosis are caused by defects in cytoskeletal proteins. These proteins are not influenced by differences between intrauterine existence and postnatal life, so the natural history of the disease starts from conception and proceeds at its own natural tempo.

In some other birth defects the fetus is completely protected in utero and illness starts only after birth. This applies in a disease like phenylketonuria, in which an enzyme defect (phenylalanine hydroxylase) in the liver, leads to accumulation of a metabolite (phenylalanine) in the bloodstream, with effects on a distant organ (the brain). Placental perfusion prevents accumulation of the phenylalanine and this allows phenylketonuria to be treated by early postnatal detection and dietary therapy. Many inborn errors of metabolism behave in this way and can be treated effectively.

Not all inborn errors of metabolism are so well 'treated' in utero. When the injurious effects of accumulation or deficiency of a metabolite are felt by each individual cell there is no protection in utero, as in the lysosomal storage disease (lipidoses, e.g. Tay-Sachs' disease and mucopolysaccharidoses, e.g. Hurler syndrome). Such diseases are generally not treatable.

FREQUENCY OF BIRTH DEFECTS

Several different figures can be quoted to describe the frequency of birth defects. Physical abnormalities are present in 4–5% of babies at birth. This figure includes abnormalities like heart defects which may not be recognized until a few weeks or months of age. Approximately half of this figure comprises defects of substantial functional importance (like neural tube defects, heart defects or cleft palate) and about half are relatively trivial defects (like syndactyly, accessory auricles, etc.) Another figure which is often quoted is that 2–3% of all babies have a serious persisting defect. In deriving this figure, the physical abnormalities which were present at birth, but were completely and readily corrected, have been eliminated and functional defects like mental retardation, cystic fibrosis, and muscular dystrophy have been added in to the figure.

Birth defects constitute the most important class of serious chronic disease in childhood. Birth defects follow second to prematurity among the principal causes of death in the remainder of childhood. Birth defects outstrip all other childhood disease in causing chronic handicap to individuals and cost to the community. Of course these statements apply to Western countries and would not be true in developing countries, where malnutrition and infections still cause far more deaths and disabilities than any other conditions.

In seeking to reduce the frequency of birth defects in Western communities, the first step must be to discover all of the individual causes. Only then can specific strategies of prevention be developed. This will be a slow process for there are thousands of different causes of birth defects, each of which is relatively rare. In the past we had just a small number of infectious diseases, each of which killed hundred or thousands of children and was prevented by a specific method, generally immunization. The future task is more difficult, although no different in logic.

Environmental causes of birth defects are more easily prevented than genetic causes and it is disappointing that so few non-genetic causes have yet been firmly identified.

The control of rubella embryopathy by immunization of young girls is a classic achievement of preventive medicine. Thalidomide was a teratogen which was unusually easy to recognize and eliminate. Abrupt introduction of the drug and stereotyped effects in most exposed fetuses made recognition easy. It was a convenient rather than essential drug. Other drugs or chemicals causing birth defects are more likely to enter the marketplace in a gradual way, to affect only an occasional susceptible fetus and be important agents not easily eliminated from use. The hydantoin anticonvulsant drugs are a good example. Suspicions of teratogenic effects have existed for over a decade, but remain unproven. Epileptic women require therapy to be continued throughout pregnancy and there are no alternative anticonvulsant drugs which are proven to be safe.

Birth defect registers

Birth defect registers have been set up in most Western countries in the hope that they may provide an early warning signal of some new teratogen in the community, but they are fairly crude instruments for this purpose. The observation of an association between sodium valproate use and neural tube defects in the Rhone-Alpes regional register in France may be cited as a success for this approach. They do provide very important background information about the frequency of each birth defect and its natural fluctuations, against which the apparent outbreaks of cases can be assessed.

Observation of clusters of cases by doctors, midwives and others in contact with newborn babies is probably the most efficient warning system, but one which creates many false alarms. A competent epidemiology group associated with a register should then evaluate each apparent cluster without alarming the general public, who become very confused and anxious when this process is carried out too publicly.

SCREENING FOR BIRTH DEFECTS

It is technically possible to test all newborn babies for some 20 rare genetic disorders and birth defects. After 20 years of experience, the criteria for community-wide screening of newborn babies have become generally accepted. The disorder should be relatively frequent and the testing programme must be cheap, sensitive and specific, detecting almost all of the affected individuals, but very few unaffected individuals. Finally, some useful consequence must follow upon detection, generally an effective form of treatment.

Phenylketonuria is the prototype. Its frequency is approximately 1 in 10 000 and treatment is very successful when started under 2 weeks of age, but much less successful if delayed until symptoms have developed. The test is very cheap and identifies only about one baby who does not need treatment for every one who does. In most countries it works out that 20 patients with PKU can be detected and treated for the cost of keeping one untreated mentally retarded individual for a lifetime.

Hypothyroidism is the second disorder for which screening is universally accepted in Western countries. There are a number of other disorders like galactosaemia, homocystinuria and maple syrup urine disease, for which screening programmes are employed in some countries, but not in others. The arguments are more balanced in these conditions because of low frequency, difficulty in detecting patients before they become severely ill and doubt about the complete effectiveness of treatment in some instances.

At present there is considerable discussion about screening programmes for cystic fibrosis and for Duchenne muscular dystrophy. Tests exist which meet the requirements of sensitivity and specificity and are economically feasible. The usefulness of early detection is debated. In muscular dystrophy the only benefit is genetic counselling for the families, with possible prevention of a few affected individuals who might have been born in the interval between diagnosis by screening and diagnosis because of symptoms. In cystic fibrosis there is a difference of opinion about the benefits of early presymptomatic treatment. The advent of prenatal diagnosis of both these conditions has changed the balance in this debate and many centres are now screening for cystic fibrosis.

DRUGS AND ENVIRONMENTAL FACTORS

In recent years there has been increasing concern over the possible effects of drugs and environmental factors in the fetus. This was triggered by the thalidomide crisis which outlined in dramatic fashion the potential for harming the fetus, a fact which had been recognized many years previously. Many new chemicals are manufactured each year but few are satisfactorily tested for their potential toxic and teratogenic effect.

Principles of teratology

Timing and dose

The timing and dose of a drug or chemical is critical in terms of teratogenesis. Agents administered during the stage of blastocyst formation usually result in the abortion or death of the fetus. Thus, the earliest part of the pregnancy is regarded as being relatively immune from teratogenic effects. The period of maximum sensitivity is during the period of organogenesis. Defects produced during this time are commonly structural and easier to detect. In humans this is from the 18 days postconception to 60 days postconception. Later in pregnancy, the effects of drugs are likely to be more subtle and not easily detected, but some agents such as Warfarin and alcohol are known to produce harmful late effects.

Genetics and drug metabolism

There is marked species difference in the sensitivity of animals to drugs. For example, certain strains of mice are much more susceptible to glucocorticoid-induced cleft lip and palate than other strains. At present there is no evidence that glucocorticoids produce cleft lip and palate in humans. This reflects a difference in the genetic make-up of animals and the metabolism of drugs. This is an important factor in an individual person's susceptibility to teratogenic agents but so far this has not been studied in any detail.

Mechanisms of teratogenicity

Teratogenic agents act by interfering with cellular metabolism. Compounds have specific effects and may interfere with cell membranes, DNA, RNA or protein synthesis. The common end point is either cell death or a failure of replication, migration or fusion. This can be organ specific or produce a generalized effect on the fetus.

Male versus female role in teratogenesis

With teratogens and environmental agents, there is a very limited number of ways in which a male can be implicated. The male largely contributes a package of DNA and most agents which result in substantial interference with DNA result in sterility. Nonetheless, this should not be taken for a licence to expose males to toxic agents.

Comparative studies

If thalidomide had been tested originally in rabbits instead of mice and rats its teratogenicity would have been established. Many agents which are known to be teratogenetic in animals, such as glucocorticoids in rats, cannot be demonstrated to be teratogenic in humans. There is difficulty in interpreting data from one animal species to another and even more difficulty in trying to apply the data to a human population. At present, the animal tests are the best possible means of screening. Where there is a precise understanding of the biochemical mechanisms of teratogenesis, specific tests can be applied to human tissues.

METHODS CURRENTLY EMPLOYED TO DETECT POTENTIAL TERATOGENS

Animal studies

Most of these studies use rats and mice. They involve administration of drugs to a pregnant animal. There are many different schedules of dosage which are in use. Obviously, the more closely the species relates to a man, the more likely it is to produce useful results in human terms. Experiments in monkeys and apes are very expensive and rarely performed.

Embryo culture studies

Administering drugs to an embryo in a culture system during the period of organogenesis provides a convenient means of assessment. This removes the effect of maternal metabolism. Human liver extracts can be added to the culture system to mimic the effects of human metabolism. Rat and mouse embryos are commonly used. This is a powerful research tool used in trying to understand and investigate further the mechanisms of teratogenesis.

Tissue culture systems

A variety of tissue culture systems has been developed to evaluate teratogens; their ultimate role remains to be established.

Human studies

Retrospective studies of human data are notoriously fallible. A number of prospective studies have been undertaken. The best known of these is the study by Heinanen et al (1977) in Boston which prospectively obtained data on over 50 000 women during pregnancy and evaluated the outcome. This study provides data on drugs commonly used in pregnant women. Although retrospective data are difficult to interpret they may provide important clues. In practice most human teratogens have been recognized by specific clinical observation. Birth defects registers provide a potential early warning system.

ESTABLISHED TERATOGENS

The list of established teratogens is perhaps surprisingly short (see Table 3.1). It is worth commenting specifically on a few agents.

Table 3.1 Teratogenic agents in humans (after Sheppard 1986)

Known teratogens	Possible teratogens	Suspected teratogens
		Not likely
Drugs and environmental chemicals	Binge drinking	Agent Orange
androgenic hormones	Cigarette smoking	Anaesthetics
aminopterin and	Heat and fever	Antinauseants
methylaminopterin	Excess vitamin A	(Debendox)
busulfan	Organic solvents	Aspartamate
chlorobiphenyls	Valium	Aspirin
coumarin anticoagulants	Varicella	Birth control pills
cyclophosphamide	Zinc deficiency	LSD
diethylstilboestrol		Marijuana
diphenylhydantoin and		Metronidazole
trimethadione		Rubella vaccine
D-penicillamine		Spermicides
goitrogens and antithyroid		
drugs		
isotretinoin		
methyl mercury		
phenytoin		
tetracyclines		
thalidomide		
valproic acid		
warfarin		
Infections		
cytomegalovirus		
herpes simplex virus I and		
II		
rubella virus		
syphillis		
toxoplasmosis		
Venezuelan equine		
encephalitis virus		
Maternal metabolic imbalance		
alcoholism		
diabetes		
endemic cretinism		
hyperthermia		
phenylketonuria		
virilizing tumours		
Radiation		
atomic weapons		
radioiodine		
therapeutic		

Thalidomide

This was introduced as the ideal sedative drug for use in pregnancy. Lenz in Germany and McBride in Australia reported an increased number of babies born with limb deficiencies, a rare birth defect. Thalidomide was quickly implicated. The incidence in doctor's families was high as they received free samples. Thalidomide awakened people's consciousness about the potentially harmful effect of drugs in pregnancy.

Warfarin

This has been shown to produce a characteristic pattern of abnormalities in about one-sixth of the pregnancies exposed to this drug. The sensitive period for the production of the characteristic Warfarin embryopathy is from the sixth to ninth week of gestation. However, exposure during the second and third trimester has resulted in severe CNS problems.

Isotretinoin

Isotretinoin has been introduced for the treatment of severe cystic acne. It is a known potent teratogen and produces craniofacial, cardiac and central nervous system defects. Great care must be taken to see that patients are not pregnant at the time of starting this drug, during therapy or for some time afterwards. The age group in which it is used is prone to unplanned pregnancies and, thus, it should be used in conjunction with contraception.

Radiation

Care should be taken to avoid unnecessary exposure of pregnant women to radiographs. Doses less than 10 rads are considered unlikely to produce any harmful effects to the fetus or embryo. Doses in excess of 10 rads are best avoided and considered by some to be an indication for termination of pregnancy. Doses in excess of 100 rads are known to produce microcephaly, general growth retardation and mental retardation. Most radiological investigation done using modern techniques including IVP, barium enemas and barium meals expose people to less than 2 rads of radiation. Considerable anxiety is aroused in women who have had such studies before their pregnancy was recognized and a number of unnecessary terminations are performed despite the low dose of radiation.

Alcohol

Alcohol had long been suspected as a teratogen but it was not until the 1970s that the seriousness and extent of the problem was recognized. The wide-spread availability of alcohol makes it the most common teratogen to which a pregnancy is likely to be exposed.

A woman who has a steady intake of two alcoholic drinks per day during pregnancy will have a babe with a slightly reduced birthweight. Mothers who are chronically alcoholic, 8–10 drinks per day, are likely to produce babies of low birthweight, with small heads, mental retardation, inco-ordination and an increased frequency of congenital heart disease. In between these extremes a graduation of effect is likely. Binge drinking in pregnancy is of particular concern. Alcohol is best avoided during pregnancy.

Virus infection

In 1941 Norman Gregg, a Sydney ophthalmologist, astutely recognized an increased number of children with eye and other defects following an epidemic of rubella. Rubella is now known to produce devastating effects on the fetus including blindness, deafness, cataracts, microphthalmos, congenital heart disease and mental retardation. The range of defects seen in a child with intrauterine rubella depend on the precise time during gestation when the infection occurred.

A number of other microbiological agents has also been implicated as teratogens, in particular toxoplasmosis, herpes, CMV, and Venezuela equine encephalitis. Syphilis was recognized as a teratogenic agent long before rubella.

Methyl mercury

The Minimata Bay disaster in Japan demonstrated the devastating effects of this compound. Methyl mercury contaminated the local bay. Fish caught were eaten by pregnant women. Babies exposed in utero had microcephaly, deafness, blindness and were severely spastic.

Phenytoin

Phenytoin and other anticonvulsants have been shown to produce an increased rate of birth defects when administered to epileptic women. The risk of producing an abnormal child is significant, but in the woman who requires anticonvulsant therapy it is substantially less than the risk of uncontrolled epilepsy during pregnancy. It is important that drug levels are carefully monitored in pregnancy as higher drug levels are more likely to be associated with abnormalities.

Maternal phenylketonuria

A woman discovered to have PKU and established on a low phenylalanine diet before pregnancy has a high likelihood that she will have a normal child. Untreated or unrecognized PKU produces children that are microcephalic, retarded and have an increased incidence of congenital heart disease.

Diethylstilboestrol (DES)

This drug was widely used about 20 years ago in the belief that it prevented miscarriage; ultimately it was proven ineffective and its use ceased. Women who had been exposed to DES in utero have been found to have an increased frequency of the very rare clear cell carcinoma of the vagina as well as other genital defects. Males exposed to DES have an increased frequency of infertility and structural genital abnormalities. All patients exposed to DES in utero require careful monitoring. This is an important lesson about the potential late teratogenic effects of an agent.

SUSPECTED TERATOGENS

Smoking

The babies of women who smoke are smaller at birth than expected. It is not known whether smoking produces any other ill-effects; it is best avoided during pregnancy. Infants of mothers who smoke have more respiratory infections in the first year of life.

Heat and fever

Retrospective studies have suggested that high temperatures in early pregnancy either as a result of an infection, sauna baths, spas, or intense prolonged exercise such as competitive squash may increase the risk of neural tube defects and other birth defects. The status of fever as a teratogen in humans remains uncertain. It has been clearly established experimentally that certain animals, such as rats and guinea pigs, are at risk from hyperthermia. As the risk remains uncertain in humans, sauna baths and spas should be avoided in pregnancy.

Agent Orange

Agent Orange was a mixture of two herbicides – 2,4-D and 2,4,5-T – with low levels of dioxine as a contaminant. There has been a great deal of concern amongst Vietnam veterans both in Australia and the United States of America that this agent might cause birth defects in the offspring of exposed males. So far, studies indicate the pattern of birth defects amongst Vietnam veterans is no different in frequency and type from that which might be expected.

Debendox (Bendectin)

This agent has been widely used in pregnancy for morning sickness over the last 20 years. Prospective studies have failed to show any increase in birth defects amongst the offspring of women who have used this drug.

A number of recent medico-legal actions in the United States have tried to implicate Bendectin as a teratogen. The cost of defending these actions has caused the manufacturers to withdraw the drug from the market. Unfortunately, this removes a well tried and apparently safe drug.

REFERENCES

Heinanen O P, Slone D, Shirpiro S 1977 Birth defects and drugs in pregnancy. Publishing Sciences Group, Massachusetts
Sheppard T H 1986 Catalog of teratogenic agents, 5th edn. The John Hopkins University Press, Baltimore

FURTHER READING

Briggs G C, Freeman K R, Yaffe S J 1986 Drugs in pregnancy and lactation, 2nd edn. Williams and Wilkins, Baltimore
Persaud T V N, Chudley A E, Skallo R G 1985 Basic concepts in teratology. Alan R Lis, New York
Wilson J G 1973 Environment and birth defects. Academic Press, New York
Wilson J G, Fraser F C (eds) 1979 Handbook of teratology 1 p 4. Plenum Press, New York

4. Genes and chromosomes

G. K. Brown

The fundamental unit in genetics is the gene. Originally genes were defined by following the distribution and frequency of readily identified characteristics (phenotypes) in individuals of successive generations. These studies were performed without any knowledge of the nature of the genetic material or of the way in which it was expressed. The first major breakthrough came when it was realized that a gene comprised a coded set of instructions for the synthesis of a particular protein molecule. With further advances in protein chemistry and genetics, the definition was refined to that part of the genome which contains the information for one polypeptide chain.

Following the identification of DNA as the genetic material, there was rapid progress in our understanding of the sequence of events in the expression of genetic information. The first step, transcription, is the process whereby the information coded in the DNA is copied into messenger RNA (mRNA). The mRNA molecule is an exact complementary copy of one strand of the DNA coding sequence except that uracil replaces thymine. The mRNA is transported from the nucleus to the cytoplasm where it acts as a template for translation. In this process, the nucleotide sequence of the mRNA determines the amino acid sequences of a protein polypeptide chain. There is a one-to-one correspondence between the genome DNA coding sequence, the mRNA sequence and the protein amino acid sequence, with a triplet of nucleotide bases (or codon) coding for each amino acid. The translation of the nucleotide code into protein requires the mediation of a family of transfer RNA molecules (tRNAs) which bind a specific codon in mRNA and a specific amino acid. Polypeptide chain assembly is carried out on large RNA-protein complexes called ribosomes.

With the discovery of the details of information transfer, the definition of the gene had to be expanded to include DNA segments which code for ribosomal and transfer RNAs – the additional components required for translating a nucleic acid sequence into a protein sequence.

In all organisms, genes are ordered in a linear sequence along an unbroken double strand of DNA. In higher organisms, including man, the total DNA is further arranged as DNA-protein complexes in a number of structural entities – the chromosomes. Man and most higher organisms are diploid, that is the chromosomes are present in pairs. This structural organization is important for the proper segregation of genetic material during cell division. In man, there are 46 chromosomes comprising 22 paired chromosomes (the autosomes) and 2 sex chromosomes, the X and Y. Normal females have the karyotype 46XX, males 46XY. One copy of each autosome plus one sex chromosome makes up the haploid chromosome set. This is the genetic constitution of the ova and sperm produced during meiosis. The chromosomes of man comprise approximately 6×10^9 base pairs of DNA and are thought to contain between 10 000 and 20 000 genes, each coding for a particular protein or RNA molecule.

CELL DIVISION

Transmission of genetic information takes place in two situations – in the replication of somatic cells and the formation of haploid germ cells.

During growth and development, individual body cells divide many times giving rise to daughter cells, each of which has the same genetic information as the parental cell. The constancy of genetic information in somatic cells is maintained by the process of mitosis. Before cell division, exact copies of the parental DNA molecules are synthesized using each strand of parental DNA as a template for the synthesis of the new DNA molecules. The stages of mitosis (Fig. 4.1) represent the changes in chromosome configuration necessary for distribution of an equal chromosome complement to each of the daughter cells.

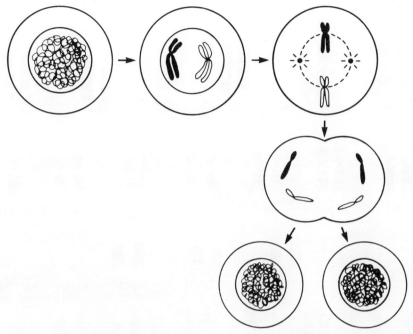

Fig. 4.1 Mitosis. Only one chromosome pair is shown to simplify the appearance of the different stages. From interphase in a single cell, mitosis proceeds through prophase, metaphase and anaphase to interphase in two daughter cells.

In non-dividing cells, the chromosomes are highly extended and cannot be recognized as separate structures. During mitosis, they become progressively contracted and distinct and by metaphase they are clearly identifiable. Each chromosome is duplicated and the two daughter strands, called chromatids, are held together by a constricted region, the centromere. The centromere structure is involved in the attachment of the chromosomes to the mitotic spindle which will result in their movement to opposite poles of the cell.

Once the chromatids are attached to the mitotic spindle they separate with one copy of each chromosome moving to one of two centrioles located at opposite poles of the cell. Following chromosome segregation, a nuclear membrane reforms around each set of chromosomes and the cell cytoplasm divides between them.

With appropriate staining techniques, the metaphase chromosomes can be seen to consist of alternate light and dark staining bands. This banding pattern is unique for each chromosome and enables its identification in metaphase preparations. Analysis of banded chromosomes is the main method used for detecting structural abnormalities of chromosomes in man (Fig. 4.2).

The mechanism for the transfer of genetic information between generations is more complex and introduces the possibility of genetic variation at several stages. The process involves setting apart some cells of the body to form germ cells – ova and sperm – in which only half of the individual's genetic information is represented. At fertilization, the two haploid gametes join to reconstitute the normal diploid state.

Genetic variation in the offspring is introduced firstly by the fact that each parent only contributes half of the genetic information. Secondly, during the formation of germ cells, random segregation of chromosome pairs and genetic recombination minimizes the probability that an offspring will inherit exactly the same haploid genome which his parents inherited from the previous generation.

The structural features of germ cell formation are the stages of meiosis as shown in Figure 4.3.

Before a cell enters the first division of meiosis, the chromosomes have replicated and each comprises two chromatids joined by the centromere. The prophase of the first meiotic division is characterized by the pairing of homologous chromosomes with crossing over and genetic recombination. During pairing, segments of the chromosomes are exchanged so that the daughter

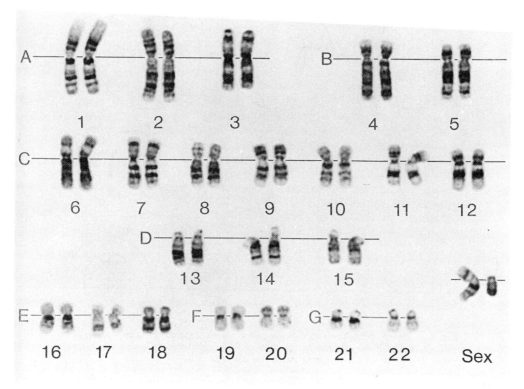

Fig. 4.2 Normal male karyotype. A G-banded preparation is shown and each chromosome pair is easily recognized. The sex chromosomes are the X and the smaller Y.

chromosomes have different arrangements of genetic material. This recombination occurs between two homologous chromatids and is a reciprocal event with an equal exchange of homologous regions of DNA (Fig. 4.4).

The products of the first division of meiosis are two cells with the diploid amount of DNA, one chromosome of each homologous pair and some chromosomal rearrangement due to recombination. In the second meiotic division, the chromatids of each duplicated chromosome separate to the two poles of the cell without further DNA replication. As a result each daughter cell receives only one of each pair of chromosomes and the produce is a haploid germ cell.

The process of meiosis is quite different in males and females. In the male, the divisions are symmetrical and from each primordial germ cell four haploid sperm are produced. After puberty this process is continuous. In the female, meiosis is asymmetric and the primordial germ cell produces only one haploid ovum. The remaining daughter cells are lost as polar bodies. In addition, the process is not continuous. At birth, the ovary of the

human female contains almost 2 million primary oocytes. These are held in the prophase of the first meiotic division. After puberty, one oocyte per menstrual cycle undergoes the remaining stages of meiosis to produce a mature ovum.

The orderly segregation of chromosomes during meiosis is of critical importance for the restoration of a normal chromosome constitution at fertilization. Anything which disturbs this process will produce an imbalance of large amounts of genetic information in the fetus, with usually marked effects on normal growth and development. The most common abnormality of meiosis is non-dysfunction. In this situation the equal segregation of chromosomes to the daughter cells does not occur and a particular gamete will receive either two copies of a particular chromosome, or none. Fertilization of these gametes will produce two new genotypes, one with three copies of the chromosome (trisomy) and another with one (monosomy). Usually, monosomy is lethal as the organism cannot tolerate such a loss of genetic information. The effect of the trisomic condition will depend on the amount of genetic information car-

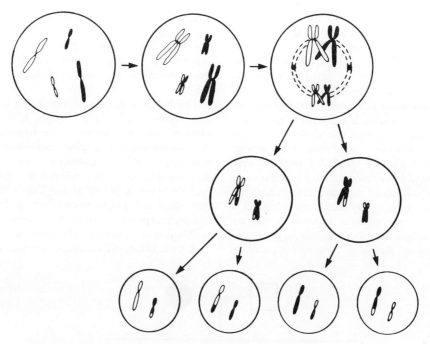

Fig. 4.3 Meiosis. In the first meiotic division, homologous chromosomes pair and crossing over and recombination occurs. In the second division, chromatids of individual chromosomes separate to generate haploid germ cells.

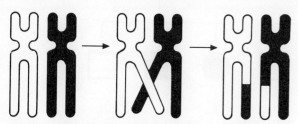

Fig. 4.4 Recombination. Crossing over and recombination in the first meiotic division is a reciprocal event between chromatids of replicated homologous chromosomes.

ried on the chromosome involved, but usually major malformations are found. The most common chromosomal rearrangement of this type found in live-born babies is trisomy of chromosome 21 in Down syndrome. These patients have a characteristic facial appearance together with mental retardation and, often, malformations in other systems, especially the heart.

GENETIC VARIATION

As defined above, a gene is considered to be a sequence of DNA which encodes the information for a protein polypeptide chain. From studies of inherited variations and genetic diseases, the molecular basis for genetic variation in particular proteins can be understood. If the DNA sequence of a particular gene is compared in a number of individuals, some will be found which differ from the common or 'normal' form. These alternative forms of the gene at a particular locus are termed alleles. The effect on the phenotype of the organism will depend on the nature and site of the alteration in the gene. Some allelic variants will have no apparent effect on the function of the protein coded for by the gene. Other allelic sequences may be so altered from the normal that either no gene product is formed or the product is structurally so abnormal that it cannot perform its normal function. These types of variants form the basis of many genetic diseases.

The existence of allelic variants, either harmless or deleterious, allows analysis of segregation of genes in successive generations. The data used for determining patterns of inheritance are the appearance of different phenotypes in the offspring and their proportions. When the transmission of genetic traits is studied in this manner, three common patterns are seen – autosomal dominant, autosomal recessive and X-linked recessive. The terms dominant and recessive refer strictly to the phenotype.

When considering patterns of gene segregation, three genetic constitutions or genotypes can be recognized. If there are two alleles at a particular locus, A and a, then individuals can have genotypes A/A, a/a or A/a. Individuals of the first two types are called homozygotes, those of the third type are heterozygotes.

In autosomal dominant inheritance, the presence of one copy of the mutant allele is sufficient to confer the phenotype. Individuals carrying this allele will express the phenotype and will pass it on to their offspring with a probability of 0.5 for each child. A typical pedigree showing this form of inheritance is shown in Figure 4.5.

In the case of autosomal recessive inheritance, the characteristic phenotype is only seen if an individual is homozygous for the mutant allele. Individuals who are heterozygous, a couple must both be heterozygous carriers of the condition. Both then form two populations

of germ cells, one with the normal allele, the other with the mutant form. At fertilization three genotypes are possible – homozygous normal (with probability 0.25), heterozygous carrier (with probability 0.5) and homozygous mutant (with probability 0.25) (see Fig. 4.6).

The X-linked pattern of inheritance is quite distinctive because males and females have different sex chromosome constitutions. In the female, there are two X chromosomes, so a given individual can again be homozygous or heterozygous for different alleles. As the male has only one X chromosome, he can only ever have one allele for X-linked genes. The Y chromosome is very small and appears to carry very little genetic information except for the testis determining factor which is involved in male sexual differentiation.

X-linked recessive conditions are seen in males when

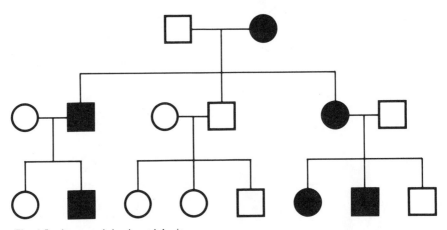

Fig. 4.5   Autosomal dominant inheritance.

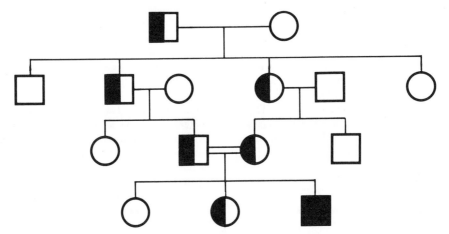

Fig. 4.6   Autosomal recessive inheritance.

they inherit a variant gene on their sole X chromosome. A female would, in general, only show the trait if she was homozygous for the same allele – a situation which is usually extremely uncommon. Also, the transmission of X-linked traits differs between the sexes. A male can only transmit the mutant allele to his daughters, all of whom will be carriers of the condition. The female can transmit the allele to both sons and daughters. In the case of her sons, each has a probability of 0.5 of being affected by the condition. In the case of her daughters, each has a probability of 0.5 of being a carrier of the trait. A typical X-linked pedigree is shown in Figure 4.7.

LINKAGE

Alleles at any given locus segregate between generations because each gamete receives only one copy of each gene. In general, genes at different loci behave as if they are independent of each other and assort between generations. The basis of this independent assortment is the random distribution of each chromosome of an homologous pair into the daughter cells during meiosis. However, the independent assortment of different genetic loci is limited by the constraints of chromosome structure. If two gene loci occupy adjacent segments of a particular chromosome, they will normally be trans-mitted together. The co-transmission of genes on one chromosome or chromosome segment is termed genetic linkage.

Rearrangement of genes on a chromosome segment can occur as a result of the genetic recombination which occurs when homologous chromosomes pair and under-go crossing over during meiosis. This means that alleles at two linked gene loci, which are usually transmitted together, will sometimes be separated by recombination

and give rise to gametes with new combinations. The probability of recombination between two gene loci is proportional to the distance between them on the chromosome and this forms the basis of gene mapping by linkage analysis. This technique was first developed

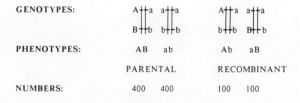

Fig. 4.8 Linkage analysis of two gene loci, A and B.

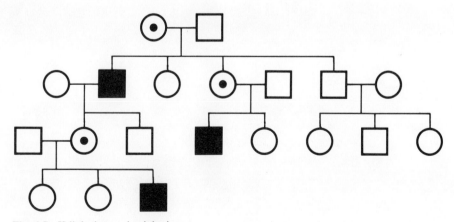

Fig. 4.7 X-linked recessive inheritance.

in organisms with short reproductive cycles, large numbers of offspring and ready availability of genetic markers. Among higher oganisms, *Drosophila* and the mouse have been most widely studied. In these species, selected matings between individuals with particular phenotypes are readily performed and the frequency of the phenotypes in the offspring easily measured. A typical linkage experiment is shown in Figure 4.8.

In man, this type of analysis is quite different because of small family sizes and long generation times. For this reason a number of mathematical methods have been devised to determine whether the pooled data from many pedigrees indicate linkage between particular traits.

The most important medical application of linkage analysis is in antenatal diagnosis of genetic disease. In this case, the genotype of the fetus must be determined in readily accessible tissues such as amniotic cells or chorionic villi. Linkage analysis is particularly useful when the basic gene defect is not known or cannot be analysed directly in these tissues.

For linkage analysis in man, it is not sufficient to identify loci which are closely linked to the disease locus. There are two additional requirements. The marker loci should exhibit a high degree of polymorphism, with multiple alleles, each present in the general population at a relatively high frequency. This condition is essential to ensure that sufficient family members will be heterozygous for different alleles of the marker locus to provide an informative pedigree. The alleles at the marker locus must also be readily detectable, either as their gene products or by direct DNA analysis.

For antenatal diagnosis, the pattern of segregation of the disease and the linked locus is determined from all available family members. The genotype of the fetus at the marker locus can be used, in conjunction with the family data, to deduce the genotype at the disease locus.

Recent advances in molecular genetics (described in the following chapter) have led to the identification of suitable linked polymorphic markers for a large number of different genetic diseases. As methods for direct analysis of the underlying mutations in these conditions have not been developed to a comparable extent, linkage analysis is, at present, the main method for antenatal diagnosis of genetic diseases which are not expressed in accessible fetal tissues.

5. Molecular genetics

G. K. Brown

Although classic genetic analysis and cytogenetic studies have contributed greatly to our understanding of human genetics, they have quite significant limitations when applied to man. There is a vast literature on the clinical features of genetic diseases, with relatively little known about the underlying basic genetic defects. However, in the past ten years there has been a remarkable increase in our knowledge of the molecular basis of human genetic disease. This has been brought about by the development of techniques for isolating and sequencing human genes, and for analysing their transcription and translation in vitro. This recombinant DNA technology overcomes many of the difficulties in applying traditional methods of genetic analysis to man.

A brief description of some of the techniques will be given in a later section after presentation of what is currently known about human gene organization and expression.

One of the most striking features of the genome of man and other higher organisms is that the chromosomes contain considerably more DNA than is required for the calculated number of genes. In man, only about half of the total of approximately 3×10^9 base pairs of DNA per haploid genome is considered to encode genetic information.

DNA nucleotide sequences in man can be divided into three classes: highly repetitive, moderately repetitive and unique. Highly repetitive sequences make up about 10% of the genome. They comprise a small group of very short DNA sequences repeated up to a million times and are preferentially located around centromeres and at the ends of chromosomes. At present their function is completely unknown, although their distribution in the chromosomes may indicate a structural role. They are not transcribed into RNA.

Moderately repetitive sequences are represented in the genome as a number of families of closely related sequences. They are interspersed between the structural genes throughout the chromosomes and account for approximately 25% of the genome. In man, the main element in this class is the ALU family which alone accounts for between 3–6% of the genome. ALU sequences are about 300 base pairs long and take their name from the presence of a site for the restriction enzyme ALU 1 in the centre of the sequence. There are between three and five hundred thousand copies of these sequences and they commonly occur between structural genes, although in some cases they are present within genes in intervening sequences (see below).

Moderately repetitive sequences are translated into RNA but are not translated into protein. Their function is at present unknown; however, they do share some properties with sequences found in many other organisms and which are termed transposable elements. These are short DNA sequences which can be moved to different sites in the genome and can affect expression of genes adjacent to their site of insertion.

The third class of DNA sequences in the genome, the unique sequences, are those which correlate with the 'genes' of classic genetics. They make up approximately 50% of the genome in man and each is represented by one or at most a few copies per haploid genome. While most of these sequences are transcribed into mRNA and translated into protein products, some encode the information for transfer and ribosomal RNAs. These unique sequences, the structural genes, are the major genetic elements in man.

ANATOMY OF THE STRUCTURAL GENE

Isolation, cloning and sequencing of human structural genes have enabled us to analyse the common elements which are important for information transfer from DNA to protein. All structural genes have a number of sequences in common and these are important for gene expression. The sequences are either identical in all genes or share considerable homology, in which case the term 'concensus sequence' is used.

The main component of a structural gene is the nucleotide sequence which codes for the amino acid sequence of the protein product. A striking feature of eukaryotic genes is that this sequence is almost never continuous but is broken up into small segments representing fragments of the final protein. These coding regions, or exons, are divided by intervening DNA sequences, or introns, which do not appear in the nature mRNA or in the protein. The number of introns varies widely between different genes. Some genes, such as the histone genes, have none, while others, such as the collagen genes, have more than 50. Most human genes sequenced so far have between 2 and 10 introns.

While the number, size and overall sequence of introns in different genes are quite variable, they do share common sequences at the junctions with coding regions. These junction sequences have been shown, particularly by analysis of the mutations in some forms of thalassaemia, to be the recognition sites for accurate splicing out of the introns during mRNA processing. The concensus sequences required for correct splicing have been determined from a large number of cloned gene sequences and are shown in Figure 5.1.

For the information in the coding regions to be expressed, additional sequences are required for transcription, processing and translation.

A number of sequences are required for transcription and, of these, the most important are the promoters (see Fig. 5.1). These are recognition sites for RNA polymerase II – the RNA polymerase responsible for structural gene transcription. A promoter sequence of the form 'TATA' is located 25-30 bases upstream from the start site for transcription. This sequence is essential for the accurate positioning of RNA polymerase II which then begins RNA synthesis approximately 25 bases downstream from the site. The CAAT sequence at a position 70-80 bases from the site of transcription and other sequences several hundred bases further along, have also been implicated as promoters. In addition, there are elements known as enhancers which can

be located at much greater distances from a structural gene, yet still influence its rate of transcription.

Although the initiation of transcription is now well understood, the DNA sequences and enzymic reactions necessary to terminate the activity of RNA polymerase II are still obscure. Unlike the promoter sequences, no uniform terminator sequences have as yet been identified. At the 3' end of the RNA molecules produced from most structural genes there is one conserved sequence of the form AAUAAA (see Fig. 5.1). This sequence directs addition of the poly-A tail (see below) approximately 11-19 nucleotides downstream, but its role in cleavage of the messenger RNA molecule to the correct length is unclear.

As well as exons, introns and promoters, most structural genes have variable lengths of DNA sequence on either side of the coding region which will be transcribed and appear in the final mRNA molecule, but will not be translated (see Fig. 5.1). Variable processing of these untranslated regions may be important in regulating the expression of some genes.

The initial transcript of a structural gene is a long RNA molecule belonging to the class of heterogeneous nuclear RNA or hnRNA. Before the information encoded in this molecule can be translated into protein, it must be processed into a mature messenger RNA molecule and transported to the ribosomes in the cell cytoplasm.

PROCESSING OF mRNA

The primary gene transcript, a molecule of the hnRNA class, must undergo considerable processing before it can be exported from nucleus to cytoplasm for translation into protein on the ribosomes. The three main reactions involved are addition of the poly-A tail, capping, and excision of introns.

The first of these reactions to occur is addition of the

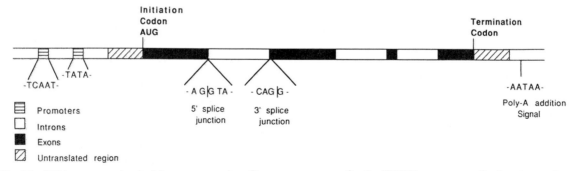

Fig. 5.1 DNA sequences involved in gene expression. Concensus sequences for the 'TATA' promoter, splice junctions and the poly-A addition site are shown.

poly-A tail. Most mRNA molecules have a 3' tail of polyadenylic acid up to several hundred residues long and this is added within 90-120 seconds of the synthesis of the primary transcript. The poly-A tail is not necessary for transport of the mRNA to the cytoplasm but is a major determinant of the life span of the molecule once it has left the nucleus.

The 5' end of mRNA molecules is also modified after transcription by a process known as capping. This involves the addition of an unusual nucleotide sequence of the form 7-methylguanine-2-O-methyladenine with the modified bases joined by a pyrophosphate group rather than the usual phosphate ester. This capping process occurs very soon after the onset of transcription. The 5' mRNA cap plays an important role in the initiation of translation by interacting with specific ribosomal proteins.

The most important processing step in the formation of mature mRNA molecules from the primary transcripts is the excision of intervening sequences. The sequence determinants of this process are the splice-junctions described above. There is considerable evidence that the splicing process is sequential with introns being removed one after the other. This suggests that the enzymes involved scan along the mRNA precursor from one end to the other, excising the introns as the splice sites are recognized.

The level of expression of a particular gene can now be seen as the overall outcome of a large number of processes, any or all of which may be subjected to some form of regulation.

Summary

The events in summary are: binding of RNA polymerase II to promoters, initiation of transcription and hnRNA biosynthesis, addition of the poly-A tail, capping, excision of intervening sequences, nuclear-cytoplasmic transport, binding of ribosomes, and interaction with cytoplasmic factors which determine stability. Mutations affecting most of these processes have been found in various genetic diseases in man and will be considered in more detail.

FUNCTIONAL ORGANIZATION OF THE GENOME

Although the expression of structural genes is regulated to some extent by intrinsic sequence components, it is also subject to higher orders of regulation. Different genes are expressed at different stages of development, in different tissues and in different metabolic states. Our knowledge of these regulatory processes is extremely poor, although we have some idea of possible mechanisms from the few systems which have been partially characterized.

In some cases, the chromosomal organization of genes indicates a particular functional requirement. This is clearly evident in the case of the histone genes, which are organized as a gene cluster. The five histones H1, H2a, H2b, H3 and H4 are basic proteins which complex with DNA to form chromatin. In the nuclei of eukaryotic cells, all of the DNA is in the form of chromatin and, as a result, histone proteins have to be synthesized at a very high rate during the short period of the cell cycle when the DNA is replicated. The new DNA molecules can then complex with histones immediately to reform the chromatin structure.

This requirement for a short, rapid burst of histone protein synthesis is reflected in the structure and organization of the histone genes. There are 10-20 copies of the structural gene for each histone protein and they are all located in a small segment of the long arm of chromosome 7. During the period of active histone protein synthesis, there is a high level of transcription from these genes and large amounts of their mRNAs are synthesized. There are also a number of other factors which contribute to the rapid burst of histone synthesis. The histone genes do not contain introns, nor are their mRNA molecules modified with poly-A tails. The primary gene transcripts do not need processing and are exported to the cytoplasm very rapidly. Although the histone mRNA molecules have a short lifespan, they are produced in large amounts and are required for only a short period. The benefits of co-ordinated transcription from closely linked genes each present in multiple copies, combined with rapid transport and translation, appear to override any disadvantage of mRNA instability.

While the gene cluster is the most extreme form of functional organization, other genes occur also in closely linked groups whose members share structural and functional properties. The best known examples of gene families in man are the globin genes. Two globin gene clusters, the α and β, are located on chromosomes 16 and 11, respectively.

The β-globin gene family is shown in Figure 5.2. It is unusual for all of the different members of a gene family to be expressed at the same time in the same cell. In the β-globin family, the genes are arranged in order of their expression during embryonic, fetal and adult life. Each β-globin-like protein has considerable amino acid sequence homology with the other members of the family and this homology also extends to the DNA sequence of the gene where the position and size of coding regions and introns are remarkably similar.

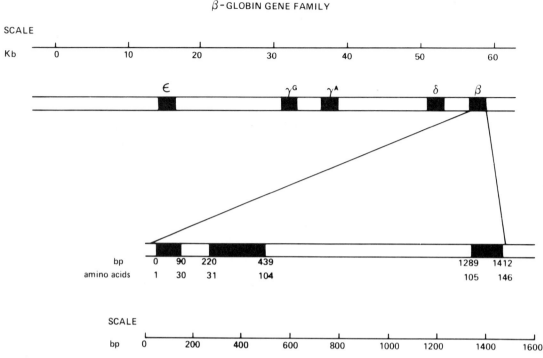

Fig. 5.2   The β-globin gene family and the structure of the β-globin gene.

It is thought that gene families arise by gene duplication due to unequal crossing over during meiosis. Once duplicated, one copy of the gene can undergo further evolution without compromising the function of the parent gene. The newly evolving gene may come to play quite a different role in the organism, depending on selective pressures.

Apart from the gene clusters and families, most structural genes are probably represented by only one copy per haploid genome. In many cases (for example multi-subunit enzymes or the enzymes in a metabolic pathway) co-ordinate expression of unique copy genes is required. The interactions between different sites in the genome which permit this co-ordinate expression are unknown.

The complexity of the information storage and retrieval system in the human genome is only now coming to be appreciated. In addition to the elements already considered, there are certainly many more to be discovered. One of the main methods for determining the biological importance of these elements is to study the consequences when they are altered by mutations. Studies of human genetic diseases have been particularly fruitful in demonstrating the most important sequences in structural genes.

MUTATION

Changes in the DNA sequence can occur by a variety of different mechanisms. These can be divided into two main groups:

1. Mutations which occur because of errors in DNA replication.
2. Mutations which are due to errors in recombination during meiosis.

Mutations due to errors in DNA replication

The semi-conservative replication of DNA is an extremely accurate process as the parental strands form exact templates for complementary strand synthesis. Of the few errors which do occur, most are recognized and removed by a complex repair system and only those which escape these processes are perpetuated as mutations. Errors of replication occur in both somatic cells and germ line cells. Somatic cell mutations accumulate in individual cells throughout life and may contribute to progressive tissue dysfunction with age. Germ line mutations are of greater importance because they can be transmitted to all of the cells of the offspring. DNA sequence changes due to errors of replication tend to involve single bases or very short sequences as they are usually due to base mismatching or errors of DNA repair. If they occur within the structural gene for a protein, the effect on protein structure and function will depend on both the site of the change and its nature.

The effect of an alteration of a nucleotide sequence is also related to the nature of the genetic code. Each amino acid is coded for by a triplet of nucleotides. As there are 4 nucleotide bases, there are 64 possible combinations of these taken 3 at a time. Only 24 combinations are needed to code for 20 amino acids which are found in proteins, an initiation codon and 3 termination codons. The difference is made up as codon redundancy, that is, several different triplet codons code for the same amino acid.

The simplest mutational change is a base substitution. This can have any one of a number of different effects. Because of the redundancy of the genetic code, some base changes will alter a triplet codon without altering the amino acid which is specified. For example, the codons GAA and GAG both code for glutamic acid. A mutation of A to G in the third position of a GAA codon would not affect the amino acid sequence of the protein. Mutations of this type have been called 'neutral' because they do not alter protein structure.

The most common effect of a single base change is to alter a codon to one for a different amino acid. In sickle cell disease, for example, the codon at position 6 of the β-globin chain, GAG (= glutamic acid), is altered by a base substitution to GTG (= valine). This has a significant effect on the structure of the haemoglobin molecule, allowing it to form a crystalline array at low oxygen tension. Patients homozygous for this mutation have a severe form of haemolytic anaemia.

Many inborn errors of metabolism are due to mutations which produce structural alterations of particular enzymes. It is likely that many of these mutations are single base substitutions.

A single base substitution can result in complete deficiency of a protein product when a codon for an amino acid is altered to a stop codon. This type of mutation, the nonsense mutation, does not usually affect mRNA synthesis, but the polypeptide is only synthesized as far as the new stop codon, then released from the ribosome. The small polypeptide is usually rapidly degraded. Some beta-thalassaemias occur because of this type of mutation – in one case a codon for lysine at position 17, AAG, is converted to the termination codon UAG. A 16 amino acid fragment of the β-globin chain is produced and there is no normal β-globin.

In all of the examples above, the mutation has been located within the coding regions of the gene. However, mutations in non-coding sequences of structural genes

which are necessary for transcription and processing can also produce defects in the protein products. Mutations of this type have now been well documented, particularly in the thalassaemias.

Several new classes of mutations due to single base substitutions have been recognized – including those which affect promoter sequences and the splicing of introns.

One form of β⁺-thalassaemia has been found to be due to a single base change in the TATA promoter. The concensus sequence of the β-globin gene promotor, CATAAAA has been changed to CATACAA and this reduces the rate of transcription dramatically. However, because all of the coding regions and processing signals are intact, a small amount of normal β-globin is synthesized.

Two types of splicing defect have been demonstrated, both in patients with β-thalassaemia. In one form, the exon-intron junction sequence has been altered, thus abolishing the signal for correct splicing. This mutated gene is transcribed into hnRNA but further normal processing is not possible.

The other form of splicing defect does not abolish the normal splice junction but introduces a new one elsewhere in the intron. This site is recognized by the processing system resulting in anomalous splicing of the mRNA precursor and reduced levels of normal mRNA. Since the normal splice site is still present, normal splicing does take place at a frequency of approximately 5%, permitting the synthesis of small amounts of normal mRNA and low levels of β-globin.

Also, errors of DNA replication and repair can result in loss or addition of bases to the DNA sequence. If the additions or deletions are in multiples of three in phase with the normal reading frame, amino acids corresponding to the codons will be added to or taken from the protein amino acid sequence. Single amino acid additions or deletions may or may not have a major effect on the function of the protein, depending on their position.

Additions or deletions of bases not in multiples of three have a much greater potential for disrupting the structure and function of the protein product. This is because these changes alter the reading frame. The effect of such a frameshift mutation is to completely change the amino acid sequence following the mutation. Transcription may proceed normally and mRNA molecules may be formed. However, when these are translated, the altered amino acid sequence is synthesized until a new termination codon is reached. The resultant protein is a hybrid of part of the normal protein and a new amino acid sequence, which is quite different. These hybrid molecules rarely function normally even when the mutation is very close to the end of the molecule.

Mutations due to errors in recombination during meiosis

Large rearrangement of genetic material can occur as a result of errors in recombination. During meiosis, homologous chromosomes pair and exchange segments of DNA by recombination. If homologous DNA sequences are not aligned accurately, duplication and deletion of DNA sequences can occur. This is more likely if closely related sequences are linked together along short lengths of the chromosome as is the case with gene families. Misalignment can occur within or between genes as shown in Figure 5.3. A defect of recombination within two gene loci is the basis of haemoglobin Lepore. The β- and δ-globin sequences are closely linked and have considerable sequence homology. A crossover event which occurs when a β and δ gene are aligned will produce two hybrid molecules, part derived from the β-globin gene, the other from the δ. Although recombination is a reciprocal event and two new chromosome rearrangements are generated during meiosis, in man only one product is recovered.

If the recombination event takes place between genes which have been misaligned, complete duplication or deletion of the gene will occur. This appears to be the basis of most cases of α-thalassaemia. The α-globin gene family contains two copies of the α-globin gene located adjacent to each other on the chromosome. This arrangement carries apparently a relatively high risk of unequal crossing over. The consequences of such an event will be to generate two new chromosomal arrangements as shown in Figure 5.3.

Repeated deletional events can lead to genomes with 3, 2, 1 or no copies of the α-globin gene and this is associated with increasingly severe α-thalassaemia (Fig. 5.4). Support for this model of gene deletion comes from the discovery that a number of normal people have a chromosome carrying three copies of the α-globin gene – this is expected because of the reciprocal nature of recombination.

MEDICAL IMPACT

Already, advances in recombinant DNA technology have greatly increased our understanding of genetic disease and this new information is now being applied in the diagnosis of particular disorders. Recombinant DNA techniques used in the diagnosis of genetic disease are relatively simple and involve digestion of cellular DNA with restriction enzymes and detection of specific sequences with cloned DNA probes.

The restriction enzymes are a large group of proteins

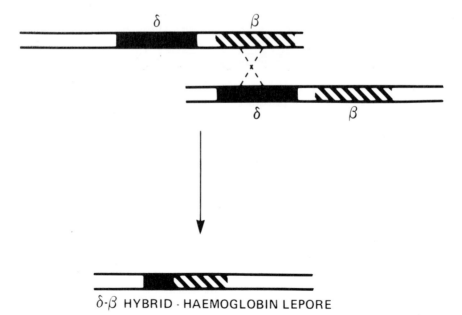

δ-β HYBRID · HAEMOGLOBIN LEPORE

Fig. 5.3 Haemoglobin Lepore. Considerable homology between the β and δ-globin genes results in occasional pairing between them. Recombination within the genes produces a hybrid globin chain.

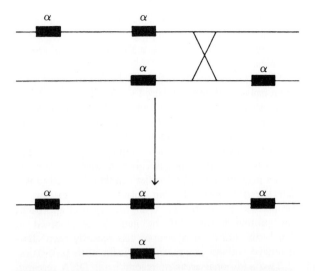

Fig. 5.4 Deletion-type α-thalassaemia. Incorrect pairing of the α-globin genes can generate two possible recombinant chromosomes with either 1 or 3 α-globin gene sequences.

of bacterial origin. Each enzyme recognizes a specific 6 or 4 nucleotide sequence of DNA and cuts across both strands of the molecule at all sites which have the sequence.

Gene probes are usually made by synthesizing a DNA copy of isolated mRNA molecules. These copy DNA or cDNA molecules are synthesized in vitro using a viral enzyme, reverse transcriptase, which uses an RNA template for DNA synthesis.

The cDNA is then inserted into a bacterial plasmid or virus and this 'recombinant' molecule is reinfected into a suitable bacterial host. Within the host, it is replicated many fold and the human DNA component can subsequently be isolated as a cloned cDNA gene probe. Incorporation of radioactive nucleotides during the procedure results in the formation of multiple labelled copies of a single DNA sequence homologous to the mRNA for a particular gene product. This can be used to detect homologous gene sequences in total cellular DNA using a variety of different hybridization techniques.

Most commonly, DNA is extracted from the patient's cells and digested with a particular restriction enzyme. The resulting DNA fragments are separated by agarose gel electrophoresis and transferred to nitrocellulose filters. Fragments bearing sequences homologous to those of a cDNA probe are identified by hybridization of the probe to the DNA on the filter and localization by autoradiography. This technique is called 'Southern Blot' analysis.

Diagnosis of specific gene defects can be made using either direct or indirect methods. Disorders which are due to gene deletions, such as most forms of α-thalassaemia, are particularly suitable for direct analysis if a cDNA probe for the gene is available. When a gene is deleted, no sequences corresponding to the gene probe will be present in the cellular DNA, so no fragments will appear in the autoradiographs.

Direct analysis can sometimes be applied to genetic diseases which are due to a single base substitution. In sickle cell disease, the mutation affecting amino acid number 6 of the β-globin chain, a change of codon GAG to GTG, results in the loss of a restriction enzyme recognition site. The normal DNA nucleotide sequence around this position is CCTGAGGAG (proline- glutamic acid-glutamic acid) and this contains the recognition sequence for the restriction enzyme Dde I (-CCTNAGG- where N is any nucleotide). In DNA from patients with sickle cell disease, the sequence is CCTGTGGAG (proline-valine-glutamic acid) and the enzyme no longer cuts the DNA at this site but cuts at the next recognition site along the sequence.

Cellular DNA digested with the restriction enzyme Dde and probed with a specific β-globin cDNA probe will produce three possible fragment patterns – a single small fragment in persons who are homozygous for the normal β-globin gene, a single, larger fragment in patients with sickle cell disease and both fragments in heterozygous carriers.

Unfortunately, most mutations cannot be detected easily with currently available methods, and indirect diagnosis by linkage analysis is often required. In this case, the presence or absence of the mutant gene is deduced from the genotype at a closely linked marker locus. The use of this approach has been stimulated by the development of simple methods for detecting polymorphisms which are suitable for linkage studies.

Genomic DNA from many individuals has been analysed with cDNA probes for various human genes. Studies of this type have revealed a significant degree of sequence variation, particularly in the DNA sequences which separate structural genes. These sequence variations are identified by the presence or absence of recognition sites for the various restriction enzymes.

When DNA is digested with a particular restriction enzyme and probed with a specific gene probe, the homologous genomic sequence will be found on fragments of different sizes in different individuals depending on the pattern of recognition sites. These restriction fragment length polymorphisms (RFLP) are inherited in families in a simple Mendelian fashion and can be used for linkage analysis. As RFLPs are really only dimorphisms (i.e. a site is either present or absent), it might be expected that their use would be quite limited. However, a number of different restriction enzymes can be used in conjunction with any gene probe and this increases the probability that diagnostically useful fragment patterns will be found in a particular family.

This approach was first developed using cDNA probes for known genes. For example, many cases of β-thalassaemia can only be diagnosed directly by isolating the β-globin genes from the patients and sequencing them. However, if there is a restriction site polymorphism near the gene, the pattern of segregation of the disease and the polymorphism can be followed in the family. This approach will provide sufficient information for antenatal diagnosis in about 80% of families.

The method can be extended to the diagnosis of genetic diseases in which the actual genes involved have not yet been identified. As long as a probe can be found for a DNA sequence which is closely linked to the disease locus, restriction fragment polymorphism analysis can be used in family studies for antenatal diagnosis. This approach has already been developed for important genetic diseases such as Huntington disease and cystic fibrosis. The main limitation to the use of linked probes in these conditions is the risk of misdiagnosis due to recombination between the marker and disease loci during meiosis. This can be minimized by isolating probes which are very closely linked to the disease locus.

In conjunction with diagnostic applications, mapping of the human genome is now proceeding extremely rapidly. Chromosomal location of cloned genes may be determined using cell hybridization techniques or by direct hybridization of the gene probes to metaphase chromosomes.

The genes involved in many important genetic diseases are as yet unknown. Recombinant DNA techniques have proved extremely powerful in identifying these genes and their protein products. The chromosomal location of the gene can be determined from linkage studies with mapped probes or by analysis of patients who have the disease as a result of a chromosome rearrangement, such as a deletion or translocation, which interrupts the gene locus. Probes for the disease locus can then be isolated by 'walking' along the chromosome using overlapping clones or from DNA libraries from the patients with chromosome abnormalities.

When probes in the region of the disease locus have been isolated, they can be used to identify unique DNA sequences which are transcribed and translated into a protein product which differs in patients and normal individuals. The amino acid sequence of the protein can be determined from the gene sequence and antibodies raised to synthetic peptides corresponding to segments of the protein. These antibodies can then be used to isolate the gene product from normal tissues so that its properties can be studied. Using this type of approach, the protein product of the gene locus involved in Duchenne muscular dystrophy has recently been characterized without any prior knowledge of its properties.

Two additional areas of recombinant DNA research hold great prospects for medical application. The first of these is the synthesis of biologically important molecules. Cloned genes for human protein products such as insulin, growth hormone, interferon and blood clotting factors can be incorporated into plasmids with sequences necessary for their expression in the host bacteria. These recombinant plasmids can be used to direct the bacteria to synthesize large quantities of the human product which can then be isolated from the cultures. Human insulin, growth hormone and interferon are already being produced in this way for clinical use.

The other area of practical application of recombinant gene technology is the development of specific gene therapy. As the basic defects in genetic diseases are defined, more and more information about human gene organization and control of gene expression is obtained. It may one day be possible to use recombinant DNA methods to replace mutant DNA sequences with normal genetic information in the appropriate tissues with the proper regulatory elements. Already, such an approach to treatment is technically possible and awaits only a better understanding of the factors which regulate expression of our genetic information in different tissues and at different stages of differentiation and development.

6. Prenatal diagnosis

L. J. Sheffield

Genetic prenatal diagnosis includes diagnosis during pregnancy of both inherited conditions and birth defects which may or may not be inherited. It aims to detect those conditions or birth defects before the fetus is viable so that parents have the option of termination of pregnancy. This of course raises a number of ethical issues as not all parents wish to proceed along these lines. It follows that structured counselling facilities must be made available so that couples can receive the appropriate information at all stages of the diagnostic process. This should include information about the limitations of any tests performed as well as the risks involved. While awaiting the results of any investigation couples require adequate support. Should termination of pregnancy be required a great deal more support will be required.

TYPE OF PRENATAL TESTING

Screening tests

There are two main screening tests in use.

Serum alphafetoprotein screening test

Alphafetoprotein is a fetal protein, i.e. it is produced by the fetus and its production is largely confined to the fetus. It is produced by the yolk sac and the liver reaching a peak in fetal serum at about 13 weeks of pregnancy and decreasing slowly to term. Amniotic alphafetoprotein levels are high in the fetus with a lesion not covered with skin, for example, an open spina bifida. This high level appears to be due to leakage from fetal serum into the amniotic fluid. Alphafetoprotein may leak into the mother's blood resulting in an elevated maternal serum level. In certain parts of the world maternal serum alphafetoprotein levels are used routinely as a screening test primarily for neural defects, but also in the diagnosis of other lesions such as an exomphalos.

It should be recognized that serum alphafetoprotein testing is purely a screening procedure and for patients with high levels other investigations are required. These include ultrasound staging, ultrasound examination for fetal abnormalities and amniocentesis if the level is beyond a certain cut-off point. There are a number of other causes of elevated maternal serum alphafetoprotein levels. These include contamination of fetal blood, microscopic fetal-maternal transfusion, twins and fetal death in utero. Serum alphafetoprotein screening is widespread in the UK, but at present is only available in some parts of Australia.

Recently, low levels of serum alphafetoprotein have been found to provide another screening test for Down syndrome. Down syndrome babies tend to be growth retarded and, therefore, have lower levels of serum alphafetoprotein on average. Again, there is quite a wide overlap between normal and abnormal and the effectiveness of this method for screening patients for Down syndrome is still being evaluated.

Ultrasound screening

Ultrasound (sonar) scanning involves either static or real-time scanning to visualize a fetus. Real-time scanning allows the movement of the fetus to be studied and better visualization as it looks at the fetus in various views. Fetal visualization and the recognition of birth defects requires an experienced ultrasonologist. It should not be confused with ultrasound scanning for gestational age which concentrates on fetal measurements – particularly the biparietal diameter.

In some centres all pregnant women have an ultrasound examination to screen for fetal abnormalities. The best time for this is at 18 weeks' gestation as the fetus is relatively large, and termination of pregnancy can still be safely done.

Amniocentesis

Amniocentesis is a well established and relatively safe technique for prenatal diagnosis. It involves abdominal puncture of the amniotic cavity at 16 weeks' gestation. Usually it is performed together with ultrasound scanning of the fetus to monitor fetal position and the movements of the needle. It is a relatively safe procedure, the only risk being that of fetal loss due to premature labour. The risk of this occurring is 0.5–1% depending upon the experience of the operator. It should be noted that amniocentesis may immunize a Rhesus-negative woman so that the blood group should be known and if Rhesus-negative, prophylactic anti-D-immunoglobulin is required for the non-immunized. There are two main uses of amniotic samples:

1. Culture of amniotic cells. This enables a karyotype to be prepared. Culture of amniocytes takes some 10 days to 4 weeks. These cells may also be used to measure enzyme levels for the diagnosis of inborn errors of metabolism.

2. Fluid analysis. This relates particularly to the determination of alphafetoprotein and acetyl-cholinesterase levels in the diagnosis of neural tube defects. Analysis of disaccharidase enzymes in amniotic fluid has been used in the prenatal diagnosis of cystic fibrosis. Occasionally other metabolites are estimated if an inborn error of metabolism is suspected e.g. methyl-malonic acidaemia.

Chorionic villus sampling (CVS)

This technique is quite recent, but allows first trimester diagnosis as it is performed between 9 and 11 weeks of pregnancy. Because direct analysis may be carried out on fetal cells, a result is obtainable whilst a patient is in the first trimester of pregnancy, thus allowing for a first trimester termination if required. Figure 6.1 illustrates the procedure of chorionic villus biopsy. This procedure was done initially through the cervix but recently the abdominal route has become popular as a method of chorionic villus sampling. The risk of the procedure is again the loss of the fetus and again is highly dependent on the operator's experience. The fetal loss risk approximates between 3 and 4%. The chorionic tissues obtained can be used for chromosome analysis, DNA analysis and biochemical analysis. For chromosome analysis short-term cultures take 1–2 days while long-term cultures take 7–14 days. It should be noted that the tissue is not precisely the fetal tissue and occasionally anomalous results are obtained in the chorion which is not reflected in the fetus. A mosaic picture would give a clue to this and such a finding should be followed by amniocentesis or fetal blood sampling. Many inborn errors of metabolism can be diagnosed prenatally by analysis of chorionic cells usually after a 1–2 week cul-

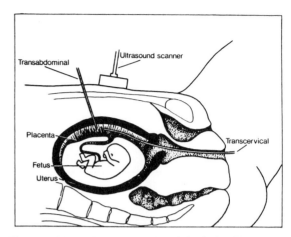

Fig. 6.1 Schematic representation of chorionic villus sampling showing transabdominal and transcervical routes. (Source: Courtesy of Sonar Department, Royal Women's Hospital, Melbourne).

ture. DNA analysis may be carried out directly on the chorionic sample if it is large enough so that a fairly rapid result (with 1–3 weeks) can be obtained.

Sonar examination

Sonar examination plays a key role in the performance of amniocentesis and chorionic villus sampling for fetal and needle localization. Also, it has a role in its own right for prenatal diagnosis of anatomical defects, especially cystic or space occupying lesions, such as cystic hygroma, hydronephrosis, exomphalos, congenital cardiac defects and shortening of the limbs.

Fetal blood sampling and fetal biopsies

Fetal blood sampling may be required for rapid cytogenetic analysis, haemoglobinopathy detection or detection of in utero infection. Fetoscopy was the main method for fetal blood sampling, but it has now been replaced in most centres by direct ultrasound guidance sampling of fetal blood through either the umbilical cord or the ductus venosus. The risk of this procedure has not been established accurately but is probably smaller than the risk of direct visualization and sampling by fetoscopy.

Fetal liver and skin biopsies may be carried out under visual control with either the fetoscope or by ultrasound guided biopsies. Direct ultrasound techniques are now replacing fetoscopy for fetal biopsy and even for fetal visualization.

DNA diagnosis

Usually, the DNA diagnosis is carried out by using restriction fragment length polymorphisms (RFLP) (see Ch. 5). It is essential for this technique that the family must be studied as early as possible before a pregnancy to note if it is suitable for DNA diagnosis. In some cases a deletion may be found in the affected individual and by tracking this deletion through the family the person being considered for prenatal diagnosis can be identified as a carrier of the gene or not. If the individual is a carrier, prenatal diagnosis is possible with little error. When no deletion is found linkage methods have to be used to track the gene through the family. Linkage methods introduce small errors due to genetic recombination. The errors involved vary according to the particular family situation. For X-linked diseases such as Duchenne muscular dystrophy it is not always possible to be certain if the intending mother is a carrier. If a person is known for genetic reasons to be a carrier the error of the test relates to a multiple of the recombination fraction. However, if the index case is an isolated case, the mother of this case may not be a carrier and the disease may be due to a new mutation. Under these circumstances calculations need to be made concerning the risk of that person being a carrier of the condition and is based both on the family structure and biochemical tests (creatine kinase). The error involved in this calculation compounds the error due to RFLP testing. Should that person have a very low risk of being a carrier, prenatal diagnosis by DNA methods may not be indicated. This is because the DNA test will only determine if the fetus has inherited the particular X chromosome that has a very low risk of having the X-linked gene on it. In this case the majority of fetuses with this X chromosome would be normal and not affected. (Assuming no deletions have been found.)

INDICATIONS FOR PRENATAL DIAGNOSES

1. Chromosomal

a. Maternal age

Late maternal age is still the main indication for prenatal diagnoses. The diagnosis is via amniocentesis or chorionic villus sampling for chromosome culture. The specific risk is for trisomies – mainly Down syndrome. The epidemiological risk figures for live-born Down syndrome babies should be used in counselling women about the risk of Down syndrome. Age-specific risks have been produced (see Table 6.1). Easily remembered risks (in round figures) are 1 in 1000 for a woman aged 30 and 1 in 100 for a woman aged 40. Most countries have suggested a minimum age for offering amniocen-

Table 6.1 Age specific risks for Down syndrome (Adapted from Sutherland et al 1979)

Maternal age (years)	Risk (1 in)
20	1 in 1850
25	1 in 1350
30	1 in 1000
34	1 in 530
35	1 in 420
36	1 in 320
37	1 in 250
38	1 in 200
39	1 in 150
40	1 in 120
42	1 in 70
44	1 in 45
46	1 in 15

tesis. This is 35 or 37 years depending upon the particular area and the facilities available for amniocentesis.

b. Parental translocation

Parents who carry a balanced translocation or a Robertsonian translocation have an increased risk of having infants with unbalanced chromosomal defects and, therefore, can be offered prenatal testing.

c. Previous trisomy

There seems to be a small increased risk of a second trisomy following a first. The risk for a live-born trisomy following a first is about 1%.

d. Mother fragile X carrier

Fragile X syndrome can be detected by careful experienced chromosome analysis via either amniocentesis or chorionic villus sampling.

e. Ultrasound examination showing an infant with exomphalos, growth retardation and other malformations make the risk of trisomy increased.

f. Low serum alphafetoprotein (in areas that screen for low serum alphafetoprotein).

2. Previous neural tube defect or high serum alphafetoprotein or suspicion of neural tube defect on ultrasound

Here amniotic alphafetoprotein is assayed. It should be noted that spina bifida cannot be detected by chorionic villus sampling.

3. Disorders detected by DNA technology

a. Duchenne and Becker muscular dystrophy
b. Myotonic dystrophy
c. Haemoglobinopathies, e.g. α- and β-thalassaemias and sickle cell disease
d. Haemophilia A or B

e. Huntington disease
f. Cystic fibrosis
g. Other rare diseases recognizable by DNA techniques such as certain enzyme deficiencies.

If DNA prenatal diagnosis is to be used, careful study of the propositus and their family should be undertaken, preferably before the pregnancy. While the haemoglobinopathies and haemophilia A may be detected by direct fetal blood sampling, DNA diagnosis offers a first trimester diagnosis and is therefore preferable.

4. Cystic fibrosis

Cystic fibrosis can be diagnosed by DNA analysis or by amniocentesis measuring disaccharidase enzyme e.g. alkaline phosphate and gamma-glutamyl transpeptidase. This test is most sensitive and specific when done at 18 weeks' gestation.

5. Specific inborn errors of metabolism

Many inborn errors of metabolism may be diagnosed prenatally by chorionic villus sampling or amniocentesis. However, an exact biochemical diagnosis is needed in the index case before these prenatal tests can be considered.

6. Previous anatomical disease

Previous congenital heart disease, X-linked hydrocephalus or certain bone dysplasias can be detected by fetal ultrasound.

COUNSELLING

The following are basic steps in prenatal counselling:

1. A careful family history must be taken and enquiries made about the reasons why prenatal diagnosis has been requested.

2. As much information as possible on the cause of death of deceased siblings must be obtained. This may involve checking postmortem records and obtaining medical reports from referring doctors.

3. Only after a firm diagnosis has been made can a risk figure be predicted and the suitability for prenatal diagnosis determined. In particular this will allow a decision to be made on the best method of prenatal diagnosis.

4. Parents need to be fully informed about the methods used and the risks involved.

5. The views of the couple on termination must be obtained. This is most important information should the fetus be affected.

6. Parents and the referring medical officer should be informed when results are available, but should recognize that there will be a delay period between performance of the test and the obtaining of a result. Also, they should know that the test may not be diagnostic and that further investigation may be necessary.

7. Should termination be indicated, a couple will need a great deal of support as most have a significant degree of depression and remorse after a second trimester termination; this probably also occurs after a first trimester termination. A review appointment should be offered after a termination when results can be reviewed, the genetic implications can be discussed, and an appreciation of the emotional status of the parents after the termination assessed. Also, discussions in respect to future pregnancies can be raised at this time.

REFERENCE

Sutherland G R, Clisby S R, Bloor G et al 1979 Down's syndrome in South Australia. Medical Journal of Australia 2: 58–61

7. Approach to the dysmorphic child

Agnes Bankier

Recognition that a child is dysmorphic, or looks unusual, is the first step towards making a diagnosis which may determine management. The unusual appearance may be noted incidentally when the child presents with an acute illness, or in the course of investigation for a birth defect, e.g. mental retardation, short stature, or an organ defect such as congenital heart disease. A diagnosis is rarely made on a single dysmorphic feature; it is the pattern of features which is diagnostic. The association of features or birth defects, which can be recognized as belonging to the one entity, constitute a syndrome. Care should be taken not to overinterpret physical features which may simply reflect a harmless family trait and which is striking in the young child. Less than half the known syndromes are associated with mental retardation and many are not known to be inherited.

Recognizing a syndrome allows a more precise definition of the natural history, management and sometimes the cause of the disorder. It also helps the parents adjust to the needs of their child, as it is often much more difficult to live with the anxieties of an uncertain prognosis. Precise definition of an entity is necessary before studying its aetiology.

The diagnosis of a syndrome relies on the recognition of a pattern of malformations and is often associated with a distinctive facial appearance.

The chromosomal localization of many syndromes is now known. Often this has been achieved by the finding of a chromosomal deletion or a translocation involving the site of the gene in the patient. The clinician may be alerted to this possibility by the finding of two syndromes in the patient or by the combination of a syndrome as well as mental retardation. For example, mental retardation in a patient with adenomatous polyposis coli led to the finding of a deletion of chromosome 5. Such deletions may be identifiable either by cytogenetics or by molecular genetic techniques, depending on the size of the deletion.

THE DIAGNOSTIC PROCEDURE

Most syndrome diagnoses made by the expert are made by inspection, often 'from the foot of the bed'. For example, a child with Down syndrome can be recognized as having Down syndrome when walking down the street, without individual dysmorphic features being analysed. There are already over 1400 recognizable patterns of malformations which may be diagnosed in this way and new syndromes are being reported at the rate of 2 per week. Such a flood of knowledge may appear overwhelming unless a rational plan of approach is adopted with each dysmorphic child. When a spot diagnosis of a dysmorphic child is not made the following procedure should be adopted.

Documentation

A detailed history is necessary for diagnosis. The history should include information about other family members with the same, or some of the same features. It should also contain pedigree details, pregnancy history – particularly asking for exposure to possible teratogens – perinatal history and the child's pattern of growth and development (namely progress or regression). If there is a history of exposure to a potential teratogenic agent, the dosage and timing of exposure must be documented. Some maternal diseases can have a teratogenic effect, e.g. maternal diabetes mellitus.

The child should be observed before being undressed and disturbed but examination can never be complete unless the child is completely undressed. In the physical examination the following aspects need to be emphasized: the alertness, the body size and proportions, the height, any asymmetry, the relative size of the head and the spinal curvature. Height, arm span, and upper and lower body segments must be measured and compared to standard normal charts for a child of that age. Charts are available for height, head circumference,

45

hand, foot and ear length, size of palpebral fissures, set of the eyes and testicular size.

An analysis should be made of the features of the facies: the shape of head and face, the set and size of eyes (upward/downward slant, hyper- or hypotelorism), shape and size of nose and mouth, modelling and position of the ears. Some experts advocate documentation of features by measurement. Tables for normal ranges are not available for all features at all ages and the available measurements do not take into consideration the ability of the human eye to assess changes related to racial background and relative changes in the size of features, e.g. length of the ears in a child with a large head. Accurate measurement of facial features is difficult in a young child and in our experience measurements do not improve the likelihood of making a diagnosis.

It is necessary to describe the facial features and we have found the following lines of reference useful (see Fig. 7.1a and b) and the resulting descriptions are in line with the available anthropometric data. In the normal person, the space between the inner canthi is approximately equivalent to the width of the palpebral fissures (inner to outer canthal distance). In hypotelorism (close set eyes or orbits) this space is reduced and in hypertelorism (widely spaced eyes or orbits) this space is significantly greater. The width of the mouth can be compared to other features of the face. The limits of the mouth in macrostomia fall outside the interpupillary lines and in microstomia come within the nasal width in infants. In assessing whether the proportion of the nasal length and philtrum length is normal, we have found that the nose becomes longer with age (2:1 in the infant, 3:1 in the older child).

In assessing the facial profile (see Fig. 7.1b) it is helpful to relate features to an imaginary line which normally intercepts the forehead, upper and lower lips and chin. Thus a bulging or receding forehead, protrudes or recedes from this line. A high nasal bridge is in line and appears to follow from the supraorbital margin. The premaxillary region may be prominent or recessed and prognathism or retrognathia may be assessed in relation to it. The set and size of the ears can be assessed by comparison to lines of reference (see Fig. 7.1a).

Height and body proportions should be measured and compared to normal range for the age of the patient. Note the proportion of the limbs, muscle bulk and tone, joint contractures and mobility, structure of the hands and feet, i.e. shape and length of digits, dermal ridges and structure of nails. The skin should be examined for vascular or pigmentary changes and the external genitalia checked. Evidence of birth defect in specific organs should be sought. A photographic record is helpful.

When facial abnormalities are noted, the parents and siblings (and their photographs at a younger age) should be examined to establish whether this is a family trait.

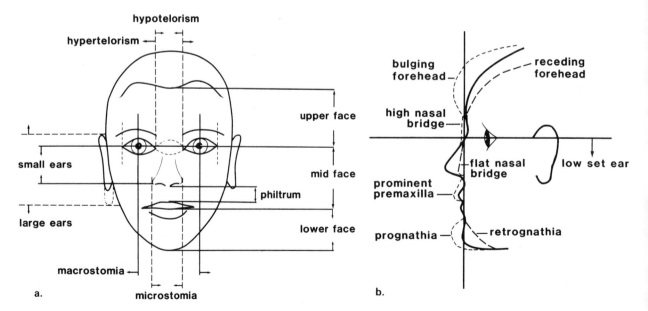

Fig. 7.1 Lines of reference for describing facial features. **a.** Full face. **b.** Profile.

Where the child has a specific syndrome the family need to be examined for characteristics of the same syndrome. Familial traits are not necessarily insignificant.

Consultation

A diagnosis may be made by looking at the catalogues of published syndromes under the key dysmorphic features and comparing the child with photographs of possible syndromes (see further reading list).

If a 'spot diagnosis' is not made, a more experienced doctor should be consulted. Paediatricians can confirm the more common syndromes, e.g. Down syndrome. Clinical geneticists have particular skills in identifying many more syndromes. A diagnosis can be made in approximately half of the children with malformations. This field is called dysmorphology.

A number of computerized databases for syndrome diagnosis are now available. The best known are the London Dysmorphology Database and the POSSUM system. POSSUM (Pictures of Standard Syndromes and Undiagnosed Malformations) is the only system which uses pictures as well as information, combining the skill of the human eye in recognizing patterns with the ability of the computer to store and sort information about syndromes.

POSSUM was produced by the Department of Genetics at the Royal Children's Hospital in Melbourne. POSSUM uses a microcomputer to store and retrieve information about syndromes and a laser videodisk system to store the corresponding illustrations which include photographs and radiographs. The doctor keys in the most striking features in the patient and POSSUM produces a list of differential diagnoses. The clinician can assess these syndromes by examining the data and on visual comparison of the case with pictures of the proposed syndrome, retrieved from the laser disk by the computer. If the features match, a diagnosis is achieved. Many syndromes will remain undiagnosed, but by careful recording of features and review a year or two later, a diagnosis may be made subsequently in many cases.

Investigations

Apart from rare chromosomal disorders, few syndromes are identified by investigations alone, and in fact most syndromes have no confirmatory text. Investigations may be useful in providing additional features, or to confirm a syndrome suspected by the clinician, e.g. lysosomal storage disorder. Radiological investigation is essential to distinguish specific types of bone dysplasia in a short child. Two investigations are commonly undertaken.

Chromosomal analysis

This is indicated in a retarded male or moderate-severely retarded female, particularly when dysmorphic features and birth defects are present. Parental chromosomal analysis is indicated when the child has a translocation or a deletion to clarify whether or not the abnormality is de novo or inherited. It should be appreciated that chromosomal analysis is a complex and expensive test and should not be ordered without careful consideration. The changes detectable on a karyotype, i.e. the smallest detectable insertion or deletion, involve hundreds of genes. Single gene defects, which are the cause of most metabolic disorders and known syndromes cannot be detected by this test.

Metabolic studies

A urine metabolic screen can detect a number of inborn errors of metabolism which may result in mental retardation. Metabolic defects may also cause dysmorphism and birth defects, e.g. Zellweger (cerebrohepatorenal) syndrome. Metabolic studies may need to be performed on blood or other tissues in special circumstances.

SOME SPECIFIC SYNDROMES

The following are some of the more common syndromes, as they present.

The multiply malformed child

Most of these children are small, dysmorphic and mentally retarded.

1. Trisomy 21 (Down syndrome)

Down syndrome is by far the commonest chromosomal disorder and the commonest cause of mental retardation (Figs 7.2 and 7.3). The incidence in liveborn is 1 in 600, but the incidence increases sharply with maternal age. The facies is characteristically flat with crowding of facial features. Note the mongoloid slant of eyes with epicanthic folds, repeated protrusion of the tongue, small low-set ears and flat occiput. The facial grimacing and gait are characteristic. There is brachydactyly with single palmar creases, hypoplasia of the middle phalanx of the fifth finger and increased space between first and second toes. Associated birth defects may be present,

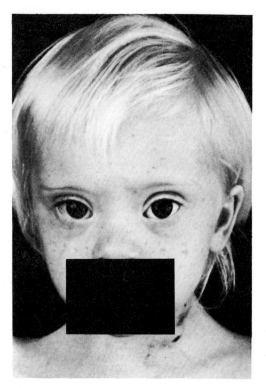 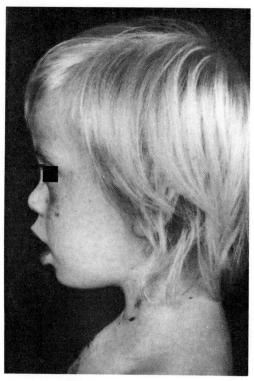

Figs 7.2 and **7.3** Trisomy 21: note the brachycephaly, flat face, mongoloid slant of eyes, epicanthic folds and straight hair.

e.g. congenital heart disease, duodenal atresia and imperforate anus.

Prognosis. Mental retardation with slightly reduced life span (60 years) in the absence of organ defects.

Genetics. In trisomy 21 the risk of recurrence is low although 10 times the population risk. A chromosomal translocation or mosaicism occurs in 3% of Down syndrome babies. Parental chromosomes need only be examined if a translocation is found in the baby. Even young mothers are most likely to have a trisomic child. If either parent carries the translocation, there is an increased risk of recurrence and prenatal diagnosis by amniocentesis or chorion villus sampling is available in subsequent pregnancies.

2. Fra X q27

This is the most common inherited form of mental retardation which can be confirmed by a chromosome analysis. The frequency in mentally retarded males has been estimated to be as high as 1:1000.

The characteristic phenotype (present in most but not all the affected males) is a long face with high forehead, large jaw, large ears, large testes and hyperextensible fingers. Females may also show some of the facial features.

Prognosis. Most males have moderate intellectual disability and some may show autistic features in childhood. Normal transmitting males have also been reported. Only 35% of females are mentally retarded.

Genetics. The fragile site is only demonstrated under special culture conditions. It is not demonstrated in all cells and is only expressed in less than half of heterozygous females. Therefore, genetic counselling is not straight forward and all families should be referred to a geneticist. The chromosome analysis is detectable in the fetus by chorion villus sampling.

3. Trisomy 18

These babies are small. The head has a prominent occiput, low set and dysplastic ears, short palpebral fissures, small mouth and micrognathia. Clenched, overlapping fingers, abnormal dermatoglyphics, dorsiflexed great toes and prominent heels are present.

Prognosis. 30% of babies die in the first month and less than 10% survive the first year.

Genetics. The risk of recurrence is low. Antenatal diagnosis by amniocentesis or chorion villus sampling is available.

4. Trisomy 13

The characteristic appearance is of microcephaly with a sloping forehead and scalp defects, microphthalmia, cleft lip and/or palate, broad flat nose and polydactyly.

Prognosis. 50% of babies die in the first month.

Genetics. The risk of recurrence is low. Antenatal diagnosis is available.

Lysosomal storage disorders

There are a number of inborn errors of metabolism, in which, because of deficiency enzyme activity, high molecular weight complexes (e.g. mucopolysaccharides) accumulate in the lysosomes, resulting in a characteristic facies and body build. The facial features are coarse with dark eye brows, broad fleshy nose, thick lips, ear lobes and skin and cloudy corneas. The hands and feet are broad with stiff joints and the abdomen is protruberant because of hepatosplenomegaly. Progressive mental retardation is characteristic in some types (Hurler, Hunter, San Filippo), whilst in others skeletal problems are prominent and mental development is normal (Maroteaux-Lamy).

Prognosis. This depends on the particular type of storage disorder. In Hurler syndrome there is decline in growth and development delay by the second year and death occurs by the second decade from cardiac or respiratory complications.

Genetics. Most types have autosomal recessive inheritance. Hunter syndrome (as above but with clear corneas) has X-linked inheritance. Specific enzyme assay of fibroblasts is essential to establish a precise diagnosis in each child. Antenatal diagnosis is available.

In the lipid storage disorders the facies is not as striking and early brain involvement and reticuloendothelial storage predominate.

Fetal alcohol syndrome

This is a variable syndrome. The features of note are those of a small, dull baby with mild to moderate microcephaly, short palpebral fissures, short nose with featureless philtrum and posteriorly rotated ears (Fig. 7.4). Congenital heart disease is present in up to 50% of cases.

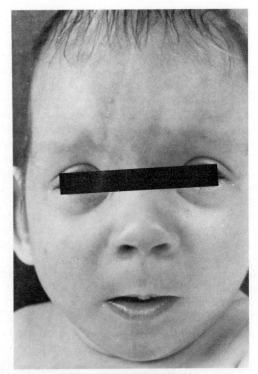

Fig. 7.4 Fetal alcohol syndrome: note short palpebral fissures, short nose with long featureless philtrum. The baby is microcephalic and developmentally delayed.

Prognosis. There is mild to moderate retardation and fine motor dysfunction.

Aetiology. This condition is due to the teratogenic effect of maternal alcohol in pregnancy. The teratogenic effects appear to be dose related above a critical intake of alcohol. Counselling is necessary if recurrence is to be prevented.

VATER association

VATER is the acronym of birth defects which occur together sufficiently frequently to warrant joint consideration. These defects include Vertebral anomalies, Anal malformations, TE-tracheo-oesophageal fistula/atresia and Radial and Renal anomalies. Cardiac malformations are common and digital anomalies include polydactyly, syndactyly and abnormal thumbs. At least three of the components must be present to make the diagnosis.

Prognosis. The outlook for mental development is good. Operative corrections are necessary for birth defects and catch-up growth occurs in most children.

Genetics. These cases have been sporadic. The intrauterine event leading to maldevelopment is not known and the recurrence risk is low.

The short child

Turner syndrome

These are short girls with normal body proportions. They have some of the following: webbed neck, cubitus valgus, shield chest, pigmented naevi and narrow deep-set hyperconvex nails (Fig. 7.5). In babies, lymphoedema and loose neck skin folds may be present. Coarctation of the aorta, idiopathic hypertension and renal anomalies may be present.

Prognosis. These girls are usually not fertile and have primary amenorrhoea and short statute (adult height less than 144 cm). Mental development is good but specific learning difficulties are common.

Genetics. The syndrome results from a sporadic chromosomal abnormality. In 60% of cases only one X chromosome is present, karyotype 45XO. In the others a portion of the second X chromosome is missing or

there is mosaicism, e.g. 46XX/45XO. Risk of recurrence is low.

Noonan syndrome

The children are short (of either sex) with abnormal body proportions, cubitus valgus and webbed neck (Fig. 7.6). The appearance needs to be distinguished from Turner syndrome in females. The facies is characteristic with broad forehead, hypertelorism, ptosis, epicanthic folds and down-slanting eyes, flat nasal bridge and low-set ears. There is pectus carinatum, kyphoscoliosis and congenital heart disease (involving the right side of the heart). Cryopochidism is common and there may be lower limb lymphoedema.

Prognosis. Variable fertility and mild to moderate mental retardation may be present. The cardiac status determines the life expectancy.

Genetics. This is autosomal dominant but many cases are sporadic and arise as a new mutation. The parents should be examined for features of Noonan syndrome by an expert. Antenatal diagnosis is not possible.

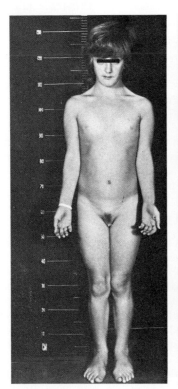 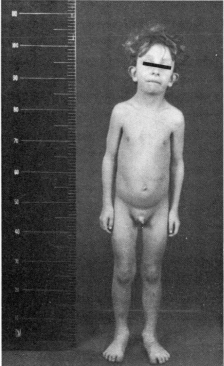

Figs 7.5 and **7.6**   Turner's syndrome (left) and Noonan syndrome (right). The phenotypes are similar: short stature, webbed neck, broad chest and cubitus valgus.

Bone dysplasia

There are more than 150 bone dysplasias which, traditionally, have been distinguished on clinical and radiological features. Increasingly, histochemical and ultrastructural studies have been used to differentiate these (particularly in the lethal skeletal dysplasias) and there is early promising progress towards the definition of the biochemical basis. Most bone dysplasias are single gene defects.

The term dysplasia refers to a generalized developmental disorder of bone resulting in abnormal organization. This in turn alters the growth potential and usually the modelling and shape of the bones rather than their strength or ability to heal. Osteogenesis imperfecta is an obvious exception. The term dysplasia is preferred to the term 'dwarfism'. Dysostosis is used when only individual bones are involved.

Bone dysplasia may predominantly affect the limbs (short-limbed short stature) or the spine. In the long bones the involvement may be *epiphyseal* leading to radiological changes and decreased growth; *metaphyseal* leading to bulky, poorly modelled ends of shafts; or *diaphyseal* leading to thickening of the mid-shaft cortex (Fig. 7.7). Often many parts of the bone are disorganized. It is the resulting appearances of long bones, spine, pelvis and skull which enables the experts to make a specific diagnosis. Intelligence is generally normal.

Whilst there is no specific treatment for bone dysplasia, early diagnosis is important in influencing management. Early counselling of the parents allows for the development of a positive approach which helps adjustment and acceptance of the child. This is of great importance for the child's well-being and self respect. Knowledge of the natural history of these disorders allows the doctor to anticipate problems, for example, diarrhoea and ear infections in the mucopolysaccharidoses, deafness in osteogenesis imperfecta and arthritis in particular bone dysplasias. Medical management, whilst not curative, can improve the quality of life of these children.

Achondroplasia. The short stature, short limbs and relatively large head, exaggerated lumbar lordosis and genu varum which are characteristic need to be distinguished from the 120 other types of skeletal dysplasia by radiological examination (Figs 7.8 and 7.9). Brachycephaly mid-facial hypoplasia with narrow nasal passages and relative prognathism are also present. There is brachydactyly with trident appearance of the hands.

Prognosis. Early motor development is often slow because of the large head and poor leverage resulting from short limbs. Growth of the head in the first year may

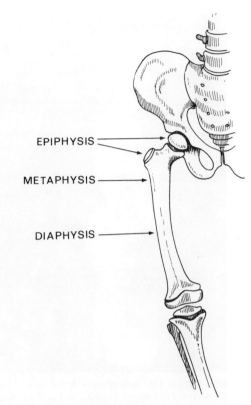

Fig. 7.7 Bone dysplasia in the long bones may involve the epiphysis, metaphysis or diaphysis.

be rapid and careful monitoring by cerebral ultrasound is necessary as hydrocephalus requiring treatment occurs in 1–2%. Mental development is generally normal. Spinal canal stenosis is present in most patients and may lead to neurological impairment in later life unless treated. Adult height is short (males approximately 131 cm, females 124 cm) and females in pregnancy require delivery by Caesarian section.

Genetics. This is autosomal dominant but most cases are as a result of new mutation (1:2 recurrence risk to offspring of an affected parent). Diagnosis by ultrasound is possible in the second trimester.

Osteogenesis imperfecta. This is a clinically and genetically heterogeneous group of disorders in which there is increased bone fragility.

In the common form (type I) fractures develop in childhood, there may be blue sclera and deafness and the inheritance is autosomal dominant. Those with dentinogenesis imperfecta have a greater likelihood of early fractures, deformity and short stature.

Type II is the lethal neonatal form. Multiple fractures occur in utero, result in 'crumpled' appearance of long

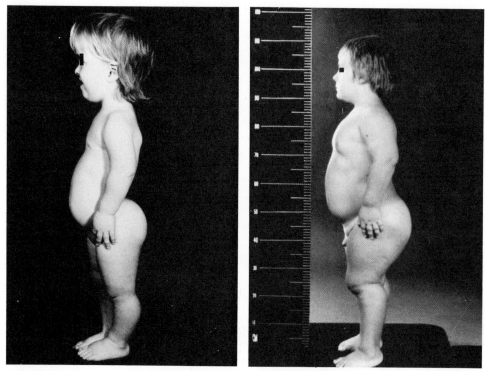

Figs. 7.8 and **7.9**   Achondroplasia (left) and spondyloepiphyseal dysplasia (right): note the similar phenotype, i.e. body proportions and posture. Radiographs are needed to differentiate these cases.

bones and beaded ribs. The skull is poorly ossified and the sclerae are blue.

In the severe deforming variety (type III) the child may be born with fractures and the skull is well ossified. The sclerae are white in the older child and dentinogenesis imperfecta may be present. Repeated fractures during childhood lead to variable short stature, deformity and kyphoscoliosis which if severe will result in chest disease and shortened survival. This type has autosomal recessive inheritance.

Type IV is distinguished from type I by having white sclerae and vary from fractures at birth to very few in childhood. Inheritance is autosomal dominant.

The tall child

Marfan syndrome

The children are tall with narrow build and long limbs (arm span greater than height, lower segment greater than upper segment) with arachnodactyly and often increased ligamentous laxity (Fig. 7.10). Upward dislocation of the lens and myopia, aortic root dilatation and mitral incompetence and kyphoscoliosis are associated features.

Prognosis. This depends on the cardiac status of the person. Aortic root dilatation may progress to fatal aortic dissection if not treated. Mental development is normal. The classic Marfan syndrome is easily recognized but more subtle degrees may not be so obvious and require considerable expertise. The management should include regular ophthalmology and cardiology review. Early treatment with B-adrenergic blocking agents and careful echocardiographics review may slow aortic root dilatation and allow prophylactic aortic root replacement before dissections occur.

Genetics. This connective tissue disorder is inherited in an autosomal dominant fashion. The risk of recurrence with normal parents is low; the risk to offspring of affected is 1:2. Antenatal diagnosis is not yet available.

Homocystinuria

The phenotype of this metabolic disorder may be clinically indistinguishable from the Marfan syndrome, exhibiting the same body proportions, scoliosis and (downward) lens dislocation. Heart disease is not a feature, but there is a risk of arterial thrombosis especially if there is dehydration or after angiography (Fig. 7.11).

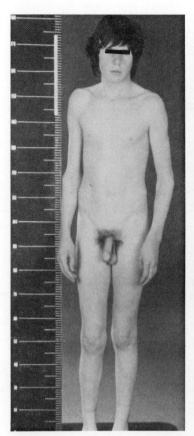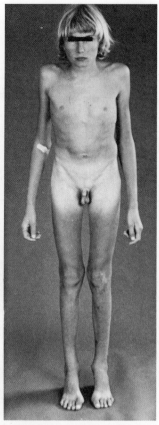

Figs 7.10 and **7.11** Homocystinuria (left) and Marfan syndrome (right). Both boys have a similar phenotype with long limbs and tall stature.

Prognosis. Mental retardation may be preventable by early diagnosis and dietary treatment. The diagnosis can be made by metabolic screening of the urine. All persons with marfanoid habitus should be screened.

Genetics. This inborn error of metabolism is inherited in an autosomal recessive fashion. Risk to offspring of an affected person is low. Prenatal diagnosis is available.

Klinefelter syndrome

This has a variable phenotype. The child may be tall with long limbs developing a female fat distribution with age, but the body build may be normal male. Testes are small.

Prognosis. These boys may present as delayed puberty or infertility. Virilization is often incomplete without testosterone treatment. Mental development is dull to normal.

Genetics. This is a chromosomal abnormality with karyotype 47XXY. The risk of recurrence is low.

The child with microcephaly

Microcephaly is seen in a heterogeneous group of disorders (Fig. 7.12a, b and c). The causes can range from viral and toxic insults to a single gene defect. The following syndrome examples are worth noting:

1. Autosomal recessive microcephaly

Note the sloping forehead, flat occiput, normal-sized face with a prominent nose and protruding ears.

Prognosis. The prognosis is for moderate to severe mental retardation. Early motor development may be within normal limits for age.

Genetics. This has a 1:4 recurrence risk. It may be diagnosable by careful serial ultrasound examinations in pregnancy.

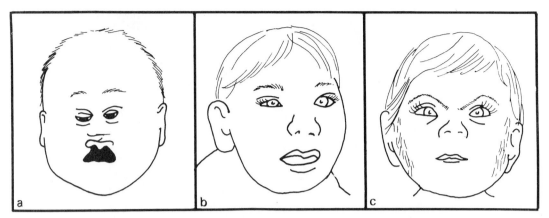

Fig. 7.12 **a** Holoprosencephaly. **b** Autosomal recessive microcephaly. **c** Brachmann-de Lange syndrome.

2. *Holoprosencephaly*

This is a defect in brain development in which there is failure to form paired cerebral hemispheres. Note the hypotelorism with oblique palpebral fissures, variable premaxillary agenesis and underdeveloped nasal bones (appearing as a soft tissue proboscis in the extreme).

Prognosis. Severe intellect handicap usually accompanied by motor defects are apparent quite early. These children rarely survive infancy.

Genetics. The aetiology is heterogeneous. May be seen as part of chromosome abnormalities e.g. trisomy 13 which has a low recurrence risk and syndromes with autosomal recessive inheritance have been described (1:4 recurrence risk).

3. *Brachmann-de Lange syndrome*

These are small hirsute babies with microcephaly. The facies is characteristic with synophrys (thick confluent eyebrows) and long eyelashes, small upturned nose, long and featureless philtrum, thin downturned lips and micrognathia. The limbs may be short with digital anomalies and congenital heart disease is not uncommon.

Prognosis. There is usually severe mental retardation and failure to thrive. Most die in the first year or two but survival into the second decade has been documented. The full spectrum of the condition is not as yet established.

Genetics. This is usually sporadic. The empiric recurrence risk is 1:30.

FURTHER READING

Goodman R M, Gorlin R J 1983 The malformed infant and child. Oxford University Press, Oxford

Gorlin R J, Pindborg J J, Cohen M M 1976 Syndromes of the head and neck. McGraw Hill, New York

Jones K L 1988 Recognizable patterns of human malformation. W B Saunders, Philadelphia

McKusick V A 1988 Mendelian inheritance in man. Catalogs of autosomal dominant, autosomal recessive, and X-linked phenotypes. The Johns Hopkins University Press, Baltimore

Spranger J W, Langer L O, Wiedemann R 1974 Bone dysplasia. An atlas of constitutional disorders of skeletal development. W B Saunders, Philadelphia   .

8. Genetic counselling

John G. Rogers

DEFINITION

Genetic counselling aims to provide sufficient information for an individual or couple to make an informed decision about their reproductive options and to assist them in coming to terms with the issues they face.

Genetic counselling is not always provided by geneticists. It is appropriate for paediatricians and disease-oriented specialists to undertake counselling in their own area of expertise. In most children's hospitals families who have a child with cystic fibrosis, a neural tube defect, or muscular dystrophy, will be counselled by their own specialist. Other family members not in direct contact with clinics are generally referred to geneticists. Medical genetics has been slow to penetrate the world of adult medicine and most adults will need referral for their counselling.

INDICATIONS OF GENETIC COUNSELLING

Anybody who has reason to suspect that there might be an increased risk of producing a child with a birth defect should at some stage receive formal genetic counselling. This would include:

1. Couples who have a stillbirth
2. A child with a birth defect
3. Mental retardation
4. Family history of any of the above
5. Relatives with known genetic disorders such as Huntington's chorea, muscular dystrophy
6. Multiple miscarriages
7. Exposure to radiation or drugs during pregnancy
8. Advanced maternal age
9. Consanguinity
10. Chromosome translocations
11. Psychiatric disorder.

For appropriate genetic counselling (Fig. 8.1) the following are essential:

1. Diagnostic precision

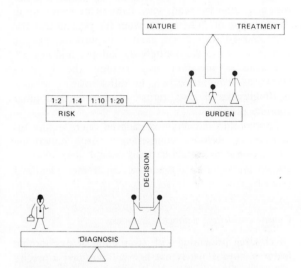

Fig. 8.1 Genetic counselling. Note that all is balanced against diagnosis – the remainder is in the parents' hands.

2. Knowledge of risk
3. Knowledge of burden
4. Knowledge of reproductive options
5. Counselling skills.

Diagnostic precision

The most important element in genetic counselling is establishing the correct diagnosis. The degree of diagnostic precision required for genetic counselling is greater than in any other field of clinical medicine. For example, a patient with muscular dystrophy can be correctly managed, without knowing precisely the type of muscular dystrophy, with the use of splints, wheelchairs and physiotherapy. Genetic counselling in such a patient or family will require a precise diagnosis confirmed by the appropriate blood, EMG and muscle biopsy studies. When considering the need for investigations a precise diagnosis may not influence treatment, but appropriate genetic counselling may be of extreme importance to the patient and his family.

Postmortem is one way of establishing a precise diagnosis. This can be of particular importance in a child with malformation or retardation in situations when a clinical diagnosis is not possible, and in adults with neurological disorders. Postmortems need to be planned in advance so that specific tissues can be obtained for biochemical study, electronmicroscopy or histochemistry. When death can be anticipated, it is best to raise the issue of a postmortem before death occurs. In practice it works better than asking permission immediately after the death when families are bound up in their own grief. When permission for postmortem has been granted, it is of the greatest importance that the parents return to discuss fully the autopsy findings.

Diagnostic precision may require the help of specialists who are expert in differentiating various neuromuscular disease, retinal dystrophies and other complex problems.

Dysmorphic and retarded children often require investigation before counselling. An underlying chromosomal or metabolic basis should always be excluded and specific dysmorphic syndromes identified (see Ch. 7).

Genetic counselling without a diagnosis

Of children presenting with retardation or dysmorphic features, approximately one-half will not have a precise diagnosis. There is a large body of empiric data that can be used for counselling in this group. The only caveat is that appropriate investigation and experienced clinicians have excluded known disorders.

While an inability to label a child with a specific diagnosis is disappointing and frustrating to both parents and doctors, it should not disadvantage the child as management can be based on periodic assessment and planning.

The evolution of knowledge and new techniques make necessary the restudy of old problems. Thus patient review is of the greatest importance. For example, when the fragile X chromosome became recognized as a major cause of retardation, many families required further study. Also, new approaches to diagnosis using DNA will require recall and storage of DNA from patients who die. In addition, the clinical features making up a syndrome may become more apparent with increasing age and thus allow for better diagnostic precision.

Estimation of risk

Following diagnostic evaluation, an estimate of risk can be made. Risk is a numerical estimate of the likelihood of a particular disorder occurring in a subsequent child. This probability may be based on a Mendelian pattern of inheritance with a recurrence risk of 1:2 or 1:4. Some 34 000 Mendelian disorders have been described in man.

There are many common disorders in which there is a genetic component and where the inheritance pattern cannot be explained simply in terms of Mendelian inheritance or chromosomal rearrangement. It appears that in these disorders it is due to the cumulative action of a number of genes together with environmental influences. This is called polygenic or multifactorial inheritance and numerically is the commonest pattern of inheritance responsible for the family tendency or predisposition to various disorders. The recurrence risk on multifactorial disorders after a single affected child is 3–5%. The following are examples of multifactorial inheritance:

1. Congenital cardiac anomalies
2. Neural tube defects – spina bifida and anencephaly
3. Club foot
4. Cleft lip ± cleft palate
5. Congenital dislocation of the hip
6. Pyloric stenosis
7. Diabetes mellitus.

Many families do not have a good grasp of probability and need a careful discussion to give meaning to any risk estimate. Whilst it might be clear in our mind what is meant by a 1 in 4 risk, many people believe that if they have had the 1 abnormal child they can have another 3 before they need worry again. It is important to emphasize to families that chance has no memory. Simple illustrations and a concrete example such as tossing two coins are often helpful.

Families often want to know how their risk compares with that of other families. In Australia there is approximately a 1 in 25 risk that any child will be born with a major defect. This is the risk that any family either accepts or ignores and is a useful point of comparison. It is reasonable to tell families that we consider risks of 1 in 2 and 1 in 4 are high; risks of less than 1 in 100 are low; and other risks are intermediate. Whilst genetic counselling does not aim to tell a person what to do, it is important for a counsellor to see that they understand the meaning of any numbers used.

Once a disorder has been identified within a family, e.g. a chromosome translocation, a dominant disorder such as Marfan syndrome, or a sex-linked disorder such as Duchenne muscular dystrophy, all family members at risk should be studied and counselled. The risk with chromosome translocations varies according to the chromosome involved. Advances in the technique of chromosome staining now enables many more transloca-tions to be identified; some involve only small pieces of a chromosome. The estimation of risk requires an ap-preciation of the possible gametes that can be produced as a result of segregation of the chromosomes at meiosis.

Collection of samples for DNA

With advances in DNA technology it has become essen-tial to store samples of DNA from probands who are likely to die and relatives such as grandparents. This enables subsequent family members to take advantage of advancing knowledge.

The burden

This is of great importance in genetic counselling. Parents of a baby recently diagnosed as having cystic fibrosis or mental retardation may have little idea of what lies ahead for the child and themselves. It is neces-sary to give the parents an understanding of what is going to be involved in the care of a child with that particular disorder including the length of life, the quality of life, treatment and variability which exists for that disorder. For instance, with tuberose sclerosis, a child may present with hypsarrhythmia and profound retardation, or alternatively may be normal. A further comparison can be made between cleft lip and palate, which can be repaired with excellent results, and Duchenne muscular dystrophy, which is incurable and produces increasing handicap until death. These condi-tions have quite different burdens for affected children and their families. A 4% risk of producing a child with a cleft lip and palate may not be acceptable to a family; the same risk of a child with Duchenne muscular dystrophy may not be either. Many parents are prepared to accept a 1 in 4 risk of producing a child with a lethal metabolic disease knowing that the child will either die soon after birth or be normal. The initial impact of a birth defect such as cleft lip and palate on a family should be equated with the doctor's concept of burden.

Alternatives for families at risk

Childless lifestyle

A family may choose not to risk another pregnancy. This has become more socially acceptable in recent years.

Adoption

The supply of young babies is very limited because of the increase in single parent families and termination of pregnancy and no longer offers a practical alternative in Australia.

Intrauterine diagnosis

Intrauterine diagnosis provides an option for many couples. This can be offered to families who feel that termination of pregnancy is an acceptable approach. The range of disorders which can be recognized by in-trauterine diagnosis is constantly increasing (see Ch. 6).

Artificial insemination by donor

Artificial insemination by donor is of limited appeal; many couples and ethnic groups find it unacceptable. However, it can provide an alternative when the father has an autosomal dominant disorder, carries a chromosome translocation or produces a child with an autosomal recessive disorder.

In vitro fertilization using donor ovum

This can be offered when a mother carries a sex-linked disorder, has a dominant disorder, carries a chromosome translocation or produces a child with an autosomal recessive disorder.

EMOTIONAL IMPACT OF GENETIC COUNSELLING

Patients often feel very vulnerable when referred for genetic counselling. This may be because of the recent arrival of a child with a birth defect, a stillbirth or a neonatal death. People might be concerned about details of their family history and worry that they might be blamed for any abnormality.

In counselling, the emotional impact of a birth defect, or the risk of producing a child with a birth defect, is carefully explored. People need an opportunity to ven-tilate their fears and anxieties. Discussion of emotional issues are of equal importance to discussion of risk, bur-den and alternative. Families who have recently lost a child may need understanding and reassurance about the process of mourning and may need to allow time before a further pregnancy.

What does the geneticist do

The geneticist allows each family one hour in quiet sur-roundings. Medical records and doctors reports should be obtained before the consultation – this will make counselling more efficient.

Detailed history or records of probands need to be obtained. A pedigree is drawn with a minimum of three generations. This should include information about stillbirths, deaths and health problems. Probands and other members of the family are examined and investigated as necessary. Only then can counselling be properly undertaken.

A geneticist will not tell the family what they should do, but help them reach a reasoned decision based on their own set of values. Thus when a family asks 'Should I have another child?', instead of a direct answer the geneticist might ask 'How would you feel about having another child with cystic fibrosis?'. In this way families are encouraged to explore their own feelings.

Whilst it is possible for a family to be counselled in a single visit, some families need to return for further discussions.

Letter to patients

It is excellent practice to write to all families seen for counselling, restating the advice given to them at the time. This letter should restate in simple clear language an outline of the discussion that has taken place. A copy of this letter must be sent to the family doctor so that everybody starts with the same information. This document then serves as a valuable family record, and can be shown to other professionals and thus overcomes the problem of selective recall.

Timing of referral

In a family where there is a risk of producing a child with a birth defect, counselling should be offered at the time the individual at risk becomes concerned about the family history or is contemplating having children. Families who have just produced a child with a birth defect should be informed of the availability of genetic counselling, but may require some time to come to terms with the problem before they can enter into the genetic counselling process.

All States of Australia have genetic counselling services. Often these are based at several different hospitals, but can usually be located through a paediatric hospital.

FURTHER READING

Harper P S 1984 Practical genetic counselling, 2nd edn. Wright, Bristol
McKusick V A 1987 Mendelian inheritance in man, 7th edn. The John Hopkins University Press, Baltimore
Emery A E, Rimoin D C 1983 Principles and practice of medical genetics, Vols 1 and 2. Churchill Livingstone, Edinburgh
Vogel F, Motulsky A G 1986 Human genetics: problems and approaches, 2nd edn. Springer Verlag, Berlin

SECTION 3

Clinical assessment

9. The clinical history and physical examination

M. J. Robinson

In the diagnostic process the importance of the clinical history is assessed as 80%, the physical examination as 15% and special investigations as 5%; therefore, no apology is necessary for this chapter.

The paediatric history differs from the history taken in internal medicine in that it is given by a second person – usually the mother, but occasionally the father, aunt, grandmother or even some unrelated person who may be caring for the child at the time. When presenting with their sick child, most parents will be anxious, but some may also be angry or hostile, excessively garrulous, evasive or even uninterested. It is important that your initial impression of the parent does not cloud your judgement. This will particularly apply to the unintelligent parent who may be a poor observer. Remember that everybody does not have your level of intelligence or the training to observe. Also, it is important to assess the parents' perception of their child's illness. For example, the parent may fear that the child's pallor is due to a serious blood disorder that had occurred in a relative or friend. When these anxieties have been identified and when the child is found to be in no danger, reassurance can be much more positive and meaningful. The best way for the student to learn is to be present when an experienced clinician is consulting.

PRELIMINARY INTRODUCTION

It is very important that you introduce yourself properly to the parents and child and ask the child what he/she likes to be called. It is very good practice to make some complimentary remark about the child, for example, small girls and boys like to be complimented on their dress. Often children will bring along a doll or a favourite toy and you should make some comment about these possessions. A few words of general conversation with a child will work wonders and make the subsequent physical examination so much more pleasant for all. For example, it is good strategy to ask a preschool child about the kindergarten and the teacher; ask a school child about friends, games and the schoolteacher. Older children can be engaged in conversation about hobbies, sporting activities, etc. Children talk of the things they know best. After this you may direct young children to a tray of toys or set of books so that they are occupied and do not continually interrupt the interview. Any person who is involved in the care of children should always have an ample supply of toys and picture books available (Fig. 9.1).

THE HISTORY

The history should commence with an enquiry into the current problem. Unless this is done first, parents tend to become irritated about questions directed towards past illnesses, family history, social activities of the family and so on. The sequence of the history will vary depending upon the age and the general condition of the child. For example, much of the history in a neonate will have to do with the pregnancy and the labour, whereas in the toddler with a convulsion the present complaint will be all important, although a past history of convulsions and a family history of seizures will be very relevant. Unfortunately, there is a tendency in emergency situations to treat symptoms without paying sufficient attention to the sequence of events that led up to the emergency.

Present complaint

In most clinical situations you will begin by noting the child's date of birth, sex and date of onset of the symptoms. Then the parents should be allowed to tell the clinical story in their own words and, if possible, in chronological order. At times it may be necessary to interrupt the garrulous parent who dwells too much on one aspect or attempts to interpret the symptoms, but in general this should be done as little as possible. If you interrupt too much you are likely to irritate the parent and compromise relationships. Learn to be a lis-

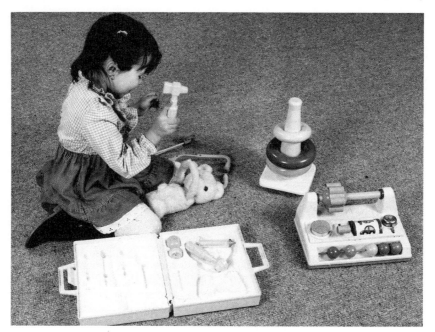

Fig. 9.1 Essential equipment for all doctors who look after children.

tener and, in general, believe what you are told. Often parents exaggerate, but only because they are anxious. Many more mistakes are made by doubting the parents' history than by believing it.

The history should bring out the state of health of the child immediately before the onset of the current illness. Relevant epidemiological information possibly related to the child's problems should be obtained, for example, the health of other members of the family and the health of other children in the same class at school. Any treatment that the child may be having should also be noted. For example, a history may read as follows:

> Sara, aged 18 months, was in good health until four days ago when she developed a fever and a dry cough. Over the next few days her appetite deteriorated and the cough became productive. The fever persisted and she appeared lethargic, wanting to sleep rather more than usual. Today her breathing has become quite rapid and the fever more pronounced. Her brother aged 4.5 years is recovering from a cold.

Past history

Once the current problem has been dealt with, the past history should be explored. This part of the history may allow for proper interpretation of the current illness. For example, in an 8-month-old child who has had several admissions to hospital with cough and fever, the pos-

sibility of cystic fibrosis will need to be considered. Generally, the past history should involve an appraisal of the mother's pregnancy although this will usually be irrelevant in older children of normal physical and intellectual development. Positive statements in respect to maternal illness during pregnancy, particularly those of fever and a rash, must be obtained. A history of smoking during pregnancy may explain low birthweight. Excessive alcohol ingestion in pregnancy may result in the fetal alcohol syndrome. The birth history becomes more relevant the younger the child and in the neonatal period it frequently provides the most useful information for the current behaviour of the infant. Thus the labour, the type of presentation, the mode of delivery – forceps, Caesarean section, etc. – must be known. Also the birthweight and the infant's general condition at birth is of great importance. Low birthweight may imply prematurity, dysmaturity, or both. Often a good idea of the infant's neonatal condition is obtained by asking the mother when she first saw her baby and when she gave the first feed. She may be asked if the baby was kept in the nursery or placed in an isolette for any period of time after birth. It is also important to ask if any bruising, jaundice, convulsions, lethargy or hyperactivity was noted in the neonatal period. However, do not be surprised if many mothers are unable to recall these events. It may be necessary to check the records of the obstetric hospital for details. Subsequently, it is important to know if there were good weight gains. This can be most accurately obtained from the infant's health centre book which most mothers bring along with them. For older sick children it is less important and may be irrelevant to the illness in question.

The type and frequency of feeding, the time of weaning and whether or not vitamin and iron supplements were given may be relevant. Next a thorough enquiry should be made into the child's previous illnesses and, in particular, if there has been any period of hospitalization. A history of past surgery may be important. Many parents forget to mention a past tonsillectomy, adenoidectomy or appendicectomy. The immunization status must be noted and, should the child not be immunized, plans should be formulated to have this done as soon as possible as it is only in this way that the level of immunization in the community will be kept at its current high level.

Family history

In no other branch of medicine is the family history as important. Although individually few, genetically determined disorders are collectively considerable in number and account for some 5% of admissions to paediatric hospitals. Many heritable disorders and particularly metabolic disorders exert their major effects soon after birth. Thus, the history should positively state the age and current health of each parent and, in the case of death of a parent, the cause. Pregnancies should be listed in order and the result of each recorded. The age and state of health of each sibling should be noted, and in the case of a death the cause recorded if possible. A positive statement should also be made in respect to any familial disease and parental consanguinity.

System review

When the history of the current illness has been obtained, a brief system review is made to ensure that important and relevant information has not been forgotten. This should include an enquiry into vision and hearing. Habits should be explored so that an understanding of the child's personality is obtained. Thus it is necessary to ask about the sleep routine, bowel and bladder training, attendance at kindergarten, school, etc, and the ability to make relationships with peers and family. The ability to relate to other members of the home is important – is the child co-operative or disruptive? These and other questions related to the child's emotional status will usually best be dealt with in the absence of the child. Sometimes a child can be separated and taken into another room, but on other occasions this

may be impossible, so these sensitive issues will need to be taken up at a subsequent interview in the absence of the child.

Developmental history

A developmental history will be required, the details depending upon the age of the chid and the underlying problem. In the case of the school child it is often sufficient to ascertain that the child is in the appropriate class for age and is able to cope adequately. This information is usually readily obtained through regular teacher/parent contact. In the small infant, particularly where there is a risk factor to normal development, the enquiry will need to be full and a proper developmental assessment performed (see Ch. 11).

The age of onset of puberty and its progression may be important in problems of growth.

Social history

As illness is often modified and influenced by social factors, these must be brought out. The occupation of the mother and father are relevant. Is there unemployment? Do the parents live in their own home and what type of dwelling is it? Does the child have a personal bedroom and is there adequate room for play, both inside and outside the house? The problems of high rise apartments are well known.

Thus, the paediatric history should not only bring out the circumstances relating to the particular illness under question, but should also provide a background of the child's past medical history, development, personality and the ability to relate satisfactorily to family and the community.

PHYSICAL EXAMINATION

It is convenient to discuss 2 groups of children.

1. The infant and small child up to about the age of 3 years. While the technique of physical examination of the newly born infant is similar to that of the older infant, there are certain areas where the emphasis is different. These differences are discussed at the end of this section.

2. The older child from about 3 years to adolescence.

Examination of the infant

The physical examination of children is a skill acquired only after considerable practice. Some infants, particularly between the ages of 1 and 2 years, may totally refuse examination, even by the most experienced doctor. Under these circumstances one can only make the best of the situation. Fortunately, such infants are rarely seriously ill; the seriously ill toddler will usually not protest and examination will be no problem.

Usually infants permit a physical examination for a short period before becoming bored and upset. Distraction with toys and other interesting objects (part of the doctor's armamentarium, and a must for any surgery), will prolong this period somewhat, but if the examination is unduly prolonged, all infants will object. The physical examination in infancy should be performed with care, but completed as quickly as possible. During the period of history taking, a great amount of information can be obtained by simple observation. For example, the general condition of the infant, any peculiarity of appearance (dysmorphism), colour, type and rate of breathing, the presence and type of any cough, the state of alertness and an appraisal of the state of development will be noted. Of great importance is the relationship between mother and baby – does mother interact with the baby in a confident and affectionate manner. It is also possible to be fairly certain that most of the cranial nerves are intact, that all limbs are moving and that vision is reasonable simply by observation.

Abdomen

It is impossible to assess the abdomen, the cardio-vascular system and to a lesser extent the respiratory system, in a crying infant. For this reason the abdomen is best examined first in the young infant, preferably with the infant on a couch with the napkin removed and the chest covered. The abdomen of the infant up to 2.5 years of age is normally full and the umbilicus slightly everted. Provided that the tip of the small finger cannot be inserted through the umbilical ring there is no hernia present and parents can be reassured that this protrusion will disappear by the time the child is 3 or 4 years of age. The abdomen should be carefully inspected and its movement with respiration noted. Next it is palpated with a warm hand, each quadrant being felt sequentially commencing in the left iliac fossa. Superficial gentle palpation is performed to assess any tenderness and rigidity and of course to avoid frightening the baby. This will also enable large masses and very large organs to be delineated. Next, deep palpation will be necessary to feel small and more deeply lying masses. Again, each quadrant is palpated sequentially. Finally one feels specifically for the liver, spleen and kidneys. A large spleen and a large liver can be missed if palpation is not commenced in the right iliac fossa and continued up-

wards to the ribs. A spleen which is just palpable in a small infant may not be significant; often the liver is palpable in the normal infant to 1 or 2 cm below the right costal margin. Occasionally one can feel the lower pole of the right kidney, but generally, except in the newborn, the kidneys are not palpable. The bladder should also be specifically palpated. Note if there is any dribbling of urine on compressing the bladder and seepage of faecal material from anus which appears patulous. These signs indicate a low spinal cord lesion.

Cardiovascular system

The physical examination of the cardiovascular system is fully covered in Chapter 39 and will not be repeated in this section.

An attempt should be made to take the blood pressure using a cuff which extends over two-thirds of the upper arm. With practice it is possible to record the blood pressure in almost every infant. The peripheral pulses should be noted, both in respect to their presence or absence, their volume and how distally they can be felt. For example, in a large patent ductus arteriosus, the pulses are full and bounding in the palms. In coarctation of the aorta the femoral pulses are either absent or diminished and delayed.

The signs of cardiac failure in infancy differ from those of older children and adults. In particular, oedema in heart disease in infancy is difficult to appreciate clinically as the oedema fluid is distributed throughout the whole of the body and, as the infant is normally in the recumbent position, oedema of the ankles will be unusual. Usually, however, there will be some puffiness around the face in heart failure of infancy. The most important sign of heart failure in infancy is hepatomegaly. The liver is enlarged, be the failure predominantly right or left sided. The liver enlargement is quite marked and usually to the level of the umbilicus. The association of tachypnoea with laboured respirations, cardiomegaly and hepatomegaly almost certainly implies heart failure. Crepitations at the lung bases are usually difficult to hear because of the reduced respiratory excursion which occurs in heart failure in infancy. Cervical venous congestion is almost never noted because of the thick and short neck of the infant.

Respiratory system

Initial observation of the chest should take into account the rate and character of respiration and any asymmetry of chest movement with breathing. In upper airways obstruction a high-pitched sound during inspiration – stridor – may be obvious. If the obstruction is severe, dyspnoea will be present and there may be suprasternal, sternal and/or intercostal retraction. In lower airways obstruction the chest will be hyperinflated (barrel shaped) and there may be associated lower intercostal retraction. The presence of any chest deformity should be noted. Chronic pulmonary or cardiac disease associated with dyspnoea will often result in permanent indrawing of the ribs at the insertion of the diaphragm – Harrison's sulci. Other chest deformities which may be associated with chronic cardiac and pulmonary disease include funnel chest and pigeon chest, but more often deformities are primary, and not secondary to lung or heart disease.

After inspection, the chest is percussed; percussion should proceed from normally resonant to dull areas. The percussion note on each side of the chest is compared. The breath sounds of the small infant are rather harsher and of higher pitch than those of the older child. The length of expiration tends more closely to approximate the length of inspiration, which gives the impression that the breath sounds are bronchial in type. The fact that they are normal breath sounds of infancy and not the bronchial breathing of pulmonary consolidation will be confirmed when the area is percussed and found to be normally resonant. Adventitious sounds should be listened for and localized. High-pitched sounds, particularly in expiration and associated with prolongation of expiration, are termed rhonchi or wheezes. Coarse or fine crackling noises – crepitations or crackles – will be heard at the end of inspiration. In the older child and adult patient fine crepitations will usually indicate the presence of alveolar exudate. Identical sounds will be heard in the small infant when the lesion is in the smaller bronchi and bronchioles, e.g. bronchitis and bronchiolitis.

The examination should now revert to the head and neck and proceed in a caudal direction. Although it is not very important now from the point of the examination if the infant becomes restless or cries, experienced doctors try to avoid making a baby cry.

Head and neck

The fontanelles should be felt remembering that the posterior fontanelle is triangular and the anterior fontanelle diamond shaped. The posterior fontanelle closes between the sixth and eighth week, whereas the anterior fontanelle remains open until at least 18 months. The anterior fontanelle is normally felt slightly below the plane of the skull bones. Clearly the tension will increase with increased intracranial pressure and will be reduced in states of dehydration. The head circumference should always be measured, i.e. the greatest fronto-occipital circumference, and the measurement compared with normal values. The shape of the head should be noted.

The neck is inspected and then palpated for any obvious lump. An assessment of the cervical lymph nodes is particularly important because of the frequency of upper respiratory tract infection in children. Other lymph nodes are palpated at this time and a general inspection of the baby made to note any birth marks, pigmented naevi, scars, burns, bruises or rashes.

Musculoskeletal system

The extremities will be noted and compared for the degree of movement, size and inequality. Any bony deformity or bony tenderness should be noted and all joints gently put through their normal range of movement. Thus any joint swelling or restriction of joint movement will be appreciated. The deformities of rickets will usually not be apparent until the age of walking. Should there be bowing of the limbs, care should be taken to assess the wrists and ankles for bony flaring and the costochondral junctions for beading – the rickety rosary.

Nervous system

Assessment of the central nervous system in infancy essentially involves the motor system and the cranial nerves. Isolated disorders of sensation are very rare in infancy and unless there are other features which would suggest a sensory deficit, e.g. spinal cord lesion, hemiplegia, etc., testing for sensation need not be routine. The limbs are inspected and any decrease in movement should be noted. It should be appreciated that one of the early signs of an upper motor neurone lesion is paucity of movement of a limb. With experience, assessment of the tone and power of each limb can be made. The reflexes are then elicited. In infancy it is usually very easy to demonstrate the biceps, triceps, brachialis, knee and ankle jerks. The plantar reflex is of no value in infancy and probably of no value until the child is at least walking. Superficial abdominal reflexes and the cremasteric reflex in the male are also easy to elicit. The anus should be inspected. The presence of a naevus or growth of hair over the lumbar or sacral spine will usually indicate an underlying spina bifida. A dark brown or black stain over the sacrum, the mongolian patch, is a normal finding in many ethnic groups. The cranial nerves can usually be assessed by inspection as mentioned earlier. Hearing may be assessed by report from the mother, but if there is any doubt hearing should be formally tested. The 9th, 10th and 12th cranial nerves can be assessed when the oral cavity is examined. It is important in infancy to assess the so-called primitive reflexes (see below).

Genitalia

Examination of the genitalia can usually be performed quite quickly in either sex and a positive statement made about normality or otherwise. In the female infant at term the labia minora are relatively large compared to the labia majora. The urethra and vaginal orifices will be noted. In the male the site of the urethra must be identified. However, if the child is uncircumcised, prepuce should not be retracted until about 4 years of age. In the presence of a hypospadias the prepuce will be deficient and the urethral orifice visible. In this situation the orifice may be located at any site from the tip of the glans to the base of the penile shaft. The testes should be identified.

Should the genitalia be ambiguous, appropriate specialist help should be obtained. Under no circumstances should the practitioner make a guess at the sex from the external appearance alone.

Finally, examination of the oral cavity, the ears and hips is undertaken. These three areas are left to the end of the examination because they all cause the infant some discomfort no matter how gentle the examination.

Oral cavity

It is best to examine the oral cavity with the help of the parent or an assistant who will extend the arms against the sides of the head. The colour of the buccal mucosa and the presence of any ulceration or exudate should be noted. The gums are examined similarly and the presence and number of teeth established. The size and mobility of the tongue is appreciated and any ulceration of epithelial denudation noted. The hard and soft palate are inspected and finally, by pressing firmly on the dorsum of the tongue with a spatula so that the infant gags, the pharynx and tonsils will be seen.

The ears

The pinna of the ear should be inspected – abnormalities of the external ear may be associated with abnormalities elsewhere, e.g. the kidneys. The auditory meatus is inspected by grasping the pinna between the thumb and finger and drawing it slightly backwards to straighten the external auditory canal. If the infant experiences pain when the pinna is pulled backwards otitis externa is likely and the external auditory canal will be noted to be inflamed. When the speculum is pushed a little further the tympanic membrane will come into view. It should normally be glistening and pearly grey. The cone

of light radiates downwards and forwards from the long handle of the malleus. A translucent tympanic membrane, normal cone of light and an obvious handle of the malleus will largely exclude middle ear disease.

Hips

The hips are assessed for congenital dislocation and are discussed in detail in Chapter 10.

Developmental assessment

Formal and detailed developmental assessment is not done as a routine as it requires the services of a multidisciplinary team which may include a paediatrician, neurologist, ophthalmologist, otorhinologist, audiologist and psychologist. Developmental assessment by the clinician will be indicated in any infant where there are risk factors to normal development. This aspect is covered in Chapter 11. Should there be no real reasons for suspecting developmental delay this part of the examination may be omitted.

Examination of the older child

Examination after the age of about 3 years and until puberty rarely causes significant problems. If the individual is approached in a friendly manner, co-operation will usually be excellent. However, this does not always apply to the adolescent who must be handled with great sensitivity; in particular there should be no feeling of loss of dignity. The examination should be preceded by accurate measurements of length and weight. Ideally, the results should be plotted on appropriate growth charts or at least be checked against normal standards for age (see Ch. 54). The nutritional status should be noted, i.e. under-or overweight.

The examination routine suggested is to begin at the head and work downwards and should be no different from that used in examining an adult patient. The question of what clothing to remove will vary with age. Occasionally the 3- to 5-year-old may resist removal of clothing. Usually, this is the result of poor preparation both on the part of the doctor and of the parents. From 5 years until puberty children will be quite happy to strip to the undergarments. The pubertal girl should be allowed to retain the bra or singlet. Problems of growth around the time of puberty will involve an assessment of the genitalia and scoring according to the method of Tanner (see Ch. 56). This can be done without causing offense if a proper explanation is given. Rectal examination will be reserved for specific indications.

It is a good plan in all prepubertal children to leave the examination of the throat and ears to the end. The urine should always be examined for blood, glucose and albumin.

Examination of the newly born infant

As soon as is practicable after birth, the newborn infant should be physically examined so that the new parents can be reassured at the earliest possible moment if all is normal and appropriate early management and referral instituted should any abnormality be detected.

If possible, the examination should be performed in front of the parents. All parents wish to know everything that they can about their newborn infant. In the first instance the infant's posture is noted and in the term infant the attitude is one of flexion of the trunk and limbs. The infant should move all limbs equally although movements will be purposeless. It is advised to count the fingers and toes. Accessory digits are not rare. The colour, respiratory rate and cry should be noted. A healthy neonate is active, pink and cries lustily when disturbed. If jaundice is present, the time of onset should be noted as this alone will provide valuable clues as to its aetiology. Birthmarks should be sought – salmon patches at the base of the nose and over the eyelids are common and disappear in time. The skull of the newborn is distorted by passage through the birth canal. This is termed moulding. Oedema of the scalp over the presenting part – caput succedaneum is also normal and disappears in a few days. A cephalhaematoma – due to bleeding under the periosteum of the skull is a soft fluctuant swelling which is limited in size by the attachments of the opponeurosis to the suture lines. The anterior and posterior fontanelle need to be identified, their size and shape noted and the skull circumference measured and compared with available standards. The general appearance of the infant must also be appraised and any dysmorphic appearance noted and described as mentiond above (see Ch. 7). Examination of the mouth will exclude a cleft palate; clefts of the gums, cysts and deciduous teeth are occasionally present at birth. The genitals are then inspected and if abnormal must be carefully described, the parents informed and consultation with an appropriate specialist arranged as soon as possible.

The spine is examined for any deformity, for example, a meningomyelocele. A hairy patch over the lumbo-sacral region will almost certainly imply an underlying spina bifida. The anus is noted, firstly, to ensure that it is patent and, secondly, to note its tone. When these preliminary observations are made the infant is systematically examined as described earlier in this chapter.

Examination of the central nervous system should include assessment of primitive reflexes. There are a number of these described, but it is not necessary to remember them all. Primitive reflexes are normally present at birth and disappear by the age of about the fifth month. Their presence at birth suggests an intact nervous system; their absence implies brain dysfunction. Persistence of primitive reflexes beyond six months of age in the term infant suggests a lesion of the central nervous system. Some of the commonly described primitive reflexes are:

1. Grasp reflex
When an object, e.g. a pencil is placed on the infant's palm from the ulnar side, automatic grasping of the pencil takes place. Sometimes the grasp is so strong that the infant may be lifted from the examination table.

2. Sucking reflex
Stimulation of the lips will produce sucking movements.

3. Walking reflex
Supporting the infant in the erect position with the feet on a flat surface will promote walking movements. Should the dorsum of the feet be placed under the edge of a table, the feet will be lifted up and placed firmly on the top of the table – the placing reflex.

4. Moro reflex
This can be elicited in the following manner – the infant is placed on a flat surface in the supine position. One hand is placed under the infant's shoulders to steady the baby. With the other hand the head is flexed on the body. When the infant is quiet and symmetrical and moderately relaxed the head is suddenly released when the infant will abduct the arms at the shoulders and flex the arms at the elbows and wrists – the abduction phase. At times there will be adduction at the hips. The abduction stage of the arms may be followed by an adduction phase. Usually this reflex produces a cry.

Finally, the hips should be assessed to exclude congenital dislocation (see Ch. 10). Gestational age assessment should be undertaken if there is doubt of the gestational age of the infant. This is described in Chapter 24.

THE CHILD IN HOSPITAL

Admission to hospital is a traumatic event for everyone, and particularly for children. Most children find hospital frightening – they meet strange people who take them to strange places (radiology department, operating theatres, etc.) and do unpleasant things to them such as taking blood, giving them injections and enemas. That mummy and/or daddy leaves them for hours, or a day, or a night at a time, and perhaps for the first time, is the ultimate trauma. Therefore, it follows that children should be admitted to hospital only when absolutely necessary and should be discharged home as soon as possible. Children can convalesce from most illnesses at home much more satisfactorily than in hospital.

Children react to hospitalization according to their age. The infant under 6 months may refuse to eat and sleep poorly. The older infant and particularly those between 9 months and 3 years are usually completely distraught – they cry incessantly, refuse to eat and sleep little. This phase may be followed by one of withdrawal when the infant may simply lie in the cot, gaze at the ceiling, and show little or no interest in people or surroundings. Young children feel abandoned, protest and constantly call for the parents; finally they become silent and begin to show signs of despair and depression. From the age of 4 to 8 years most children are anxious and fearful about what is going to be done and concerned about the sophisticated apparatus that surrounds them.

There is a small group who react differently. They are children who have lacked a constant parent figure and because of neglect or failure of the parent to cope, have frequently been separated from their parents. These children do not exhibit the usual signs of separation anxiety – rather they appear overtly friendly, they make friends with anyone and, in fact, to the uninitiated they are delightful children. They are emotionally deprived and have never had the opportunity of making a permanent and satisfactory relationship with an adult. Many of them have spent periods of time in institutions as wards of the State.

If the problem of the child in hospital is taken seriously, the answers are fairly obvious. In the first instance admission should be avoided if at all possible and particularly between the ages of 9 months and 3 years. Admissions should be as brief as possible and for this reason day-stay wards have been established in a number of paediatric hospitals. This has proven very satisfactory for minor surgery and for some children who require investigation. The child arrives in the morning, the surgical procedure is performed and discharge home follows in the latter part of the day. An increasing number of more complex surgical procedures are now being performed in day surgical units.

It must also be clear that when hospital is essential, one or both parents should accompany the child to hospital and remain throughout the whole period if at all possible. Clearly problems will arise when there are other young children in the family, or in the case of a single parent. Nonetheless, every effort should be made to have somebody well known to the child at the bedside as much as possible. When this is not possible, a paediatric hospital should have a group of caring people who are trained to meet the physical, emotional and intellectual needs of these children. These personnel will include a paediatric nurse, occupational therapist, schoolteacher or a trained volunteer. There must also be facilities in hospitals for play, e.g. toys, drawing materials, painting materials and suitable television.

When admission is elective the child must be prepared for hospitalization. Many hospitals provide booklets for parents which will indicate how children should be prepared for admission. These booklets should be well illustrated so that the child will know exactly what to expect. It may be advantageous for some children to visit the ward, the radiology department and even the operating theatre before admission.

For children who require long-term stay in hospital, the experience should be made as enriching as possible; a host of pleasant activities can be provided. School work can be continued by many, so that the child does not feel left behind on returning to school. Many children can go home on 'weekend leave' so that home and friendships are not forgotten. Visitors should not be restricted and the visiting of young siblings should be encouraged.

Recently, care by parent wards have been opened in some paediatric hospitals. In these areas nursing duties are performed entirely by parents under supervision. Apart from the psychological benefits, requirements for nursing staff are reduced, and of course the cost of hospitalization. Finally, medical and nursing staff must see to it that the total needs of the child are met – not just the physical care which has demanded the admission. Hospitals should revolve around patients and their parents and not simply around doctors, nurses and other hospital personnel, a situation which in the past has all too often been the case.

10. Posture and common orthopaedic problems

Malcolm Menelaus

POSTURE AND ITS VARIATIONS DURING GROWTH

Adult posture should not be used as a criterion for the proper posture in infancy and childhood. During this period of development a number of different limb shapes (or postures) may be noted and cause parental anxiety. These transitory postures include positions of the limbs secondary to intrauterine posture and these may be described as 'package defects'. Other postures, which are not present at birth, may appear, then spontaneously disappear. The latter group includes bow legs, knock knees, flat feet, out-toeing, in-toeing, in-toe stance and in-toe gait. These conditions seldom require active treatment for the posture itself but the parents do require informed reassurance which can only be based on accurate knowledge of the natural history of the variations of posture of infants and children.

POSITION OF THE FETUS IN UTERO AND PACKAGING DEFECTS

The position of the child before birth is normally one of flexion. The spine is flexed so that it forms a long curve with a concavity forward, the arms and legs are flexed, and the feet may assume a variety of postures. In the newborn the intrauterine posture can be readily reconstructed by 'folding' the baby into his most comfortable position and this may indicate any postural abnormality present.

Posture of the spine

After birth, as the child stretches out, there are two primary curves in the spine – both convex backwards: one is in the dorsal region and the other at the sacrum.

On the assumption of the erect posture two secondary curves appear, both convex forward: one in the cervical region and one in the lumbar region (which appears after the child stands).

Sometimes children display an increase in the normal thoracic and lumbar curves: this may merely reflect ligamentous laxity, poor muscle tone, fatigue and a listless mood. These curves do not tend to become fixed and generally no action is called for.

When the newborn infant is viewed from behind, the spine is generally quite straight. However, some babies are seen who have a persistent scoliosis in the form of a long curve which extends from the base of the neck to the sacrum. This is generally a packaging defect and like other packaging defects will correct itself spontaneously. It is merely necessary to note the curvature and to confirm, at subsequent examinations, that this spontaneous correction is taking place. Very rarely will one encounter progressive scoliosis in infancy and generally the curve is over a short length of the spine. Further comments on spinal posture are made under the heading Scoliosis (see page 74).

Foot posture in the newborn

Many babies are born with the foot turned upwards at the ankle so that the toes lie close to the front of the shin – talipes calcaneovalgus. This posture can be passively corrected so that the foot can be brought down to a plantigrade position or even into a little equinus. The condition has a strong tendency to correct itself spontaneously over a period of two to three months.

Some babies are born with one or both feet in a position of plantar flexion at the ankles and inversion of the remainder of the foot so that the sole of the foot faces the opposite foot. This is postural talipes equinovarus and may be distinguished from true talipes equinovarus by the fact that the former condition is easily correctable, either actively by the baby's movement or passively by the attendant. The foot can be readily held in normal alignment to the leg or even in a position of calcaneovalgus whereas in true congenital talipes equinovarus (club foot) the deformity is rigid. All mobile foot postures correct themselves spontaneously whereas fixed deformities require treatment (see Congenital talipes equinovarus (congenital club foot) – page 74).

Bow legs

Bow legs (Fig. 10.1), occurring as an isolated condition, is due to bowing of the tibia, so that the lower articular surface is directed down and inwards. In addition, the tibia is also twisted inwards so that, with the upper end of the tibia pointing forward, the ankle joint is directed inwards. This twist is referred to as internal tibial torsion.

Bulky nappies are not causative because the bowing is in the tibiae. It is possible that the internal torsion of the tibiae may be aggravated by the child sleeping on the face with the feet turned inwards. This posture is common from the age of walking to the age of three years and seldom requires treatment. Even if the child's internal tibial torsion is marked it is not necessary to turn the child onto his back at night as the condition will correct itself spontaneously. Very rarely a Denis Browne boot and bar night splint is applied to correct this condition. A bar joins the heels of the two boots which are set in a position of out-toeing. Adults who have bow legs do not have a persistence of this childhood tibial bowing and internal torsion.

Knock knees

A high proportion of the population between the ages of 2.5 and 7 years have knock knees (Fig. 10.2). This has a very strong tendency to correct itself by the age of seven years and generally the only management necessary is parental reassurance that improvement will occur.

There is a rare form of knock knees which presents in obese children over the age of twelve years and which does require treatment.

Out-toeing

Between the ages of 6 and 10 months some infants have a tendency to lie or stand with the toes of one foot

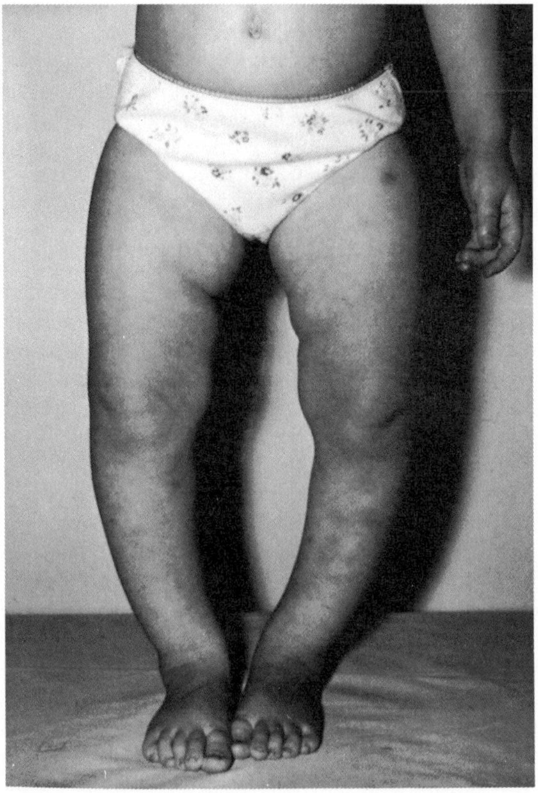

Fig. 10.1 Bow-legs in a toddler – a normal phenomenon.

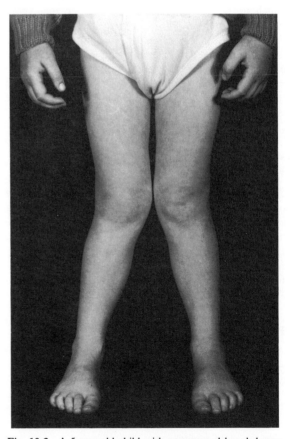

Fig. 10.2 A 5-year-old child with pronounced knock knees.

directed outward from the midline. The condition is usually unilateral and is most commonly seen in the left leg. Closer inspection reveals that not only is the foot turned out but the knee on that side lies in an externally rotated position also. When the child is examined on the couch one finds that the hip on the affected side has an excessive range of external rotation and a limited range of internal rotation. These children lie or stand with the foot turned out because that is the comfortable position for that limb: it is the position halfway between full internal and full external rotation of the hip joint. When the baby is folded into the most comfortable position the leg with the out-toe posture folds high onto the chest with the hip in a position of 90% of external rotation. This was the posture assumed by this leg whilst the child was in utero. The opposite leg lay more caudally on the trunk and in a less externally rotated position.

Children who have this form of out-toeing will tend to walk with an out-toe gait at first. The condition has invariably corrected itself by the age of 14 months.

Flat feet

The four propositions on which a logical attitude to this problem is based are as follows:

1. Foot posture varies with age.
2. Whilst the majority of the population develop a medial longitudinal arch, there are others who, for reasons that are presumably genetically determined, do not.
3. It is very doubtful whether the ultimate shape of the foot can be altered any more than the colour of a patient's eyes or any other genetically determined feature.
4. Those people who remain flat footed seldom have trouble resulting from the flat shape of their feet. In some parts of the world it is the normal foot shape. The Australian Aboriginal tends to have very flat feet.

THE NATURAL HISTORY OF FOOT POSTURE

When children commence walking they do so on feet that appear flat, partly because there is true flatness of the medial longitudinal arch and partly because the arch is filled in by a fat pad, which like the sucking pad, inevitably disappears. Between the ages of 2 and 8 years, mothers are often concerned because 'a second ankle bone appears on the medial aspect of the foot'. They are referring to a prominence of the navicular bone which is present in most children who have flat feet. Unless the prominence of this bone is causing symptoms it can be ignored. Children with flat feet generally have some

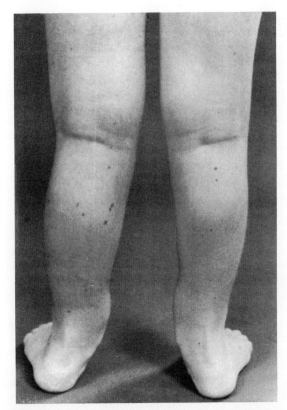

Fig. 10.3 Child with flat feet at age 6 years. Note the valgus heels.

valgus deformity of the heel – when viewed from behind the heels do not point straight up and down but tend to slope outwards and downwards (Fig. 10.3). This seldom persists into adult life.

During the first 7 or 8 years of life the majority of children develop a medial longitudinal arch but approximately 15% do not. Clearly the results of any form of treatment for flat feet are going to be excellent as some 85% will get better whether or not they are treated. Flat feet may be ignored unless the feet are quickly distorting the child's shoes. If this is the case then arch supports may be worn for a period in order to preserve the footwear, but this is seldom necessary. The child with a prominent navicular may have some temporary discomfort which may be relieved by wearing arch supports for a period of a year or two.

Toe posture

It is common for one or two toes to be out of line with the others. Most commonly the third toe curls inwards under the second toe so that the second toe tends to lie above the level of the first and third toes. Parents are generally concerned with the abnormal posture of the second toe, but it is the third toe which is the cause of the problem. Sometimes the lesser toes have a flexed posture (hammer toe). All of these toe deformities can be safely ignored until the child is at least 18 months old; this applies also to syndactyly of the toes. If the deformity of curly and hammer toes is so gross that symptoms appear likely, division of the long flexor tendon will readily correct either deformity.

In-toe gait

An in-toe gait in children may have one or more of the following three causes:

1. Inset hips – that is hips which have internal rotation in excess of the range of external rotation, and this is common between the ages of 3 and 8 years.

2. Internal torsion of the tibia – this had already been discussed under the heading of 'Bow legs'. It is commonly present from the age of walking to the age of 3 years.

3. Metatarsus adductus – commonly present from birth to the age of 5 years (see Fig. 10.4).

Children with inset hips commonly sit between their feet with their hips in full internal rotation, the knees flexed and the legs splayed outwards. This is the only

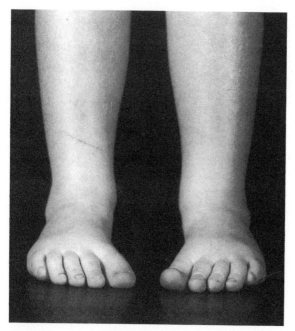

Fig. 10.4   A 3-year-old child with metatarsus adductus.

way they can sit comfortably as they cannot externally rotate their hips sufficiently to sit in a cross-legged fashion. There is no evidence that this sitting posture should be discouraged in children and it is worthwhile remembering that it is almost unknown for an adult to present with a complaint of in-toeing.

Metatarsus adductus is a condition in which the feet are banana shaped with the convexity of the banana outwards and the toes directed towards each other. These children are not seen to be in-toed until they take their shoes off. This foot shape is common from birth to the age of 5 years. It is passively correctable and slowly rights itself over a number of years of observation. Very rarely is manipulation and plaster immobilization, or a period in night splints necessary.

CHILDREN'S FOOTWEAR AND MODIFICATIONS TO FOOTWEAR

The only essential is that children's shoes should be roomy enough. Shoes themselves are not necessary to promote normal foot growth and development; they are only worn for protection and need not be worn until activities demand this protection. Boots are no better than shoes though in toddlers, boots may be more satisfactory in that they are less likely to fall off or be taken off.

It is not harmful to use 'hand down' shoes from older children in the family provided they are roomy enough. There is no evidence that sandals, thongs, or sneakers have any harmful influence on the feet.

Footwear modifications

Whilst wedging of the soles and heels have long been employed for in-toeing and out-toeing, such footwear modifications have no influence either on the gait itself or on the natural history. Thomas heels are of little or no value in the management of flat feet and are less effective than properly designed arch supports; and as has been indicated, few children require these.

CONGENITAL ABNORMALITIES

Congenital dislocation of the hip (CDH)

The incidence of this condition in Australia and North America is usually quoted as 4 per 1000 live births. In some regions of Europe it is more common. These figures would be much increased if every child who had a 'clunking' hip at birth were diagnosed as having a congenitally dislocated hip. Many of these 'clunking' hips do so for a few days only and it is doubtful if they should be included. The CDH is 5 to 10 times more common in girls. When diagnosed and treated from birth it is possible to produce a normal hip joint after a few months in an abduction splint. However, if the diagnosis is not made until after the child begins to walk, the treatment is long and tedious and often ends with an imperfect joint.

Diagnosis in the newborn

Every baby should be examined for hip dislocation during the first day of life and again before discharge from the maternity hospital. The baby is stripped and examined on a large firm bench. If the baby is crying a bottle or bottle teat is offered. With the legs extended, any asymmetry of the legs or adductor creases is noted. The examiner then holds the leg to be examined in his hand (his hand is the opposite hand to the side of the hip to be examined). With the knee flexed, the thumb is placed over the lesser trochanter and the middle finger over the greater trochanter (Fig. 10.5). The pelvis is steadied by the other hand and the flexed thigh is abducted and adducted and any 'clunk' or jerk is noted (Ortolani's sign). With the hip abducted about 45 degrees the femur is gently rocked backwards and forwards on the pelvis and again any jerk or clunk is noted. The findings on this examination may be of four kinds:

1. A fine click in the hip joint not associated with any laxity or abnormal movement between the femur and the pelvis. This is very common and of no significance.

2. A laxity in the hip joint not associated with any jerk on abduction of the hip. The hip can be felt to dislocate smoothly without any 'clunk'. This is common in the first two or three days of life especially in prema-

ture and shocked babies. Those who have temporary laxity of this kind (disappearing within a week) should be subjected to re-examination and radiology at the age of three months.

3. A palpable and visible jerk forwards of the upper end of the femur when the flexed thigh is abducted to approximately 45 degrees; the thigh can then be fully abducted. When the thigh is then adducted the upper end of the femur jerks backwards; this distinctive sign is palpable and visible but rarely audible. If untreated these hips are likely to progress to congenital dislocation as seen in young children.

4. There is considerable restriction of abduction in flexion usually on both sides but the 'clunk' sign cannot be elucidated. This usually means that the hips are dislocated and irreducible – a group referred to as teratological dislocations because the hip has been manufactured in the dislocated position. These hips require operative reduction at a later date.

Radiography has no place in the diagnosis of congenital dislocation of the hip in the neonatal period. The diagnosis is clinical and treatment is dictated by the clinical findings. All children who have been suspected at birth of having any hip abnormality at all should have an antero-posterior radiograph of the pelvis at the age of three months. Also, all siblings and first degree relatives of children with congenital dislocation of the hip should have radiographs at this time to rule out the possibility of symptomless dysplasia.

If the dislocated hip is held in a flexed and abducted position, for 8–12 weeks, it will usually develop normally. The Pavlik harness is the most satisfactory orthosis for maintaining this position and should be supplemented by the use of double nappies. Mother is instructed to lie the baby either prone or supine but not on the side. If the hip is clinically stable after a month then the harness may be removed daily for bathing.

Diagnosis in the older infant

Palpable dislocation and reduction becomes more difficult to elicit during the first few weeks of life but it sometimes presents up to the age of six months. As this physical sign disappears, new signs appear because the head of the femur is never in the acetabulum; there is now limited abduction of the flexed hip. This sign is not diagnostic but a radiograph is indicated when there is asymmetry in the range of the abduction of the hips or when the range of abduction of both hips is inappropriate for the age of the child. In the first year of life the range of abduction in flexion should be approximately 60 degrees; this arc lessens with age.

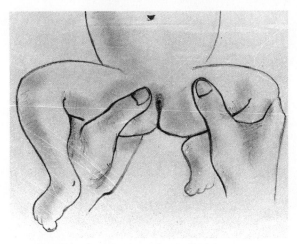

Fig. 10.5 How to demonstrate Ortolani's sign.

With the hips extended, the relationship of the tip of the greater trochanter to the anterior superior iliac spine should be palpated on both sides simultaneously. Elevation of the tip of the trochanter indicated hip dislocation or coxa vara. In addition, there may be difficulty in palpating the pulsations of the femoral artery at the groin, broadening of the perineum, or asymmetry of the gluteal or adductor creases: telescoping may be present and in unilateral cases there is shortening of the affected leg. Over the age of one year the child may present because of delay in walking or because of an abnormal gait.

Congenital talipes equinovarus (congenital club foot)

Congenital talipes equinovarus is the commonest congenital abnormality of the foot, occurring in about 1 per 1000 live births. It is twice as common in boys and may be unilateral or bilateral.

The deformity is a combination of equinus, varus, adductus and cavus (Fig. 10.6). The degree of each deformity is variable but all are rigid and incapable of being corrected manually.

Club feet should be treated from the first day of life. Treatment may involve the application of Denis Browne splints or serial plaster casting. Failure to correct the deformity in the first few months or relapse after correction indicates that surgical intervention is required; the majority of patients do require such surgery.

SCOLIOSIS

Scoliosis (lateral curvature of the spine) most commonly appears in early adolescence. However, there are 3 other forms of scoliosis. These are as follows:

1. Infantile idiopathic scoliosis – most commonly seen in males and may be seen in association with congenital dislocation of the hip and other congenital anomalies. The natural history is for the curve to resolve in a high proportion of cases.

2. Congenital scoliosis – vertebral anomalies are responsible for the curvature. Usually the deformity is minor and may be present at birth or develop during growth. In only 5% is the deformity progressive.

3. Juvenile idiopathic scoliosis – a curve in children between the age of 3 years and the onset of puberty; it is uncommon.

Adolescent scoliosis

Although there are many causes for scoliosis, adolescent idiopathic scoliosis makes up 55%; 90% occurs in girls and progresses during the rapid growth spurt. Recently, screening has been carried out in schools in an attempt to detect cases at an early stage. Treatment is undertaken to avoid cosmetic impairment.

As a general rule, curves of more than 20 degrees require conservative treatment. Once the curve has

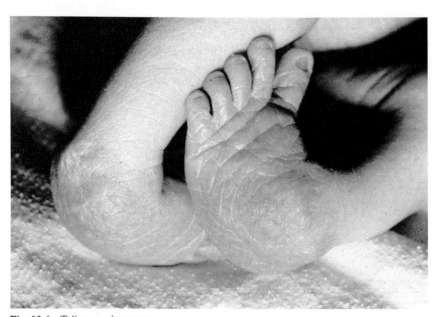

Fig. 10.6   Talipes equino varus.

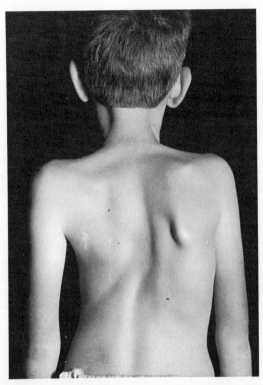

Fig. 10.7   Adolescent scoliosis in a male – 90% occur in females.

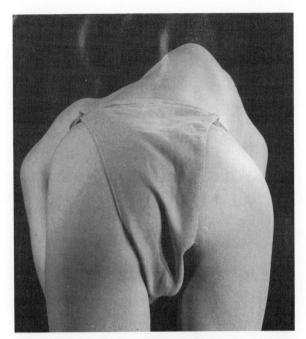

Fig. 10.8   On flexion a rib hump becomes readily visible.

progressed beyond 40 degrees surgical correction must be carried out. Conservative treatment involves the use of a brace; physiotherapy is valueless for this condition.

For diagnosis, the child must remove all clothing above the waist and stand with the back facing the examiner (Fig. 10.7). In all but very minor curves the deformity will be readily apparent. When the child bends forwards the curve may disappear completely, in which case it can be labelled postural and treatment is not required. Should the curve remain the same or a rib hump become visible due to rotation occurring at the site of the curvature (Fig. 10.8) the curve is labelled 'idiopathic'; the implication is that at least observation is required and at most surgical treatment may become necessary. Minor degrees of rib hump may be better seen if the examiner faces the bending child; those screening adolescent girls for scoliosis should be instructed to examine in this way.

Sternomastoid torticollis

Torticollis presents most commonly in the first 3 years of life when the characteristic deformity is noted. The head is held with a lateral flexion toward the shoulder with rotation of the face towards the opposite side (Fig. 10.9). The face is smaller and the eye lower on the side of the tight sternomastoid. Some patients will have presented in the first few months of life with a sternomastoid tumour; i.e. a palpable lump in the middle of the sternomastoid muscle. The cause of this tumour and of torticollis is unknown. Because the condition may resolve it is not necessary to treat cases seen in infancy but if the condition persists over the age of two years, or is progressive, then surgical correction is required. At operation, the muscle is divided transversely and the corrected position maintained by the use of a collar.

Osteochondroses (Osteochondritis)

These are a group of conditions involving the epiphysis. The pathology consists of localized areas of ischaemic bone necrosis and oedema of adjacent soft tissues. The tendency is for healing to occur, but this is dependent on a number of factors which include age, the site of the lesion, its blood supply and perhaps the method of treatment. Any bone having a cartilaginous area at the site of either the primary or secondary centre of ossification may be affected. The aetiology is uncertain.

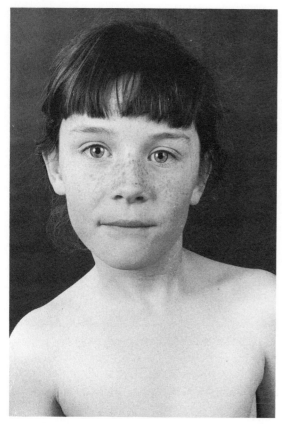

Fig. 10.9 Left-sided sternomastoid torticollis in a
6-year-old girl. Note the characteristic posture and facial
asymmetry.

Scheuermann's disease

The epiphyseal plates of the vertebral bodies are involved. Usually it is seen in the thoracic vertebrae but
occasionally in the lumbar spine. It almost always occurs
in the adolescent. Usually children present in early
adolescence because of an increase in the normal
thoracic kyphosis so that the child appears round-
shouldered. Many do not progress much and merely
require observation whereas others progress rapidly and
require management in a brace.

Slipped femoral epiphysis

This is primarily a disorder of the adolescent between
the ages of 10 and 15 years. Approximately 20% of cases
are bilateral. Its aetiology is unknown but recently work
suggests that hormonal factors may be of importance.
Most cases present with pain and limp – pain is often
referred to the knee. Varying degrees of limitation of
movement of the hip joint will be found depending upon
the extent of the slip. The diagnosis is confirmed
radiologically, and all cases of slipped upper femoral
epiphysis require surgery to prevent further slip.

Chondromalacia patellae

This is particularly common over the age of 12 years. It
is characterized by pain in the knee after activities which
involve the quadriceps muscle. This syndrome is sometimes associated with an effusion into the knee. The
diagnosis is based upon obtaining the relevant history;
it rapidly responds to rest.

Injuries in infancy and childhood

Children are susceptible to injury because of their
carefree play habits and skeletal injuries are extremely
common. For practical purposes sprains do not occur in
children so that post traumatic pain, swelling, and loss
of function are nearly always the result of a fracture or
growth plate separation. Therefore, radiographs are
obligatory. Dislocations are also rare in childhood. The
type of injury which may produce dislocation of an adult
joint usually gives rise to a fracture or growth plate
separation in a child.

   Thus, fractures are the commonest type of skeletal injury in childhood; these generally unite in less than half
the time the equivalent injury would take to heal in an
adult; non-union is almost unknown. Furthermore,
childhood fractures may unite in a position of deformity
with the deformity correcting itself spontaneously over
the ensuing 6–12 months. Some shortening of bones can
also be expected to correct spontaneously following
childhood fractures.

   Child abuse is an important cause of childhood injury;
it is important because, if unrecognized, further abuse
is likely to occur and might even be fatal. Child abuse
is discussed in Chapter 21.

FURTHER READING

Williams P F (ed) 1982 Orthopaedic management in
   childhood. Blackwell Scientific Publications, Oxford

ACKNOWLEDGEMENT

The material in this chapter is similar to that which the
author prepared for, and was published in Clements A (ed)
1986 Infant and family health in Australia. Churchill
Livingstone. We are grateful for permission to include it here.

11. Developmental screening and assessment

Kim Oates

Developmental screening

Developmental screening is different from developmental assessment. Developmental assessment refers to assessing the development of particular children in relation to the developmental milestones for their age. In contrast, developmental screening looks at groups of children to see if there are any developmental handicaps which would require early intervention.

In 1966 a Report on a Working Party (WHO 1967) stated that:

Screening implies the application to all children of certain procedures which can be carried out in a short time by less specialized members of staff and which will give an indication of the presence or absence of certain disabilities. If the result of the test is positive, including the actual or probable presence of a disability, the child is referred for specialist investigation and care.

The scope of developmental screening can be very broad such as looking for the presence of handicaps, visual and hearing impairment and developmental delay.

The tests used for screening need to be simple, quick to use and to give reproducible results. They should have a high sensitivity (producing very few false negative results) and be highly specific (producing very few false positives). Potential problems with screening programmes include variable skills in those doing the screening and perhaps more importantly, the fact that those groups which have the highest level of developmental problems are often the least likely to avail themselves of screening services.

Developmental screening can of course be done on individual children to see whether a developmental problem is likely. Popular tools for developmental screening are the Denver Developmental Screening Test (DDST) and the Developmental Record for Infants and Young Children (DRIYC) which was developed in South Australia. These tests are useful for children up to five years of age. Children who are suspected of having a developmental problem, either as a result of being detected by a screening test or by the doctor being aware that the child's pattern of development does not fall within the usual developmental milestones should be referred for a full developmental assessment.

Developmental assessment

A complete developmental assessment is a complex procedure requiring a paediatrician with special training in this area. In this assessment the paediatrician uses the skills of others such as psychologists, physiotherapists, speech pathologists, occupational therapists, social workers, audiologists and ophthalmologists to obtain a thorough understanding of the child's abilities. Not all of these people would be required for every developmental assessment, the features of the delay often suggesting which specialty groups need to be involved. In a good, close working assessment team there is also an overlap and sharing of skills with team members learning from each other so that there is some flexibility of roles. It is evident that a complete assessment is expensive and time-consuming so that it is only appropriate for children where a developmental problem is already suspected.

NORMAL DEVELOPMENT

An assessment of a child's development, in contrast to a full developmental assessment, is an essential part of the examination of any child. In the same way that the examination of a child would be incomplete if the history and examination of the respiratory system or the genito-urinary system were omitted, the assessment of the child's development, by history and examination, is required before it can be said that the child has been completely evaluated. Enquiries should be made about the child's skills and abilities, the child should be observed, skills tested and the findings accurately recorded. This chapter describes how this sort of assessment may be done.

Why learn normal development?

As well as allowing significant deviations from the normal to be detected, so that appropriate intervention can be commenced, knowledge of normal developmental patterns will allow the doctor to recognize those patterns which are a variation on the normal, or within the normal range so that parents can be reassured. Being able to assess a child's level of development and knowing what the developmental progress over the next few months is likely to be is valuable for informing parents what sort of behaviours to expect. This will enable guidance about child management and accident prevention to be given. For example an infant of nine months will be starting to crawl and will be beginning to develop a pincer (finger-thumb) grip so that small objects can be picked up. At this age all objects will still be automatically tested by putting them into the mouth. This mobile infant will also be interested in exploring the environment. It is helpful to be able to predict these behaviours for parents so that they can take precautions to make their homes safer. Examples of this include putting railings at the top of a staircase, reminding them of the dangers of small, sharp objects or tablets which the mobile, inquisitive child now has the ability to pick up precisely and to deposit quickly into the mouth.

The best time to assess development

In contrast to a physical examination, the child is not a passive part of the developmental examination. The child should be given the opportunity to perform optimally. If ill, or just woken, or miserable for some other reason, it may be better to do the developmental assessment at a more opportune time. For example, it would be foolish to try to do a developmental assessment on a 22-month-old admitted to hospital with asthma who was in respiratory distress as well as being 'high' from Salbutamol medication. While the developmental part of the history can still be taken at the same time as the general history, the assessment of development is best kept until the child has improved and is able to give the best performance. The child's co-operation must be obtained if the developmental assessment is to be successful. This is best done by relating to the child in a friendly, enthusiastic way, praising the child for good performances, giving new challenges and supporting the child with encouragement during the assessment. This is why an important part of paediatric training is to develop skills in playing with and relating to children.

The developmental history

This should include general factors about the child's health and environment and specific information about developmental milestones. It is important to know about the child's family and environment as well as about past health. The parents should be questioned about unusual patterns of family development and about any stillbirths or deaths in infancy.

In taking a developmental history it is helpful to remember that the information obtained will only be as good as the questions asked. The question 'When did your baby sit?' will have different meanings for different parents. For some this may mean the baby being able to get into the sitting position without assistance (usually at about 10 months) while for others it may mean being able to sit up in the stroller with the aid of several pillows for support at the back and sides (this could be achieved at two or three months). The more precise question is 'How old was your baby when able to be put in the sitting position and to remain there unsupported?'. This is likely to yield a much more useful answer of about six or seven months for the average baby.

When asking about language development remember to distinguish between expressive and receptive language. Expressive language is what the child can say. Ask whether the child's words have consistent meaning. The clarity of pronunciation in the first year after speech develops is less important than the extent of the vocabulary and the consistent use of the same sounds for the same object or person. Receptive language is how many words the child can understand and is usually well in advance of expressive language. A child of 18 months who only says four or five distinctive words with meaning may have a receptive language of 200 words or more.

Because smiling is an important early milestone which should have developed by six weeks, it is important to determine whether this is social smiling. The grimace which a baby makes associated with bringing up wind is quite different from the social smile which is made in response to a parent smiling and talking to the child.

Parents should be given credit for their observations. Although some studies suggest that parents do not always remember normal milestones accurately, when there is parental concern about a milestone, such as onset of walking, being reached, the memory for this milestone is likely to be reasonably accurate. Surveys of childhood deafness have shown that a parent is usually the first to suspect a hearing problem. Any parent who expresses concern that her child may not be able to hear must be taken seriously, whatever the child's age, and the child should be promptly referred for formal audiology testing.

The accuracy of the history can be improved by asking about the child's development in relation to that of the siblings. Asking parents to remember whether specific milestones had been reached by the child's first birthday or first Christmas, checking on family photographs and asking parents to check milestones recorded in the child's baby book, are other ways of improving recall. Another useful source is the infant health clinic booklet which will contain past measurements of weight, length and head circumference so that percentiles can be plotted to give a picture of the child's growth pattern.

The history should also reveal factors which may have influenced the child's development. Allowance has to be made for prematurity. If birth was at 32 weeks' gestation, eight weeks should be subtracted from the chronological age when assessing development, so that milestones would be expected to be reached two months later than in a baby born at full term. Environmental factors may also influence development. Children who are emotionally deprived, who receive little verbal stimulation, or who do not have the opportunity to practise walking or crawling when they are ready to achieve these milestones will be delayed in their development. In contrast, children who live in a stimulating environment, who receive good quality language stimulation and opportunities for a wide variety of play experiences may develop in advance of average milestones.

Developmental milestones

Developmental milestones can be conveniently grouped into four main areas:

- body mastery (gross motor skills)
- manipulative skills and vision (fine motor function)
- language and hearing
- social skills and understanding.

It is daunting to try to learn all of the developmental milestones but it is important to try to learn one or two in each of these four main categories at key ages. A summary of some of the main milestones is listed in Example 11.1. More complete lists can be found in the references listed at the end of this chapter.

Although the milestones are important, there are other less tangible factors which are also valuable in the assessment. The main one is the quality of the child's behaviour and interaction with the examiner. In the absence of physical illness, the child who shows lack of interest, who is lethargic, does not relate to the examiner and is disinterested in the surroundings is a cause for concern whatever the traditional developmental milestones show. In contrast, the child who is alert, interested in new objects, keen to explore and who re-

lates to a friendly examiner is giving useful information. A developmental problem in this child is more likely because of an isolated condition rather than to global retardation. The child's home environment and the amount of stimulation given there have to be taken into consideration. A 2-year-old whose parent is enthusiastic about early stimulation is likely to be more advanced than a child who may have the same potential but who rarely receives any verbal stimulation and who spends most of the day in a room with few toys.

When describing a child's developmental milestones, it is helpful to use the four main areas described above. However, the order in which the child is tested does not particularly matter, as long as all of these areas are covered. It is important to use the information which the child presents spontaneously. For example, if a 10-month-old child is put on the floor in the crawling position with a small, interesting object not far away and the child crawls towards the object (9–10 months), picks it up in a finger-thumb pincer grip (9–10 months), automatically mouths it (6–12 months), gets into the sitting position to play with it more readily (10 months), spontaneously lets it go when the examiner's hand is held out for it (11 months) and then waves goodbye in response to the examiner's wave (10 months), the developmental assessment is almost complete. The child has just demonstrated age-appropriate body mastery, fine motor and social skills. There is little point in now trying to get the child to go through a variety of developmental milestones to prove what has just been observed. All that remains to complete the developmental examination in this case is to assess the child's hearing and language.

As young infants and children have fairly short attention spans, the developmental assessment has to be done efficiently. A useful approach is to see first if the child can pass a skill in each of the four main areas appropriate to the age. If the child is able to demonstrate that milestone, see if a skill in the next higher age bracket can be performed until you find the developmental age at which skills are passed and the next nearest developmental age at which the skill cannot be achieved. Similarly, if the child cannot achieve a skill appropriate to the age, move down quickly until you find skills which the child can pass. The child's developmental age will be somewhere between the age at which skills can be passed and the next highest age at which other skills are failed. If the child is obviously a long way behind in development, it is better to come down quickly to the appropriate developmental age of the child rather than laboriously come down in one or two months' steps. This will avoid the child becoming irritable and bored with the assessment before there has been time to complete it.

Example 11.1 Main developmental milestones

Age	Body mastery	Manipulative skills and vision	Language and hearing	Social skills and understanding
Newborn	Prone: pelvis high, knees under abdomen. Turns face to one side.	Can fixate on a visual object about 20 cm away and follows it horizontally for 90°.	Blinks or becomes quiet in response to sound.	Sleeps and feeds. Elicits affection from others.
1 month	Lifts head momentarily when held in ventral suspension. Prone: raises head momentarily.	Watches examiner intently when speaking. Regularly follows objects through 90–180°.	Soft, guttural noises when content.	May smile back at parent or examiner.
2 months	In ventral suspension keeps head in same horizontal plane as body. Holds head erect when held upright.	Hands mostly open, grasp reflex weak. Follows moving person with eyes.	Vocalizes when talked to.	Smiles readily. Starts to respond more readily to parent than to others.
3 months	Prone: lifts chest off bed, taking weight on forearms. Only slight head lag when pulled to sit.	Holds rattle placed in hand. Reaches towards objects, but unable to grasp. Starts to look at own hands.	Consistently turns to soft sound at ear level. Squeals in delight.	Pleasurable response to familiar, enjoyable situations (bottle, bath).
4 months	Rolls from front to back. Pulled to sit, only slight head lag.	Hands start to come together in midline.	Spontaneous vocalizing to self, people and toys. Laughs.	Initiates social contact with smile or vocalization.
5 months	Rolls from back to front. No head lag when pulled to sit.	Reaches out for and grasps toys.	Babbling more tuneful.	Smiles at self in mirror.
6 months	Prone: lifts chest on extended arms. Spontaneously lifts head when supine.	Transfers objects between hands. Picks up wooden block in palmar grasp.	Turns towards soft sound at 40–50 cm on ear level.	Laughs, squeals and chuckles. May imitate sounds (cough). Fear of strangers.
9 months	Crawls. Sits unsupported for 10 min. or more. Stands holding onto support.	Pincer grip developing.	Localizes soft sounds at 1 metre above and below ear level.	Looks for toy fallen out of sight. Plays pat-a-cake, peek-a-boo.
12 months	Walks alone or with one hand held.	Repeatedly throws objects onto floor. Less likely to take all objects to mouth.	Says 2 or 3 words with meaning.	Drinks from cup with help. Knows and turns to own name.
18 months	Jumps with both feet together. Walks backwards.	Builds tower of 3 or 4 blocks. Scribbles spontaneously.	Uses 5–20 words (recognizes many more).	Points to 2 or more parts of body. Indicates toilet needs.
2 years	Runs well. Kicks ball without overbalancing.	Builds tower of 6 or 7 blocks. Copies vertical and circular strokes.	Uses 2 and 3 word phrases. Starts to use pronouns.	Behaviour becoming negative. Gives first name. Begins fantasy play.
3 years	Rides tricycle. Stands on 1 foot momentarily.	Builds tower of blocks. Copies circle.	3 to 5 word sentences. Uses plurals. May count to 10.	Gives full name and sex. Competent with fork and spoon.
4 years	Hops on 1 foot.	Copies cross. Draws person with three parts.	Asks many questions. Tells fanciful stories.	Gives age and address. Knows and names 4 primary colours. Very imaginative play.
5 years	Can skip.	Copies square. Draws person with 6 parts.	Fluent speech; good articulation.	Dresses with assistance.

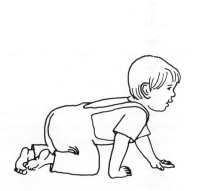
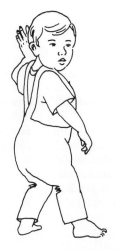
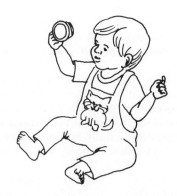

Equipment for developmental assessment

The basic equipment used is listed in Example 11.2. (For other tests refer to Holt 1977; Sheridan 1968.)

Example 11.2 Basic equipment for developmental assessment

12 Wooden cubes (approximately 2.5 cm in primary colours)
Bell, high pitched
Rattle, low pitched
Fluffy red woollen ball
Tennis ball
Pencil and paper
Selection of small, safe, interesting toys
Jelly beans, for testing pincer grip
Picture book, with simple coloured pictures (*Things We Like To Do* and *Baby's First Book* published by Ladybird are excellent)

Wooden blocks are particularly useful. They should be cubes of approximately 2.5 cm so that they can be easily manipulated by the infant. With them the examiner can test for the ability to reach for and grasp objects and can observe the development of the grasp. They are used for seeing how many can be stacked one on top of the other and by offering them to the child from the right and left sides, hand preference and peripheral vision can be checked. A strong hand preference developing under 18 months suggests that there may be a problem in the side which is not being used as readily. Also, blocks can be hidden from a child to see if a hidden object is looked for (9–10 months), to see whether the child can spontaneously release the cube into the examiner's hand (10–11 months) and for testing the recognition of primary colours (3–4 years).

The child who does not have 'normal' milestones

For a child to be quite average in all respects is unusual. Most children will show some variation from the 'average range'. It is important to remember that there is a normal range for the attainment of milestones even though most tables of milestones just give one average age. When a child shows delays in several areas there should be concern about the possibility of global delay. Also other factors should be considered. They include the need to make allowances for prematurity, family patterns of development, obesity which may delay gross motor function, and whether the child has been in a stimulating or a depriving environment.

Specific delays in some areas, with normal development in others, raises the question of isolated defects. For example, delayed speech in a child who is normal in other milestones suggests a hearing loss. Delayed motor development with normal social relationships and speech suggests a neuromuscular disorder.

Interpretation and prediction

The aim of the developmental assessment is to tell how far the child has progressed in relation to average developmental milestones for children of that age. If development is uniformly slow, this gives the child a developmental age below the chronological age. If factors such as prematurity, illness, prolonged hospitalization, emotional or environmental deprivation are not present, it is likely that the child will have continuing developmental delay. In contrast, predictions of high intelligence cannot be made based on advanced developmental milestones. Advanced gross motor milestones have little useful correlation with high intelligence and while early speech development shows some correlation, it is unwise to forecast high intelligence in an individual case. What is appropriate where milestones are either delayed or advanced, is to say where the child's development is in relation to average children of that age and then help the parents with techniques of responding appropriately to the child's developmental age.

Unless the developmental examination is markedly abnormal, it is important to be cautious in diagnosing abnormalities, as there is a wide variation in the attainment of milestones. The intellectually handicapped baby or infant will usually be behind in all areas of development. Occasionally sitting and walking may not be as far behind as other areas, but the delay is usually global and would be most marked in general understanding and language. If the developmental examination raises concerns it should be repeated later if not initially done under optimal conditions. Other appropriate investigations should be performed and the child should be referred for another opinion. To avoid undue anxiety in many cases it may be better to repeat the developmental assessment, do appropriate investigations and seek another opinion before telling the parents that you think the child is 'backward'. Although developmental assessment may look simple, it is a relatively difficult skill to acquire, but one which can be mastered with practise and which is rewarding to perform.

REFERENCES

Holt K S 1977 Developmental paediatrics, Butterworth, London

Sheridan M D 1968 The developmental progress of infants and young children, 2nd edn. Her Majesty's Stationery Office, London

World Health Organization 1967 The early detection and treatment of handicapping defects in young children. Report on a working party convened by the Regional Office for Europe and WHO (Chairman: Kershaw J D) WHO, Copenhagen

research project. Salisbury College of Advanced Education, South Australia

Egan D F, Illingworth R S, MacKeith R C 1969 Developmental screening 0–5 years. Clinics in Developmental Medicine No. 30. Spastics International Medical Publications, London

Frankenburg W K, Fandal A W, Sciarillo W, Burgess D 1981 The newly abbreviated and revised Denver Developmental Screening Test. Journal of Pediatrics 99: 995–999

Illingworth R S 1987 The development of the infant and young child, 9th edn. Churchill Livingstone, Edinburgh

FURTHER READING

Burdon B F, Teasdale G R 1978 The developmental record

Social and preventive paediatrics

12. The child and the family

M. J. Robinson

THE NEEDS OF THE CHILD AND THE FAMILY

A healthy child is one who is physically fit, emotionally stable and socially well adjusted. There is good evidence that the first years of life are vital in establishing later physical and emotional well-being and the ultimate potential for intellectual development. For these to occur a loving, secure and stimulating family environment is of the greatest importance. Many workers have documented the ill-effects of emotional deprivation through parental separation on the subsequent emotional and intellectual development of the child.

The physical needs of the child

The child's physical needs are basically met by:

1. The provision of an adequate diet to provide for nutritional needs.
2. Protection against heat and cold in early life and later against various physical dangers, e.g. fire, electricity, poisons, water, motor cars, etc.
3. Prevention of illness through satisfactory living conditions, health surveillance, immunization and certain public health measures.

Parents learn to provide for the physical needs of their children from their own parents, from doctors, child health nurses and, at times, through the media.

The emotional and social needs of the child

Of equal importance in child development is the need for children to have the opportunity for proper emotional experience and the facilities for intellectual development. In order to develop emotionally and socially, children have the following needs:

1. The opportunity of growing up in a family unit where the child is in the care of responsible adults whose primary care is the well-being of their children. In such a family, the formation of strong bonds between parents and child, commencing from the time of birth, provide the basis for a good relationship to continue throughout childhood and adolescence. Ideally the child should be the result of a planned and wanted pregnancy.
2. In cases where a family is unable to care for their child the provision of a substitute family should be made.
3. The experience of consistent parenting which allows the child to experience and express angry as well as loving feelings appropriately, rather than acting these out in an antisocial manner.
4. Reasonable limits should be set on the child's behaviour which allows for the development of inner controls.
5. Feeling of being worthwhile, which will be accompanied by a capacity for concern for the well-being of others.
6. The development of self-help skills and sense of achievement.
7. Opportunities for companionship and recreation.
8. Educational facilities appropriate to the child's particular needs.
9. Good physical health and sensitive handling of emotional needs during ill health – particularly in chronic or disabling illness.
10. Recognition of each child's individuality including personality differences and differences in physical, intellectual and ethnic attributes.
11. The recognition of the basic rights of every child as outlined by the United Nations' Declaration of the Rights of the Child.

To meet these needs for their children, parents and others who care for them also have needs of their own. These would include adequate housing in an area allowing for acceptable social ties to be established. There should be freedom from undue economic stress. Correctly sited and organized child-care social and educational facilities are of importance, as is access to and an understanding of how to better use the state health and welfare services and the voluntary agencies. Also, parents should understand through education, beginning at school and continuing through the health and welfare services, the rudiments of child development and behaviour.

The needs for proper intellectual development

The stimulus for intellectual development in a family situation is initially on a one-to-one basis with the adult (usually the mother) obtaining and sharing pleasure from the child's reaction to stimuli. The child is thus rewarded so that learning becomes a pleasurable experience. Thereafter, adequate sensory stimulation must continue if young children are to develop cognitive and problem-solving abilities.

Clearly the amount, the intensity, the variety and the complexity of the input stimuli will vary according to the age, but also to the personality of the child. Hence, the adult who cares for the child will need to be aware of this and treat each child individually. In the happy and well-adjusted family, this provides no problem as it appears to occur quite naturally.

As time goes on, a one-to-one parent-child relationship is inadequate, so, shortly after the age of 2 years, the child seeks the company of children of a similar age and play forms a most important part of the learning process. Play may be defined as that endeavour in which young children learn to exercise their physical and cognitive resources successfully with the material world and with other people, both children and adults. Such activity initially tends to occur with neighbours, but thereafter it may be more organized into play groups followed by organized preschool training until the formal education setting of school commences at about the fifth year.

Risks to the child's proper development

In the current era, many Australian, and indeed many other Western families, are unable completely to provide for the physical, emotional and intellectual needs of the child. This applies particularly to socialization of young children. There are a number of reasons for this.

1. Socioeconomic and newer cultural trends have led to the break-up of the expanded family leaving in its place the nuclear group. Here the mother and father can no longer count on the support of grandparents, maiden aunts, servants, etc., to provide additional care and stimulation for their children.

2. The family stability has been further threatened by increasing parental separation and a rising divorce rate – the latter reaching approximately 1 in 3 of current Australian marriages.

3. Differing attitudes to marriage have resulted in an increasing number of de facto relationships and, consequently, even easier separation. There is now a greater number of single parent families than ever before, as single mothers now tend to keep their babies rather than have them adopted. Society no longer frowns on this practice, rather it is condoned, if not actively encouraged.

4. The present generation of mothers no longer see themselves as purely housewives. Increasing educational opportunity has provided them with the skills necessary for job opportunity and establishing careers. Many of these young women are loathe to relinquish these skills and the social contacts at work, not only at the time of marriage, but also with the birth of children.

5. Increasing costs of living and a desire on the part of both parents to improve living standards (at least in the materialistic sense) add to the number of families where both parents are employed outside the home.

6. Efficient birth control techniques have resulted in a decreased span of adult life occupied with child rearing, and thus smaller families. A greatly reduced infant mortality has also allowed for optimism in family planning.

7. There are also groups of families within the community where special problems arise. Among these are:

a. Migrant families, Aboriginal families, children of families living in areas remote from towns and cities, single parent families and children with handicapping conditions. The latter would include those physically disabled and others with visual, hearing and with intellectual disability. These children have special needs which cannot always be met in the average family.

b. Housing has drastically changed in the last generation. Many families in the larger cities now live in high-rise flats where provision for play and other social activities are often inadequate.

c. Some families have problems because of inadequate material resources (poverty) while other families cannot cope because of a lack of adequate emotional and intellectual strengths, e.g. the emotionally immature, the intellectually dull and the psychiatrically sick.

MODERN SOCIETY'S RESPONSIBILITY TO MEET THESE NEEDS

Thus, it is recognized that many families do not have the resources to meet the total needs of young children so that additional facilities are necessary if these families are to stay together. Modern societies have had to develop systems of social, educational and medical assistance whereby parents are able to obtain additional help in bringing up their children. The needs of these individuals and groups have been recognized, partly from official statistics and partly from investigations prompted by aware and caring individuals. At times public interest and concern may be increased from media reports (newspaper, radio and television), or through the concentration of groups on particular problems. These groups have tended to comprise parents of handicapped children, such as the cerebral palsied, the blind, deaf, and intellectually handicapped. In addition to these, facilities are now being established to assist in the care of and encourage research into certain minority groups, such as cystic fibrosis, muscular dystrophy and haemophilia. The State has gradually accepted responsibility in this area on advice from expert committees and now provides funds and personnel, either wholly, or in conjunction with the particular voluntary bodies. For these services to succeed, there must be skill, enthusiasm and drive in the personnel serving them and that such personnel are acceptable to the families they serve. These services must also be used by the people with the greatest needs. Unfortunately this is not always the case, as too often the services are best used by the child of well-informed, middle-class parents and least by the socially disadvantaged, either because the parents do not know about them, or do not care. This is referred to as the Law of Inverse Care.

COMMUNITY HEALTH FACILITIES AVAILABLE TO ALL FAMILIES

These can be considered in the following categories:

1. Primary health services
2. Social services
3. Services concerned with the help to handicapped children and their families, and to certain other minority groups, e.g. migrants and Aboriginals (see Chs 17–19).

Primary health services

Infant welfare clinics

In Australia, these are conducted under the auspices of municipal councils assisted by State Government grants. A mobile service is provided by the Department of Health to provide for sparsely populated areas. Also the Department supplies an infant welfare correspondence service for those who cannot use the regular service. Infant welfare clinics are sited to be within easy reach of

parents and at present are staffed by a trained nurse with postgraduate qualifications in maternal and child health and welfare. All births in each area are notified to the sister who makes contact with the family soon after the mother arrives home from hospital. Thereafter, mothers attend the clinic at intervals of one, two or four weeks, according to the specific needs of the child and family. For example, the young mother with a premature or first infant may attend weekly whereas the experienced mother with a normal term infant may attend once each month. The aims of the infant welfare clinics are:

1. Health supervision of infants and small children up to the age of approximately five years. In respect to infant feeding, the importance of breast-feeding is stressed, but, if for any reason artificial feeding is chosen, the nurse will advise on the technique and preparation of formulae. Later advice on the introduction of solid feeding will be given.
2. Regular follow-up of all infants is made to assess physical growth in terms of length and weight. Any infant who fails to conform to normal standards is referred to the family medical practitioner or to a hospital paediatric department.
3. Regular follow-up to assess the developmental status of each infant is made. Any infant demonstrating developmental delay will be referred for further opinion.
4. To advise and assist with immunization against tetanus, diphtheria, pertussis, poliomyelitis, measles and mumps according to government health requirements.
5. To advise on minor illnesses and to refer to the family practitioner or local hospital any infant in need of medical care.
6. To arrange health educational activities with groups of parents through discussions and lectures; home visiting when necessary.

Infant welfare clinics are free and are very popular amongst all socioeconomic groups, there being a 90% enrolment rate. However, the rate of attendance falls off rapidly after the first year.

Community health centres

This comparatively new facility was developed about 12 years ago because it has become increasingly obvious that present day health problems must be tackled outside hospitals and within the community if effective and economic solutions are to be found. It is also clear that the general practitioner – the major provider of health care in the community – cannot totally carry the supportive and preventive role in medicine so essential to this era. Additional resources and personnel such as teachers, health educators, nurses, physiotherapists, social workers, psychologists and counsellors are needed to help people avoid unnecessary illness and accidents and to help them live more comfortably with any illness or handicap. This is the philosophy behind the initiation of community health programmes.

The main aims of the community health programme are to provide comprehensive health care services to the community and should include components of health education, disease prevention, primary medical care, supportive care, rehabilitation and referral where appropriate.

This service has the potential for meeting the needs of many families, particularly those in the lower socioeconomic groups. In the first instance, the centre can provide primary medical care for parents and children at low cost. In addition, advice and support are available from trained personnel in such areas as family planning, mothercraft, health education, house keeping and budgeting and for the family with matrimonial problems. Facilities for marriage counselling are also available. The availability of community health nurses and social workers to go into the homes of families with problems represents a real advance in health care. Also, the centre is available to provide support and help in obtaining the various community resources, such as disabled children's allowance, child endowment, pensions and other social service benefits. This service should be particularly beneficial to such groups as new migrant families and for single parent families. The needs of handicapped children, be they intellectual, physical or psychological, should also be more efficiently provided for from such a centre. It is not known how successful these centres have been. Also, it is still not known whether this service provides help for groups who need it most. Until this information is obtained it will not be possible to make a proper evaluation of the community health.

The school medical service

The States provide through their Departments of Health a medical service to all children attending government schools. Basically, this service aims to ensure that there are no health problems in the child that are likely to impair school performance. However, it has become apparent both in this country and elsewhere that routine physical examinations of children after infancy are rarely productive in finding undiagnosed physical disorders or malformations. The exception to this is disorders of vision and hearing. Therefore, it is likely that in the future routine physical examinations of preschool and early school children will be abandoned and replaced by regular testing of vision and hearing by school health nurses. Should a parent or teacher be concerned about the physical health of a small child, the school health nurse will be able to examine the child and refer the child to a medical officer of the School Medical Service, or should the parent prefer it, to a local medical practitioner or paediatric hospital. Obvious disorders of vision and hearing will usually be referred directly to the appropriate consultant of the Health Department. It is anticipated that in the future school medical officers will play an increasing role in the assessment of children with learning problems.

Dental health

The dental health service aims to provide free dental service for all primary and preschool children, but this is not yet possible. The service itself may involve restoration, extractions, cleaning, minor orthodontic measures and advice to parents where major orthodontic problems exist. Dental health education is a most important aspect of the service. The dental health service is also engaged in the treatment of children in institutions, including those for the physically and intellectually handicapped.

Social services

Preschool training (kindergartens)

Preschool education centres cater for children between the ages of three and five or school entry. Preschool education is sponsored both by Government and private groups. Attendance is not compulsory, but is almost the rule. However, it appears that some children for various reasons need preschool education but do not receive it. Particularly this applies to poor socioeconomic multiethnic municipalities where the attendance at kindergartens averages about 50% of those eligible.

At preschool centres children receive a planned educational programme under the direction of a trained teacher. While activities are supervised they are not structured, so the children may choose and move from one activity to the next as they wish. The preschool environment thus allows the child to meet, play and share with peers. Form, colour, drawing, painting and certain cognitive and physical skills are developed in this environment. By the end of the preschool year most children are able to concentrate on a task for a sufficient time that formal class-room teaching in schools will follow naturally. The children usually attend for half a day from two to five times weekly. Where both parents work, and for other family problems, the programmes may be extended to the whole day when the child also receives a midday meal and a supervised rest period. Kindergartens are managed by parent committees.

Toddler groups

There is a body of opinion that favours child groups even before the preschool year so that toddler groups have evolved. While there is no real evidence to suggest that these activities influence ultimate educational performance, they do at least enrich the life of the young mother who, of necessity, meets other mothers with children of similar ages. Consequently, these mothers feel less isolated, they make friendships and enhance their knowledge and skills. Playgroups and toddler groups are designed to cater for children up to the age of about three years. The parent attends with the child, who is provided with a wide range of stimulating activities appropriate to the age level. In addition, there is the opportunity to interact with other children and a limited number of adults. These groups are still not generally available to the community and most are privately organized but standards vary considerably. Again, it is unfortunate that such groups are not readily available to the particular families where the need is greatest. Toddler groups are particularly valuable to parents with handicapped children, for migrant and minority ethnic groups and for isolated units.

Child care groups

There are many of these, some conducted as private business ventures and some managed by parents. Despite the fact that registration is necessary, the standard of these centres varies considerably.

Baby sitting groups

Some families who know and trust each other make reciprocal baby sitting arrangements without involving payment of money. In this way the children become familiar with the sitters and the parents are given some relief from total care. Some parents, for example, single

parents, parents without transport and others financially disadvantaged may be unable to take part in such reciprocal arrangements, but they need this type of service even more and at a price they can afford. Some local Government agencies have been able to provide such a service, but in this country it is at present far from the rule.

Family day care

It is now well recognized that many families have difficulty in coping with the demands of bringing up children without outside help. This is more frequent where there is maternal depression, in marriage breakdown and with recent migrants. In addition, the community's perception of the mother role is changing, so that she is no longer expected to stay at home full time to care for her family. Family day care is a facility which has been evolved to provide care for children (0–12 years) in the private homes of women who are selected by trained personnel to work as care givers. The benefits of this service are not only for the young mother; the care giver also obtains much satisfaction. Many are women in their late forties or early fifties who have brought up a family but are still active, enthusiastic and possess parenting skills which the community should be able to use. Family day care is largely sponsored by municipal governments, but recipient families may pay a small fee if they are able. The care giver receives a small wage for her services. Family day care has been very successful in a number of European countries and is beginning to meet an increasing need in Australia.

FURTHER READING

Annual Report 1982–83 Institute of Family Studies, Commonwealth of Australia
Klaus M, Kennel J 1976 Maternal-infant bonding. Mosby, St Louis
Picton C, Boss P 1981 Child welfare in Australia. An introduction. Harcourt Brace Jovanovich Group (Australia)
Rutter M 1979 Maternal deprivation. Child Development 50: 283–305

13. Nutrition

John Boulton

Nutrition has a special place in child health because of the central role of food in growth and development, in the management of many childhood diseases, and in the aetiology of disorders common in later life. Food and eating have a central place in family life, and in the expression of parental love and care. A child's health is also intimately linked to the social conditions and health attitudes of the family and the available food supply. Everyone is interested in food so it is important to have a clear understanding of the science underpinning nutrition that one may be an informed counsellor for concerned parents, and an advocate in community health education.

WHAT ARE NUTRIENTS?

Nutrients provide energy, essential minerals, vitamins, and fibre. The energy from food comes from the macronutrients protein, fat, and carbohydrate (CHO) and also alcohol. Food energy is expressed in kilojoules (kJ) or kilocalories (kcal) – 1 kcal = 4.182 kJ. The amount of energy per gram of nutrient is described by the Atwater factors (Table 13.1).

Table 13.1 Atwater factors for the macronutrients

Macronutrients	kcal	kJ
Protein	4	17
Fat	9	37
CHO	3.8	16
Alcohol	7	29

The energy of our usual diet is made up from 15% protein, 35–40% fat, and 45–50% CHO. The proportion of polyunsaturated to saturated fat is expressed as the P:S ratio. The current recommendations are for protein 12–15%, fat 30%, carbohydrate 50–55%, and the P:S ratio 0.5 to 1. The source of the fat dictates its chemical composition in terms of fatty acid chain length and degree of saturation, which in turn predicates its biological effects. Carbohydrate comprises starch (complex CHO) and sugars (e.g. lactose in milk). Both are naturally occurring and are released in the gut by hydrolysis.

The term micronutrient is used to describe dietary components which are not metabolized for energy and present in milligram amounts or less. They comprise essential minerals and vitamins.

The amount of nutrients needed depends on age, size, and individual variations. Recommended Dietary Intakes (RDIs) originated as public health strategy when there was a need for clear guidelines for adequate food provision. The RDI for a nutrient is that which will provide an adequate intake for 95% of the population. The RDI says nothing about an individual's needs because these vary so widely. The RDIs for Australia have been reviewed, and those for selected nutrients are summarized as they provide levels for essential nutrients (Table 13.2). Normal values for the intake of nutrients for healthy children have been included. Table 13.3 shows the daily energy intake and how it is used during infancy.

The dietary history

Usually, parents are pleased to relate details of their child's diet and use this opportunity to express their various concerns, for example, about how little their toddler eats, how little their obese child eats, or how well they are looking after a child by giving healthy food. Keeping a structure to questions allows a brief synopsis of each typical meal through the day to be recorded in sequence so that an overall estimate can be made of food energy intake from solids and milk and other fluids. Start off by asking about breakfast, and for an infant, is a bottle taken before that? Ask specifically about the amount of milk on cereal, in the cup or bottle, and how it is made up. Go on to enquire about the next meal, but do not forget the morning snack, again asking

Table 13.2 Recommended Dietary Intakes (RDIs) in childhood for energy, protein, and various micronutrients by age group (years)

	1–3	4–7	8–11	12–15	16–18
kJ	5400	7200	b 9200 g 8000	b 12 200 g 10 400	b 12 600 g 9200
Protein (g)	20–39	25–71	36–66	b 51–87 g 52–75	b 67–90 g 60–66
Micronutrients					
Calcium (mg)	800	800	b 800 g 900	b 1200 g 1000	b 1000 g 800
Iron (mg)	6–8	6–8	6–8	10–13	10–13
Zinc (mg)	4.5–6	6–9	9–14	b 12–18 g 12–16	b 12–18 g 12–16
Sodium (mg)	320–1150	460–1730	600–2300	920–2300	920–2300
Sodium (mmol)	14–50	20–75	26–100	40–100	40–100
Potassium (mg)	980–2730	1560–3900	1950–5460	1950– 5460	1950–5460
Potassium (mmol)	25–70	40–100	50–140	50–140	50–140
Thiamine (mmol)	0.5	0.7	b 0.9 g 0.8	b 1.2 g 1.0	b 1.2 g 0.9
Riboflavin (mg)	0.8	1.1	b 1.4 g 1.3	b 1.8 g 1.6	b 1.9 g 1.4
Niacin (mg)	9–10	11–13	14–16	b 19–21 g 17–19	b 20–22 g 15–17
Vit B6 (mg)	0.6–0.9	0.8–1.3	b 1.1–1.6 g 1.0–1.5	b 1.4–2.1 g 1.2–1.8	b 1.5–2.2 g 1.1–1.6
Vit B12 (mg)	1.0	1.5	1.5	2.0	2.0
Vit C (mg)	30	30	30	b 30 g 30	b 40 g 30
Vit A retinol activity (mg)	300	350	500	725	750
Vit D	10				
Total folic acid (mg)	100	100	150	200	200

Table 13.3 The daily intake and expenditure of energy (kcal/kg) during infancy

Age	Intake	Expenditure		Thermogenesis
(months)		Basal Metab.	Increase in mass	(Activity energy cost of growth)
0–2	126	48	33	45
2–3	116	48	18	50
3–4	106	48	18	40
4–5	100	48	7	45
5–12	100	48	4	48

about amounts of food, the type of spread on biscuits and bread, as well as drinks. These questions need to be repeated for the day. The information may need to be collected in collaboration with a dietitian who will then be able to provide the parents with more detailed advice about the child's diet.

Dietary intake in healthy children

Food intake requirements increase with age, but there is a wide individual variation in food energy intake. Al-though this is accepted as everyday knowledge for adults, it is less readily recognized for infants and tod-dlers and is a common source of parental anxiety. The main reasons for this variation are heritable differences in the efficiency of energy use, and habitual or cus-tomary food intake. This in turn relates to the child's appetite setting, which is influenced by both central (hypothalamic) regulation and habits. The concept of the efficiency of food energy use is helpful in under-standing how children of similar sizes can grow normally when having different energy intakes. This supposed ex-planation comes from the presence of futile metabolic cycles (pathways) in which energy is generated and dis-sipated as heat as substrate A forms product B, and is reconverted to A using a different enzymatic action.

The most sensitive indicator of the adequacy of food energy intake is the child's growth rate. The intake can also be related to the international reference values of World Health Organization (WHO). Formulae for ener-gy intake of infants and children which have been derived from the mean value for a population from mul-tinational studies are also available.

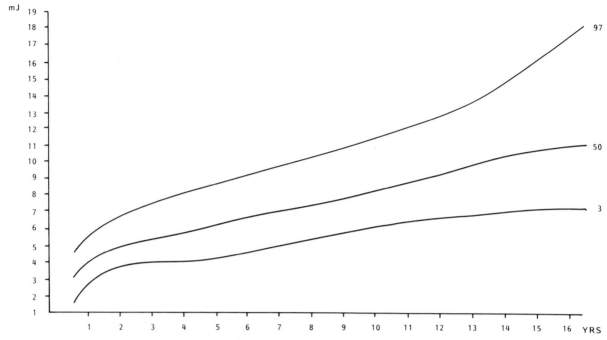

Fig. 13.1   Daily food energy intake: boys 6 months to 16.5 years.

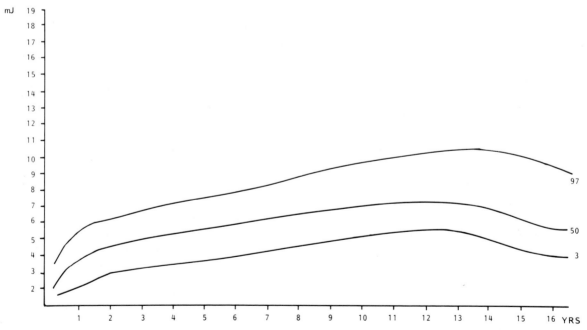

Fig. 13.2   Daily food energy intake: girls 6 months to 16.5 years.

An alternative method is to express the observed intake as a percentile, based on normative Australian data (Figs 13.1 and 13.2).

Food in the maintenance of health

The Commonwealth Department of Health has issued dietary guidelines for Australians to assist people make informed decisions about selecting a nutritious diet and help reduce the misinformation in the community about food and nutrition. Primary health care workers have an important role in individual and community education about nutrition and health. The eight dietary guidelines to improve the health of Australians comprise:

1. To promote breast-feeding
2. To choose a nutritious diet from a variety of foods
3. To control your weight
4. To avoid eating too much fat
5. To avoid eating too much sugar
6. To eat more bread and cereals (preferably whole grain and vegetables and fruit)
7. To limit alcohol consumption
8. To use less salt.

Food at different ages

For babies food comes as milk. Parents expect doctors and nurses to be able to give them help and advice about their anxieties and problems over their baby's feeding. Anxiety about 'good enough' and amount are commonplace. A mother needs to feel that the person to whom she turns for advice understands her feelings, empathizes with her, takes her concerns seriously, and is able to provide sympathetic support and encouragement. This aspect needs emphasis because parents are unlikely to be confident about advice, however appropriate, from someone who appears either to disregard their anxiety, or lack warmth towards their precious baby. The most commonplace anxieties include 'Is my milk good enough' (with the implication of being of not sufficient quality), and 'Is my baby getting enough milk'.

Babies in the newborn period and for the first 4 to 6 months can obtain all their nutritional needs from breast milk.

During the second half of infancy additional energy is needed in the form of solid food. This is also called transitional food or beikost. Fortunately, the human infant is extremely resilient to a wide variety of feeding practices which are based on fashion, culture, religion, economic and food-availability factors. Extremes of accepted practice, for example, solely breast-feeding past 18 months, or trying to give lumpy hard food before the baby can chew, may come to medical attention and gentle tact may be needed to persuade the parents that their use of food is not necessarily the best way.

Breast-feeding

Two generations ago about half of mothers breast-fed their infants fully until the age of 3 months. About 20 years ago this figure had fallen to 20%, but soon afterwards the rate increased. The present incidence of breast-feeding in Australia is over 80% on discharge from hospital, 70% at 6 weeks, 55% at 3 months, 40% at 6 months and 10% at 12 months.

Most women make the decision to breast-feed or not during pregnancy. This decision is based on an interaction on the couple's knowledge about infant feeding with perceptions from current fashion together with family and peer influences. Any event which interferes with the perinatal course, such as the baby being born by caesarian section, needing oxygen, phototherapy, or antibiotics, is likely to adversely affect the chance of the mother breast-feeding. There are many other reasons why mothers do not wish to breast-feed. Some find it technically difficult, saying that the milk comes too quickly or too slowly and that they have difficulty with attaching the infant to the nipple. Others find that breast-feeding is painful; that they worry because they do not know just how much milk their infant is taking; that their breasts will become too large; and that breast-feeding will cause them to gain weight. Others will say that they had trouble when they fed their last baby, or that they had cracked nipples or a breast abscess. Some wish to go back to work as soon as possible and will find breast-feeding inconvenient. These reasons may not seem valid from a medical viewpoint, and reflect perceptions which are not easily altered after the baby is born.

On a population basis sociodemographic factors correlate most strongly with the prevalence and duration of breast-feeding, as well as the type of milk used by the mother during weaning. A high proportion of mothers of high educational status breast-feed and for longer than those of lower status. Breast-feeding is often stopped in response to a minor setback, for example, the baby cannot suck because of a cold, or because the planned time for breast-feeding has been achieved. It is important that breast-feeding be promoted during pregnancy by doctors and other health professionals. Mothers should be properly instructed in the technique of breast-feeding on the birth of their baby. Educational programmes should be initiated and designed to inform the community of the advantages of breast-feeding and school children as well as fathers must be included in these programmes.

Breasts are prepared for lactation during pregnancy by human placental lactogen (somatomammotropin) secreted by the placenta. They are stimulated to lactation by prolactin secreted by the anterior pituitary. Sucking and skin stimulation is very important in milk production. Sucking initiates the release of oxytocin from the posterior pituitary which causes contraction of the muscular elements of the ducts and thus expulsion of the milk. The daily amount of milk produced is related proportionately to the frequency and total duration of suckling.

Technique of breast-feeding. The newborn should be put to the breast within 4 hours of birth and thereafter on demand, or at approximately 4-hourly intervals. After a few weeks most infants will settle into a routine of feeding 3- to 4-hourly through the daytime and having a long period of some 8 hours during the night when feeding is unnecessary. Adequate volumes of milk are not established until about the third day. During feeding, one breast should be totally emptied and the infant put to the other breast and allowed to feed until satisfied. The majority of stored milk is taken by the baby in the first 4 minutes. At the next feeding the breast last used at the previous feeding will be the one first used. Once breast-feeding is established a satisfactory situation results with the mother-infant dyad of a thriving and contented baby and a happy relaxed mother.

Properties of breast milk. What is there in breast milk that makes it so unique and suitable for the infant? The protein content with a range around 1% appears low compared to the 3% in cow's milk, but it includes a considerable amount of secretory IgA, lactoferrin, peroxidases, and lysozyme. These proteins are partially resistant to digestion and protect the infant from infections, IgA forming a barrier in the gut against invading bacteria, lactoferrin by depriving bacteria of their iron, lysozyme and peroxidases by their antibacterial action.

The carbohydrate of breast milk is lactose 7%, as in the milk from other mammals with the exception of marsupials. The fat content varies from being low in the beginning of a meal, then increasing towards the end of the feed with an average of 3%. The change in fat content may be important in the development of appetite control. The fatty acid content of milk reflects the diet of the mother and usually has an adequate amount of the essential unsaturated fatty acids linoleic and linolenic acid. If the mother is on low fat diet breast milk fat comprises mainly lauric acid.

Colostrum is the breast milk secreted in the first week. It is especially high in protein from immunoglobulins and has a high concentration of lymphocytes. Therefore, it is advantageous for the baby to get this product. There are mothers who are unable or unwilling to breast-feed their babies. If possible, try and persuade them to put the baby to the breast for the first week of life before changing to artificial feeding.

There are many artificial milk formulae on the market. The humanized formulae attempt to imitate breast milk as much as possible in terms of the concentration and chemical characteristics of the protein and fat. A comparison is shown in Table 13.4 between breast milk, cow's milk, modified cow's milk and humanized formulae. The latter have a reduced casein and a casein-lactalbumin ratio that mimics human milk. The profile of fatty acids is altered with an increase in unsaturates mainly from the inclusion of linoleic acid (C18:2) which comprises 10–12% of the fatty acids in human milk. However, none can supply the secretory IgA, specific for breast milk.

The infant requires about 150 ml/kg/day after the age of 5–days. This volume is divided into individual feedings, 5–6 per day during the first months, 4 or 5 after 3–6 months. The volume and number of meals should be adjusted according to the infant's appetite and growth rate. It is of importance, especially in a hot climate, to observe hygienic rules; use only clean utensils and safe water (preferably boiled).

Table 13.4   Energy (kJ) and nutrient content (gm/dl) of milk

	Breast milk		Formulae				Cow's
	Colostrum	Mature	NAN	S26	SMA	Lactogen	Milk
Energy	215	280	280	280	280	268	285
Protein	2.3	1.2	1.7	1.5	1.5	1.9	3.5
Lactalbumin/casein	80/40	60/40	60/40	60/40	18/82	18/82	18/82
Fat	2.3	4.2	3.6	3.6	3.6	3.1	3.7
Lactose	5.7	7.0	7.7	7.2	7.2	7.1	4.8
Na mmol/l	48	7	7.8	6.5	7.0	12	22
K mmol/l	74	13	21.4	16	14	24	35
Calcium mg/l	300	340	450	444	445	670	1170
Phosphorus mg/l	150	140	310	330	330	520	920

Weaning and transitional foods

Food is needed after 6 months of age in addition to milk to satisfy the increasing energy demands of the infant. By 1 year a 10 kg child who needs 3800 kJ (900 kcal) for maintenance and growth would have that provided by 1300 ml milk; this would supply over 30 gm protein (over 3 gm/kg). By comparison 700 ml milk would provide just over 20 gm of protein and 2050 kJ (490 kcal) with the remaining 1715 kJ (410 kcal) coming from either 103 gm of CHO, or 50 gm CHO and 23 gm fat.

The introduction of solid feedings initiates a decrease in breast milk production through a reduction in the secretion of prolactin from diminished suckling time. It can be a difficult time requiring patience and understanding on the part of the mother, as many infants do not immediately like the new flavours and thicker foods. Therefore, an anxious mother can easily become frustrated so that feeding becomes a problem. At this time milk is still the most important constituent of the diet and all infants from 6–12 months need 600 ml of milk each day to provide an adequate protein and kJ intake. Orange juice is best introduced at about 3 months of age as this will ensure an adequate intake of vitamin C by 6 months. Initially, it requires dilution with boiled water but should never be heated. The introduction of foods into the diet accustoms the infant to new tastes and consistencies. Also, it encourages chewing and allows the infant to cope with spoon feeding and drinking from a cup. The time that chewing occurs varies from infant to infant. Transitional food should not be started before the age of about 4 months, as the infant is unable to carry them to the back of the mouth with the tongue and to swallow. If spoon feeding is attempted before this the infant reflexly protrudes the tongue and spits out the food. Therefore, the timing of the introduction of foods which require chewing is predicated by the developmental maturity of the baby. At about the age of 6 months most are making chewing movements so that lumpy foods can be accommodated. The ability to chew starts from 8 to 10 months and food given before then has to be sufficiently fluid to be swallowed whole, or finger food which can be chewed.

Commercially prepared cereals are convenient and, being iron enriched, they make a worthwhile contribution at a time when the infant's iron stores are diminishing. Initially these are made up with milk to a consistency just thicker than ordinary milk. The amount and consistency of the cereal is increased as the infant matures, and mixed foods are then added. These include various stewed fruits such as apple, pear and mashed ripe banana; at another meal finely mashed vegetables such as potato, pumpkin, marrow, mashed peas. Soft meat such as chicken and fish can then be introduced.

After 7 months the yolk of a well-boiled egg can be tried and if this is tolerated the white of the egg may be introduced. By 8 months the baby is ready to cope with foods of a courser texture, even if the front teeth have not erupted, as the gums are sufficiently strong to bite and chew these foods. This helps to promote the eruptions of strong healthy teeth and jaw development.

As solids and chewing foods are introduced at the appropriate times, breast-feeding is discontinued slowly, one feed at a time. Under these circumstances lactation will gradually fail and there will be a smooth transition to a full diet. At 8 months an eating pattern of 3 meals a day should be emerging and, if bottle fed, training to cup feeding may be initiated. By 12 months of age, the baby should be eating the same foods as the rest of the family excluding highly seasoned or tough foods, rich foods and very sweet foods.

Diseases caused by specific deficiencies of micronutrients

For details of these conditions the reader is referred to one of the listed textbooks of nutrition. Specific nutritional deficiencies of essential minerals and vitamins are uncommon in Australia, although children with disorders of absorption from the small bowel are at risk, as are pre-term neonates. It is important to have a global perspective on the significance of such nutritional deficiencies because they contribute to an enormous load of morbidity. For example, a quarter of a million children are blinded each year by xerophthalmia brought on by severe *vitamin A deficiency*. In population based UNICEF studies in Indonesia vitamin A deficiency was found to relate causally to early childhood mortality as well as the incidence of diarrhoeal and respiratory disease, particularly in children less than 3 years of age. In developing countries vitamin deficiencies are usually multiple, and the physical signs seen are due to a combination of deficiency of the vitamins A and B group.

This aspect of malnutrition sadly reflects the child's status in situations of political and social disadvantage. In this country those most at risk are the socially disadvantaged fringe dwellers of cities and country towns, particularly those with an Aboriginal background.

Vitamin C deficiency is the cause of scurvy. Infants who are fed cow's milk formulae without supplementary vitamin C and who are not offered citrus fruits and vegetables are at risk. Ascorbic acid deficiency results in defective and deficient collagen formation and a haemorrhagic tendency. The presentation is usually at about the age of 4 to 5 months with gross pallor and irritability. Infants with scurvy lie immobile on their back, as any movement causes severe pain from subperiosteal haemorrhages. Bruising and petechiae, sponginess and bleeding from the gums, if teeth have erupted, and a 'rickety rosary' the result of epiphyseal subluxation at the costochrondral junctions are common findings. Occasionally proptosis due to retro-orbital haemorrhages is seen. The diagnosis is readily made from radiology of the long bones which demonstrates a 'ground glass' appearance of the shaft, thinning of the cortex and dense white line at the metaphyses. Also, the epiphyseal centres have a ground glass appearance and are sharply outlined in the 'egg shell' sign. During healing, calcification of subperiosteal haemorrhages may occur. Treatment with oral vitamin C (200 mg of ascorbic acid daily) results in symptomatic cure within a week.

Vitamin D deficiency: nutritional rickets – this is described in Chapter 58.

Iron deficiency anaemia. This has been covered in Chapter 42.

PROBLEMS OF OVER AND UNDER NUTRITION

Obesity

Obesity is common. The ideal body shape is determined by society and the available food supply, and over the past four or five decades the ideal shape has changed towards thinness. This image is encouraged by the known associations between obesity in adults and the risk of hypertension, type 2 diabetes, higher levels of plasma lipids, osteoarthritis from bone and joint overuse, as well as adverse cosmetic considerations. In our society people who are obese are discriminated against in many subtle ways. This applies to children who often suffer teasing at school, as well as adolescents who have a statistically lower chance of academic success and of further education.

Obesity is a clinical diagnosis: the child looks too fat (Fig. 13.3). It can be defined more precisely in the following ways: over 20% of the expected mass for height; having a skinfold thickness (e.g. measured at the triceps at the mid upper arm) over the 90th percentile. Estimates of obesity prevalence vary up to 9.5% for teenage girls and 7% for boys. And the risk for a fat child of obesity during adult life is not known. In this country the majority of fat babies become of normal size by primary school age.

Childhood obesity is more easily understood as being of two types according to the age of onset. Infancy onset obesity starts between 4 to 6 months. There is an accelerated rate of growth for length and mass, and these

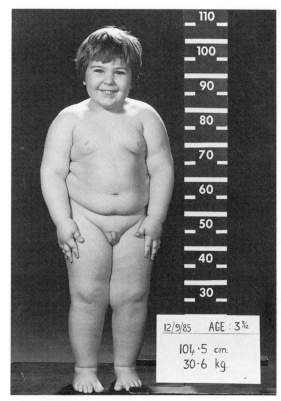

Fig. 13.3 Infancy onset obesity.

children may not look overweight for height until age 4. Their accelerated height velocity continues, they have an advanced skeletal age, and often reach puberty earlier than expected for their family. For them being fat is biologically and psychologically normal; their mass and height follow a channel parallel to the 97th line. Intervention is effective only in preschool years provided the parents are sufficiently motivated and informed.

Obesity which starts in later childhood often coincides with an emotionally traumatic event, such as a period of separation from the parents. The weight of these children fluctuates widely above the 97th percentile, whereas their height usually does not deviate from its channel. The bone age is not advanced. These children are often unhappy at school, with low self-esteem, and often they try one slimming course after another.

Management of obesity

This is very difficult in any age group so prevention is critical. Public health education directed towards eating habits and campaigns designed to promote public awareness of the risks of obesity have had limited success. Mothers should be counselled about the disadvantages of obesity at child health clinics, but some ethnic groups equate obesity in infancy with health and this folklore is very difficult to change.

Success in treatment requires a great deal of motivation from both the child and the parents. A sensible attitude to food intake is fundamental so that parents and the child should talk with an experienced dietitian about the composition of meals. A total reduction in the number of calories (kJ) taken in rather than specific food omissions is the basis of sensible weight reduction diets. Regular weighing and the charting of weights can be helpful in a well-motivated family. An enthusiastic family doctor with a good relationship with the child and family can do a great deal to improve motivation.

Exercise is more helpful than predicted from the actual energy expenditure during exercise. Walking, cycling, and skipping are good forms of exercise. It is more useful to encourage a physical activity which the child enjoys. Not only is this useful in weight reduction, but it enhances the child's self-esteem. The use of drugs to suppress appetite is not successful and their use is not recommended.

Malnutrition

On a global basis malnutrition is the major source of childhood morbidity and mortality. In 1945 world food production was insufficient to meet estimated human requirements, but at the present time over 40 years later food production is more than sufficient to feed everybody despite the vast increase in population. Therefore, malnutrition is due to social and political forces which prevent an equitable distribution of food to under-privileged people. In Africa 5 million children die from malnutrition each year, and the same number are disabled. That continent grows only half its food requirements and imports 20 million tons of grain. Poverty affected 82% of its people in 1974 but 6 years later that percentage had increased to over 90%. This has obvious implications to the plight of the world's children for whom available nutrition is less likely to meet the demands of normal metabolic functions and allow normal growth than in industrialized countries. Because children have proportionately higher nutritional requirements than adults and are less equipped to face adverse environmental conditions, they are especially susceptible to the ill-effects of under-nutrition. Malnutrition is often called protein-calorie malnutrition to highlight the importance of both inadequate total food energy intake as well as the need for adequate protein supplies for growth and development. Children growing in such an underprivileged community have slowed height growth from the second half of infancy, and have low muscle bulk and very thin subcutaneous tissue. Worsening of food supply because of further drought or war results in weight loss and failure to thrive (marasmus). Children who have a greater deficit of protein than total food energy present with kwashiorkor: they have a pot belly, muscle wasting, dependent oedema, lack lustre depigmented hair, and skin changes. These include flaking skin, which on a dark child can appear to be patchily depigmented and is often most noticeable on the face and limbs, a red sore tongue (glossitis) and cracking at the corner of the mouth (cheilosis).

Anorexia nervosa and bulimia

Anorexia nervosa is a condition in which mid to late adolescent girls (more rarely boys) pursue thinness to the degree of emaciation and sometimes death by self starvation, purging, vomiting, and continuous activity. The incidence is not accurately known, but estimated to occur to some degree in 1:250 adolescent girls. It is considered to be at the serious and opposite end of the continuum of eating disorders from bulimia. Bulimia describes the common but variably severe condition in which a cycle of binge eating is followed by remorse, sometimes vomiting, and further self-inflicted diet restriction. This occurs to some degree in several percent of women and often continues through adulthood. The aetiology of eating disorders is not known. They are further discussed in Chapter 65.

Situations and disorders where nutrition has an important place in management

Precise details of management are given in those chapters where the disorders listed below are covered. They are:

1. The preterm baby
2. Diabetes mellitus
3. Cystic fibrosis
4. Coeliac disease
5. Liver failure
6. End stage renal failure
7. Epilepsy
8. Congenital and acquired disorders of carbohydrate absorption
9. Inborn errors of metabolism.

Nutrition in the aetiology of disease

Many diseases common in later life have a long latent

period in which nutrition plays a major aetiological role. These include ischaemic heart disease, hypertension, stroke, type 2 diabetes, gall bladder disease, adenocarcinoma of the bowel, constipation and diverticulitis, dental caries and anaemia. In addition, alcohol is a most important risk factor in the development of cirrhosis of the liver. Although most of these diseases have a strong genetic influence, the nutritional environment plays a facilitatory role in their development and, therefore, offers an opportunity for primary prevention starting in childhood.

FURTHER READING

Dietary guidelines for Australians 1982 Australian Government Publishing Service, Canberra
Goldfarb J, Tibbetts E 1980 Breastfeeding handbook. Enslow Publishers, New Jersey
Jelliffe D B, Jelliffe P E F 1979 Human milk in the modern world. Oxford University Press, Oxford
McLaren D S, Burman D 1982 Textbook of paediatric nutrition. Churchill Livingstone, Melbourne
Paul A M, Southgate D A T 1978 The composition of foods. McCance and Widdowson, London HMSO
Stunkard A J (ed) 1980 Obesity. Saunders, London
Wahlqvist M L (ed) 1981 Food and nutrition in Australia. Methuen Australia, Melbourne

14. Immunization

Cliff Hosking

Whether or not a person becomes infected with a virulent microorganism depends, firstly, on the presence of the microorganism and, secondly, on the resistance of the potential host.

Great strides have been made in public health over the past 100 years aimed at preventing the population coming in contact with pathogenic microorganisms. Thus, the provision of a pathogen-free water supply has been a major force in removing microorganisms from the environment.

However, not all microorganisms are water borne. Quarantine is another means of preventing the spread of microorganisms. Australia is free of rabies due to great care being taken in the importation of live stock and other animals from countries where rabies is endemic. Yellow fever can be controlled by eliminating the mosquito *Aedes aegypti* which acts as the vector for the virus.

The incidence and severity of many infections has dropped for ill defined reasons. Between 1900 and 1950, the death rate from measles in the UK fell from about 300 to 2.0 per million population. This is probably related to higher living standards resulting in improved general health giving greater resistance to the severe effects of infection. In support of this relationship was the report of the Registrar General for Health in the UK which showed that the mortality from measles in children aged 1 year in social class 5 was about 20 times greater than those in social class 1.

However, for some diseases the microorganism cannot be readily controlled or eliminated and immunization may be the most cost-effective way of managing the problem.

IMMUNIZATION

Costs and benefits of immunization

Before a vaccine is produced and used, the following factors should be weighed against each other.

1. The disease must be of sufficient severity
2. The frequency must be sufficiently high prior to an immunization campaign
3. Immunity to infection and/or the important products of infection must be produced by immunization
4. The vaccine must be comparatively safe
5. The disease should not be readily treated or prevented by other means
6. The cost of the vaccine should be related to the economic and social disability caused by the infection.

The immunological basis for immunization

The basic hypothesis which underlies immunization is to reproduce the protective immune response that occurs after natural infection. The exception to this rule is with tetanus when natural infection with the organism or near fatal toxicity may not produce antibody to the toxin because of the small amounts involved. In this instance immunization with tetanus toxoid (chemically modified toxin) aims not to prevent infection but to neutralize any neurotoxin produced.

The original vaccine to smallpox was probably a naturally modified virus. From that time have followed live attenuated mycobacteria (BCG), killed organisms (pertussin), toxoids (diphtheria and tetanus), laboratory attenuated viruses (poliomyelitis, measles and rubella), and extracted capsular polysaccharides (pneumococcus).

Most of the vaccines became available before fine dissection of the immune system was possible. Even now the nature of the epitopes (antigenic sites) and the nature of the protective immune response (B or T cell) is not well understood for virtually all vaccines. There is considerable variability in the nature and longevity of response both between individuals and between vaccines. The classic description of a primary and a booster secondary response is to killed or toxoided antigens. On initial vaccination a rise in IgM antibody is followed at about two weeks by a fall in IgM and a rise in IgG antibody. A second dose of vaccine one month or later after the first, leads to an accelerated IgG response both in time and magnitude. The IgG antibodies persist longer after a second or subsequent dose.

Attenuated vaccines tend to produce a rise in IgM which is replaced by persisting IgG. It is still too early to say whether the antibody levels produced to measles and rubella vaccination will persist throughout the life of the vaccines.

Immunity arising from natural infection or immunization is said to be *active*. *Passive* immunity is acquired when the products of the immune response (usually antibodies) are transferred to another person. This can occur naturally as in the transfer of IgG antibodies from the mother to the fetus, or artificially during whole blood transfusion or gammaglobulin therapy.

A question that is sometimes asked is whether a vaccine is still necessary once the incidence of a disease has dropped for some time. In this instance one is not sure whether this is due to the vaccination programme or to a change in the epidemiology of the microorganism or environmental changes. The only way the question can be answered is to let the immunization rate fall and see whether this produces an increase in the disease incidence in the target group. This, in fact, happened in the 1970s in the UK where publicity of the neurotoxicity of pertussis vaccine caused many parents not to permit their children to be vaccinated. During this time the incidence of the clinical disease and its complications rose considerably. An expert committee was set up by the British Government and came to the conclusion that many of the reputed cases were not due to the vaccine and that the costs and benefits of giving pertussis vaccine outweighed the costs and benefits of not giving the vaccine.

Definitions

1. An *antigen* is a substance able to induce an immunological reaction. The usual measure of an immunological reaction is the production of specific antibody.

2. *Antibody* is the B cell or humoral immune response to an antigen. The molecule has a general structure and shape similar to other antibodies but specifically binds to the antigen which stimulated its presence.

3. *Vaccine* is the general term for an antigen given to develop immune resistance to a microorganism or its products.

4. *Toxoid* is a modified toxin, usually of bacterial origin. The toxin has been altered so that it maintains its antigenicity but is no longer toxic.

5. *Immune globulin*, immunoglobulin and gammaglobulin are synonyms for the purified extract of human plasma that contains antibodies. This is administered intramuscularly but specially modified immune globulin can be given intravenously.

6. *Specific immune globulin* is immune globulin that has been prepared from high-titre plasma. It is more effective prepared in certain circumstances than immune globulin. Specific batches are used particularly for preventing chicken pox in immunosuppressed children and following needle stick injuries with hepatitis B containing blood.

7. An *attenuated microorganism* is one which has been grown for some time in vitro in an attempt to retain infectivity and antigenicity while losing virulence. Attenuated microorganisms are generally injected live. Extensive testing in the field is required of such organism to ensure maintenance of antigenicity and failure to revert to the wild virulent strain.

8. An *antitoxin* consists of antibodies able to neutralize a toxin. They are usually produced by immunization with a toxoid – a modified toxin.

9. An *antivenom* is a preparation of antibodies normally produced in animals used for the passive treatment of envenomation by snakes or other noxious animals or insects.

10. An *adjuvant* is a substance mixed with a killed or toxoided antigen to boost the immune response. The most common adjuvants are aluminium salts.

Questions commonly asked about vaccines

If a dose of triple antigen is missed, should the course be restarted?
The answer is 'no'. While the recommended spacings should be followed if possible, even a major delay of several months makes little difference to the final antibody titre.

If a child has a cold should vaccines be given?
The vaccines should not be given to a child with a febrile illness. However, an URTI where the child is neither ill nor febrile is not a contraindication.

Should more than one vaccine be given at the one time?
This of course is done with triple antigen (pertussis, diphtheria and tetanus). Live virus and killed or toxoided vaccines should not be mixed in the one syringe but can certainly be given at different sites at the one time.

Table 14.1 Recommended childhood immunization schedule (NH & MRC)

Age	Disease	Vaccine	Route
2 months	Diphtheria-tetanus-pertussis	Triple antigen 'DTP'	Intramuscular★
	Poliomyelitis	Sabin vaccine 'OPV'	Oral
4 months	Diphtheria-tetanus-pertussis	Triple antigen'DTP'	Intramuscular★
	Poliomyelitis	Sabin vaccine 'OPV'	Oral
6 months	Diphtheria-tetanus-pertussis	Triple antigen 'DTP'	Intramuscular★
	Poliomyelitis	Sabin vaccine 'OPV'	Oral
Between 12–15 months	Measles/mumps/rubella	Measles/mumps 'MMR'	Subcutaneous
18 months	Diphtheria-tetanus-pertussis	Triple antigen 'DTP'	Intramuscular
5 years or prior to school entry	Diphtheria-tetanus	Childhood diphtheria and tetanus 'CDT'	Intramuscular★
	Poliomyelitis	Sabin vaccine 'OPV'	Oral
15 years or prior to leaving school	Diphtheria-tetanus	Adult diphtheria and tetanus 'ADT'	Intramuscular★

★ See 7. Precautions and contraindications below

Notes on the schedule:
1. *Combined vaccines* are used where possible in routine immunization of infants (diphtheria, tetanus, pertussis, [DTP or triple antigen]; measles, mumps [MM].)
2. DTP should be used for primary immunization only under the age of two years.
3. A combined diphtheria and tetanus (CDT) vaccine is used:
    (a) for primary immunization of infants where the pertussis component is contraindicated (see below). (In this situation, CDT is recommended in three doses, i.e. at *two*, *four* and *eighteen* months.);
    (b) for booster doses in children to the age of seven years;
    (c) for primary immunisation of infants who have already suffered bacteriologically confirmed pertussis.
4. A combined diphtheria and tetanus vaccine suitable for adults (ADT) is used from the age of eight years for primary immunization and for intermittent booster doses (see tetanus section). This vaccine has a lower concentration of diphtheria toxoid and causes fewer side effects in older individuals.
5. Immunzation of premature infants should be commenced at two months after birth, providing there are no contraindications. These infants especially need protection, have adequate antibody responses and do not have a higher incidence of adverse, reactions.
6. Immunization is commenced at two months because of the high morbidity and established mortality of pertussis in infancy.
7. **Precautions and contraindications:**
    (a) Immunization should not be carried out during the course of an acute illness.
    (b) Any major reaction following DTP (triple antigen) is likely to be due to the pertussis component and any further DTP or single pertussis vaccine is contraindicated. In this situation there is no indication to use a smaller dose of any pertussis vaccine. Major reactions include:
    (i) fever above 40.5°C;
    (ii) convulsions (uncommon); and
    (iii) shock, anaphylaxis, thrombocytopaenia and encephalopathy (all extremely rare).
    Mild local reactions occur very frequently (up to 50 percent) following DTP and **do not** contraindicate further DTP. Rarely sterile abscesses have been observed. It is believed these are more likely to occur when the vaccine is given subcutaneously.

Should an egg allergic child be given vaccines?

Influenza and yellow fever vaccines are both grown in the allantoic fluid of eggs, and contain potentially dangerous amounts of egg protein for an egg allergic individual. While measles vaccine is grown in chick embryo cells in tissue culture the incidence of severe reactions is very low, even in egg allergic patients. If a child has a history of an anaphylactic reaction to egg protein, assessment by an allergist should be made before immunization.

Is a family history of eczema a contraindication to vaccination?

Again the answer is 'no'.

Can a patient on steroids or other immunosuppressive drugs be immunized?

Yes and no. They can be immunized with any of the non-live vaccines and usually the antibody response is close to normal. Patients on low-dose steroids may be vaccinated with any of the killed or live vaccines. However, patients on high-dose steroids or other immunosuppressive drugs should only be vaccinated with live vaccines with extreme caution. In hazardous situations protection with passive antibody (general or specific immunoglobulin) should be considered.

When should a premature baby be immunized?

The immune system of a premature baby is equivalent to that of a full-term infant. Premature infants have been shown to respond equivalently to full-term infants if immunized at the same time after birth. There is no need to wait till after the expected date of confinement before commencing triple antigen and oral polio vaccine.

SPECIFIC VACCINES

Triple antigen (diptheria, pertussis, tetanus: DPT)

The NH & MRC recommendations should be followed (see Table 14.1). However, because of the uncertainties with pertussis, recommendations on withholding the pertussis component are interpreted differently by different health givers. Nevertheless pertussis vaccination remains worthwhile. Severe neurological damage occurs in less than 1 in 100 000 injections and is irreversible in less than 1 in 300 000. The likelihood of severe neurological damage and death in unimmunized individuals is much greater than that from the vaccine.

However, the pertussis component should not be given (a) in the presence of an evolving neurological dis-

order; (b) if there is a history of a severe reaction within 48 hours following a previous dose. Severe reactions may involve:

- collapse or shock
- fever 40.5°C or above with no other obvious cause
- persistent screaming
- convulsions
- persistent drowsiness
- generalized or localized neurological signs
- systemic allergic reactions (anaphylaxis).

Rubella

The current recommendations are for immunization of all infants between 12 and 15 months of age as in the USA. The aim of this strategy is to eliminate rubella eventually. The previous recommendation was to immunize girls about 12 years.

Measles

Unfortunately, measles is considered a nuisancce disease by many parents rather than a common illness that can lead to chronic ill health or even death in some circumstances. One of the problems with measles immunization campaigns is that the vaccine should not be given too early (maternal antibody will prevent the vaccine 'taking' in a moderate proportion of children if given before 9 months). However, delay in giving the vaccine means that children are susceptible to the disease. The 'window' period is from 9 to 15 months. Studies are required to determine the most cost-effective age for giving vaccine in this range.

FURTHER READING

Dick G 1986 Practical immunization. MTP Press, Lancaster

Feery B J 1982 Incidence and type of reactions to triple antigen (DPT) and DT (CDT) vaccines. Medical Journal of Australia 2: 511–515

Miller C L 1978 Severity of notified measles. British Medical Journal 1: 1253

Miller D L, Alderstade R, Ross E M 1982 Whooping cough and whooping cough vaccine: the risks and benefits debate. Epidemiology Review 4: 1–24

National Health and Medical Research Council 1986 Immunization procedures, 3rd edn. Australian Government Printing Office, Canberra

15. Child trauma

John Pearn

After the first year of life has passed, injuries remain the biggest cause of morbidity and mortality during childhood. Many doctors who work with children have responsibilities in the clinical care and follow up of child trauma victims. Because of the magnitude of the problem, *all* doctors have an inescapable role in the prevention of such accidents in the future.

Almost 1000 children die violently in Australia each year. The child trauma problem, as a relative cause of mortality and morbidity, continues to increase. The size of this current accident problem was totally unforeseen half a century ago. Over recent decades, effective rapid-response counter measures to deal with new types of accidents as they arise have not yet been fully developed. Although accident problems change from decade to decade, one thing that shows no secular trend is the basic curiosity, daring and inquisitiveness of children. Costs associated with illness and disease generally are expected to reach 11% of the gross national product by 1990. In childhood, the costs are relatively high, as not only does one have to add in costs of therapy in its broader sense, but also the concept of 'years of living lost'. Clinical paediatricians are in a unique position to witness the costs of preventable child trauma, which remains unchecked, and to monitor accident trends and implement preventive stratagems.

CHILD TRAUMA TODAY

Fatal child trauma

Collectively, six types of childhood accidents account for 95% of violent child deaths. The rank order of current types of child fatalities is shown in Table 15.1. The patterns of violent death to which the growing child is vulnerable vary dramatically according to age. Preschool children are the most vulnerable, and toddlers in the 1 to 3-year age group manifest very high age-specific trauma rates. So far, this is the area where preventive measures have been least effective. Drowning, road

Table 15.1 Rank order of causes of violent death in children aged 0–15 years

Causes of violent deaths	Annual rate per 100 000 children at risk
Road trauma	10.3
Drowning	5.2
Burns	0.9
Falls	0.8
Non-accidental injury	0.6
Poisoning	0.3

Table 15.2 Rank order of causes of violent deaths in infants and preschool children aged 0–5 years

Causes of violent deaths	Annual rate per 100 000 children at risk
Drowning	11.1
Road trauma	9.6
Non-accidental injury	3.8
Burns	1.5
Falls	1.4
Poisoning	0.5

trauma, non-accidental injury and burns remain the major causes of violent child death in this group. Together, these four problems cause 26 annual deaths per 100 000 children at risk in the preschool years. Fatality rates in this highly mobile but vulnerable age are shown in Table 15.2.

Trauma morbidity

Fatal child accidents are only the tip of the trauma iceberg. Drowning fatalities (fresh and salt water combined) comprise less than half of all cases of children who lose consciousness in the water. For every child killed on the roads, another 20 suffer serious injury. If one examines hospital admissions for trauma, the rank order of causes is:

Head injuries   26.5%

Poisoning	20.1%
Burns	13.0%
Fractures	12.8%
Lacerations	5.3%

This progression describes the profile of child injuries coming to a doctor's surgery, or passing through the portals of the casualty department. Outcome is quite another matter, and is accident-specific. Children rarely suffer after-effects from accidental poisoning, whereas almost all children have some after-effects from burns and scalds. One-third of near-drowning survivors have some degree of minimal cerebral dysfunction.

Secular trends

Paediatric death rates are never static and manifest dramatic secular trends. Japan's low infant mortality rate of 5.5 deaths per 1000 live births would have been inconceivable even a generation ago. Secular changes in the type and severity of child trauma are no exception to this more general phenomenon. Australia's current low accidental poisoning fatality rate has been described as 'one of the success stories of the decade', illustrating that vigorous preventive campaigns can be very effective. Indeed, the overall rates for accidental child trauma have continued to fall in Australia, as in other parts of the world, as part of the non-specific trend towards healthier societies. Unfortunately, this decline has been less than that seen in other areas of childhood ill health. In Australia and New Zealand, if one considers some special types of severe childhood accidents in particular local geographic areas (e.g. drowning, recreational accidents and bicycle accidents), the rate has continued to increase.

Child trauma has always been a significant cause of morbidity. Only the type changes. Trauma rates vary according to:

1. The overall secular trends in health
2. The vigour and effect of preventive campaigns
3. Safety legislation and safety design
4. Changes in consumer fashions in hardware (cars, swimming pools, mowers, barbecues, etc.).

The history of trauma prevention in childhood is that of a balance between concerned individuals campaigning to reduce hazards on the one hand, and the late recognition of new environmental dangers on the other. New environment hazards occur as the result of the affluent consumer society, of changed lifestyles and of new cultural mores superimposed on children living in societies hitherto in danger-safety equilibrium. Secular trends in the death rates for Australian children are shown in Fig-

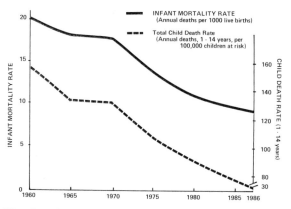

Fig. 15.1   Secular trends (1960–1986) for infant mortality rates, and total child death rates (1–14 years) Australia.

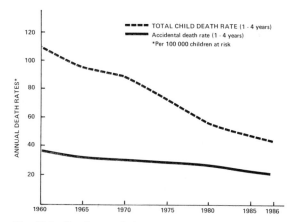

Fig. 15.2   Secular trends (1960–1986) for preschool children (1–4 years). Total child death rate, and total accidental death rate; both given as annual rates, per 100 000 age-specific children at risk, Australia.

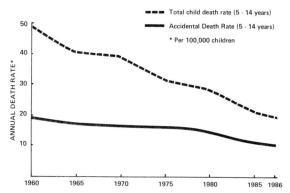

Fig. 15.3   Secular trends (1960–1986) for mortality among school-age children (5–14 years). Total child death rate, and total accidental death rate; both given as annual rates, per 100 000 age-specific children at risk, Australia.

ure 15.1, and for death specifically due to accidents, in Figures 15.2 and 15.3.

As infection has become increasingly controllable, as genetic counselling has reduced the number of deaths of children with genetic disease and as the treatment of childhood neoplasms has been so successful over the last two decades, accidents as a relative cause of child deaths have risen inexorably from one-third of all deaths in 1960, to one-half in 1983. Road trauma and drownings have continued to rank first and second as causes of accident fatalities involving Australian children, over the last two decades. Secular trends for these two specific

types of important accident are shown in Figures 15.4 and 15.5.

At present, fatality rates for both drowning and road trauma in preschool children remain above their 1960–1965 levels. So far, the only evidence of real success in trauma prevention is the reduction of accidental drowning in the school-age child (see Fig. 15.5).

A probable recent reduction in trauma to very young children on the roads is a heartening secular trend. It is worrying that there is no sign of any reduction in the rate of road deaths to school-age children and there is evidence to suggest that, particularly in the case of girls, road trauma rates are continuing to rise. Studies of secular trends relating to road trauma in Australia showed a dramatic increase in the 1950s and 1960s, not only in accident rates themselves, but in the severity of the injuries sustained. This was noted by Jamieson & Yelland in 1972. It has been stressed that the major threat to society in general and to children in particular is increased levels of kinetic energy to which they are exposed. This is seen on the roads, in sport and in recreation.

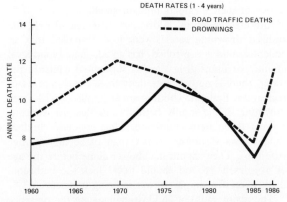

Fig. 15.4 Secular trends (1960–1986) for accident-specific death rates – Australia; children aged 1–4 years. Road traffic deaths and drowning fatalities; age-specific rates per 100 000 population at risk.

SOME SPECIFIC ACCIDENTS

Road trauma

Analyses of secular trends in childhood road traumas in Australia have shown that 15% of all fatal road trauma victims are children, with a peak vulnerable period (involving both sexes) of 5 years of age. Children are injured (a) as occupants of cars in intervehicle crashes; (b) as pedestrians in run-down accidents; and (c) as bicyclists who fall or are knocked from their cycles.

Of the road trauma related causes, child pedestrian run-downs comprise the biggest group. The peak age of risk is 5 years and approximately 7% of those injured die from this type of run-down accident. The majority of young chidren who are killed or injured as pedestrians sustain their injury close to their home, on relatively 'low speed' streets. Some 45% of children who are injured as pedestrians, are actually in their own street. The peak time of such pedestrian accidents is between 3.00 and 4.00 p.m. Child run-downs occur because young children run on to, or attempt to cross the road without control, or walk out from behind or between parked vehicles. It is rare for children to be run down whilst they are playing on the roadway, or when they are near or on pedestrian crossings (less than 10% of all child pedestrian run-downs fall into these three groups). Of the three types of road trauma, severity rates (measured as the percentage of children killed from such accidents) are highest for pedestrian run-downs.

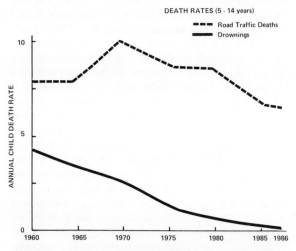

Fig. 15.5 Secular trends (1960–1986) for accident-specific death rates – Australia; children aged 5–14 years. Road traffic deaths and drowning fatalities; age-specific rates per 100 000 population at risk.

This rate is more than double the severity rates for both passengers and for cyclists who sustain injuries from road trauma.

At present, bicycle accidents in Australia, as elsewhere, comprise a problem of considerable proportion. If all bicycle accidents are considered, the victims are largely male (3:1) and are in their middle childhood years. They fall from their bicycles because of inexperience, doubling, striking holes or objects, or are playing bicycle 'games'. Studies in Brisbane, Australia, have shown that if one considers serious bicycle accidents (those causing hospital admission, or death), the typical profile is that of a male schoolboy who is struck by a sober motorist on a well-lit street, often on a straight stretch of road, within 3 kilometres of his home or school, and between 3.00 and 5.00 p.m. on a weekday.

Children may be killed or injured as occupants of cars, although the secular trends are changing in this regard. However, there are wide interstate and international differences in these statistics. Young children and unrestrained infants are known to be at special risk. Almost all such accidents occur to children who are riding in closed sedans. Head, or head and combined chest injuries account for almost all of the deaths. Drink-driving does not seem to be a major cause of this type of childhood injury.

Drowning

Accidental drowning is a significant cause of mortality in the toddler age group. If there is an exposed water hazard within 50 metres of a toddler's home, there is a very material risk of drowning, or near-drowning. The principle risks apply to fresh water hazards. Salt water drownings in Australia (involving children) are comparatively rare. This is not due to any intrinsic difference in water osmolality (which might be thought to influence the pathophysiology of drowning), but rather to the geographic closeness of the hazard. A problem with accident preventive approaches is that it is almost impossible to quantify the degree of hazard exposure as it applies to the individual child. Two studies (one in Australia and one in New Zealand) have given some estimate of the degree of the drowning threat to modern children. The Royal Plunket Society of New Zealand (in a 1 in 8 sample of New Zealand's 67 000 children between the ages of 1 and 3 years) showed that 10% of children at present have a swimming pool (53% unfenced) in their garden and that another 26% live beside a neighbour with a pool (66% unfenced). Australian estimates show that 1 in 9 homes have a pool erected for at least part of the year; this figure applies equally to homes in temperate parts of the country where winters may be freezing. Current best estimates for exposure risks to children from accidental swimming pool drownings are zero for properly fenced pools, rising to a rate of 1 child death in 800 pool years if there is no effective safety barrier.

There are a small number of older school-age children who drown, but these are almost all boys, the accident usually occurring in a setting of disobedience or clandestine swimming, well away from potential help if a child gets into difficulties in the water. Boating accidents involving children are not uncommon and are usually the result of adult inexperience and are often alcohol-related. In spite of this, the actual number of children who drown in such accidents remains small.

Although epileptic children are at increased risk, the realized drowning rate is very low. Provided that an epileptic child is controlled, has an adequate blood level of anticonvulsant drugs, and is supervised whilst in the water, there is no reason to deny them the joys of water recreation. Epileptic children are at significant risk from drowning in the family bathtub and this risk remains present throughout childhood. Thus epileptic children should always shower (rather than bathe in a plunge type tub). They should not shower alone before the age of 6 years or so and should never lock the bathroom door, even if a simple shower is being undertaken.

The major cause of child drownings are the presence of unprotected fresh water hazards, usually swimming pools, dams, trenches or drains which are close to domestic homes. No drowning is a single event and studies of large numbers of such accidents have demonstrated that the final tragedy is always the end result of a chain of disparate but sequentially linked events. Such a chain comprises a number of identifiable links. A typical linked chain might be: an unfenced in-ground swimming pool in the back garden; a fit and well, intelligent toddler playing on the rear porch of a low-set home; the telephone rings or a visitor calls at the front door; mother's attention is momentarily distracted and the adventurous and curious toddler crawls or toddles to the pool edge; a toy on the bottom, or leaves, or a ball floating on the surface attracts attention and the child simply walks into the water. Toddlers have a high head-mass versus body-mass ratio, and the head is dependent if a toddler is in water deeper than his/her height; under these circumstances cries cannot be heard. Anecdotal evidence suggests that such infants simply go to the bottom without struggles and drown. The parent or custodian (usually the mother) discovers the child, but in 10% of cases such parents are ineffective in rescue or resuscitation because of hysterical behaviour. Although trained resuscitation and first aid can turn some 30% of potentially fatal cases into survivors, most parents are not trained in such techniques. In practice, only approximately 50% of children apparently dead when rescued from the water actually survive. In theory, the potential drowning can be averted at any point along this linked chain. Studies have shown that there is an average of four such links in every drowning accident which involves children.

Children who survive near-drowning accidents tend to do well clinically. It is known that, as a group, toddlers who drown are more intelligent than average and that survivors have an average IQ of approximately 110. Some one-third have selective loss of some islands of mental functioning (the minimum brain dysfunction syndrome), but only 5% live in a total vegetative state. Children who survive near-drowning accidents are at significant risk of the same accident happening a second time.

Burns

Burns and scalds remain significant causes of child mortality and morbidity. Conflagrations are the commonest cause of death from burns, but scalds are the commonest causes of hospital admissions following thermal injury. Children's skins are burnt by moist heat hotter than 45°C. This problem is particularly relevant in the 0 to 4-year age group, and children under 2 years of age are particularly at risk. Burnt children are not representative of the normal child population in any community, and are not 'randomly' involved in such accidents. Children from socially disadvantaged groups are always over-represented in all thermal injury series. (The rates of childhood burns are high, for example, in the Northern Territory, and are low in the Australian Capital Territory, an area where the population is skewed to middle and upper socioeconomic status groups.) Most burns occur indoors, with some 37% occurring in the kitchen. Of those children who are scalded, 37% are injured by spilled cups and teapots and 14% are scalded in the family bathtub. In the case of flame burns, 29% are due to open outdoor barbecues and incinerators, 14% are involved in flash conflagrations from fuel cans, and some 13% of children are still burnt on radiators and heating appliances.

Poisoning

Accidental poisoning in childhood is a worldwide problem. Patterns of ingested substances change from time to time and with the vigour of preventive programmes, such as safety packaging. Fashions in prescribing also change and, therefore, types of drugs kept in homes, also show significant secular trends. Although the ingestion of potentially toxic substances is a significant cause of hospital admission through the casualty or emergency department, child deaths are now very uncommon from accidental poisoning.

The current age-corrected rate of poisoning is 393 per 100 000 children per year (0 to 5-year olds). The rank order of poisons, drugs and chemicals which cause hospital admission and death is:

Petroleum distillates	13%
Antihistamines	9%
Benzodiazepines	9%
Bleach and detergents	7%
Aspirin	6%

Recent studies have identified the practical risk of death, following the ingestion of various common substances. The rank order of danger, and the absolute risk of death following ingestion of unknown amounts of the toxin, are shown in Table 15.3.

Table 15.3 Rank order of danger following ingestion of poisonous substances by children aged 0–4 years (after Pearn 1982)

Poisonous substances	Rates of fatality to ingestion
Digoxin, quinine	1 to 25
Tricyclic antidepressants	1 to 44
Sympathomimetic drugs	1 to 54
Caustic soda	1 to 68
Paracetamol, aspirin	1 to 350
Petroleum distillates	1 to >750

Although the types of agent which cause accidental child poisoning vary from time to time and from place to place, the modal ages for poisoning fatalities remain in the second and third years of life and this pattern has never shown any secular trend. Toddlers ingest everything from dog repellant to caustic soda out of curiosity. In clinical practice, a noxious taste or burning sensation in the mouth produces one or two reflex actions – a spitting out or a reflex swallow, often with dire results.

The crusade against childhood fatalities from poisoning is one of the success stories of modern preventive medicine and is due largely to the combination of voluntary and legislative approach to the safety packaging of drugs and medicines which are dispensed through pharmaceutical outlets. At a time when some types of childhood accidents are increasing, deaths from accidental poisoning have shown one of the most heartening falls. It is probable that children living in rural areas are at greater risk. The intentional poisoning of children is a now recognized form of child abuse. With the fall in the rate of serious poisoning, intentional poisoning of children leading to death or near-death is assuming greater importance.

Sporting and recreational injuries

Children injured during recreation is a subject of topical concern and one which will have to be addressed with courage and pragmatism. Doctors are increasingly accepting their responsibilities as advocates for the reduction of the current high rate of sporting trauma, particularly involving adolescents. Spinal injuries from football are of current concern. The bulk of such injuries can be prevented by on-field rule changes and by more vigorous enforcement of current laws. Permission to participate in high risk sports should be conditional on the use of certain safety features. It is now well established that students will wear protective helmets, mitts and shinguards if they cannot play on school teams without them. As a result of mandatory facial protection of ice-hockey goalies in the USA and Canada, these high-risk players now have fewer facial injuries than other team members.

It is appropriate that doctors keep a 'watching brief' of playground injuries and trauma from recreational hardware. Vigorous advocacy by medical practitioners is one of the best ways of ensuring that dangerous equipment is either repaired, or withdrawn. At present, newer types of metal slippery slides, new high-suction pool filters and high energy ride-on mowers are all causing severe and permanent injuries to Australian children.

Injuries from animals

Although injuries from animals are now trivial as far as mortality is concerned, significant morbidity still occurs. Childhood injuries from dogs in contemporary society are not trivial. One dog in every 40 causes an injury requiring a child's attendance at hospital, and one-third of bites to children are on the face. Children in Australia have died in the past from snakebites (the first survivor from a Taipan bite was in 1955 when specific antivenom was first used), but deaths are now rare. Only one child death has been recorded over a recent 5-year period in south-eastern Queensland, although during this period some 90 children have sustained snakebites.

Follow-up

The management of trauma victims includes follow-up both in the clinical and preventive contexts. Children who have sustained serious or near-fatal trauma remain at risk of the incident occurring again. Follow-up studies of near-drowned children have shown that some 5% sustain a second similar life-threatening accident. All experienced casualty officers are familiar with the syndrome of the second near-fatal accidental ingestion of toxic chemicals or drugs after a primary event several months before.

Follow-up is required also on clinical grounds. The child who has sustained a head injury is at risk of developing epilepsy, and children who have survived partial strangulation from rope games, or partial suffocation from collapsed cubby-houses, or who have been rescued from near-drowning situations are at risk of being left with the residuum of long-term subtle psychological problems.

IDENTIFYING THE CAUSES OF CHILD TRAUMA

Subcultures accept passively that accidents are part of life and that trends cannot be reversed. Some contemporary Aboriginal cultures and a number of Third World societies accept that accidents may be supernatural visitations, or are due to spirit influence. This passive approach can be seen also in modern Western communities; for example, the difficulties there have been in introducing legislation to protect children from flammable nightwear, to have seat belts in motor cars and helmets for bicycle users, and to enclose swimming pools with a fence.

Identifying causes of different types of accidents is an essential step if prevention is to be effective. No experienced worker now subscribes to the concept of the 'fault doctrine' in the field of child trauma. Although human agency, or lack of it, can be identified as one of several links in the accident chain, from the pragmatic point of view there is nothing to be gained by ascribing 'fault' or 'blame'. The Child Accident Prevention Foundation of Australia, and similar bodies in the UK and in the USA emphasize the fact that preventive approaches should be aimed at altering the potentially hazardous environment, rather than attempting to alter human behaviour. Proven successes with safety packaging of drugs, safety legislation relating to heating appliances in homes, to the introduciton of non-flammable nightwear and to legislation relating to safety barriers around water hazards, all illustrate this point.

PREVENTION

All who work with children have a responsibility for the prevention of child trauma. This theme comprises one of the greatest current practical problems in paediatrics. Preventive counselling and advocacy should be pursued

(a) at the clinical level with individual families, e.g. at well-baby clinics; (b) as part of follow-up of individual clinical cases after trauma; (c) in media and publicity campaigns which are in the public interest; and (d) in advocacy situations relating to safer practices and the achievement of a less dangerous environment for children, through safety legislation. There are three portals through which doctors can make effective preventive thrusts – education, design improvement and safety legislation. These three approaches are mutually inclusive.

Education

It is now recognized that education of vulnerable families may be successful if (a) the target 'at risk' population is identified with great specificity; (b) the safety and preventive message is formulated appropriately; and (c) the carrier medium is appropriate to the 'at risk' group. Reception and acceptance of a safety message is only the first step; behaviour modification remains a demanding but not impossible task. Experience with antismoking campaigns (especially in members of professional class families) has shown that education can be very effective. Also, the same has been found with respect to the voluntary fencing of swimming pools where toddlers are at risk.

Education aimed at reducing child vehicle occupant fatalities should be aimed at eight points listed in Example 15.1.

Example 15.1 Scope for safety education concerning child – vehicle safety

1. Every infant, toddler and child should be restrained at all times when a car is in motion.
2. Children should not ride in the front seat of a moving vehicle and should never travel in the back of an open vehicle.
3. If it is necessary to leave children in a car:
   a. leave the doors unlocked with all windows partly open.
   b. remove the ignition key, and take all precautions to ensure that the child is unable (as far as practicable) to put the car in motion.
4. Children should never be left in a car in the sun in hot weather (temperatures reach 60°C in dark coloured cars in subtropical Australia within 15 minutes, even if the windows are wound down to a 5 cm gap).
5. Children should have no access to matches, cigarettes or lighters whilst they are in the car.
6. Door-lock and 'buckle-up' ('clinck-clunk') drills should always be undertaken and taught to children from the age of 2 years.
7. Children should be trained to get out of a vehicle only by the kerbside.

This educational approach should be directed at parents, at school children themselves and at the general public. At present, there is an average of only 4 minutes of safety instruction each week in the primary school curriculum in classes in Australia. Doctors have an important advocacy role to increase the time and scope of safety education in schools (see Example 15.2).

Example 15.2 Safety education themes relating to child drowning

1. Children should be protected from water hazards within 50 m of a dwelling by a safety barrier. Unprotected in-ground pools are particularly dangerous.
2. A safety barrier is effective and will protect children at risk if it conforms to the Australian Standard, i.e. has a fence 1.4 m in height and the gate is self-closing and self-latching, with a high hidden lock.
3. The bath tub is dangerous for unsupervised children under 18 months of age.
4. No child should be left in the care of other children in the face of a water hazard.
5. Children should not play in a potential water hazard, or swim unsupervised, under the age of 10 years.
6. Swimming skills should be taught to all children from the age of 3 years and resuscitation skills to all children from the age of 9 years.

There is continued debate about the efficiency of safety education and media campaigns, and several studies of broad-based campaigns, which are not selectively aimed or specifically tailed to the 'at risk' population, have not shown these to be effective in behaviour modification. However, one important point is the potential transgeneration effect. At the centre of this theme is the belief that children themselves, if given a safety message, will retain part of this information and modify the life-style of their future families when they are parents themselves.

Design improvement

Ergonomic approaches to safety are important. Improving design is a relatively unexploited stratagem when it comes to the prevention of trauma. Head injuries sustained in the home, or at play, contribute some 11% of all visits to hospital casualty departments, and furnishings and household fittings and fixtures are the major cause of these. Aesthetic appeal and functional safety go hand in hand in a surprisingly large number of instances – an important medical role here is to act as an advocate for safety and to encourage fashion in hardware design which may have safety spin-offs. Setting household thermostats to deliver water at not more than 50°C is a current topical example (some solar hot water systems can deliver water at 75°C), which will cause instantaneous, permanent thermal damage to young children. Since 1980 double-packaging and foil wrapping of tablets has been a major cause of the dramatic reduction in accidental child poisonings in Australa. Self-closing and self-latching gates for swimming pool enclosures, and the change from clothes wringers to enclosed spin driers are other important examples of heartening developments in this area. The doctor must be able to advise on safety equipment for children. All Western countries now have consumer committees in the form of Standards Associations. The Australian Standards Association sets rigorous criteria for hardware (such as child seat restraints and motor cycle helmets) which have safety implications. The setting of such standards ensures that effectiveness, practicability and aesthetic acceptability can go hand in hand.

Safety legislation

Safety legislation is very effective in reversing upward secular trends in child trauma. The sociological basis of safety legislation is community acceptance of one fundamental principle – that children's lives cannot be discretionary at the will or behest of their parents. This means rejecting the philosophy that 'it's up to the parents to protect their own children'. Sadly, this is still a source of bitter debate even in sophisticated Western communities in the 1980s. In practice, it takes on average between 5 and 15 years for effective safety legislation to be introduced after the identification and acceptance by the medical profession that a real safety threat exists. Historically the difficulties of introducing safety legislation is illustrated by the following example: the protection of machinery in factories where children were working in the UK in the last century; the introduction of lead-free paints in Australia; seat restraints for children under the age of 8 years; safety barriers around water hazards. These important battles have only been won by informed advocates for children's safety carrying the message repeatedly not only into the public arena, but to concerned and responsible legislators.

FURTHER READING

Jackson R H (ed) 1977 Children, the environment and accidents. Pitman Medical, London
Jamieson K G, Yelland J D 1972 Traumatic intracerebral haematoma. Journal of Neurosurgery 37: 528–532
O'Connor P J 1982 An analysis of Australian child accidents statistics, vol 1 Child Accident Foundation of Australia, Melbourne
Pearn J 1982 The prevention of childhood accidents. Design, education and legislation. Australasian Medical Publishing Company, Sydney
Pearn J 1983 Accidents to children – their incidence, causes and effects. Child Accident Prevention Foundation of Australia, Melbourne
Pearn J 1984 Drowning. In: Dickerman J D, Lucey J F (eds) The critically ill child. W B Saunders, Chicago
Rivara F P 1984 Childhood injuries, III: epidemiology of non-motor vehicle head trauma. Developmental Medicine and Child Neurology 26: 81–87

16. The child with school problems

Frank Oberklaid

Many terms have been used to describe children who do not succeed at school – dyslexia, minimal brain dysfunction, perceptual disorder and congenital word blindness. These terms are difficult to define objectively and cause much confusion among both parents and professionals.

As well as labelling children inappropriately, they make it more difficult for professions from different disciplines to communicate clearly with each other. In addition, the use of terms which do not have widespread acceptance and understanding are not helpful in either understanding the causes of the child's problems or in developing an effective intervention plan. It is preferable to develop a broad description of these children in terms of their developmental strengths and weaknesses. This takes into account the unique individual characteristics of each child, avoids labelling them with terms that have little validity or meaning, and makes it easier to develop management strategies that specifically address the child's problems.

EXTENT OF THE PROBLEM

The number of children with learning problems is impossible to estimate accurately. Figures ranging from 5 to 50% have been quoted, depending on what one considers to be a learning disability. In this chapter we will be considering those children who have normal intelligence, do not have gross physical or sensory handicapping conditions, yet who fail to reach their expected academic potential. Such a broad definition excludes children with high severity low incidence conditions such as cerebral palsy, mental retardation, deafness and blindness.

Learning disabilities have been described as being part of the low severity high incidence spectrum of handicapping conditions. Children with school problems are at risk of developing a number of associated or secondary problems. Sometimes these children may present to the medical practitioner with various psychosomatic complaints such as abdominal pain, headache, withdrawn behaviour, depression, or any number of vague or ill-defined complaints for which no organic cause can be found. They may be accused of being lazy or disinterested in their school work. Often parents and teachers will observe that they have increasing difficulty with peer relations, tending either to be 'loners' and withdraw from social situations or to seek out children who have similar problems and subsequently exhibit acting-out and difficult behaviours. Many children with learning difficulties have problems with attention and motivation, and in all of these children there is a fall in self-esteem and self-confidence which may spill over into many other facets of their life.

AETIOLOGY

Most children with school problems do not have a single identifiable cause. From the history obtained from the parents, the physical examination and neurodevelopmental testing, it is usual to identify a number of factors that are likely to be contributing to a child's problems. These can include constitutional or intrinsic factors within the child or factors within the environment. It is the interaction of these constitutional and environmental factors which over time leads to the dysfunction which presents as school learning difficulties.

Environmental factors

Examples of environmental factors include inappropriate schooling, inadequate stimulation, family disruption and upheaval, while constitutional factors would include developmental weaknesses, organic disease, and physical or sensory handicaps (Example 16.1). These are detailed below, and will be further discussed in the section on assessment.

Example 16.1 Constitutional and environmental factors which may contribute to school problems

Environmental
    Cultural, e.g. bilingual child
    Socioeconomic status
    Family – structure and dynamics
    Parental expectations – role models
    Early stimulation and experiences
    Peer contacts and relationships
    Preschool experience
    Other environmental stresses
    Classroom/school environment

Constitutional
    General health
    Vision/hearing deficits
    Genetic/familial
    Perinatal stresses
    Intelligence
    Temperament/personality
    Developmental strengths and weaknesses

Constitutional factors

Developmental weaknesses

A large number of children who experience school problems have as the major contributing factor weaknesses in one or more areas of development which are often subtle, and are only elicited by neurodevelopmental assessment. These are children who look, walk and talk normally, and it is not until they are asked to perform specific age appropriate developmental items that their weaknesses become apparent. Areas of development that are important for the achievement of school competence and which may be assessed as part of the paediatric examination include the following.

Language. Competence in language is an essential component of school success. Children may have receptive or expressive language difficulties. Those with receptive language problems have difficulty understanding auditory commands, especially if these are lengthy or complex. They may have difficulty following the meaning of explanations, and have subsequent problems in academic areas such as reading. Children with expressive language problems have difficulties with organizing, narrative, with articulation, or with word finding. They have problems expressing what they want to say, and often have difficulty with peer relationships because of their weakness in verbal communication. Subtle language problems can sometimes be limited to recurrent ear infections and fluctuating hearing loss in the toddler and preschool periods.

Auditory and visual sequencing. Children with auditory sequencing problems have difficulty remembering information that is presented to them as a verbal sequence. Parents and teachers may say that they seem to have difficulty in following instructions, or need to have things repeated before they can understand. Children with visual sequencing difficulties have problems with aspects of spelling and reading. Sequencing problems may cause difficulties in any academic area because so much instruction and retention of meaning depends on the ability to integrate sequential information. Children with sequencing difficulties also have problems with time concepts such as days of the week, months of the year and learning to tell the time.

Youngsters with sequencing problems commonly are described as not being able to concentrate, or being easily distracted, or even disruptive in class – often this is secondary to their inability to retain sequences of instructions.

Visual perceptual motor function. Children with weaknesses in this area are at risk of problems with writing, reading, spelling, and the organization of material on a page. Weaknesses may be in visual perception, in fine motor function, or in the integration of the two. They may become apparent at an early stage when a child exhibits problems in discriminating between similar letters and words, as well as copying letters or numbers. Letter reversals may continue well into school.

Motor function. Children with weaknesses in gross motor function appear inco-ordinated and clumsy, and often are isolated from their peer group. This may then have a secondary affect on self-esteem which may then affect their classroom motivation and performance. Difficulties in fine motor function on the other hand may cause difficulty with shoelaces, zippers, and using a pencil. Writing may be poor and very slow. Subtle fine motor problems may not become apparent until the child approaches adolescence when the demands for written output increase.

Attention. A number of children have problems in focusing attention and maintaining concentration. In addition, many are described as being overactive, fidgety, impulsive and distractible – all of these behaviours may contribute to problems learning in the classroom as well as social difficulties.

While some children will have these behaviours as part of their intrinsic make-up, in others there are underlying emotional problems or anxiety. There is another group in whom these difficulties with concentration and attention are secondary to hearing deficits or developmental weaknesses such as auditory sequencing or language deficits.

A neurodevelopmental assessment is an important part of the evaluation of children who are thought to be 'hyperactive' in order to exclude developmental weaknesses.

Health problems. Children who have had a serious illness and make an apparent normal recovery may have subsequent school problems. For example, any child who has had bacterial meningitis should be followed closely to ensure that there are no subtle neurological deficits causing learning difficulties. Children with any form of chronic disease may have school problems. The reasons for these are multiple (see Example 16.2). The disease itself may be responsible (e.g. seizure disorder) or in some instances the treatment of the disease may contribute (e.g. side effects of medications). There may be frequent absences from school because of hospitalizations or episodes of illness. A child with chronic disease may have diminished self-confidence and self-esteem resulting in decreased motivation. Peer relationships may be affected because of the child's self-esteem and also because the child may be perceived as being different in some way by his or her peer group. He or she may be less active and not able to participate in regular classroom activities. Sometimes parents and teachers reinforce unwittingly the sick role in some of these children.

However, there are many children with chronic or disabling illnesses who do not appear to suffer any school problems, and a number who in fact seem to be spurred on to later achievement as a result of their illness.

Hearing and vision problems. In recent years it has been increasingly recognized that children with subtle hearing problems are at major risk of school dysfunction. This applies not only to those with a sensorineural hearing loss, but particularly those who have repeated ear infections as toddlers, leading to chronic otitis media and a fluctuating conductive hearing loss which often goes unsuspected and undetected. These children may develop subtle language and academic problems, as well as problems with attention and behaviour. Children with

any form of visual problems which affect acuity or eye movements will similarly be at risk of school dysfunction.

Perinatal stress. Whereas any form of perinatal stress must be regarded as a potential contributor to subsequent school problems, there is by no means a clear one to one relationship. It is true that prematurity, hypoxia, and other perinatal factors are sometimes associated with subsequent developmental difficulties. However, the majority of children with school problems do not have any abnormal perinatal history, and conversely a significant number of children with perinatal stress subsequently have normal academic achievement. In an individual child, environmental factors are important in modifying the outcome of perinatal stress; the potential of a poor outcome resulting from perinatal stress may be altered significantly by the beneficial effects of a favourable environment.

Genetic factors. While it is commonly said that cognitive ability, intelligence and other personality traits are inherited, no one to one relationship can be demonstrated. Often a family history of school problems is obtained and in some children does seem to be an inherited basis for their problems. However, it is only in a minority of children that a specific genetic cause or diagnosis can be entertained. On the other hand, there are identifiable syndromes which in addition to their dysmorphic features have limited cognitive ability or learning difficulties as an associated feature.

Socioeconomic factors

Many factors in the child's environment may contribute significantly to school problems. Children from different cultural backgrounds may have problems with language, with adapting to a new culture, and coping with attitudinal differences between their peer group and family. Children from deprived socioeconomic circumstances are at risk of school dysfunction; there are multiple factors responsible, including family disruptions, sub-optimal medical care and nutrition, the lack of early stimulation, poor role models, and low parental education and expectations. For some children the educational experience may not have been a positive one – for example class size and facilities in schools vary considerably. A particular child may have been put in a classroom where needs are not met, leading to alienation from the learning process and a decrease in motivation.

There are children in whom multiple environmental stresses seem to have a compounding effect in contributing to their school problems – poverty is associated with sub-optimal health, housing, and attending schools which are disadvantaged in terms of resources.

Example 16.2 The impact of ill-health of chronic disease on a child's school functioning

1. The condition itself, e.g. epilepsy, cyanotic heart disease
2. The treatment of the condition – e.g. side effects of medications such as anticonvulsants, antihistamines, cytotoxics
3. Absences from school because of illness of hospitalization
4. Lowered self-confidence and self-esteem, distorted body image
5. Perception of child by parents and teachers altered – the 'vulnerable child syndrome'
6. Difficulties with peer relationships – unable to partake in normal activities, low self-esteem, altered perception of child by peer group

ASSESSMENT

Evaluation of a child with school problems is time consuming and usually takes more than one session. Close communication with the child's school and sometimes with other professionals is essential. The assessment needs to be broadly based so as to take into account all the possible constitutional and environmental factors that may be playing a part in the genesis of the child's problems. The process of evaluation is outlined in Example 16.3.

A careful history is taken from the parents, paying particular attention to the child's early health, development and behaviour and when the parents first became aware of problems. The family situation including its composition, social circumstances, education and expectations of the parents are particularly relevant. Parent questionnaires are often useful in terms of providing a standard structure for obtaining a history and also as a means of saving time. Any points or issues raised either in the history or in the questionnaire should be explored in detail. The results of any previous evaluations should be obtained.

At the earliest opportunity the medical practitioner must communicate with the child's school either by telephone or letter. It is useful to obtain copies of the child's reports, and a written communication from the school is often helpful. A detailed teacher questionnaire is useful as a means of obtaining a considerable amount of information in a standard form, and also serves the purpose of involving the child's teachers in the assessment process. The school is asked to share the results of any previous assessments, and the physician ascertains whether other agencies are involved with the child. It is useful to ask the teachers for their perception of a

---

Example 16.3 Steps in the assessment process of the child with school problems

1.* History from parents – parent questionnaire useful
2.* Information/report from school – use of teacher questionnaire
3.* Physical and neurological examination
4.* Sensory examination – vision and hearing
5.* Neurodevelopmental assessment to elicit individual profile of developmental strengths and weaknesses
6. Educational assessment
7. Psychiatric/pyschological assessment
8. Other special assessment/investigations, e.g. speech pathologist

* These parts of the assessment process are within the domain of the medical practitioner. Steps 1–6 are regarded as a minimum evaluation of a child with school problems; steps 7–8 are optional and depend on the issues present in a particular child.

---

child's academic and developmental strengths and weaknesses, peer relationships and classroom behaviours. This information is then integrated with the findings obtained from the physician's assessment.

A careful physical and neurological examination is performed on every child. It is important to exclude any acute or chronic disease, and also to check carefully for any neurological signs indicating either neuromaturational delay, or a specific neurological lesion. While it is not common for serious neurological disease to present for the first time as learning difficulties, this should nevertheless be excluded. Any dysmorphic features are carefully documented, and if it is suspected that the child may have an identifiable syndrome, referral for consultation should be considered. The majority of children with school problems do not benefit from any investigations unless these are clearly indicated, either from the history or from the physical or neurological examination. In particular investigations such as an EEG or CT scan are rarely, if ever, indicated.

The child's vision and hearing are screened using standard techniques. For a school-aged child visual acuity is tested relatively easily using a standard eye chart. If there are any doubts about either visual acuity or any other aspect of visual functioning, the child should be referred for further assessment. The child's hearing acuity should be tested using pure tone audiometry. The medical practitioner can easily administer such a test if facilities are available, as both administration and interpretation are relatively straightforward. However, if such facilities are not available, and especially if there is anything in the history to suggest the possibility of past or present hearing difficulties (for example recurrent ear infections, difficulty understanding directions, etc.) then a formal hearing screening test should be obtained.

Neurodevelopmental testing should then be administered to determine whether there are subtle developmental weaknesses contributing to problems. Such an assessment takes between 20 to 30 minutes to administer, and leads to a descriptive account of the child's developmental strengths and weaknesses. Any identified weaknesses can then be interpreted in light of the child's academic difficulties. As previously mentioned, many children with learning problems have as a significant contributing factor one or more developmental weaknesses.

The neurodevelopmental assessment consists of the administration to the child of age-appropriate tasks in each of the developmental areas previously outlined. This may be done formally or informally. Items are drawn from standardized developmental or psychological tests. They are administered to the child whose performance on each of the items is carefully observed. For example, gross motor tasks will include standing on one leg for a five-year-old, hopping in a straight line for a six- or seven-year-old, catching and throwing a ball with one hand for a ten- to twelve-year-old, etc.

Examples of neurodevelopmental assessment procedures can be found in various texts (see Levine et al 1980). While some general practitioners who are interested in this area will be able to administer neurodevelopmental testing, it is more commonly a task for the consultant paediatrician, school doctor or other professionals who work closely with children who have school difficulties.

All children with school problems should at some stage have an educational assessment administered by a skilled educator, preferably with training and expertise in special education. This may be done at a school level, in the community, or at a hospital-based multidisciplinary clinic. The educator administers a variety of specific psychoeducational tests in order to determine the child's present academic level of functioning and preferred learning styles, together with motivation, concentration, sensitivity to his performance, and ability to be taught specific strategies for overcoming weaknesses. In many instances it is most helpful for the educator to be aware of the physician's assessment, in particular the findings on the neurodevelopmental assessment.

Other assessments are then organized as indicated. For example, in some children there may be indications from the history or the assessment process that there are significant emotional issues, either within the child himself or in the family context which may be contributing to the problems. A referral to a psychologist or psychiatrist may serve to clarify these issues and lead to a recommendation for specific intervention. In some instances it is appropriate for a child with language weaknesses as elicited on the neurodevelopmental examination to be referred to a speech pathologist for a formal speech and language assessment. The child who fails a screening examination of auditory acuity should be referred for formal audiological assessment. Subsequent referrals such as these should be individualized for each child according to the findings of the assessment.

MANAGEMENT

Physician

Medical practitioners have an important role to play in the management of children with school problems. While rarely called upon to provide ongoing 'treatment'

in the traditional sense, they will co-ordinate ongoing management, help obtain appropriate services for the child, and continue to be available to support the child and the family throughout his schooling.

Any health problems either newly found or ongoing will need to be treated. The child who has difficulty with auditory acuity or auditory discrimination problems needs preferential seating in the classroom in an area free from distractions and near the front of the class. Where there are family disruptions and other environmental factors, specific support will need to be organized.

The child's developmental weaknesses need to be addressed. The child who has problems with attention will need a structured classroom, given preferential seating towards the front of the class, and specific strategies formulated to improve the concentration and reduce distractibility. The child who has difficulty with auditory sequencing will benefit from having verbal instructions kept simple, given in small sequences, and repeated as necessary. Wherever possible, instructions should be written down as well as spoken, so the child may have the opportunity of visual reinforcement. Medical practitioners should communicate to the school the results of their assessment, interpreting any biomedical findings for the teachers, and making clear the child's developmental strengths and weaknesses.

Parents

It is important that the parents be involved both in the assessment process and in any plan for management. The child's difficulties and strengths should be explained to the parents as simply as possible. They should be encouraged to create an atmosphere at home that is conducive to learning and they can be counselled regarding the most appropriate way to motivate and encourage their child. In general, it is not a good idea for parents to coach their children at home or to spend much time going over homework with them in a rote fashion, because of tensions that may result. Parents should keep in close contact with the school, discussing the child's progress with teachers. Often teachers will suggest ways in which parents can assist the child in maintaining motivation and encouraging the child's interest in learning.

Educational programmes

The majority of children with school problems will need specific educational programmes organized for them. These will vary considerably both in intensity and breadth. In some instances it is sufficient for the regular classroom teacher, aware of the child's needs, to modify a teaching curriculum or otherwise make some compensations for the child's difficulties. In other cases a remedial teacher or a teaching assistant may work in the child's classroom either on a one-to-one basis or in a small group. In a number of instances the child is actually taken from the classroom for set periods per week for intensive remediation in a one-to-one or small group situation.

For some children, the measures described above are still not sufficient because of the severity and extent of the learning problems. In these instances a child may attend a special classroom full time, or even a special school. Educational programmes will vary according to the resources available to the school and the severity and nature of the child's problems.

There are a large number of specific educational remedial strategies available to assist children, depending on their particular needs. Many of these are commercially available as teaching kits, and are well known to remedial teachers and those working in the educational field. Medical practitioners cannot be expected to have more than a very superficial knowledge of them, and it is best that they work closely with an educator in these instances.

Repetition of grade

Generally it is unusual for repetition of a grade to solve any problems that the child may have. Retention may well allow the child to consolidate skills before being promoted, but to be of maximum value to the child retention must be associated with an intensive remedial education programme to correct apparent weaknesses.

At times the medical practitioner may be asked about the benefits of a child being retained in a particular classroom, receiving a particular educational programme, switching to a different school, having private tutoring, or other non-medical questions. Doctors should exercise caution in answering parent or teacher requests in this regard. Often they will find themselves unwillingly asked to take sides where there is disagreement, and otherwise being asked to give an opinion in an area that is generally foreign to them. Generally, such decisions are best made at a local educational level, with medical practitioners contributing to the discussion as appropriate and according to the level of their expertise and interest.

Often parents are reassured by teachers (as well as medical practitioners) that their child is 'immature' and if left alone will grow out of his problems. Such statements should be avoided. In fact, the vast majority of children do not grow out of their problems, and an assertion that the child is immature is often a way of avoiding dealing with the problem.

REFERENCE

Levine M D, Brooks R, Shonkoff J P 1980 A pediatric approach to learning disorders. Wiley, New York

FURTHER READING

Kinsbourne M 1975 Models of learning disability: their relevance to remediation. CMA Journal 113: 1066–1068
Lerner J W 1976 Children with learning disabilities. Houghton Mifflin, Boston
Levine M D, Oberklaid F, Meltzer L 1981 Developmental output failure: a study of low productivity in school-aged children. Pediatrics 67: 18–25
Oberklaid F 1984 The child with school problems; an expanding role for paediatricians. Australian Paediatric Journal 20: 271–275
Oberklaid F, Levine M D 1980 Precursors of school failure. Pediatrics in Review 2: 5–11
Senf G M 1973 Learning disabilities. The Pediatric Clinics of North America 20: 607–640

17. The physically disabled child

A. C. L. Clark

Although there is now good evidence of declining childhood mortality in developed countries, measurement of morbidity is much more difficult, so that we often cannot say with certainty whether the frequency of chronic disease is changing. However, it is certain that changing patterns of disease and health care are such that doctors caring for children spend an increasing amount of their time in the management of those with chronic disease, and that increasingly their work is in collaboration with other professionals in health, education and community roles.

The World Health Organization has distinguished between *impairment*, which is a pathological process affecting organ structure or function, *disability* which is the impaired ability to undertake tasks resulting from an impairment, and *handicap*, which is the social consequence of an impairment or disability. The perception of handicap depends upon attitudes of society and upon the response of the individual to the disability. In some settings, a disability may so impair the fulfilment of a chosen role as to constitute a significant handicap, whereas in others the same disability can be overcome, and role fulfilment achieved. For young children, judgements about future handicap are made by those who care for them, and may prove to be quite wrong when the child reaches adult life and makes his own judgement in the setting of that time.

In our efforts to understand the causes of disability and hence to prevent it, there is a clear need to document population frequencies and trends. Because it depends on societal attitudes and individual responses, handicap can never be precisely quantitated, but approximate estimates can be made of the frequency of disability, while impairments can often be quite precisely enumerated. For these reasons, comparisons between frequencies of disabilities in different countries, or over different periods of time, must be interpreted with great caution.

CATEGORIES OF DISABILITY

Disability may be categorized as physical, intellectual or emotional. This chapter will be largely concerned with physical disability, but it must be realized that multiple disabilities are very common. Thus, a child with cerebral palsy may have auditory, intellectual and emotional disabilities in addition to the motor impairment. Not surprisingly, those physical disabilities most commonly associated with intellectual disability are those in which the impairment affects the nervous system. The common groups are:

1. Motor
   a. cerebral palsy
   b. spina bifida
   c. traumatic brain injuries
   d. epilepsy
2. Sensory
   a. deafness, especially nerve deafness
   b. blindness. In general, the more anteriorly the visual impairment is located, the less likely it is to be associated with other nervous system abnormalities, but there are many exceptions.

Common physical disabilities in which the impairment does not usually lie in the nervous system, and is therefore less often associated with intellectual disability, include:

1. Muscular dystrophy (but note a significant incidence of intellectual disability (see Ch. 48).
2. Congenital heart disease
3. Chronic respiratory disease – cystic fibrosis, severe asthma
4. Diabetes mellitus
5. Childhood malignancy and its sequelae
6. Juvenile chronic arthritis
7. Chronic renal failure
8. Skeletal abnormalities, e.g. arthrogryposis, amputations.

It will be apparent that almost any chronic disorder in childhood may result in disability. The conditions listed above are considered in relevant chapters, which should be consulted for specific aspects of management. Many parent support groups and societies deal with specific disorders, and can provide useful information on locally available resources.

Recognition of disability

There are several settings in which disability may be recognized, and in each the effect on the family and the counselling required of the doctor may be different.

1. Disability recognized at birth

For parents who have anticipated the birth of a healthy child, the recognition of a defect is inevitably shocking. They will, of course, vary in their reaction, but all will undergo a period of mourning. There may be denial, or an angry reaction, with which medical and nursing staff will have to cope. Most parents will at some stage have guilt feelings and these will need to be dispelled. Some may reject the child, others over-indulge and thus increase the potential for handicap.

Breaking the news of disability requires the greatest sensitivity of the doctor. Both parents should be present, and the interview should be conducted in private, though other professionals who may be in continuing contact with the family should be included if possible. A second interview should follow within a day or two, and several may be needed.

The recent development of imaging techniques allowing the recognition of impairment before birth has complicated the process of informing parents, and many examples have occurred of incorrect advice being given before the birth of a child.

When active intervention, such as emergency surgery, is required in the newborn period, parents often cope well because of the perception that something is being done for their child. However, if disability remains after surgery, the effect on the family may more closely resemble that of the second setting described below.

2. Disability recognized gradually

There is a large number of infants whose disability is not apparent at birth, although the risk of disability may be evident in many.

Examples are the premature infant, especially the very low birthweight group, those with a family history of genetic disorders lacking clear-cut laboratory markers, and infants asphyxiated at birth.

It is important that disabilities should be recognized early. This applies particularly in the deaf and the blind, where early intervention programmes are of the utmost importance. On the other hand, the labelling of a child as 'at risk' can imperil family and social relationships. A balance must be struck, and judgement made about the timing of communication of concern to the parents. Perhaps because there is no clear-cut time at which the grief reaction occurs and is resolved, the gradual recognition of disability may more often be followed by long drawn-out adverse parental reactions than in those cases recognized at birth. Expert paediatric opinion should be sought when the question of possible disability is raised by parents.

3. Development of disability in a previously normal child

In some respects, this setting resembles that of the child disabled at birth, in that a defined grief reaction is likely to occur, although often modified by the anxieties surrounding an active treatment period. The situation is made more complex by the anger felt at the loss of a loved and healthy child, and family breakdown may occur. The risks of super-added emotional disturbance are particularly high in the adolescent, and great skills are required to manage impairments occurring at that time.

Diagnosis

In the past, the diagnosis of disability has sometimes consisted in the labelling of the underlying impairment, and the medical profession has often been criticized for not proceeding beyond that point. That is not to say that precise diagnosis of the impairment is unimportant. It is essential for accurate genetic counselling and often required for proper therapeutic interventions, and not least may end the otherwise endless search undertaken by some parents for an explanation of their child's disability. Nevertheless, the second component of diagnosis, the identification and assessment of disability, is equally important, and has been greatly enhanced by the evolution of multidisciplinary assessment and management teams.

AUDITORY HANDICAP (DEAFNESS)

The extent to which an auditory impairment results in handicap depends upon the ability to hear and understand normal speech, for this is a prerequisite for language development. At birth, hearing is reflexic, so that a moderately intense sound elicits a startle response. Progressively, from about two to four months a less intense sound, such as the mother's voice, elicits learned responses, and by about eight months the infant turns head and eyes to localize a sound.

For the reasons outlined above, the frequency of auditory handicap in children is not precisely established. Mild degrees of hearing loss are very common and are due to chronic otitis media with effusion, or glue ear. There is much controversy about the effects of this condition on hearing and speech development, and about its treatment. These aspects are discussed in Chapter 71. More severe degrees of auditory impairment which undoubtedly affect language development and communication are much less common, with a frequency of about 2 children per 1000.

Significant risk factors for deafness are as follows:

1. Family history of deafness
2. Congenital anomalies of the ear, nose and throat
3. Antenatal virus infections, especially rubella and cytomegalovirus
4. Low birthweight
5. Neonatal jaundice
6. Apgar score at birth less than 5
7. Administration of toxic drugs
8. Cerebral palsy, especially athetoid.

Despite the length of this list, attempts to detect deafness early by the establishment of 'at risk registers' have been unsuccessful. A large proportion of those ultimately found to be deaf come from groups not listed above.

The most important advice for those concerned to detect deafness early is never to ignore the suspicion of a parent that their child may be deaf.

Causes of deafness and techniques for its detection are discussed in Chapter 71. In Australia routine hearing testing is conducted in infant welfare centres at about eight months of age, making use of the expected turning of the infant's head and eyes to familiar sound at that age. Useful though such screening may be, there is a high rate of false results, both positive and negative. For this reason, it is essential that the routine infant welfare centre test not be relied upon as evidence of normal hearing if there is any reason to suspect impairment, such as parents' concern or delayed or disordered speech development. Skilled audiological testing is available through the National Acoustic Laboratories Hearing Centres and through major paediatric institutions. Even in such centres, repeated testing may be required to exclude important degrees of hearing loss in infants and young children.

Management

In many cases of conductive deafness, treatment of the cause is available (see Ch. 71). For most other forms of deafness, treatment of the cause is not possible, although cochlear implants have been developed which may prove useful in selected cases. For most children reliance must be placed on hearing aids, which are supplied by the Commonwealth free of charge.

Auditory training

Even in the most severe cases of deafness, residual hearing can be used to enable some instruction in speech. With the use of hearing aids very early, in the first two months of life, there is every possibility that some speech will be learned.

Speech training

Speech is normally learned by auditory, kinaesthetic and tactile feedback mechanisms. When the auditory loop is impaired, the other mechanisms have to be used. Speech pathologists are highly trained professionals whose skills are essential in the management of the deaf child.

General measures

The ultimate aim of training is to enable the child to take an effective place in a hearing society. Usually, the mother is the key person in this and her role must be clearly and fully explained to her. Most deaf children can and should be educated in a normal school, supported by necessary educational aids. A child should not be excluded from a normal school simply because of deafness, although attendance at a special school may be necessary on a short-term or ancillary basis. For children with multiple impairments, special schools may still be required. Such schools and preschools are conducted by the various State Governments and also by other groups throughout the country. Some are residential, to provide for the needs of country children, or the multiply disabled, but residential requirements should not provide an excuse for exclusion of deaf children from normal schools.

Speech therapy is available through State education departments, through larger hospitals and by private speech pathologists. Other important needs of the deaf such as dissemination of information, social action and advocacy are provided by centres and associations for the deaf.

VISUAL HANDICAP (BLINDNESS)

Vision is a primary mode of learning. It is not fully developed at birth, although the full-term infant sustains momentary eye contact and tracks a light source briefly. Prolonged eye contact and responsive smiling occur during the second month, but visual attention to small detail is not evident until about eight months.

Definition and prevalence

Various definitions of blindness have been used. WHO defines blindness as 'best visual acuity less than 3/60'. In Australia, a legal definition used for determination of eligibility for government benefits is 'bilateral corrected visual acuity less than 6/60; if visual acuity is better than this then collateral visual impairments (e.g. visual field defects) may be included'.

Given the variations and lack of precision in definitions, it is hardly surprising that the reported prevalence of visual impairment in childhood varies considerably. A figure of 1 in 2500 for Victorian children is similar to that quoted in the UK. In third world countries, potentially preventable nutritional and infective causes of blindness lead to a much higher prevalence.

Aetiology

Diseases of the eye are considered in Chapter 70. It should be noted that about 40% of blind children have an associated impairment, most usually intellectual, motor or both, and exclusion of the multiply impaired often distorts published data. An approximate order of frequency of causes of blindness in children is:

1. Cortical blindness
2. Optic atrophy
3. Choroidoretinal degenerations
4. Cataracts
5. Retinopathy of prematurity.

Almost half of the causes of blindness in developed countries are genetically determined, in contrast to the nutritional and infective causes which predominate in much of the third world.

Diagnosis

In general, the diagnosis of blindness is less often made late as occurs with deafness. Exceptions are those cases where blindness is part of multiple handicap, and where the visual impairment is not of severe degree or is progressive.

Most often, visual impairments are recognized when the developmental pattern outlined above fails to occur, but the presence of risk factors such as family history, extreme prematurity and perinatal asphyxia are indicators for early formal assessment of visual function.

Wandering nystagmus or cataracts may be obvious, and later, rocking movements of the head and eyeball poking may be clues to the diagnosis. Congenital glaucoma, although rare, requires early expert intervention, and the appearance of a large eye in a newborn is an indication for immediate ophthalmological consultation.

Management

The intimate relationship of mother to infant necessary for normal development requires that in the blind child the missing visual stimuli be replaced by voice and touch, and that any residual visual function be used to the full. All members of the family must be alerted to the need for alternative stimuli. Home visiting services are available through the various state organizations to counsel families in this process, and they should be used even when the diagnosis of visual impairment is only suspected. Nothing is lost if vision turns out to be adequate, but a great deal is lost if early stimulation is not provided.

In some cases, ophthalmological interventions such as correction of refractive errors, squint surgery and cataract extraction can correct the impairment and early specialist referral should be made. Amblyopia, a reduction in central visual acuity, may occur if a visual impairment is not corrected. This is thought to be due to poor retinal images during the critical early years leading to impairment of neuronal development of visual pathways.

Education

Home-based services and parent support systems should lead on to kindergarten and preschool placements. Increasingly such placements are made in normal kindergartens, supported by counsellors from State education departments and associations for the blind, but in some cases special preschools are required. At school age too, placement in a normal school with teaching aids is preferred to placement in a special school but, for the multiply impaired, special schools, often residential, are available and are sometimes required. Although most blind children transfer from formal education to job training after about year 9, a significant number complete secondary and tertiary education and take their place as independent members of society.

The doctor's role in the care of handicapped children

Whatever the nature of the impairment, there are certain principles which apply to the care of handicapped children and their families, many of which will be apparent from the discussions above. These may be summarized as follows:

1. Early identification of the impairment.

2. Diagnosis, which includes precise classification of the impairment, usually requiring consultant paediatric opinion, and definition of the resulting disability.

3. Review of the family and social setting to identify potential strengths and weaknesses.

4. Recruitment of necessary immediate practical support measures usually through a social worker.

5. Treatment of those components of the impairment which are treatable, and the establishment of a management programme for residual disabilities, usually by a specialist team.

6. Provision of normal medical services such as immunizations and management of intercurrent illness.

7. Regular reassessment of disability and the management resources required.

The application of these principles requires a team approach, using personnel and resources from many agencies. The central role of the family doctor may be impaired unless a conscious effort at communication is made by all parties.

Special resources for the handicapped child

Although emphasis has been placed on the desirability of use of mainstream facilities for the handicapped child, many special resources are required. These include:

1. Provision of special equipment, such as splints, wheelchairs and surgical appliances. The Commonwealth provides annual funding for the Programme of Aids for Disabled People (PADP) administered by the States through PADP agencies at a number of public hospitals, available for disabled children living at home.

2. Home help. Many local councils provide subsidized home help.

3. Genetic counselling. In the past this has been provided by members of the management team. Increasingly, geneticists from major paediatric hospitals are providing regionally based services, and the importance of accurate diagnosis and skilled counselling has been emphasized.

4. Special schools. It will be evident from the foregoing discussion that the trend is away from segregation of the disabled, whether for education or residential care. However, with certain severe or multiple disabilities the child cannot attend a normal school and special schools are provided. These are usually run by private non-profit societies receiving varying degrees of government support, and often provide residential accommodation for the geographically isolated.

5. Parent discussion groups. Groups which began simply to allow parents to meet each other, discuss their difficulties and obtain mutual support, have assumed an important advocacy role, and many of the improvements in services for the handicapped can be attributed to the political effectiveness of parent groups.

6. Child disability allowance. An allowance is paid by the Commonwealth Department of Community Services and Health to parents or guardians of handicapped children under the age of 16 years living in the family home and needing constant attention, and to dependent students aged 16 to 25. It is intended to supplement normal family allowances, and help with education, training, transport and general welfare of the handicapped child.

7. Invalid pensions. A pension is paid by the Commonwealth Government Department of Social Security to those handicapped individuals over the age of 16 years on advice from a medical practitioner.

The decision to recommend a handicapped children's allowance or invalid pension requires sensitive consideration. Once the pension is provided, it is difficult for the disabled individual to regard himself as other than handicapped, and its recommendation should be the occasion for appropriate counselling, often by a skilled social worker.

The law in Australia recognizes the needs of the handicapped, and the Equal Opportunity (Discrimination Against Disabled Persons) Act 1982 makes it an offence to discriminate against a handicapped person.

FURTHER READING

Forfar J O (ed) 1988 Child health in a changing society. Oxford University Press, Oxford

Haggerty R J (ed) 1984 Chronic disease in children. The Pediatric Clinics of North America 31:1. W B Saunders

Scheiner A P, Moonaw M 1982 Care of the visually handicapped child. Paediatrics in Review 4: 3, 74–81

World Health Organization 1980 International classification of impairments, disabilities, and handicaps. WHO, Geneva

18. The intellectually disabled child

Philip Graves

DEFINITION

Children who have intellectual disabilities share with all children a potential for growth and development, individual aspirations and susceptibility to environmental factors. They need even more nurturing, tolerance and education from their parents, caregivers and society than their non-disabled peers. Their intellectual impairments manifest as delays in psychomotor development, behavioural problems or difficulties with schooling. Intellectual function cannot be measured directly but can be deduced from assessment of skills in a number of different areas. The most reliable indirect measure is the IQ test, although results are not consistent and are influenced by cultural and environmental factors.

In the past IQ tests have been misused by people more concerned with reinforcing social and racial prejudices. The original purpose of IQ tests and still their only valid use is in the identification of children who would benefit from additional assistance (Gould 1984).

Application of an IQ test to a population produces the standard bell-shaped normal distribution curve (Fig. 18.1).

The mean is set at 100 and 2 standard deviations below the mean (70 on most tests) is usually defined as the lower limit of 'normality'.

The definition of intellectual disability used by the American Association of Mental Deficiency reflects these issues: 'Significantly subaverage general intellectual functioning, existing concurrently with deficits inadaptive behaviour and manifested during the developmental period' (Grossman 1977). 'Significantly subaverage' is usually interpreted as more than two standard deviations below the mean. 'Existing concurrently with deficits in adaptive behaviour' reflects the limitations of IQ testing and the need to take into account how a person functions in everyday life. 'Manifested during the developmental period' excludes disabilities that result from cerebral insults occurring in adult life.

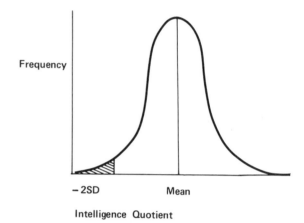

Fig. 18.1   Frequency distribution of IQ.

Intellectual disability is further subdivided by the World Health Organization into mild (IQ 50–70); moderate (IQ 35–49); severe (IQ 20–34) and profound (IQ below 20) categories.

PREVALENCE

Prevalence estimates for intellectual disabilities vary from 1–7% with most figures being in the range of 1.5–3%. (Table 18.1; Kiely 1987). The range is due to differences in the definition of intellectual disability, differences in methodology and true differences in prevalence. Some studies use 75 rather than 70 as the lower limit of normal. Examination of the normal distribution curve illustrates that this variation will dramatically increase the number of children included. Case detection may be by notification, registration of children enrolled for a service (both of which are likely to underestimate true prevalence) or by population screening using an IQ test. The latter method is most reliable, but because of financial, practical and ethical considerations, is not often used.

Table 18.1 Prevalence estimates for intellectual disability

Source	Location	Age	Prevalence (%) IQ 0–49	IQ 50–70
Rutter et al	Isle of Wight United Kingdom	5–14	0.34	2.53
Hagberg et al 1981	Gothenburg Sweden	8–12	0.3	0.37
Rantakallio & von Wendt 1986	Northern Finland	14	0.63	0.56
McQueen et al 1986	Maritime provinces, Canada	7–10	0.32	

Prevalence estimates often indicate higher rates for school-age children than for older or younger children. This fact is more likely to reflect difficulties of detection rather than true variation. Children with intellectual disabilities are more likely to present with problems at school than as preschoolers or school leavers. The studies summarized in Table 18.1 are based on total population surveys.

AETIOLOGY

Early discussion on causation focused on the organic versus non-organic aspects and on the effects of environmental factors (Penrose 1972). Some children may be classified as intellectually disabled simply because they fall, naturally, at the lower end of the normal distribution curve (see Fig. 18.1), whilst others are intellectually disabled as a result of malformation, organic injury or social environmental factors. Social and environmental factors are normally associated with mild

intellectual disability although they may be a contributing factor in more severely affected children. A specific organic cause can be found in 70–90% of children with moderate and severe intellectual disability and in up to 45% of children with mild intellectual disability (Mackay 1977). Mackay highlights the importance of aetiology because it provides a basis for accurate genetic counselling, prediction of outcome, preventive strategies and parent support. It is helpful to grieving families to know why their child is disabled. The data summarized in Figure 18.2 is based on Swedish epidemiological studies (Hagberg et al 1981).

The more common associations with intellectual disability are listed in Example 18.1.

The same range of factors are implicated in the aetiology of mild intellectual disability although the proportion in which a specific cause can be identified is much lower (see Fig. 18.2).

DIAGNOSIS

There are two tasks:

1. To establish that an intellectual disability is present, and
2. To identify the cause.

Does the child have an intellectual disability?

Children with intellectual disabilities may present in the following four ways:

1. In the neonatal period with recognizable malformations which are usually associated with intellectual disability (e.g. Down syndrome).
2. With developmental delay. The more severe the delay the earlier these children are likely to present.

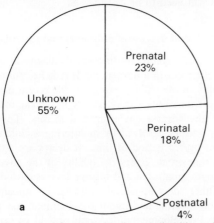

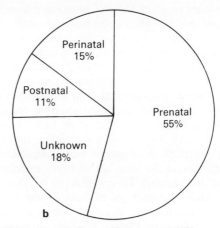

Fig. 18.2 Aetiological factors in intellectual disability: **a** IQ 50–70; **b** IQ less than 50. *Source*: Hagberg et al 1981.

Example 18.1 Aetiology of intellectual disability

Prenatal factors

Genetic
Fragile-X syndrome
Tuberous sclerosis
Neurofibromatosis
Metabolic and storage disorders
Chromosome abnormalities
Down syndrome
Trisomy 18
Cri du Chat syndrome
Sex chromosome abnormalities
Dysmorphic syndromes
Prenatal infections
Drugs and toxins

Perinatal factors

Hypoxia
Trauma
Infections
Biochemical abnormalities

Postnatal factors

Trauma
Hypoxia
Meningitis
Encephalitis
Poisons

---

3. As a result of surveillance of infants at increased risk of developmental problems (e.g. infants with a very low birthweight).

4. With feeding or behavioural problems which on investigation are found to be associated with intellectal disability.

Often parents of children with intellectual disabilities suffer unnecessary hardship as a result of inappropriate reassurance. Diagnosis of the presence of intellectual disability relies on a high index of suspicion followed by comparison of the child's performance with age-appropriate norms. Retrospective recollections of developmental milestones are seldom useful, but milestones recorded at the time (often in infant welfare books) and comparisons with siblings at similar ages are valuable. Once a developmental delay is suspected it is appropriate to use a developmental screening test such as the Denver Developmental Screening Test (Frankenburg et al 1971). These tests are useful in that they compare the child's development with a population of normal children at the same age and they examine all aspects of development. Their limitations are that they are not precise and they are of limited value once a specific disability has been identified. They are no more than a screening test. Once a disability is suspected

more detailed and specific testing and investigation is required.

Aetiological diagnosis

The history should include a family pedigree, details of the pregnancy, birth and neonatal history (including birthweight, length and head circumference), early feeding, psychomotor development and any specific illnesses.

The examination should record growth – especially head circumference. In a child with microcephaly, serial head circumference measurements may indicate the stage in the child's life when the cerebral insult occurred. The child's general responsiveness, the presence of dysmorphic features and any abnormalities of skin pigmentation should be noted. Full neurological examination should include assessment of vision and hearing. If there is a significant developmental delay it may be preferable to obtain specialist assessment of these functions. General physical examination should particularly include a search for other congenital abnormalities.

The history and examination will often lead to a specific aetiological diagnosis or at least limit the range of possibilities. Most children with moderate or severe intellectual disability warrant a chromosome analysis (which should include examination for fragile-X syndrome) cranial computerized tomography (CT) and screening tests on the urine for metabolic abnormalities. In many countries, including Australia, all newborn infants are routinely tested for phenylketonuria and hypothyroidism. In specific instances serology for congenital infections, tests of thyroid function, urinalysis for mucopolysaccharides, serum creatine phosphokinase, a maternal Guthrie test for maternal phenylketonuria and other specific tests for rare disorders will need to be considered.

Differential diagnosis of intellectual disability

The most common differential diagnosis is delayed development in a normal child. It is helpful to note the quality of the child's responses, the recent developmental progress, any family history of developmental delay and any adverse environmental factors. This dilemma may only be resolved by monitoring a child's development over a period of time. If delays are attributed to environmental factors the quality of the environmental changes monitored and organic factors excluded.

Other developmental disabilities; impairments of vision, hearing and motor development may present as global developmental delay and should be excluded.

Disorders associated with ongoing disease and deteriorating function such as muscular dystrophy, the mucopolysaccharide storage disorders, hypothyroidism, craniopharyngioma, and the neurodegenerative disorders may all present with delayed development. These conditions warrant consideration in any child who presents after a period of normal development or who has lost developmental skills.

SOME SPECIFIC CONDITIONS

Down syndrome

Down syndrome (Fig. 18.3) is the most common abnormality associated with intellectual disability and accounts for approximately 25% of children with an IQ less than 50. The incidence in Australia is approximately 1:1000 births. This is lower than in the past because of the reduced number of older women having babies and the availability of intrauterine diagnosis (see Table 18.2).

Approximately 95% of children with Down syndrome have standard trisomy 21; the remainder have additional

Table 18.2 Common neonatal characteristics of Down syndrome (Hall 1966)

Clinical features	Incidence (%)
Hypotonia	80
Poor Moro reflex	85
Hyperflexibility of the joints	80
Excess skin on the back of the neck	80
Flat facial profile	90
Slanted palpebral fissures	80
Anomalous auricles	60
Dysplasia of midphalanx of fifth finger	60
Single palmar crease	45

chromosome 21 material as translocation – D/G or G/G – or trisomy/normal mosaicism. The extra chromosome may be of maternal or paternal origin. In approximately one-third of cases it can be traced to the father and in two-thirds to the mother. The incidence of Down syndrome increases with increasing maternal age, rising to 1% over 40 years of age. Despite the higher incidence of Down syndrome in older women, the vast majority of mothers of children born with Down syndrome are aged 20–30 years.

The spectrum of intellectual disability in Down syndrome varies from mild to profound with most performances being in the moderate and severely disabled range. With active early education programmes some children are functioning at or above age-appropriate level. Despite this it is likely that the majority of children born with Down syndrome will have a significant intellectual disability.

Children with Down syndrome have increased susceptibility to infection. Congenital heart disease occurs in 60% of infants – one-third of whom have an atrioventricular canal and one-third a ventricular septal defect. Conductive deafness occurs in 60–80%, and many may benefit from hearing aids in early life. Visual impairments, hypothyroidism due to autoimmune thyroiditis are common as is duodenal atresia. Haematological abnormalities including leukaemias are approximately 20 times more common in Down syndrome than in the general population. Estimates of mean life expectancy at birth vary from 30–45 years although children who survive the infectious and cardiac hazards of infancy can be expected to live longer than this.

Fragile-X syndrome

Fragile-X syndrome is the second most common cause of intellectual disability (after Down syndrome). It occurs in 2–10 per 10 000 males. Intellectual disability may be mild, moderate or severe. In most cases there

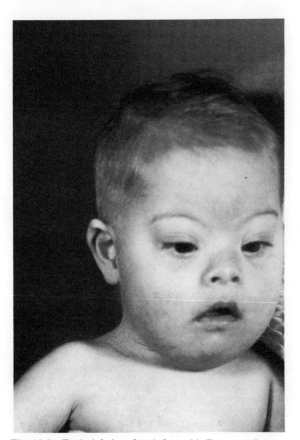

Fig. 18.3 Typical facies of an infant with Down syndrome.

are craniofacial characteristics (prominent forehead, large jaw and prominent ears) and orchidomegaly. Chromosome analysis, using a special culture medium, reveals a fragile site on the long arm of the X chromosome. The disorder is inherited as an X-linked recessive condition. Most but not all carrier females show the fragile site and up to 35% have a mild intellectual disability. The chromosome abnormality is not always apparent in carrier females and a few females inherit the abnormality from asymptomatic fathers with the abnormal X chromosome. In some cases there is the typical family history with or without the physical characteristics, but no chromosome abnormality (Hsiu-Zu et al 1988).

Autism

Autism is a developmental disability in which the principle impairments are in social communication. The prevalence is 2–4 per 10 000 and it is 2–4 times more common in males than in females. The diagnosis is made when there are characteristic abnormalities in each of the following areas:

1. Language: delay, minimal use of speech, echolalia.
2. Social interaction: poor eye contact, aloneness, difficulties in relating to peers.
3. Unusual pre-occupations or stereotypic behaviours: postural mannerisms, 'insistence on sameness', pre-occupations with objects or issues.
4. Onset before the age of 30 months.

Most children with autism are also intellectually disabled with the causes being similar to those listed for intellectual disabilities. Significant improvements are noted as these children grow older, but most retain specific communication and intellectual impairments.

Duchenne muscular dystrophy

10–15% of boys with muscular dystrophy have an intellectual disability which may cloud the clinical presentation. A serum creatinine phosphokinase estimation should be considered in all boys not walking by 18 months (see Ch. 48).

Neurofibromatosis and tuberous sclerosis

These conditions are both caused by autosomal dominant genes. They vary considerably in severity, have dermatological manifestations (see Ch. 69), and may be associated with intellectual disability.

Dysmorphic syndromes

There are a large number of rare, sporadic conditions in which characteristic patterns of malformation are usually associated with intellectual disability. The commoner of these are: Cornelia de Lange syndrome; Prader-Willi syndrome; Sotos syndrome (see Ch. 7).

THE EFFECTS OF INTELLECTUAL DISABILITY

For the affected child

Intellectual disability is associated with developmental delays, difficulties in acquiring new skills, communication impairments and social adjustment problems.

Children with mild intellectual disability often do not present until school age when they have major problems with learning to read and write and difficulties with social and interpersonal skills. As adults they can be expected to be capable of living independently and maintaining a job in open employment. Difficulties with reading, writing, handling money and interpersonal relationships are likely to persist.

Children with moderate intellectual disabilities will usually present with developmental delays in the pre-school years. They can be expected to have greater difficulties with educational learning and will require specific teaching to master basic social skills such as dressing, feeding, preparing food, using public transport and living independently. As adults they will be capable of productive employment and independent living although some ongoing support is likely to be needed.

Children with severe and profound intellectual disabilities will often have little or no speech and may require considerable assistance with dressing and feeding. They are capable of mastering new skills but progress will be very slow.

Approximately two-thirds of all children with intellectual disabilities have additional impairments of vision, hearing or motor function. Epilepsy is common and is often difficult to control. For all these children family stress, limited education, social rejection and sensory deficits may result in additional secondary disabilities.

For the family

The realization that their child has a disability is a major grief stress. Among the common manifestations of their grief are guilt and denial. These are often manifested by seeking multiple opinions and unorthodox treatments. Anger is common and often directed at doctors and hospitals. Occasionally there may be rejection of the child. Parents have to come to terms with their grief whilst simultaneously coping with a difficult child. Friends, relatives, doctors and other professionals are not always sensitive to their needs and coping with these is an additional burden. Many families will be forced to change their lifestyle and career plans. Usually, mothers are expected to carry the major caring burden and find it difficult to pursue a career and at the same time care for a child with an intellectual disability.

For the wider community

A prevalence rate of 1–3% and the move away from segregated services means that most people will have some contact with a person with an intellectual disability. Consumer pressure and public conscience increasingly demand tolerance, acceptance and material contributions from all sections of the community. Human services such as child care, kindergartens, schools, transport, libraries, and recreation facilities which are established for all children and families are expected to adapt to meet the needs of people with intellectual disabilities.

MANAGEMENT

Family support

Parents need to be told that their child has an intellectual disability openly, accurately and sensitively. Where doubt exists this should be discussed and, where appropriate, a second opinion sought. Often parents seek a second opinion and this should be supported. Stressful information should be given with both parents present. Written material should be provided and the information repeated at follow-up meetings with the family. Many parents find it helpful to talk with other families who have a disabled child and there are 'parent to parent' programmes to facilitate this. Later, drop-in centres, toy libraries, disability support and advocacy groups, and respite care will be used. Programmes which facilitate interaction between families who have a disabled child and other families in the community are available to provide further support.

Income support, assistance with health care costs and subsidized home support will be available to many families. In Australia, most families who have a child with a significant intellectual disability are eligible for the child disability allowance. Transport subsidies, in-home assistance, free or heavily subsidized orthotic equipment, wheelchairs and special seating are also available.

Children's services

The pattern of service provision to children with intellectual disabilities is changing. Increasingly playgroups, kindergartens and schools which encourage integration of children with intellectual disabilities with non-disabled children are replacing segregated facilities. Integration is based on philosophies of human rights and normalization. Normalization evolved in Scandinavia in the 1960s. It stresses individual dignity, choice and the value of the same everyday life activities and routines for disabled people as are experienced by non-disabled people (Nirje 1985). Segregated services which offer more specialized intervention, a more tolerant environment and higher staff ratios are still seen as more appropriate for some children.

Few data based principles are available to guide families in the selection of appropriate services. It is helpful to look at the philosophies and professional standards of the service.

In general, services which (a) are sufficiently flexible to respond to the child and family's needs; (b) acknowledge the value of normal life experiences, the importance of the family and interaction with non-disabled children; (c) establish management aims and monitor progress, are the most likely to be helpful.

Residential care

Many families will benefit from short-term residential care and a few will need long-term residential care for their child. If parents feel they cannot care for their child at home it is seldom effective or helpful to attempt to persuade them otherwise. Parents should be assisted to find the option that best suits their needs. Foster care (both short and long term), adoption, small community based residential houses, nursing homes and larger residential units may be available to meet these needs.

The doctor's role

Many professionals, including teachers, therapists, social workers and psychologists have useful contributions to make to children with intellectual disabilities. Doctors, who are usually the pivotal figures in the early diagnostic phases, should be well informed about child and family services so that they can properly advise families. They will need to be aware of associated conditions such as epilepsy, sensory deficits and cardiac anomalies and ensure that these are detected early. As the child grows older the doctor's role will become more peripheral. However, there will still be a need to treat associated conditions and intercurrent illnesses, and provide information and advice to families. The family doctor may also be asked to assist the child and family as an advocate for appropriate services.

PREVENTION

The cornerstone of prevention is accurate understanding of the causes of intellectual disability in the community. Without this data, prevention planning must be based on assumptions drawn from studies on populations that may or may not be similar. Thus monitoring the efficacy of prevention strategies will be difficult. Detection of families at high risk of genetic abnormalities, followed by genetic counselling and intrauterine diagnosis will prevent a small number of cases. However, it must be appreciated that the majority of infants with genetic abnormalities are born of families who were not considered to be at high risk. Measures to reduce alcohol and cigarette consumption are likely to reduce mild intellectual disability. Further research and continued monitoring of birth defects and potential environmental teratogens are needed to identify new and unknown causes. Immunization programmes, particularly those against measles and rubella will reduce cases due to these agents. Improvements in antenatal and neonatal care and measures to ensure that these services are accessible to all sections of the community are likely to have a small effect. Further reductions in this area must await research leading to the prevention of prematurity. Neonatal screening for treatable conditions is already preventing most cases of intellectual disability due to phenylketonuria and hypothyroidism. Traffic management, bicycle helmets, seat restraints, drink-driving legislation, swimming pool safety regulations, and measures to reduce child abuse, will reduce intellectual disability due to brain injury. Continued improvements in community education and standards of living are likely to be associated with a reduction in incidence, particularly of mild intellectual disability (Ministerial Review 1986).

REFERENCES

Frankenburg W K, Goldstein A D, Camp B W 1971 The revised Denver developmental screening test: its accuracy as a screening instrument. Journal of Paediatrics 79: 988–995

Gould S J 1984 The mismeasure of man. Penguin, London

Grossman H J 1977 Manual on terminology and classification in mental retardation. American Association of Mental Deficiency, Washington DC p 5

Hagberg B, Hagberg G, Lewerth A et al 1981 Mild mental retardation in Swedish school children I: prevalence. Acta Paediatrica Scandinavica 70: 441–444

Hall B 1966 Mongolism in newborn infants. Clinical Pediatrics (Philadelphia) 5: 4

Hsiu-Zu H, Glahn T J, Ju-Chang H 1988 The fragile-X syndrome. Developmental Medicine and Child Neurology 30: 257–261

Kiely M 1987 The prevalence of mental retardation. Epidemiologic Reviews 9: 194–218

Mackay R I 1977 The causes of mental handicap. Developmental Medicine and Child Neurology 24: 386–388

McQueen P C, Spence M W, Winsor E J T, Garner J B, Pereira L H 1986 Causal origins of major mental handicap in the Canadian maritime provinces. Developmental Medicine and Child Neurology 28: 697–707

Ministerial Review 1986 Health education and promotion in Victoria. Government Printer, Melbourne p 59–63

Nirje B 1985 The basis and logic of the normalization principle. Australia and New Zealand Journal of Developmental Disabilities II: 65–68

Penrose L S 1972 The biology of mental defect. Sidgwick and Jackson, London Chapter IV

Rantakallio P, von Wendt L 1986 Mental retardation in a birth cohort of 12 000 children in northern Finland. American Journal of Mental Deficiency 90: 380–387

Rutter M, Tizard J, Whitmore K 1970 Education health and behaviour. Longman, London

FURTHER READING

Frankenburg W K, Dodds J B 1967 The Denver developmental screening test. Journal of Paediatrics 71: 181

Jenkinson J C 1987 School and disability: research and practice in integration. Australian Education Review No. 26

Lane D, Stratford B 1985 Current approaches to Down's syndrome. Praeger, New York

19. The family in difficulty

M. J. Robinson

In our society, a loving, secure and happy family life is by no means the rule. Perhaps the rate of divorce provides the best evidence for this. The divorce rate in Australia in 1971 was 14%, but has risen to 35% in 1987. Part, but by no means all, of this increase is explained by the ease of obtaining divorces in this country. Prior to 1976 the Matrimonial Causes Act required five years separation as a minimum period for 'no fault' divorce. Fault divorce could be obtained in a shorter time. After January 1976, the sole requirement became 12 months separation. The percentage of marriages that end in divorce is even greater when one or both of the partners has been married previously. Family break-up is now such that 16% of children can expect to experience the divorce of their parents before they reach the age of 16 years. Many other marriages end in separation without divorce, and an even greater number of marriages exist in name only. Other at risk families include single parent families, de facto relationships, migrant families and families of minority ethnic groups, such as Aboriginals.

The causes of marital disharmony are many – some couples cannot cope with family life because they are either emotionally and/or intellectually inadequate or because they are just too immature. Others may find the financial commitments of family life are beyond their ability to cope. Other marriages break up because of alcoholism, drug dependence or, at the present time, because of unemployment. Some parents become so involved in their separate careers that they are either unwilling or unable to meet the needs of their children. In lower socio-economic groups the remaining parent will have difficulty providing for the physical needs of their children. In all social groups where there is family break-up the children will suffer emotional deprivation. Many will suffer from lack of intellectual stimulation particularly if the mother is depressed.

IDENTIFICATION OF THE FAMILY IN DIFFICULTY

The family in difficulty may be identified in various ways:

1. In cases where there is actual deprivation because of financial hardship, a parent may apply directly to a community agency for help.

2. On occasions neighbours may report the situation to the community welfare services department or even to the police.

3. A more subtle presentation, and one which should alert the doctor or health professional, is the development of certain organic symptoms in the child. Children react to stress in a variety of ways, and, depending upon the age of the child, the symptoms vary. Symptoms suggesting stress in the small infant are difficulties with feeding and sleep. Recurrent abdominal pain, headache, school failure and difficulty in making peer relationships should alert the doctor to stress and anxiety in the older child. In adolescence antisocial behaviour, school refusal, the taking of drugs, and deliquency are common symptoms.

4. A not uncommon presentation is for an isolated and frequently depressed mother to take her child repeatedly to the health centre, to a hospital, or to the local practitioner for trivial complaints – the mother being either unwilling or unable to directly admit to the underlying problem.

5. An increasingly frequent mode of presentation is one of child abuse (see Ch. 21).

The following discussion identifies certain family groups at risk for breakdown, e.g. single parent, migrant and Aboriginal families. However, it should not be inferred that these families invariably have problems. Many of these groups cope very well indeed and provide optimal conditions for the health of their children.

SOLE-PARENT FAMILIES

At present, 12.7% of Australia's 2 042 727 families with dependent children are sole-parent families (Fig. 19.1). Recent surveys have suggested that in the near future upwards of 1 in 5 children born in Australia will spend a significant part of their childhood in a one-parent family. While the majority of lone parents are mothers, a significant number of fathers are now undertaking full responsibility for families. Clearly, one-parent families must now be regarded as a legitimate variation of traditional Australian family life.

Desertion of the family and divorce comprises the largest group of one-parent families. Other causes are death of a parent, voluntary separation, father in prison or in mental institutions and unmarried mothers wishing to keep their babies rather than have them adopted.

The lifestyle of one-parent families varies a great deal. A minority of single parents, through superior intelligence, drive, energy, help from relatives and friends, together with an intense love for their children, cope very well, so that the needs of the children are met in every way. Much more often the mother finds it difficult to cope through lack of financial and other types of support, intellectual inadequacy, immaturity, etc. The result, of course, is family malfunction.

Problems of the sole parent

Financial

Inadequate finance is the most obvious problem and occurs most often. Very few fatherless families are securely economically and at least 30% have an income below the poverty line. Where the husband has died, the widow may benefit from insurance, worker's compensation or superannuation payments, but more often these are either not available or very small and the widow has to face debts accumulated during her husband's terminal illness. Also, in cases of divorce and voluntary separation, the woman is financially disadvantaged, but not to the same extent as the deserted wife or the wife whose husband is in prison or in a mental institution. The unmarried mother is invariably in a poor financial position. The widow is more likely to receive sympathy and assistance from relatives, friends and the community. However, in the other sole-parent categories there is usually less sympathy and assistance and very often a critical community attitude. Few fatherless families will have private means and only a minority of these mothers will be able to obtain employment outside the home. Even if employment is obtained, pensions tend to be reduced on the income earned, so that many sole parents believe it is not worth their while to take on outside employment. Therefore, it is not surprising that the majority of sole parents will largely be dependent upon social service benefits (Fig. 19.2).

Housing

Sole-partner families have problems in obtaining satisfactory housing. About 18% of fatherless families are

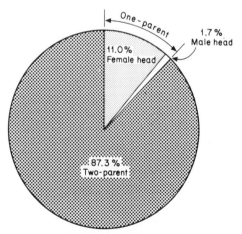

Fig. 19.1   Families with dependent children 1981. Notes: (a) Dependent children 0–15 years and full time students 16–20 years. (b) To overcome inflation of the proportion of one-parent families at the expense of two-parent families, one-parent families cross-classified as 'now married' have been counted as two-parent families. *Source*: ABS Census of Population & Housing, 1981.

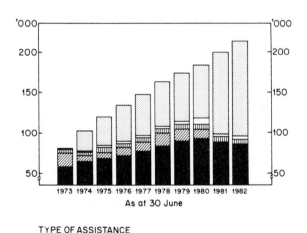

Fig. 19.2   Sole mothers in receipt of income support 1973–1982. *Source*: Department of Social Security (DSS) Annual Report 1982.

living as boarders in the households of others. This is compared with 2% of two-parent families. Although most are living with relatives, a valued freedom – the ability to live as a family in one's own house – is lost. Tenancy is far more common in sole-parent families as few are able to purchase their own homes. Housing commissions, through the provision of cheap rents, have made a very important contribution to the housing of many needy families and this certainly includes sole-parent families. Unfortunately, not all sole-parent families who wish to, can obtain accommodation through housing commissions, so that many will live in expensive, but sub-standard homes in overcrowded areas with inadequate space for child recreation. At present, it is estimated that some 30% of fatherless families are so accommodated.

Social problems

A large number of sole parents suffer considerable social isolation. Some will have severed relations with families and old friends, but for those who have not, maintaining contact with relatives and former friends may be difficult, not the least because of the costs of transport involved. Also, lack of funds will produce problems in respect to other social activities, for example, taking children to parks, zoo, theatres, etc. Because of the persistence of old community attitudes, many unmarried and some deserted mothers will be oppressed by feelings of guilt and shame, so that, in addition to loneliness, periods of apathy and overt depression will be common. This will compound the difficulties in child rearing and the stresses will be such that there is less time to devote to the children, less patience and a consequent reduction in the quality of parenting in many instances. It is not surprising that the incidence of child abuse in single-parent families is disproportionately high.

Problems for the child in sole-parent families

Often, the problems faced by the mother as a single parent affect the children. Thus, intellectual and emotional stimulation cannot always be adequately provided.

For example, children of one-parent families are generally less likely to be given adequate books and toys in their early years and extracurricular activities such as ballet, music and sporting opportunities during schooling. Children of sole parents are also less likely to obtain postsecondary school education. Therefore, many will grow up poorly prepared for adult life and it is not surprising that this cycle of poverty, deprivation and underachievement is maintained in the next generation. Additional assistance from government and the community must be provided to this large and increasing population if the current situation is to improve.

ALCOHOL AND THE FAMILY

Alcohol is the most widely used and abused drug in our society and its consumption is steadily increasing. Australia is the tenth largest consumer of alcohol per head. It seems that the drinking of alcohol is not only accepted, but is expected social behaviour in Australia. The amounts of alcohol consumed by Australians in 1970 and 1976 are shown in Table 19.1. There are good reasons to believe that the amount of alcohol consumed at present has increased.

Adult drinking patterns are related to sex, age, socioeconomic class and to the ethnic group. The Australia-wide survey on alcohol (1977) showed that three-quarters of all adult men over the age of 18, and one-half of all adult females are drinkers. Some 18% of men and 2% of women drink more than an average of 40 grams of alcohol per day. The survey reported also that 4% of men and 0.2% of women consume over 80 grams of alcohol a day – a level widely regarded as damaging to health. The number of persons drinking, the frequency and the amount drunk, reaches its highest level between the mid–20s and the mid–40s.

Recent surveys in Australia have shown that the number of adolescents drinking has increased since 1970. In one survey (1985) 56% of year 7 students (aged 12–13 years), 80% of year 9 students (14–15 years) and 92% of year 11 students (16–17 years) had taken alcohol on at least one occasion (see Fig. 19.3). The same survey noted that the frequency of adolescent drinking in-

Table 19.1 Consumption of alcoholic beverages

Year	Beer	Wine	Spirits	Estimated total
Total consumption ('000 litres)				
1970	1 532 328	110 856	12 657	102 837
1976	1 903 040	180 765	15 901	134 362
Consumption per head of population (litres)				
1970	123.5	8.9	1.0	9.3
1976	137.4	13.1	1.2	9.9*

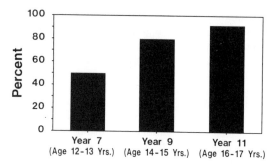

Fig. 19.3 Frequency of alcohol use amongst groups of students.

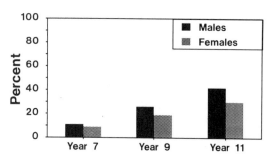

Fig. 19.4 Percentage of males, females who had at least five drinks in a row in the previous two weeks.

creased with age, and amongst year 11 students 45% had taken alcohol in the previous week. Figure 19.4 indicated the percentage of males and females at each level studied who had taken at least five alcoholic drinks in a row in the previous two weeks.

Amongst tertiary students, 90% admit that they drink alcohol and about 7% drink every day or on most days. Amongst male apprentices, 93% take alcohol and about 43% drink alcohol at least several times per week. More young males drink than females, but the difference is small. However, the incidence of heavy drinking is greatly increased in males compared to females. In all age groups the incidence of drinking is greatest in the lower socioeconomic classes. Australians originating from Western and Central Europe generally consume more alcohol than those of Southern European extraction and from South East Asia.

Alcohol and health

The Commonwealth Department of Health has estimated that alcohol is a major factor in about 3% of all deaths in Australia each year. This amounts to some 30 000 deaths over the last 10 years. Some 10% of ad-

missions to mental health institutions are due to alcohol and at least 10% of admissions to public hospitals are the result of alcohol intake. The physical complications of alcohol tend to occur in a minority of adolescent alcoholics; for example, alcoholism may be present for 10 to 15 years before evidence of definite liver disease becomes apparent. The systems chiefly affected in chronic alcoholism are the alimentary tract with gastritis, peptic ulceration, pancreatitis and liver disease and the central nervous system. Also, it is well known that heavy drinking during pregnancy adversely affects the physical and mental development of the fetus – the fetal alcohol syndrome.

Alcohol and antisocial behaviour

There is a high correlation between alcohol abuse, crime and violence. Domestic violence – wife and child battering – very often related to heavy alcohol use and abuse. All available evidence suggests that driving under the influence of alcohol is the major factor causing death and injury on Australian roads. The major cause of death in young men aged 15–24 years is the combination of drinking and driving.

In industry, surveys have shown that the majority of alcoholics at work are performing jobs below the level of their training and experience. And, it has been estimated that by the age of 45 years nearly 50% of alcoholics will be unemployed.

Effects of alcoholism on the family

In the early stages the problem is usually denied both by the alcoholic and the family. When it is accepted, social isolation results because of feelings of guilt and shame. Disorganization of family life soon follows with consequent neglect of specific roles by the alcoholic which are then taken on by the spouse. The children suffer tremendous anxieties and unhappiness and many are severely emotionally disturbed as unpredictable and erratic behaviour and even neglect by parents engenders a cycle of mutual distrust, suspicion, resentment, bitterness and frustration. In many cases this results in antisocial activities in the children leading ultimately to alcoholism, drug-taking and criminal activities. Families of alcoholics move frequently, often to distant locations which results in further social isolation, often associated with a decline in the husband's occupational status. Financial stress is almost invariable, either because of loss of employment, or reduction in the husband's earning capacity. Thus, debts accumulate and legal problems arise. Also, these latter are often associated with minor nuisance charges, traffic offences, etc. Periodic or chronic illness or premature death of the breadwinner may further complicate the situation. Gradual deterioration of family relationships leading to separation or divorce is a common end result.

Management of the alcoholic

The treatment of alcoholism is both difficult and complex and will not be detailed here. A team approach is essential, and the team should consist of physicians supported by medical social workers, welfare officers, occupational therapists, clergymen, etc. Specialized medical and surgical expertise should be available when required. The treatment programme must involve the spouse and the family, as the whole family is profoundly affected. A tremendous amount of support and counselling to the alcoholic and family is basic to the management.

Facilities for the treatment of the alcoholic and family

The alcohol and drug services section of the health departments provide clinics for management and are located in all capital cities. Most community health centres have facilities for counselling alcoholics. Emergency accommodation is provided by State governments and certain religious groups. Alcoholics Anonymous is widely located throughout the country and can be consulted through the telephone directory. Also, some public hospitals provide counselling and treatment facilities.

THE ABORIGINAL FAMILY

The Aboriginal population of Australia, including Torres Strait Islanders, is at present about 205 000. This is equivalent to 1.5% of the total population of Australia.

The distribution by age groups of Aboriginals as a percentage, and compared to that of the Australian population, is shown in Table 19.2.

It can be seen that the percentage of Aboriginal children under the age of 14 years is 46.4% compared to 28.8% for the total Australian population. A similar population distribution is seen in the majority of underdeveloped societies through the world. It will also be apparent that there are fewer adult Aboriginal people so that less support will be available for dependents both young and old. These figures suggest that the Aboriginal family is large and households often overcrowded. Other surveys have shown that the distribution of occupation between Aboriginal people and other Australians is very different – only 3% are employed in professional, technical, administrative, executive or managerial positions; the figure for the remainder of the Australian population is about 17%. Only 3% of Aboriginal people occupy clerical positions as compared to almost 16% for other Australians.

The educational status of the Aboriginal people is also vastly inferior to that of the Australian population as a whole – only 5% between the ages of 20 and 24 years have been educated up to year 10 compared to 50% of the white population. A significant proportion of adult Aboriginal people have had little or no formal education whatsoever.

Overall housing conditions are poor for the Aboriginal family, for example, 30% of Aboriginal dwellings are without gas and electricity and 19% of Aboriginal homes do not contain a bathroom or a kitchen. This compares to 0.4% of the remainder of the Australian homes thus situated.

The health status of the Aboriginal is very much inferior. Infant mortality rates for Aboriginal people in the Northern Territory is some 3 times that of the Australian average of 10.3 per 1000 live births (1982) mainly because of gastroenteritis and pneumonia.

Dobbin (1977) surveyed the nutritional status of a group of Aboriginal children. He found the percentage of mild to moderate malnutrition to be 20.7% in urban areas and 50.6% in rural areas. Anaemia in the 6 to 23-month-old Aboriginal age group was noted in 25% of urban and 44.4% of rural dwellers. Birthweights too are significantly lower and the high incidence of morbidity in Aboriginal children is well known. Of particular importance is middle ear disease, chronic chest disease, bowel infections, parasitic infestations, skin disease and trachomas. Inadequately treated middle ear disease has resulted in hearing loss in many instances with subsequent language impairment and learning disability.

In the past the Aboriginal people have been at a significant disadvantage in law and, although the Commonwealth Government provides funds for an Aboriginal legal service in each State, there is adequate evidence that the Aboriginal people are still at a disadvantage; fortunately, this position is now improving

Table 19.2 Age groups of Aboriginals compared with the total Australian population (both expressed as percentages)

Age group	Aboriginal (%)	Total Australian population (%)
0–4	17.1	9.6
5–9	15.4	9.6
10–14	13.3	9.6
Total less than 14	45.8	28.8
15+	54.2	71.2
Total	100	100

following deliberations of the Australian Law Reform Commission.

Thus, it is obvious that the Aboriginal family are at a great disadvantage in virtually every respect. As mentioned, they have large families, they live in crowded and substandard homes, their educational status is low and their nutrition, hygiene, dental health and general health are substandard. In addition, the consumption of alcohol and substance abuse has now become a major problem with them. Aboriginal adults and children are grossly over-represented in corrective institutions.

Services available to the Aboriginal people

The following services are available:

1. The Federal Government, through its Department of Aboriginal and Ethnic Affairs, has made many significant grants to aid the Aboriginal people. These grants are directed to the various State Health Departments in the main.

2. The State governments are basically responsible for health care of the Aboriginal people through their departments of health. The most enlightened approach is that the problems of health educational programmes are directed by the Aboriginal people themselves. It is quite certain that curative medicine alone will never solve the Aboriginal health situation.

3. Services provided by Aboriginals – the Aboriginal people themselves conduct health services, child care agencies and legal aid for their own people.

4. There are a number of hostels – both Government and non-Government – to provide emergency accommodation.

THE MIGRANT FAMILY

Migration has been responsible for the majority of the Australian population increase since World War I. The birthplace of the Australian people from 1947 to 1981 and the places of origin of migrants are shown in Figure 19.5. From 1955 to 1976 migration from Continental Europe has outnumbered that from the British Isles. There has been some decrease in migration since a peak was reached in 1974. The current aim of the Federal Government is to maintain an intake of about 72 000 migrants per year which will include approximately

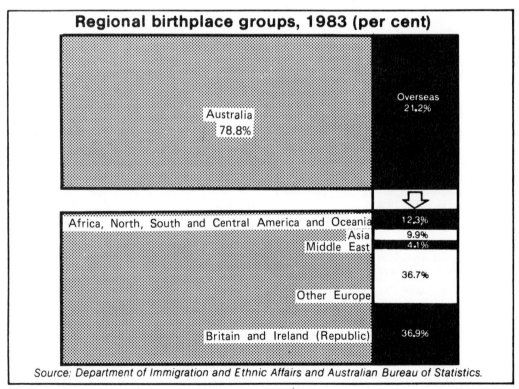

Fig. 19.5   Percentage of migrants in Australia and their places of origin.

15 000 people admitted as refugees and under other humanitarian programmes. These latter groups arrive largely from Indo-China, the Middle East, Latin America and Africa.

Settlement in a new country is a complex process of adjusting to a new environment. All migrants are affected but those coming from cultures different from that dominant in Australia and those without a well-established ethnic group here are particularly at risk. Its end point is the acceptance by and the feeling of belonging to the receiving society. Settlement takes a variable period of time from months to years. Difficulties for migrants are greatest immediately after arrival and these will be accentuated if inadequate arrangements for their initial settlement are made. There is good reason to believe that such arrangements have been less than adequate in the past in Australia.

Problems of migrants

Settlement

There is no doubt that many of the problems encountered by migrants and their families arise from inadequate arrangements for their initial settlement here. This may well explain why migrants tend to move from place to place, are more likely to be unemployed, change jobs often and are employed in jobs which are at a level below their true capacities. It is not surprising that many migrants suffer disillusionment and discontent soon after arriving in this country and that about 25% of them return to their country of origin. In addition, migrants accumulate often large debts through their passage to Australia, high rents and purchases of furniture and other household items immediately required. The majority of families migrating to this country come from lower socioeconomic groups and often the wife has to go out to work soon after arrival. It is easy to imagine the stresses placed upon the family if there are very young children involved.

Language

A lack of knowledge of English compounds the problems of migrant families. In particular this will result in:

1. Problems of finding employment, shopping and travelling to and from work.
2. Major problems of education of the children.
3. An ignorance of rights, duties and entitlements in health, in law and in income security.
4. A low level of community involvement due to ignorance through an inadequate orientation. This will lead to social isolation. A lack of representation, particularly in Government, will further disadvantage.
5. Isolation. Most migrants will have few or no friends on whom they can rely and in cases where families are available, they usually live some distance away. Depression is common among recently arrived migrant women.

Education

In 1974 a Government enquiry was made into the educational needs of migrant children in Australia. The enquiry indicated that there was little incorporation of the cultural heritage of migrant students into the learning process and few attempts made to allow students to identify with their own culture. There was a high incidence of educational failure, reading retardation and dropout rates amongst migrant children. In general, teachers were found to have a low expectation of migrants and the teachers themselves had received little special training for the teaching of migrant children. Often, non-migrant pupils in the class were bored because of repetitions of explanations given to migrant children with limited English. Taking migrant children out of classes for remedial English tuition had not been a great success and had intended to increase their sense of isolation. And migrant children were found to be self-conscious; there was a high absentee rate and a high transfer rate from school to school. Also, prejudices existed between the various ethnic groups, with alienation and discrimination. Because of this some parents even refused to send their children to school. Also there was a serious problem of communication between school and parents. Parents did not attend school functions, could not read notices sent out and they could not cope with the different system of education in this country compared to the one they had experienced. Extracurricular activities such as scouts, clubs, etc. were regarded with suspicion and rejected.

Sociocultural aspects

Migrants, while wishing to start a new life and improve the lot of their families, still wish to retain much of the culture of their former society. Therefore, they will tend to segregate and form ghettos. While this may resolve the cultural problem and help to relieve the loneliness, particularly of the wives, it is counter-productive in terms of learning English and integrating into the new society. This throws a particular strain on the children who are brought up only speaking their mother tongue. Because of a lack of knowledge of community facilities, a great number of migrant children do not attend infant health centres and preschool centres and commence their schooling with little or no English. This places a great strain on them, particularly when parents have high expectations for their future. In this country schools encourage the students to pursue personal goals. This may conflict with the role the Southern European families have placed on their children – that of strengthening the family and leaving it in a better position, both economically and socially, for the next generation. When children cannot realize these expectations, frustration occurs in the parents and a sense of failure in the children. Because of an inability to cope with the educational system, many migrant children develop personality problems and antisocial behaviour and ultimately gravitate to non-skilled occupations. Thus, at least in the first generation, the low socioeconomic status of the migrant is perpetuated. Strong cultural ties of some ethnic groups make it difficult for the children to make good social relationships outside their own ethnic group. Many ethnic groups actually discourage children from making such friends. These aspects must be appreciated if migrants are to be given meaningful assistance.

Often children are used as interpreters, which is clearly wrong, because parents are prone to become dependent on them with loss of face and authority. The children in turn often become impatient of their parents inability to learn English and tend to forget their native tongue so that interfamily relationships suffer even more. Many teachers express concern about what happens to children after school in cases where both parents work and such children have often been labelled as 'latch key' children. In addition, transition of migrant children from primary to secondary school has caused difficulties. Since 1974, the situation has improved, but much is still needed in the area of migrant education.

Community facilities to assist migrants

On arrival in Australia migrants may either go to one of a number of migrant hostels or directly into the community. Those going to hostels are usually those migrants who have come to Australia on assisted passages. Those migrants going directly into the community will be particularly those whose migration is self-motivated or has been sponsored by relatives or friends.

Within migrant hostels settlement officers co-ordinate the various activities of the initial settlement programme. These include:

1. An optional full-time six-week course in English.
2. An orientation programme designed to provide migrants with the necessary information for them to live in and cope in their new community.
3. Information in respect to housing through housing officers.

On leaving hostels, migrants are given a list of the community facilities available in the area where they will live.

Migrants who go directly into the community are contacted by an officer of the State Department of Immigration and Ethnic Affairs and provided with the essential information as discussed above.

Community settlement centres

The centres are sited in areas of high migrant density. They provide community based services for those who wish to participate in orientation and settlement programmes by daily attendance, and may provide: initial accommodation; an intensive course in English; and information about Australia, its Constitution and services.

Telephone interpreter service

This is an important facility which is available in all capital cities and many larger country centres. Through this service, interpreters who are fluent in a wide range of languages, can assist migrants during emergencies; for example, obtaining a doctor, an ambulance, the fire brigade or the police. They are also available to advise on housing, legal and personal problems.

Ethnic supporting services to migrants

Many ethnic groups provide welfare services to people who need them, for example, the Greek, Italian, Turkish and Cypriot communities, etc.

Media dissemination

Ethnic radio, a commercial enterprise has been available for quite some time, and ethnic television also provides a valuable service, maintaining at least in part cultural ties and relieving loneliness.

Despite the services available at present much needs to be done to help migrants. A major need is the provision of many more trained welfare personnel. Many of these will ultimately be recruited from the various ethnic groups already in this country. Of course, they will need to be multilingual and have empathy and understanding of the social, cultural and economic needs of the migrant and his family.

It should be appreciated that the problems of settlement of refugees and families brought to Australia under various humanitarian programmes are usually accentuated.

SERVICES AVAILABLE FOR THE FAMILY IN DIFFICULTY

State governments

Family support units

There are a number of these centres scattered throughout the metropolitan area and in certain country areas of each State. Each of these centres has on its staff a number of family aids. These are mature women, most of whom have had families of their own. Although they do not possess a formal academic qualification, they have been selected and trained because of their personality and character. They receive payment for this service and would in general support about three families each. Their work is supervised by social workers attached to each unit. These women go into the homes of families at risk and provide supportive care in respect to mothercraft, house-keeping and family budgeting. In this way, and through the general support they give, a further parent figure is provided for the home. Occasionally, the family support units are able to provide a little additional financial help, but in general these centres prefer not to act as distributors of money. A number of other non-statutory agencies also provide family support services.

Financial grants

All separated wives (including de facto and prisoners' wives), single mothers and lone fathers who are bringing up their children on their own, may be eligible for Family Assistance Payments. These may also be available to a person who is bringing up a child other than their own with insufficient financial means. They are sponsored by the State Government Community Welfare Departments. Such payments may continue for six months, after which time they may be continued through the Commonwealth Department of Social Security.

Emergency grants

These are available to families who are experiencing hardship because of money shortage. Emergency grants involve sums of money given by the State community welfare departments to such families in order to purchase essential facilities such as accommodation, household maintenance, household equipment and the payment of outstanding debts. Many non-statutory organizations, both church and others, are alo involved in providing financial assistance, either as grants of money or goods.

Commonwealth government

Family allowance

These are regular payments made to all people bringing up children or with dependent full-time students. The family allowance increases with the number of children or students in the family. At present, the allowance for the first child is $22.80 per month. This rate increases with each subsequent child to $133.35 per month for four children. For each additional child the rate is increased by $45.55 per month.

Orphans pension

This is payment to a guardian of an orphan under the age of 16 years, or a dependent full-time student under the age of 25 years. For the purpose of payment of this pension, an orphan is defined as a child, both of whose parents are dead or one of whose parents is dead and the other is missing. The child whose only surviving parent is a long-term inmate of a prison or mental hospital is also regarded as an orphan. The pension is paid in addition to the family allowance. There is no income test for it and it is not subject to income tax.

Widows pension

These are regular payments made by the Commonwealth Government through the Department of Social Security to widows who have lost the support of their partner. The term widow includes a de facto wife who has lived with a man for at least three years immediately before his death. They are also available to wives who have been deserted by their husbands for six months or more, divorcees, women whose husbands have been in prison for at least six months or are in a mental hospital. These payments include an allowance for each child under the age of 16 years or for a dependent full-time student aged 16 to 25 years. Payment depends on an income test and income tax may be payable if certain additional income is received.

Widows may also be eligible for additional benefits such as free hearing aids, medical care, discounts on telephone rentals, rail and travel, mail redirection and purchases from Government bookshops.

Supporting parents benefit

These are regular payments made by the Commonwealth Government through the Department of Social Security to:

1. A man who supports a child and is a male divorcee (a woman who is divorced may be eligible for a widows' pension).
2. A widower.
3. A separated husband or wife or separated de facto husband or wife including people whose partner is in a prison or mental hospital). In this situation the supporting wife is eligible for a widows' pension (see above).
4. An unmarried parent.
5. A sole parent who supports a child for any other reason and who does not qualify for a widows' pension.

Special benefit

This is a benefit paid by the Commonwealth Government through the Department of Social Security to any person not entitled to other assistance or who is in need. For example, a single woman expecting a child may be paid from 12 weeks before the expected birth and until 6 weeks after the actual birth of the child. A supporting father may receive this benefit provided that he is not receiving it from another source.

Invalid pension

This is paid by the Commonwealth Government to persons who are permanently blind or who are not able to work because of permanent incapacity. It is available to any person over the age of 16 years.

Unemployment benefits

Through the Department of Social Security of the Commonwealth Government, unemployment benefits are available for people who are temporarily out of work, who are willing and able to undertake suitable work and are looking for such work. It is available to any person over the age of 16 years, provided that they have lived continuously in Australia for at least one year before applying, or intend to live in Australia permanently.

Family counselling and information service

These services are provided by state governments, by many local government authorities and by various voluntary organizations. These facilities are designed to make contact with families in need and to inform them of their various entitlements.

Child care services

Emergency care

Facilities for emergency care of the children of families in difficulty are required regularly. Both the Community Welfare Department and a number of voluntary agencies can arrange emergency accommodation for children requiring a temporary home. Such children are returned to their own homes as soon as possible after the crisis has passed. These services also provide daytime nursery care for such families.

Foster care

This implies that a child lives away from home and with another family until the child's parents can take him/her back again. Foster care may be short-lived or for a period of months to years depending upon the family's circumstances. Unfortunately, at this time the demand for foster care placement exceeds the supply of fostering families.

Children's homes and family group homes

These are less satisfactory alternatives to foster care. Here the Community Welfare Department or voluntary agencies take over the case of children who are unable to live at home. The children live in family groups and are cared for my cottage parents. These cottages are gradually replacing larger children's homes to avoid the old institutional atmosphere. However, a number of large children's homes catering for about 30 children are still operational. These are conducted by both the Community Welfare Department and voluntary organizations. It is of the greatest importance that these homes are close to the homes of the parents for visiting purposes and, when circumstances permit, the child is returned to the parents. It is of equal importance that the parents are helped and supported in every way to be able to cope when the child or children are returned to them. Social and welfare workers work closely with the parents while the child is in care.

Adoption

In the event of total family breakdown, parents may agree to adoption. Most adoptions have involved babies and children under school age, but there has been a dramatic decrease in the number of babies now available for adoption and hence there is a long waiting list for couples requesting this group of children. Fortunately, there has been an increasing trend towards adoption of children with special needs, for example, the baby with moderate to severe medical problems or the child who has suffered emotional deprivation or other emotional trauma. A particular need is for placement for adoption of school-aged children or children with significant handicap in carefully selected private homes. Some progress is being made in this field through the establishment of a special needs unit of the Community Welfare Department, but much needs to be done. All adoptions are arranged by the Community Welfare Department or staff of approved private adoption agencies.

Marriage counselling

A number of marriages break up because of certain interpersonal problems of the husband and wife. Some of these problems can be resolved by discussion with a marriage counselling expert. For these to be successful it is obvious that both partners need to be present at the interviews. Usually, initial interviews only involve the couple, but subsequent sessions may involve groups of couples. There is also a need for many young couples to receive counselling before marriage. A good case could be made for marriage to be discussed at secondary schools and at tertiary education centres, but so far little is organized in this area. Marriage counselling is readily available in the community. Some centres are conducted by religious voluntary bodies, a number of voluntary bodies without any religious affiliation; the community welfare departments also provide marriage guidance facilities.

The Family Court has a simple form which is available at no charge to any person seeking marriage counselling. If the form is filed the other spouse will be contacted and the parties referred to the appropriate marriage guidance organization.

Family planning

Many couples will have difficulty in producing children. Others for a variety of reasons, but in particular for financial reasons, will wish to avoid large families. A great deal of ignorance surrounds the understanding of conception, contraception and human sexuality in general. In addition, moral issues confront certain religious groups who may wish to limit the size of their families. Therefore, it is important that family planning facilities be available to educate couples before marriage and to assist their various needs in family planning after marriage. State Governments through their health departments provide family planning clinics in both metropolitan and country areas. In general, these are conducted by medical officers trained in this field. And also voluntary and religious organizations conduct family planning programmes.

REFERENCE

Dobbin M 1977 The health and nutritional status of Victorian Aboriginal children. PhD thesis, Monash University, Melbourne

FURTHER READING

Bain C 1977 Lone fathers: an unnoticed group. Australian Social Welfare 3:4–17
Burns A 1980 Breaking up: separation and divorce in Australia. Nelson, Melbourne
Galbally Report 1978 The review of post-arrival programmes and services to migrants. Commonwealth Expert Committee
Henderson R, Harcourt A, Harper R A 1970 People in poverty – a Melbourne survey. F O Cheshire, Melbourne
Hollingworth P 1979 Australians in poverty. Nelson, Melbourne

20. Failure to thrive

M. J. Robinson

Failure to thrive is the term used to describe failure of somatic growth. Traditionally, it implies failure to gain weight normally, but when there is a concomitant failure of linear growth the problem is usually a long standing one. Severe reduction in head circumference suggests that there has been intrauterine growth retardation.

Growth is a complex process and is discussed in Chapter 54. For normal growth the following conditions are necessary:

- a proper physical and emotional environment
- adequate nutrition
- correct tissue utilization
- a proper genotype, i.e. one compatible with normal growth.

When these conditions are not met normal growth will not occur and the child will fail to thrive. Standards for normal growth (growth charts) are available for most Western societies and in many developing countries. It is of the greatest importance that doctors caring for children have ready access to and use these charts. Growth charts plot length, weight and head circumference from birth to the end of adolescence; one such set is illustrated in Chapter 54. Optimally all children should have their length and weight recorded at birth and serially thereafter at child health clinics so that deviations from the normal will soon become apparent. Growth failure may occur from birth, as in cystic fibrosis, whereas in coeliac disease, for example, growth failure occurs after a period of normal growth.

Often doctors are consulted by anxious parents who believe that their child is not growing to their expectations. This is particularly the case in the second year of life when appetite deteriorates and activity increases. Weight gains are slow at this time and unless parents fully understand this phenomenon, unsatisfactory feeding practices will develop with all the behavioural problems that these bring. Reference to growth charts will rapidly define a growth problem and allow for reassurance to those parents who mistakenly believe that their child is not thriving. Properly kept growth charts

also quickly identify the child whose height and weight is below the third percentile and thus requires further investigation. However, it should be recognized that while the third percentile is taken as an indication for further investigation, 3% of normal children will fall within these limits. Despite reference to growth charts and much reassurance, some parents will continue to worry about their child's physical development. The doctor will need a great deal of patience in managing this situation; in some cases there will be an underlying psychosocial problem within the family which will have to be identified and treated.

There are a large number of reasons why an infant may fail to thrive. Most can be solved by the basic methods of clinical paediatrics – a complete history, observation of the interaction between mother and baby and a thorough physical examination. Often a few simple laboratory tests will be necessary. The need for extensive investigation of failure to thrive is not commonly required in this society but when necessary it will generally be indicated on the basis of obvious dysfunction in one or more body systems; for example, bowel disturbance and abdominal distension will suggest investigation for malabsorption, whereas dehydration in the absence of bowel losses may suggest renal or adrenal disease.

NON-ORGANIC FAILURE TO THRIVE

There have been a number of studies to indicate that the commonest cause of failure to thrive in this society does not have an organic basis but is the result of inadequate mothering and poor nutrition. Often such infants are admitted to hospital for investigation, when they will usually feed well and gain weight. When investigations do not provide an organic basis for the growth failure, closer enquiry will usually reveal a number of psychosocial problems. For example, it is common for the family to be in the lower socioeconomic group, the pregnancy often unplanned and unwanted, and the infant born within 18 months of a sibling. The mother is often young, single, or deserted and very frequently depressed. Obstetrical complications are not infrequent in this group and satisfactory bonding between mother and baby has never been established. These infants are almost always bottle fed, formulae often poorly prepared, immunization schedules incomplete and minor infections very frequent. The cause of the growth failure in these infants is multiple. Poor physical care due to ignorance or indifference is an important factor. Poor care may be closely associated with stress within the home and often with maternal depression. Neglect may be of sufficient degree to constitute frank child abuse (see Ch. 21). Some babies are difficult behaviourally and, when this is added to the socioeconomic and psychological problems, the growth problem is compounded.

The diagnosis of non-organic failure to thrive can only be made after a thorough enquiry into the psychosocial background. The physical examination must be thorough and a few simple tests such as microscopy and culture of urine, chest radiograph and blood examination are advisable.

Management is difficult because of the multiple factors involved and the inadequate facilities within our society for the care of these families. Long-term studies are now available on several groups of these infants and indicate that they grow up to have significant psychosocial problems in their adult life. It is not surprising to find that the non-organic failure to thrive syndrome is often perpetuated to the next generation at least. Management is supportive, involving much reassurance, home help and other support systems, e.g. community nurses, infant and maternal welfare personnel, medical social workers, etc. (see Ch. 19).

ORGANIC CAUSES OF FAILURE TO THRIVE

The organic causes of failure to thrive may be classified in many ways. The following approach is suggested and is essentially a clinical one:

Failure of intake from
  underfeeding
  congenital abnormalities
  dyspnoea
  neurological lesions
  behavioural factors

Abnormal losses through
  vomiting
  stools
  urine

Failure of utilization from
  chronic infection
  metabolic disorders
  endocrine disorders
  constitutional, genetic, chromosomal abnormalities and intrauterine lesions.

Failure of intake

Underfeeding

This may occur in the breast-fed baby if the breasts are large and engorged and particularly if the nipples are inverted. A young mother with her first baby may not realize that her breast supply is inadequate; the lusty baby will avoid underfeeding in this situation by showing obvious signs of hunger, but the small and rather weak infant may not and become sleepy and disinterested. Regular weighing will detect inadequate intake. In the bottle-fed infant the teat may be defective or the baby may be too sleepy or too irritable to feed, the milk mixture may be qualitatively deficient (too weak), or insufficient in amount. It is a simple matter to calculate the total daily milk intake of a bottle-fed infant and relate it to the weight of the infant (see Ch. 13). This fundamental calculation is all too often omitted in assessing infants who are failing to thrive. Additional fluid must be offered in warm climates. It must also be pointed out that failure of intake may be the result of anorexia through organic disease, which must always be considered and excluded by a proper physical examination.

Congenital abnormalities

Those interfering with feeding include cleft palate, the Pierre-Robin syndrome (micrognathia, cleft palate and glossoptosis), pharyngeal inco-ordination and, very rarely, bilateral facial nerve palsy (Moebius syndrome).

Dyspnoea

If dyspnoea is severe intake will be reduced. Failure to thrive is not a rare mode of presentation of severe congenital heart disease and the rule in chronic heart failure. With cardiac surgery now performed early in life, such problems are now much less common. Dyspnoea due to pulmonary disease is seen in chronic asthma and in cystic fibrosis, both of which limit growth if poorly controlled. Failure to thrive in cystic fibrosis is in part due to persisting chest infection.

Neurological lesions

Those which produce severe neurological deficit, e.g. pseudobulbar palsy and pharyngeal inco-ordination, are associated frequently with feeding difficulties. Causes include very low birthweight and other causes of cerebral anoxia, cerebral birth injuries and some rare cerebral degenerative disorders. Often Werdnig-Hoffman spinal muscular atrophy presents as a problem of failure to thrive through severe muscle weakness and thus inadequate intake. Some acquired lesions of the central nervous system may result in developmental delay sufficient to prevent adequate feeding: examples include meningitis, encephalitis and hypoglycaemia.

Behavioural factors

Some infants are hyper-alert, restless, feed poorly, sleep fitfully and do not suck steadily or contentedly. The reasons for this behaviour are obscure, but genetic factors, maternal anxiety and inadequate mothering may play a part.

Abnormal losses

Vomiting

The causes of vomiting have been discussed in Chapter 59. For vomiting to result in failure to thrive it must be severe and persistent. Clinically, vomiting may be recognized as primarily a mechanical problem or the result of toxic or chronic infective causes.

Gastrointestinal disorders. Mechanical causes in the oesophagus include stricture, duplication, achalasia and, most commonly, gastro-oesophageal reflux. Congenital hypertrophic pyloric stenosis and pylorospasm may result in failure to thrive through vomiting. Similar effects are seen in infants with incomplete or recurring intestinal obstruction such as in Hirschsprung's disease or with midgut volvulus.

Renal disorders. Renal tract infection in infancy may present solely as vomiting together with growth failure. Fever and leucocytosis may be absent and the diagnosis will only be made if the index of suspicion is high and the urine examined. Renal insufficiency may present solely as a problem of growth failure. Under these circumstances the urine will usually contain albumin and blood and the serum creatinine will be elevated. Usually, renal ultrasonography and micturating cystourothrography will define the lesion. However, it should be noted that a single negative urinalysis does not rule out renal disease. Renal tubular lesions, although uncommon, present with vomiting and growth failure (see Ch. 52).

Metabolic disorders. There are a number of metabolic disorders which present because of failure to thrive. The failure to thrive is not infrequently the result of vomiting. Hypercalcaemia, galactosaemia and hereditary fructose intolerance are examples. The clinical features of these disorders are described in Chapters 28 and 58.

Toxic agents. It is now well established that the excessive ingestion of alcohol during pregnancy may result in intrauterine growth retardation, intellectual handicap and a typical facial appearance. This latter consists of narrow palpebral fissures, a short nose with a broad low nasal bridge, facial hypoplasia, a shallow philtrum and small upper lip. Infants with the fetal alcohol syndrome continue to grow poorly in extrauterine life and often present because of failure to thrive. Also, cleft palate and congenital heart disease may be associated with the fetal alcohol syndrome.

Lead poisoning is now an infrequent cause of unexplained vomiting and growth failure. It should be suspected in association with an unexplained anaemia and convulsions. Sutural separation of the skull bones and dense lines at the metaphyses of the long bones may be demonstrated radiologically. Sometimes opaque material (lead flakes) may be seen on a plain radiograph of the abdomen. The diagnosis is confirmed by estimation of lead levels in blood and urine.

Stools

Failure to thrive may be associated with persistent diarrhoea or steatorrhoea. When taking the history, the characteristics of the stools need to be defined. The approach to the diagnosis of persistent diarrhoea and malabsorption has been discussed in Chapter 61 and will not be further discussed here.

Urine

Failure to thrive due to renal disease is by no means always associated with vomiting. Growth failure, anorexia and lack of energy may be the presenting symptoms. Also, an obscure anaemia or evidence of rickets may be present. A metabolic acidosis and polyuria which characterizes renal failure is invariably associated with growth failure. Losses from the urine which result in failure to thrive are:

Sugar. Usually, diabetes mellitus in childhood is an acute illness so it is quite uncommon for it to present as a chronic problem of failure to thrive. Nonetheless, the urine must always be checked for sugar and the blood glucose measured if there is doubt.

Water. Polyuria with osmolality of less than 300 mosmols/kg is a feature of chronic renal failure. The diagnosis will be established by urinalysis, renal function studies, renal ultrasound, radiology of the renal tract, and at times, renal biopsy.

Diabetes insipidus is associated with the passage of

large volumes of dilute urine of osmolality less than 50–200 mosmols/kg (SG 1.001–1.005). Usually the serum electrolytes are elevated. Response to pitressin will differentiate pituitary from renal diabetes insipidus.

Water and salt. Water and salt cannot be retained in adrenal insufficiency, which, in infancy, is associated most commonly with congenital adrenal hyperplasia. The presentation is usually in the second week of life with collapse and dehydration, or, before that, in the female with ambiguous genitalia. Congenital adrenal hyperplasia may be difficult to recognize in infancy in the male in the absence of salt wasting. By the age of about 18 months excessive androgenic production results in rapid growth and early masculinization. Congenital adrenal hyperplasia is discussed in Chapter 56.

Base. Base may be lost in the urine in certain renal tubular defects (see Ch. 52).

Failure of utilization

Infection

Here, failure to thrive may be the result of anorexia, vomiting and increase in metabolic rate. Although infection is usually obvious, this is not always the case in tuberculosis, anicteric hepatitis, Crohn's disease and ulcerative colitis. Again the renal tract should be considered. Recurrent or persisting respiratory infection is a frequent mode of presentation of cystic fibrosis. A collapsed and infected lobe or segment of lung, which may not be apparent clinically, can behave similarly. Usually, chronic lower airways obstruction associated with failure to thrive is due to asthma, even in infancy, but occasionally may be the result of persisting viral infection or immunological lung disease.

Severe chronic infection or recurrent severe infections is the common mode of presentation of an infant with an immunological deficiency disorder. Although individually rare, there are a number of such syndromes and, in most, failure to thrive is an associated feature (see Ch. 22). Many of these disorders are genetic so that establishing the diagnosis is of particular importance for genetic counselling. Congenital AIDS is now well documented in the African continent and in the USA. Infants with congenital AIDS suffer persisting infection and failure to grow. This disorder will occur with increased frequency in the paediatric age group through the world in the next few years.

Metabolic disorders

There are a number of disturbances of metabolism which may present as growth failure, and they have been discussed in Chapter 28. In cases where a metabolic disorder is suspected as the cause of failure to thrive, chromatography of the urine for organic acids and high voltage electrophoresis of urine for amino acids are the key investigations. Phenylketonuria is the commonest of the metabolic disorders, but is no longer a clinical problem because of neonatal screening when cases are identified and a low phenylalanine diet is instituted immediately.

Endocrine causes

Hypothyroidism, formerly the commonest endocrine cause of failure to thrive through growth failure, is no longer seen in infancy because of neonatal screening. Of the other endocrine causes, isolated human growth hormone deficiency is only occasionally recognized in infancy (see Ch. 54).

Constitutional, genetic and chromosomal causes

Some infants have a genotype of small stature and a growth rate which is slower than the average. Such a diagnosis is a presumptive one, but will be suspected if one or both parents are small, or if there is a family history of short stature. These infants, although small, are otherwise perfectly healthy, active and normal in all respects. In addition, they have normal levels of growth hormone. Some in this group may show low levels of somatomedin. There is now evidence to suggest that at least in the short term these children respond to large doses of human growth hormone.

Intrauterine growth retardation may be followed by failure to grow postnatally. So far no endocrine basis or metabolic derangement has been found responsible for this syndrome and it is presumed that the tissues of these individuals have a diminished capacity for growth. They are referred to as primordial dwarfs. In some cases there are associated abnormalities, such as mental retardation, mandibular facial dysostosis, limb abnormalities and premature senility.

Chromosomal abnormalities may need to be considered in infants who fail to thrive; the index of suspicion for these is the presence of multiple congenital abnormalities. The commonest is Down syndrome (trisomy 21). Other less common abnormalities include trisomy 13 and trisomy 18. Intrauterine infections – rubella, cytomegalovirus and toxoplasmosis will alter potential for growth and may present as a problem in infancy.

In small girls, Turner's syndrome should always be considered and a karyotype performed. This syndrome may be recognized in the neonatal period because of peripheral oedema and the various associated skeletal abnormalities. However, these are by no means always present so that all females whose height is below the third percentile require karyotyping.

Finally, there will be a group of patients who will remain undiagnosed even after investigation. Some remain small and some quite suddenly, and for no apparent reason, will commence to grow normally.

FURTHER READING

Berwick D M, Levy J, Klinerman R 1982 Failure to thrive: diagnostic field of hospitalisation. Archives of Disease of Childhood 57: 347–351

Goldbloom R B 1982 Failure to thrive. The Pediatric Clinics of North America 29: 151–166

Groll A et al 1980 Short stature as the primary manifestation of coeliac disease. Lancet ii: 1097–1099

Oates R K 1984 Non organic failure to thrive. Australian Paediatric Journal 20: 95–100

Rodriguez-Soriano 1971 Acid-base balance and renal tubular acidosis. The Pediatric Clinics of North America 18: 529–546

Stanbury J B, Wyngaarden J B, Fredrickson D S (eds) 1978 The metabolic basis of inherited disease, McGraw Hill, New York

21. Child abuse

Allan Carmichael

While abuse, neglect and exploitation of children has been recognized throughout history and continues in the form of child labour and prostitution in parts of the developing world today, the prevalence of child abuse in the 20th century industrialized societies has been acknowledged only since the 1950s. In 1946 and 1953, two American radiologists Caffey and Silverman raised the possibility of non-accidental injury to children. In 1962 Henry Kempe coined the term 'battered child syndrome' and forced reluctant professionals and communities to acknowledge the problem. The first Australian reports on physical child abuse were from Birrell & Birrell in 1966. Bialestock (1966) reported on neglect of children resulting in non-organic failure to thrive. Oates & Yu (1971) reported non-organic failure to thrive in children admitted to hospital and its sequelae in the form of emotional and learning difficulties in teenagers. Since the 1970s child sexual abuse has become increasingly recognized, as has emotional abuse with behavioural and developmental sequelae (Oates 1985).

DEFINITION

Child abuse may be defined as involving physical injury, sexual abuse, or deprivation of nutrition, care and affection in circumstances which indicate that injury or deprivation may not be accidental or may have occurred through neglect.

INCIDENCE

Comprehensive data for Australia are not available. In recent years the State of Victoria (with a population approximately five million) has recorded 4–6 deaths per year, due to abuse, some 30–50 cases of serious injury resulting in permanent disability and many hundreds of cases of lesser severity requiring investigation and intervention. In New South Wales with a somewhat larger population, almost 1000 sexually abused children are presenting to the three major metropolitan sexual assault centres each year. At present, estimates of incidence of child abuse in Western societies range between 10 and 20 cases per 1000 live births.

Current understanding acknowledges that child abuse and neglect exists as a spectrum of conditions as shown in Figure 21.1. Abnormalities in the child may range from death through physical injuries, failure to thrive, developmental, emotional and behavioural problems to normality. Corresponding labels which relate to these disorders are indicated in the diagram. Sexual abuse (described in detail later) may be added with findings including emotional and behavioural disorders and in rare cases injury. The concept of a spectrum is useful in that it recognizes overlap between various types of abuse, e.g. developmental and behavioural disturbances due to emotional abuse or neglect will often be present in children who are physically abused. Furthermore, it indicates that in some families there is a progression of abuse from more minor degrees of abnormality to more serious injuries thus emphasizing the importance of early identification and intervention. The diagnosis of child abuse may be clearcut towards the righthand end of the spectrum (failure to thrive and physical injury) while at the lefthand side firm categorization is difficult. This is especially in differentiating 'at risk' situations from extremes of normal child rearing practices which are particularly complex in a multicultural society such as Australia.

CLINICAL PRESENTATION OF ABUSED OR 'AT RISK' CHILDREN

The clinical approach to children who may be abused or neglected is no different from the approach to children who present with other medical problems. A thorough history and examination are mandatory and investigations are performed as indicated to confirm or elaborate on the diagnosis.

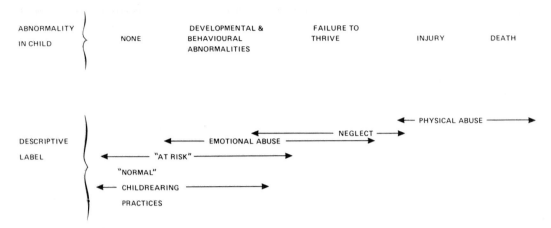

Fig. 21.1   Spectrum of child abuse.

Features of history suggestive of child abuse

1. Inappropriate parental concern

This may relate to late presentation for an injury or other problem or alternatively it may alert to an 'at risk' situation. This may apply to the parent who presents repeatedly for what may be seen as a minor medical problem or 'over-anxiety' in the face of medical reassurance that no serious illness exists. This latter circumstance may represent a cry for help on the part of the parent and is a point of early identification and intervention.

2. Frequent accidents

While some children, by virtue of their different temperament and personalities, seem more accident-prone than others, the child presenting with frequent accidents should be carefully evaluated for potential non-accidental injury. Consideration should be given to the quantity of care and supervision exercised within the home as studies of children presenting with frequent accidents have shown overlap between accidental and non-accidental injury.

3. Previous injury or abuse in other siblings

It has been established that within some families only one child of a number may be subject to abuse, perhaps by virtue of temperament, personality or parental expectation. Nonetheless, in other families, particularly those where there is violence, alcoholism or multiple problems, there is more likelihood that abuse may affect all children.

4. Inconsistent histories

The explanation of the event or incident causing the injury or presentation may vary when histories are taken at different times or when two care givers give different explanations in relation to the same event. It is important not to overlook the history given by the child, as even children of three or four years of age may give a very straightforward account of what has happened to them.

5. Acute disturbance or crisis in the social situation

While this is not a necessary or consistent feature in child abuse, it may indicate a precipitating or exacerbating factor leading to child abuse. It also acknowledges that physical abuse and neglect are more often found in families of lower socioeconomic groups where such stress factors as unemployment, poverty and limited access to resources are more prevalent.

Features on examination indicative of child abuse

1. Injuries inconsistent with events described or with the child's developmental level

The presence of a skull fracture in a six-week infant who is alleged to have rolled off a bed, represents a classic example in this category. The gross motor development of a six-week infant is such that rolling is not yet achieved. Similarly the presentation in a toddler of a complete fracture through the shaft of the humerus, allegedly as a result of falling over, would lead to suspicion that an injury of much greater force has occurred.

2. Bruising or other injuries at unusual sites

The normal toddler or preschool child will often sustain bruises over the anterior tibiae, extensor surfaces of the forearms or even on the forehead from normal activity and minor accidents. However, bruises over the flexor surfaces of the arms or legs or on the back should raise questions about non-accidental injury. A young infant with bruising around the mouth or a torn frenulum may have been repeatedly fed subjected with undue force.

3. Burns and scalds

These are usually accidental in origin, although in the past decade or so large burns units have reported between 5 and 10% of their admissions are a result of child abuse. Small burns at unusual sites without adequate explanation, especially cigarette burns, are pathognomonic of child abuse.

4. Non-organic failure to thrive, developmental delay, emotional and behavioural disturbances

These findings may be manifestations of child abuse and neglect and may present alone as the main problem leading to diagnosis (see Ch. 20).

5. Fear or apathy in the child

The toddler who seems unduly wary of parents or strangers may be exhibiting a sign of past abuse. Kempe has coined the term 'frozen awareness' for this apprehensive response in toddlers.

6. Subdural haematoma and retinal haemorrhages

These central nervous system signs should be regarded as pathognomonic of child abuse unless proved otherwise. Subdural haematoma may be caused by direct trauma but retinal haemorrhages are indicative of vigorous shaking of small children.

Precise documentation of history and examination findings in children suspected of being abused are essential. Detailed descriptions together with clearly marked diagrams and photographs are recommended to record the extent and evolution of physical injury including bruising.

INVESTIGATIONS WHEN CHILD ABUSE IS SUSPECTED

In common with many paediatric conditions, some 80 to 90% of the information on which diagnosis is based is obtained from the history and examination. Investigations are required to confirm or extend diagnoses and in some instances for medico-legal purposes. When physical injury is present, a skeletal survey is required to seek current and past evidence of bony injury. Initial imaging is best done by a skull radiograph and a total scan of the body and long bones (Fig. 21.2). Further radiographs may then be taken to further define 'hot spots' on the bone scan (Figs. 21.3, 21.4). In addition to the clinical information, radiographs will also exclude rare conditions such as osteogenesis imperfecta as a cause of frequent or early fractures.

A full blood examination including platelet count and clotting studies are more relevant for medico-legal purposes than for clinical diagnosis. Most presentations of bleeding and bruising, the result of a bleeding or coagulation disorder, should be suspected on the basis of clinical findings and merely confirmed by investigation.

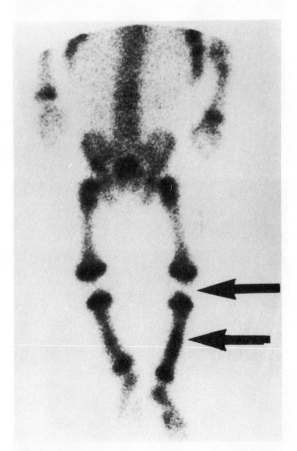

Fig. 21.2 Bone scan – lower limbs of 6-week infant showing increased radio-pharmaceutical uptake at both knees and midshaft left tibia.

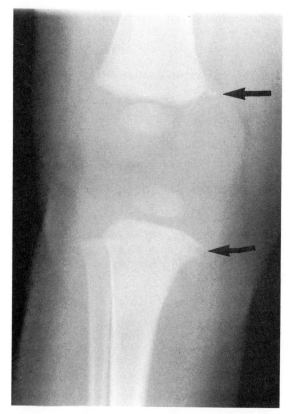

Fig. 21.3 Radiograph – left knee of same infant showing chip metaphyseal fractures to lower femur and upper tibia.

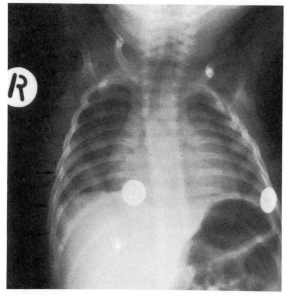

Fig. 21.4 Chest radiograph showing fracture of right 8th, 9th, 10th ribs in left axillary region.

Specific organic causes of failure-to-thrive should be excluded by appropriate investigation when indicated by the clinical findings (see Ch. 20). A confirmatory finding in children with non-organic failure to thrive due to abuse and neglect is their documented weight gain with normal feeding in a hospital or residential care environment.

CHILD SEXUAL ABUSE (CSA)

Kempe (1978) has defined this as the 'involvement of dependent, developmentally immature children and adolescents in sexual activities that they do not fully comprehend, to which they are unable to give informed consent, or that violate the social taboos or family roles'. Most centres dealing with child sexual abuse report that while almost all perpetrators are male, 20% of victims are also male. In contrast to adult sexual assault, 80% of cases involve chronic incest with only approximately 20% resulting from a single episode of sexual assault or rape. Further, the mean age of presentation in many CSA centres is 7 years or less with the likelihood of penetration or intercourse increasing with increasing age of the victim. In many incestuous families, sexual abuse of all children, especially girls, may occur. Those commonly involved are the father, stepfather, de facto, grandfather or other male relative.

Based on history and examination and having regard to the epidemiology of reported cases, it is again possible to list indicators (see Example 21.1). These may be considered presumptive evidence of sexual abuse (1–4), possible indicators (5–9) and other conditions (10–12) which may occasionally be manifestations of child sexual abuse.

The following comments elaborate on some of the listed indicators.

Direct reports from children (1)

It is now generally believed that the child's report

Example 21.1 Indicators of sexual abuse

1. Direct reports from children
2. Pregnancy in adolescents
3. Prepubescent venereal disease
4. Genital or rectal trauma
5. Precocious sexual interest or preoccupation
6. Indiscreet masturbatory activity
7. Sexual abuse of other family members
8. Repeated absconding from home in adolescent girls
9. Social withdrawal and isolation
10. Fear and distrust of authorities
11. Negative self-esteem, depression, suicidal behaviour, substance abuse
12. Somatic complaints including abdominal, pelvic pain.

should be believed unless it can be proved inaccurate. Past teachings and certainly the early work of Freud and others, have attributed children's reports of sexual activities to fantasy. This has resulted in the slow acceptance of the validity of most reports of incidence by children.

Adolescent pregnancy (2)

Here it is important to rule out premature but peer appropriate sexual activity.

Prepubescent venereal disease (3)

Prepubescent venereal disease when discovered is pathognomonic of CSA. However, non-specific vaginal discharge may also be a presentation of CSA. The child with recurrent vaginal discharge, in particular, requires careful evaluation.

Genital or rectal trauma (4)

A thorough general examination and particularly close inspection of the external genitalia and anus is important in all cases of suspected CSA. The absence of abnormal findings, however, does not exclude child sexual abuse, especially in the young child. In particular the presence or absence of a hymen is non-specific to sexual abuse. It should be noted that in one series a prepubescent vaginal introitus greater than 4 mm was correlated with child sexual abuse in 80% of cases. Nonetheless, the examination findings alone should not be relied on for diagnosis, as has seemed to be the case in the recent unfortunate and widely publicized cases in Cleveland, United Kingdom.

Possible indicators (5-9)

Should any of the possible indicators (5-9) be present, child sexual abuse should be seriously considered as a cause and appropriate history and examination performed.

Non-specific behaviour (10-12)

Non-specific behavioural and other clinical associations (10-12) are less frequently manifestations of CSA than the preceding indicators, but CSA should always be considered in the differential diagnosis. It should also be noted that CSA can be present in children who exhibit normal peer appropriate behaviour and achievement; many children may carefully conceal any sign of sexual victimization.

MANAGEMENT OF ABUSED AND NEGLECTED CHILDREN

When child abuse is suspected, the safety and protection of the child is of paramount importance. In the first instance for cases of physical abuse and neglect this usually involves admission to hospital. Child sexual abuse is best managed by referral to hospital or community based sexual assault centres with ability to manage child victims. Protection of the child in these cases often involves removal of the perpetrator from the home, rather than admission to hospital. Admission to hospital in other cases of child abuse allows more effective treatment of the presenting problem, for example, reduction of fractures, repair of lacerations, observation and management of head injuries, or appropriate feeding if the infant is suspected of non-organic failure to thrive. Investigation will also be facilitated by hospital admission. These aspects will usually be dealt with under the guidance of an experienced paediatrician with consultation from an orthopaedic surgeon, neurosurgeon, ophthalmologist and paediatric gynaecologist when appropriate. Also admission allows for thorough assessment of the child and the family. For this to be properly achieved a multidisciplinary team is required as the initial assessment and later therapeutic intervention must involve professionals such as social workers, psychologists and child psychiatrists who are competent in emotional and social assessment of children and families. Expertise is also required in the areas of physical development and emotional problems of children, as these areas must be assessed in any child with evidence of physical or sexual abuse or neglect.

Once child abuse is suspected on initial assessment, a multidisciplinary planning meeting is required to formulate a management plan for the child and family, but in particular, to consider the need for protective intervention. Health professionals in most, but not all states of Australia, are compelled to report suspected child abuse to a protective authority, namely a government social department or the police. Notification, whether mandatory or not is usually followed by further assessment culminating in a case conference at which a plan for ongoing management is formulated. Decisions will be influenced by the nature of the abuse, the family circumstances and in particular the continuing risk to the child. There are usually two main options:

1. The parents may voluntarily agree to enter into a counselling and therapeutic programme.

2. The case may be brought before the Children's Court for safe custody through a care and protection application. Should the care and protection application be granted, the case will usually be adjourned to be heard

in the Children's Court within a matter of a few weeks. A number of options are available to the Children's Court:

1. The case may be dismissed.

2. The child may be allowed to return home with the parents, but under supervision of an officer of the Social Welfare Department. Under these circumstances the parents will often be required to accept counselling and support.

3. The child may be removed from the parents' care and placed in the care of the State. The child will remain in care as long as the Protective Authority is determined that the child remains at risk. An obvious prerequisite will be a change in the home environment after counselling and social support to the parents.

In CSA, therapy for the child victim is required, together with support and counselling for other family members. Treatment of the perpetrator is essential to the reconstitution of the family and in some states pretrial diversion treatment options are being developed following their successful use in overseas centres.

The management of child abuse is not easy. Parents almost invariably deny accusations of child abuse so that anger and hostility are often occurring, particularly when a safe custody order is granted. Often facilities for parent counselling are inadequate and many abused children are returned to their parents before the home situation is a safe one and parents have been adequately counselled. Follow-up of families who have abused their children is difficult because such families move often and give no forwarding addresses. This makes appraisal of therapeutic techniques difficult. Despite this there are many families who are rehabilitated and subsequently care for their children in an exemplary fashion.

PREVENTION OF CHILD ABUSE

Although the larger part of this discussion has been devoted to the management of abused children, it is generally agreed that the most effective strategy for management is prevention. A number of overseas studies have documented the merit of identification of high risk families in the antenatal and perinatal period, followed by selective home visiting by child health nurses. The Maternal and Child Health Services in Australia maintain contact with approximately 90% of infants in the first year of life providing preventive and supportive programmes. Therefore, it would seem that this service is well placed to play a preventive role in child abuse. Further preventive strategies include education for parenthood both within schools and during pregnancy. The use of programmes such as 'protection behaviours' have been developed to assist prevention of child sexual abuse. The philosophy underlying such programmes is that children are encouraged to accept that they have a right to feel safe at all times and that if they do not feel safe, they are able to seek help from supportive adults. Finally, measures which reduce stresses on families such as those caused by unemployment and poverty, together with positive family support and child care programmes, while not expected to eliminate child abuse are likely to reduce its incidence.

REFERENCES

Bialestock D 1966 Neglected babies: a study of 289 babies admitted consecutively to a reception centre. The Medical Journal of Australia 2: 1129–1133

Birrell R G, Birrell J H W 1966 The 'maltreatment syndrome' in children. The Medical Journal of Australia 2: 1134–1138

Boss P 1980 On the side of the child — an Australian perspective on child abuse. Fontana Collins, Melbourne

Carmichael A 1983 The needs of the abused child in the community. Australian Paediatric Journal 19: 143–146

Kempe C H 1978 Sexual abuse: another hidden pediatric problem. Pediatrics 62: 382

Kempe C H, Silverman F N, Steele B F, Droegemueller W, Silver H K 1962 Battered child syndrome. Journal of the American Medical Association 181: 17

MacFarlane K, Waterman J, Connerly S et al 1986 Sexual abuse of young children: evaluation and treatment. Guildford Press, New York

Oates R K 1982 Child abuse — a community concern. Butterworth, Sydney

Oates R K 1985 Child abuse and neglect: what eventually happens. Brunner Mazel, New York

Oates R K, Yu J S 1971 Children with non-organic failure to thrive – a community problem. Medical Journal of Australia 2: 199–203

Allergy and immunity

22. Factors involved in resistance to infection

D. M. Roberton

RESISTANCE TO INFECTION

The ability to resist infection is dependent upon the relationship between host immunity and the challenge produced by the microbiological environment. Throughout life infection occurs when there is an alteration in either or both of these factors. Examples of infection due to a change in the microbiological environment are seen during epidemics (influenza), with travel (gastroenteritis, malaria), during hospitalization (hospital-acquired infection) and even during the administration of broad-spectrum antibiotics (candidiasis). Variation in host immunity occurs with age, both the very young and the old being relatively immunodeficient, and in a number of disease states.

HOST IMMUNITY

The intrinsic ability of the host to resist infection involves a complex interaction of non-specific and specific mechanisms. Non-specific immunity refers to the ability to provide protection against invasion by any pathogen; specific immunity refers to an adaptive and highly antigen-specific response resulting from prior exposure to that antigen.

Non-specific immunity

1. Epithelial surfaces

One of the most important determinants in the prevention of infection is the provision of an intact barrier which prevents access of microorganisms to body tissues. The skin is the largest single organ system in the body and its role in preventing infection becomes apparent when the skin is damaged as in burns, abrasions or major lacerations. Epithelial surfaces in the respiratory tract, gastrointestinal tract and urinary tract also have an important barrier function. Each of these epithelial surfaces have developed specialized cell types such as mucus-secreting cells or cells which secrete specific chemicals which enhance their protective role.

2. Secretions

Mucus secreted by goblet cells and cells in mucus glands provides a barrier to adherence by microorganisms, thus preventing cell invasion by preventing attachment of organisms to cell surfaces.

Secretions at mucosal surfaces also contain chemical substances which are important in defence against infection; examples of these are lysozyme, proteases, and lactoferrin. Oligosaccharides in mucosal secretions may act as substitute ligands, preventing adherence of microorganisms to epithelial cells.

The pH of secretions has an effect on the survival of invading pathogens. The low pH of the stomach protects the upper gastrointestinal tract from many forms of infection and the pH of the skin may have a bacteriostatic effect.

3. Flow

Flow of secretions and fluids removes pathogens from potential sites of infection. Coughing and ciliary activity in the respiratory tract produce continual passage of mucus from the airways. Salivary flow removes organisms from the orthopharynx. The importance of flow in removing pathogens from the urinary tract and the gastrointestinal tract is seen when these organ systems become obstructed, with subsequent stasis and bacterial infection.

4. Normal flora

Commensal microorganisms living in or on the skin and in the gastrointestinal tract have a beneficial effect by excluding other microorganisms which may be pathogenic. Alteration of the normal flora of the

gastrointestinal tract during the administration of antibiotics may permit the overgrowth of *Candida albicans*
or other organisms with subsequent alteration in
gastrointestinal function.

5. Phagocytic cells

Phagocytic cells are capable of ingesting microorganisms
non-specifically although the efficiency of ingestion and
microbial killing is enhanced by specific antibody and
complement, both of which act as opsonins. There are
two types of specialized phagocytic cell – the polymorphonuclear leucocyte and the macrophage. Macrophages
and closely related mononuclear antigen-presenting cells
are found in almost all body tissues. They line the
sinusoids of the liver, spleen and lymph nodes; they are
also found at mucosal surfaces, in the pulmonary alveoli,
and specialized forms exist in the skin and in the central
nervous system. Polymorphonuclear phagocytes include
neutrophils and eosinophils. These phagocytic cells use
a variety of oxygen-dependent microbicidal mechanisms
to kill ingested organisms.

6. Complement

The complement system is composed of two pathways.
The classical pathway consists of nine numbered components; three further proteins are involved in the
alternative pathway. There are also a number of
regulatory proteins. Complement proteins interact in a
predetermined sequence; the result of their interaction
is to either deposit C3b on the surface of organisms and
thus enhance phagocytosis by acting as an opsonin, or
to cause direct lysis of the organism or cell. During the
sequence of complement activation further proteins are
generated which enhance the inflammatory response by
acting as vasodilators and as chemoattractants for
phagocytic cells.

Specific immunity

Specific immunity is lymphocyte dependent. Lymphocytes undergo a complex process of proliferation and
differentiation during which they develop the ability to
respond to particular antigens either by producing
specific antibody or by initiating a specific cell-mediated
immune response. After the initial contact with an invading pathogen a small number of lymphocytes survive
as long-lived 'memory' lymphocytes and these antigen-
specific lymphocytes are able to mount a rapid
protective response on future contact with the same organism. It is this adaptive response which provides
immunity by preventing reinfection.

There are many different types of lymphocytes which
can be distinguished by specialized techniques. A useful
broad categorization is division into cells responsible for
cell-mediated immune responses (T cells) and cells
which lead to the production of specific antibodies (B
cells).

Lymphocytes are produced from stem cells resident
in the bone marrow (Fig. 22.1). Some pass to the
thymus and here they differentiate into cells which have
the surface membrane characteristics and functional
characteristics of T lymphocytes. T lymphocytes are important in the recognition of foreign antigens, in the
amplification and regulation of the immune response,
and in the first killing of certain pathogens. T lymphocytes and T lymphocyte subpopulations are
recognized in vitro by monoclonal antibodies directed
against cell membrane components. These surface structures are related to cell maturation and cell function.

B lymphocytes also arise from the bone marrow but
they do not depend directly on the thymus for maturation. B cells produce immunoglobulin of which there are
five different classes: IgG, IgA, IgM, IgD and IgE.
There are four IgG subclasses (IgG1, 2, 3 and 4) and
two IgA subclasses (IgA1 and IgA2). Following stimulation by antigen a clone of B cells is generated which
mature into plasma cells producing antibody directed
against the stimulating antigen. Specific IgM antibody
is produced in the early phase of infection, with IgG
antibody production being seen after about ten days.
IgA is the predominant immunoglobulin class in secretions, where it is present largely in dimeric form in
association with another protein, secretory component,
which confers resistance to proteolysis.

Each B cell can produce antibody of one specificity
only. Antibody production by B cells is controlled by
regulatory T cells. B cells are recognized as lymphocytes
carrying surface membrane immunoglobulin, or by
specific monoclonal antibodies. There are also
laboratory techniques available which allow detection of
specific antibody produced by B cells.

The initiation and regulation of the immune response
is dependent upon a large number of complex intercellular reactions. Subpopulations of T lymphocytes have
a major role in the control of B cell differentiation after
exposure to antigen and in the later cessation of specific
antibody production once adequate antibody levels have
been achieved. Soluble mediators known as lymphokines (e.g. IL1, IL2) are produced by
antigen-presenting cells and T and B lymphocytes and
play an important role in the regulation of the interactions of the immune response.

Abnormal immune regulation forms the basis of certain autoimmune disorders in which immune reactions

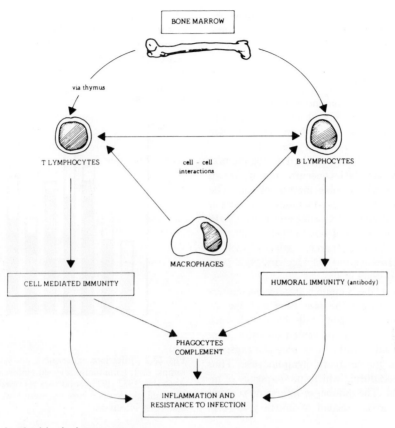

Fig. 22.1   Pathways involved in the immune response.

occur against the host's own tissues as in systemic lupus erythematosus or autoimmune haemolytic anaemia. Defective immune surveillance or immune regulation may also have a role in the development of some malignancies. Oncogene effects on immune regulation may be important in this regard.

DEVELOPMENT OF IMMUNITY

Fetus

The fetus develops immunological capabilities at a very early stage in gestation. Lymphocytes are present in the thymus by the eighth week of pregnancy, and are able to produce antigen-specific responses by the middle of the second trimester. IgM appears in hepatic cells by nine weeks. However, the normal fetus exists in an environment which is effectively free of extrinsic antigen and thus no specific immune responses develop until exposure to the microbial environment begins at the time of birth. To afford some protection in the early neonatal period there is active placental transport of IgG, but no IgA or IgM, from the maternal circulation during the third trimester. This provides the term neonate with passively acquired antibody which has an important role in preventing infection during the first weeks of life. The premature neonate may fail to acquire some of this maternally derived antibody.

Neonate

Although capable of normal lymphocyte responses from an early stage of gestation the neonate is functionally immunodeficient because of lack of prior exposure to infecting organisms. Some complement components are present in only low concentrations at birth and neutrophil migration may be deficient in the newborn. At birth there is very little IgM and no IgA in either serum or secretions. These abnormalities, in combination with physiological immaturity of the gut, lungs and skin, make the newborn highly susceptible to infection. Breast-feeding is an important source of passively acquired secretory IgA and helps to protect the newborn from gastrointestinal infections and possibly some respiratory tract infections.

Infancy and later childhood

Whereas there is a relative immunodeficiency at birth, it is the immunological naivety of infancy and early childhood that is responsible for the increased incidence of infection seen in comparison with later life.

Maternally acquired IgA is catabolized during the first few months of life and IgG concentrations in serum reach their lowest levels at three months of age. The infant's own immunoglobulin production commences at birth with IgM reaching adult concentrations by 18 months, IgG by 5–6 years and IgA by 9–10 years. Antibody formation to polysaccharide antigens, such as Pheumococcal or Haemophilus polysaccharides, is poor during the first two years of life.

During childhood the immune system encounters many infecting agents for the first time and specific primary immunological responses develop with each new infection. Reinfection is prevented on subsequent challenge by the rapid recruitment of secondary responses, a function of the 'memory' lymphocytes. Thus childhood is a period during which the frequency of infections is increased. The number of infections per year of life is maximal in the second to fourth year (Fig.

22.2); during the first 12 years of life the mean number of infections experienced per child by a sample of urban Australian children studied in a cross-sectional survey was 67 (Fig. 22.3).

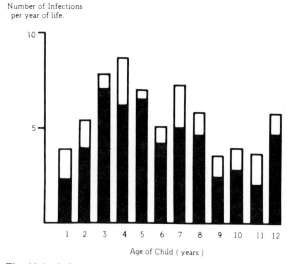

Fig. 22.2   Infections experienced per year of life for a sample of 131 randomly selected children in Melbourne, Australia, 1977–1979. Solid bars represent upper respiratory tract infections; open bars represent lower respiratory tract and other infections.

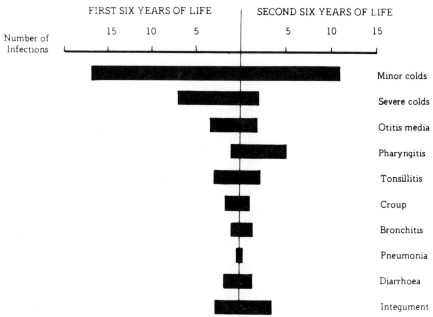

Fig. 22.3   Mean number of specific infections experienced per child during the first 12 years of life for the same study group.

INVESTIGATION FOR IMMUNODEFICIENCY

Indications for investigation

Immunodeficiency in childhood presents with infection. Infections occur in all children and thus the indications for investigation for the presence of a primary immunodeficiency disorder cannot be defined absolutely. In the primary immunodeficiency disorders affected children have frequent or persistent infections, often due to organisms which are usually of low pathogenicity (e.g. *Candida sp.*, *Pneumocystis carinii*). The infections lead to tissue damage in organs such as the respiratory tract or the gut. Growth failure secondary to recurrent infection is common. Investigation should be considered in children with frequent infections, in children with persistent diarrhoea and/or growth failure of undetermined cause, and in children with associated abnormalities characteristic of some of the immunodeficiency syndromes as described below.

Investigation

Tests for immunodeficiency are often complex and many are indicated only in special circumstances. Quantitative assays determine whether particular components of the immune system are present in normal concentrations or numbers with respect to the age of the child; functional assays determine whether these components are effective (Table 22.1).

A simple approach to initial investigation for a suspected immunodeficiency disorder is to determine total lymphocyte and neutrophil numbers from a peripheral blood sample, measure IgC, IgA and IgM concentrations, and assess lymphocyte responses to the mitogen phytohaemagglutinin (PHA). These assays can be performed on as little as 1 ml of blood and will, if normal, exclude the majority of the primary immunodeficiency disorders.

IMMUNODEFICIENCY DISORDERS

Immunodeficiency disorders include primary disorders, often congenital and sometimes familial, in which there is a defect of the immune system itself, and secondary disorders in which immune function is compromised because of abnormalities of other body systems.

Primary immunodeficiency disorders

These disorders are listed in Example 22.1. Most are rare. The first of the primary immunodeficiency disorders was recognized in 1952 when the association of hypogammaglobulinaemia and recurrent infections was discovered. The incidence of the more commonly recog-

Table 22.1 Investigation for suspected immunodeficiency (peripheral blood sample)

Immune component	Quantitative	Functional
Phagocytic cells	Neutrophil numbers Eosinophil numbers	Chemotaxis Phagocytosis Metabolic activation: NBT reduction O_2 consumption superoxide production iodination Bacterial killing
Complement	Measurement of individual components of classical and alternative pathways	Opsonization CH_{50}/CH_{100}
Immunoglobulin and antibody formation	Immunoglobulin and immunoglobulin subclass concentrations Specific antibody titres	Opsonization Agglutination Neutralization
Lymphocytes	Lymphocyte count Cell surface antigens (sheep red cell rosettes, surface membrane immunoglobulin, antigens defined by monoclonal antibodies)	Proliferative responses (mitogens, allogeneic cells, specific antigens) Regulatory function: suppressor assays helper assays lymphokine production Skin testing (SK/SD), ppd, mumps

Abbreviations: NBT = nitroblue tetrazolium; CH_{50}/CH_{100} = lysis of sensitized red cells by complement; SK/SD = streptokinase/streptodornase.

Example 22.1 Primary immunodeficiency disorders (WHO Committee classification)

Predominantly antibody defects
  X-linked agammaglobulinaemia
  X-linked hypogammaglobulineamia with growth hormone
    deficiency
  Autosomal recessive agammaglobulinaemia
  Immunoglobulin deficiency with increased IgM
  IgA deficiency
  Selective deficiency of other immunoglobulin isotypes
  Transient hypogammaglobulineamia of infancy
  Antibody deficiency with normal/elevated
    immunoglobulins

Immunodeficiency associated with other major defects
  Wiskott-Aldrich syndrome
  Ataxia telangiectasia
  3rd and 4th arch syndrome (Di George anomalad)
  Transcobalamin 2 deficiency

Complement disorders
  Hereditary angioneurotic oedema
  Isolated complement component deficiencies

Combined immunodeficiency
  Common variable immunodeficiency with predominant
    antibody deficiency with predominant cell mediated
    immunity defect
  Severe combined immunodeficiency reticular dysgenesis
    low T and B cell numbers low T, normal B cell
    numbers
  MHC class I deficiency (bare lymphocyte syndrome)
  MHC class II deficiency
  Adenosine deaminase deficiency
  Purine nucleoside phosphorylase deficiency
  Chronic mucocutaneous candidiasis

Phagocytic cell disorders
  Neutropenia
  Chronic granulomatous disease
  Chediak-Higashi syndrome
  Schwachman disease
  Phagocyte membrane defects

Table 22.2 Incidence of selected primary immunodeficiency disorders in Victoria, Australia, 1970–1982

Immunodeficiency disorders	Incidence per million live births
X-linked agammaglobulinaemia (including normal/elevated IgM)	10
Common variable immunodeficiency	12
Severe combined immunodeficiency	15
3rd and 4th arch syndrome (Di George anomalad)	15
Chronic granulomatous disease	5.5

nized primary immunodeficiency disorders in Victoria, Australia, is shown in Table 22.2.

Predominantly antibody defects

X-linked agammoglobulinaemia. Boys with this disorder begin to suffer from recurrent bacterial infections between 3 and 6 months of age as passively acquired maternal IgG concentrations fall. Sites involved most commonly are the nose, middle ear and the lower respiratory tract; the usual organisms are *Streptococcus pneumoniae*, *Staphylococcus aureus* and *Haemophilus influenzae*. Bacterial meningitis, septicaemia and osteomyelitis occur with increased frequency, and affected boys also are susceptible to ureaplasma arthritis and a progressive meningoencephalitis due to ECHO viruses and other enteroviruses. Tissue destruction as-

sociated with lower respiratory tract infections gives rise to bronchiectasis.

Tonsils, adenoidal tissue and lymph nodes are small or absent. B cells are absent from the peripheral blood, bone marrow and lymphoid tissues. Immunoglobulin concentrations in serum are very low; usually no IgA, IgM, or IgE can be detected although small amounts of IgG may be present. IgA is absent from secretions. No specific antibody is formed.

Treatment involves the early and adequate treatment of infections with appropriate antibiotics, and the administration of immunoglobulin. Gammaglobulin, consisting almost entirely of IgG, is available in forms suitable for either intramuscular or intravenous administration and is very effective at preventing infection. Intravenous immunoglobulin administration is preferable as larger amounts can be given. It is given at monthly intervals, the half-life of IgG in the circulation being between 21 and 28 days. Extra gammoglobulin should be given during severe infections. Plasma, containing IgG, IgA and IgM, can also be used as an adjunct in the treatment of infection.

The diagnosis of X-linked agammaglobulinaemia has important genetic implications for the family. As yet there is no widely available method for carrier-detection, although RFLP analyses may be informative in some families. Some families may elect to terminate pregnancies which result in male children. Early diagnosis and treatment of subsequent male children helps to prevent the destructive sequelae of infections.

Immunoglobulin deficiency with increased IgM. Some boys fail to make IgG and IgA but have high serum concentrations of IgM. This may be due to a defect in genomic 'switch' mechanisms responsible for sequential immunoglobulin heavy chain gene expression. These children may have an associated neutropenia and they have a high incidence of pneumocystis pneumonia for reasons which are not yet understood. In this condition tonsils are usually present and B cells bearing surface IgM are present in the peripheral blood, but their ability to form functional antibody is deficient. Treatment is with replacement immunoglobulin as for X-linked agammaglobulinaemia.

IgA deficiency. This is the commonest primary immunodeficiency, occurring once in every 500 to 700 members of the population. IgA is absent from both serum and secretions. The great majority of affected individuals are asymptomatic, but in some there is an increased frequency of infections, particularly respiratory tract infections. It has been shown that many of those with symptomatic IgA deficiency also have a deficiency of the IgG2 subclass of IgG, and sometimes also a deficiency of IgG4. IgA deficiency is found with greater than expected frequency in patients with allergic or autoimmune disease. Isolated IgA deficiency does not require treatment, but symptomatic patients with associated IgG2 deficiency may benefit from intravenous immunoglobulin therapy.

Transient hypogammaglobulinaemia of infancy. In this condition there is a delay in the ability to produce normal concentrations of immunoglobulin. B cells are present and immunoglobulin concentrations become normal by 18 months to 2 years; before this, affected children are susceptible to infections which are similar to those seen in X-linked agammaglobulinaemia. Treatment with gammaglobulin is necessary until intrinsic immunoglobulin production becomes normal. There is no evidence for familial occurrence.

Antibody deficiency with normal/elevated immunoglobulins. It seldom occurs that some children have normal immunoglobulin concentrations but are not able to form antigen-specific antibody. Diagnosis of this condition is dependent upon assays of specific antibody formation to antigens such as tetanus toxoid. Treatment is with replacement gammaglobulin which provides passively acquired antibody from a large pool of donors.

Combined immunodeficiency

This term encompasses a heterogeneous group of non-hereditary disorders whose aetiology is largely unknown. Patients with common variable immunodeficiency have in common an inability to make useful antibody. This defect may involve all immunoglobulin classes or only some classes. Generally there are associated abnor-malities of T cell function, often involving regulatory T cells. The onset is after the age of 2 years. Most patients do not suffer from recurrent infections until later childhood or adult life, and it is thought that the hypogammaglobulinaemia is an acquired defect. The most common infections are those involving the respiratory tract although there is also a high incidence of gastrointestinal infections, giardiasis being frequent. Atrophic gastritis and nodular lymphoid hyperplasia of the gut are common in adult patients. Neutropenia may occur and malignancies, particularly lymphomas, are seen with increased frequency. Patients with common variable immunodeficiency have lymph nodes and tonsils, and B cells are present in the blood and bone marrow in normal or low-normal numbers. T cell numbers may be either normal or decreased, and often there are abnormalities of T cell subpopulations.

Treatment is again dependent upon vigorous treatment of infections and the use of replacement gammaglobulin.

Severe combined immunodeficiency. T cell dysfunction is the predominant defect in this disorder. Antibody formation is also defective, and affected children are extremely susceptible to infection. Most die before the age of one year if untreated. There are several recognizable variants of severe combined immunodeficiency (see Example 22.1). Pneumocystis pneumonia is frequent (Fig. 22.4) and respiratory tract infections due to

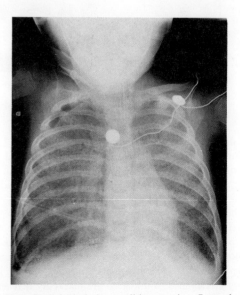

Fig. 22.4 Radiological abnormalities seen in a 7-month-old child with severe combined immunodeficiency and pneumocystis pneumonia. There is diffuse pulmonary consolidation and a pneumothorax is present.

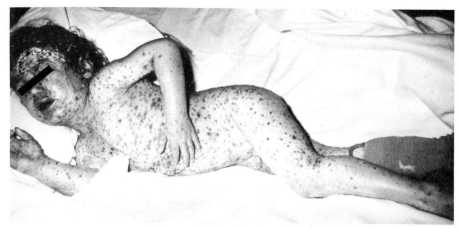

Fig. 22.5   Disseminated varicella infection in a child with severe combined immunodeficiency.

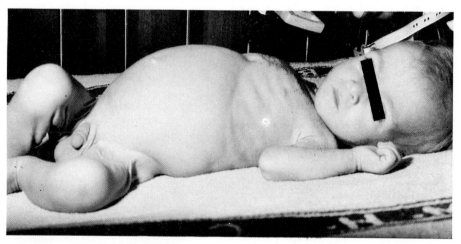

Fig. 22.6   A child with severe combined immunodeficiency and severe wasting due to recurrent infection.

measles and chickenpox are usually fatal (Fig. 22.5). Failure to thrive is due to repeated infections and persistent diarrhoea (Fig. 22.6). Many affected children have a widespread seborrhoeiform rash and candidiasis is common.

The thymus is hypoplastic and T cells are either absent from the peripheral blood or are present in very low numbers. B cells are usually absent and immunoglobulin levels are low, with the occasional exception of IgE. Many patients are lymphopenic; lymphocyte responses to mitogens are markedly deficient.

The primary defects leading to the severe combined immunodeficiency syndromes remain unknown; the most likely explanation is a failure of lymphoid stem cells to mature and differentiate. In some families an autosomal recessive or X-linked pattern of inheritance has been shown. Antenatal diagnosis is possible by examining fetal cord blood lymphocytes for the presence of T cells and determining their mitogen responsiveness.

Marrow transplantation is curative if a tissue-matched sibling donor is available. Antibiotics and intravenous immunoglobulin are used to treat infections prior to marrow transplantation.

Combined immunodeficiency and enzyme defects. Two forms of combined immunodeficiency have been shown to be associated with inherited enzyme abnormalities. Adenosine deaminase (ADA) deficiency accounts for 20% of cases of severe combined immunodeficiency and is an autosomal recessive disorder. Some children have improved clinically with infusions of frozen irradiated red cells which contain ADA but marrow transplantation is indicated if a suitable donor is available. Purine nucleoside phosphorylase deficiency is also associated with a form of progressive combined immunodeficiency.

Chronic mucocutaneous candidiasis. Some children have lymphocyte defects which are specific for one antigen only. In chronic mucocutaneous candidiasis immunity is normal for all antigens except *Candida* sp. Affected children have gastrointestinal, and skin and nail infections with *Candida albicans*. In some there may be an associated endocrinopathy such as hypoparathyroidism or Addison's disease. Long-term therapy with ketoconazole, an imidazole antifungal agent, has been very effective.

Phagocytic cell disorders

Chronic granulomatous disease. This disorder results in a metabolic abnormality of neutrophils which impairs their ability to kill microorganisms. Inheritance is usually as an X-linked recessive disorder although an autosomal recessive form has been described. The primary abnormality has been shown to be a defect of cytochrome – b_{245}, which is absent in the X-linked form of the disorder and functionally deficient in the autosomal recessive form.

Affected children suffer from recurrent abscesses. Lymph nodes are a common site of involvement, and hepatic abscesses may occur. Osteomyelitis is frequent. The organism isolated most frequently is *S. aureus*; *Serratia* sp. and *Aspergillus* sp. are also common infecting agents.

Laboratory tests demonstrate deficient oxidative metabolism within neutrophils (e.g. NBT test) and deficient microbial killing by phagocytic cells. Treatment involves the use of appropriate antibiotics particularly those with an intracellular mode of action (e.g. rifampicin), granulocyte transfusions during acute infection, and prophylactic co-trimoxazole.

Complement disorders

Disorders of complement function are recognized only rarely. Deficiencies of each of the complement pathway components and each of the control proteins have been described. Most result in recurrent infections. C2 deficiency is seen in some patients with systemic lupus erythematosus and other autoimmune disorders. C1 esterase inhibitor deficiency results in the frequently life-threatening episodes of hereditary angioneurotic

oedema during which there may be obstruction of the proximal airways.

Immunodeficiency associated with other major defects

Some immunodeficiency disorders are not classified readily as defects of the immune system alone, but have other abnormalities associated with them which allow their recognition as specific syndromes.

Wiskott-Aldrich syndrome. This X-linked disorder encompasses thrombocytopenia associated with small platelet size, impaired antibody responses to bacterial polysaccharide antigens, progressive impairment of lymphocyte function, low IgM concentrations and eczema. A defect in platelet and leucocyte membrane sialophorin production has been described in these patients. Affected boys present with bleeding, often involving the gastrointestinal tract, eczema, and recurrent infections. Usually the disease is fatal within the first two decades of life unless treated by bone marrow transplantation.

Ataxia-telangiectasia. Affected children develop telangiectases of the bulbar conjunctivae and over the ears. There is a progressive cerebellar ataxia and respiratory tract and other infections are common. IgA and IgE concentrations are low and cell-mediated immunity becomes deficient in later life. Serum levels of alpha-fetoprotein are often elevated and there is abnormal chromosomal fragility. There is a high incidence of malignancies, with many patients developing lymphomas. The primary cause is unknown but the disorder is inherited in an autosomal recessive fashion.

3rd and 4th arch syndrome (Di George anomalad). Thymic hypoplasia, hypoparathyroidism, congenital cardiac defects (interrupted aortic arch, Fallots tetralogy, truncus arteriosus or ventricular septal defect) form the triad of abnormalities recognized as the Di George anomalad. Most affected infants present in the early weeks of life with signs of congenital heart disease and hypocalcaemia. The supposedly typical facial appearance is often difficult to recognize. There is a variable T cell defect with low T cell numbers and poor lymphocyte responses to mitogens.

Secondary immunodeficiency disorders

Secondary abnormalities of the immune system occur in many disorders of childhood. They may occur as part of the disease process itself or may be due to treatment.

Nutrition

Malnutrition is responsible for deficient cell-mediated immune responses. Deficiencies of specific substances such as zinc may also lead to a secondary immunodeficient state.

Infection

Some infections cause a temporary immunodeficiency. Neutropenia is common after some infections, and measles and tuberculosis cause depressed lymphocyte function.

Infection with human immunodeficiency virus (HIV-1) causes progressive immunological dysfunction and is termed the acquired immunodeficiency syndrome (AIDS). Maternal infection with HIV-1, often as a result of intravenous drug use, may lead to infection of the neonate in utero or at birth. Retroviral transmission by breast-feeding may have caused infection in rare instances. Some children, particularly haemophiliacs, have become infected after the administration of blood products collected before the introduction of blood bank screening procedures. Other possible sources of infection in childhood are sexual abuse and intravenous drug use.

There may be a latent period of many years between initial infection and the development of symptoms of the acquired immunodeficiency syndrome (AIDS). Presentation may be with opportunistic infections (*Pneumocystis carinii* pneumonia; candidiasis; persisting cryptosporidial enteritis; atypical mycobacterial infection), failure to thrive, lymphoid interstitial pneumonitis or pulmonary lymphoid hypoplasia, encephalopathy, and severe bacterial infections. Diagnosis of AIDS is supported by positive antibody tests (e.g. by ELISA or Western blot) or by tests for HIV serum antigen, culture or in situ hybridization using a nucleic acid probe. Some infants may have maternally acquired antibody present for up to 15 months after birth but may not be infected. There is a gradual reduction in the number of T4-positive cells, associated with lymphocyte dysfunction. The initial hypogammaglobulinaemia is followed by low immunoglobulin concentrations.

Management of AIDS in children consists of treatment of the secondary infections, and immunoglobulin replacement therapy. Azidothymidine (AZT) administration may slow progression of the disorder, but no curative therapy is yet available.

Loss of immunological mediators

IgG is lost in the urine in the nephrotic syndrome. Severe burns lead to protein loss from the affected skin. Lymphocytes are lost from the gut in gastrointestinal lymphangiectasia, and splenectomy removes large numbers of macrophages. There is a high risk of Pneumococcal and *H. influenzae* sepsis after total splenectomy and prophylactic antibiotics and immunization with Pneumococcal polysaccharide vaccine is recommended.

Immunosuppressive therapy

Corticosteroids alter lymphocyte function when given in high doses over prolonged periods. Cytotoxic therapy for malignancies is responsible for neutropenia and altered lymphocyte function.

FURTHER READING

Mims C A 1982 The pathogenesis of infectious disease, 2nd edn. Academic Press, London

Primary Immunodeficiency Diseases: Report of a WHO Scientific Group 1986. Journal of Clinical Immunology and Immunopathology 40: 166–196

Revision of the CDC Surveillance Case Definition for Acquired Immunodeficiency Syndrome 1987. MMWR supplement (Aug 14) 35, no 1

Roitt I 1984 Essential immunology, 5th edn. Blackwell Scientific Publications, Oxford

Roitt I, Brostoff J, Male D 1985 Immunology. Churchill Livingstone, London

Skvaril F, Morell A, Perret B 1988 Clinical aspects of IgG subclasses and therapeutic implications. Monographs in Allerby, 20 (Karger AG)

Soothill J F, Hayward A R, Wood C B S 1983 Paediatric immunology. Blackwell Scientific Publications, Oxford

Stiehm E R, Fulginiti V A 1988 Immunologic disorders in infants and children, 3rd edn. Saunders, Philadelphia

23. The atopic child

Andrew Kemp

PRINCIPLES OF ATOPY

Atopy is defined as the predisposition to produce IgE antibodies in response to the ordinary exposure to allergens in the environment. Diseases associated with atopy, such as asthma, atopic eczema and allergic rhinitis, are called atopic diseases. These diseases are very common affecting 10–20% of the total population and often commencing in childhood. In atopic subjects IgE antibodies bound to mast cells can trigger the release of a number of inflammatory mediators after reaction with the appropriate allergen. Skin-prick testing and radioimmunoassay (RAST) provide evidence of sensitization by IgE antibodies (Table 23.1). It is often assumed that all the symptoms of atopic diseases are due to the release of mast cell mediators. This is not necessarily the case and in some situations it is more likely that IgE antibodies are produced in association with atopic diseases without necessarily being the fundamental cause of the symptoms (Table 23.2).

Table 23.1 Demonstration of specific IgE in atopic disease

RAST	Skin prick test
Expensive	Cheap
Delayed result	Immediate result
Widely available	Less available
Error ++	Error +
Interference (IgG and IgE)	Interference (antihistamine)

Table 23.2 Atopic disease

Symptoms usually produced by allergen mast cell reactions	Symptoms usually produced by other mechanisms
Seasonal allergic rhinitis	Perennial rhinitis
Allergic conjunctivitis	Asthma
Immediate hypersensitivity food reactions	Atopic dermatitis
	Spastmodic croup
	Delayed food reactions

ATOPIC SYMPTOMS

Atopic diseases often involve the respiratory tract, both upper and lower, the eyes, the skin and the gastrointestinal tract. These sites are exposed to the environment and contain relatively large concentrations of mast cells. About three-quarters of the atopic children will suffer from nasal symptoms, three-quarters from respiratory symptoms of cough and/or wheeze and one-third from atopic dermatitis. Symptoms in atopic children are frequently multiple and it is important to consider all the symptoms in the assessment of any atopic child. Atopic symptoms can occur at any age; however, certain patterns are often observed. Atopic dermatitis often begins early in infancy at about 2 months of age. The pattern of involvement changes from extensor surface involvement to involvement of the flexures at about 2–3 years of age. Alternatively the dermatitis may remit by 2–3 years of age. Subsequently these children may develop wheezing and perennial rhinitis in the preschool period and these symptoms improve as the child enters the teens to be replaced by seasonal rhinitis or hay fever.

Allergic rhinitis

Allergic rhinitis in children may be seasonal or perennial. Perennial rhinitis is associated with symptoms throughout the year. Seasonal rhinitis is commonly known as hay fever and occurs in spring and summer time. Perennial rhinitis is more common than seasonal rhinitis in childhood. Seasonal rhinitis is rarely seen in preschool children, but the incidence increases with age and in the teenage years is more common than perennial rhinitis.

Perennial rhinitis

In children under the age of ten years, perennial rhinitis accounts for the great majority of cases of allergic rhinitis. Symptoms are nasal obstruction, nasal discharge or both. Nasal obstruction due to a combination of oedematous nasal mucosa and mucus secretion can lead to snuffiness, mouth breathing and snoring at night. The parents may state that the child 'always has a cold'. Sneezing occurs particularly on awakening in the morning. The child may be observed to rub his nose and may give the 'allergic salute', an upward motion with the palm of the hand across the nose. On examination, a transverse nasal crease and 'allergic shiners', dark areas under the lower eye lids due to venous congestion, may be seen. These features are only found in a proportion of cases. The nasal airways should be assessed for air flow and this is best done by holding a metal object under the nose with the child breathing through a closed mouth, and observing the area of condensation on expiration. The nasal mucosa should then be inspected. The mucosa may appear pale and swollen. In more severe cases a marked mucosal swelling over the inferior turbinates can lead to complete obstruction to both nasal airways. The typical appearance of the mucosa is not always seen.

Investigation. There is little evidence that skin prick or RAST test can be used to identify allergens which provoke perennial rhinitis. The extent to which symptoms of perennial rhinitis are provoked by allergens is unclear. One possible provoking allergen is the house dust mite, but the role of this allergen has yet to be proven. Therefore, the identification of specific IgE antibodies is not particularly helpful in the management. Examination of a wiped nasal smear for the presence of mast cells, mucous cells and eosinophils may help, particularly when the diagnosis is in doubt or there is confusion between perennial rhinitis and recurrent infective rhinitis.

Management. Persistent snuffliness or nasal obstruction in infants is most appropriately treated by the regular application of normal saline nose drops three to four times daily. In older children the most effective treatment is a topical steroid nasal spray. A suitable regime is one puff of spray up each nostril three times daily for one week, twice daily for the next week, and daily thereafter. Daily treatment is continued for six to eight weeks. Antihistamines are usually not helpful and have been demonstrated to be ineffective in relieving nasal obstruction. Topical sodium cromoglycate is less helpful than topical steroids.

Over three-quarters of cases of perennial allergic rhinitis will respond to topical steroids and failure to respond should lead to consideration that the diagnosis is either a vasomotor or recurrent infective rhinitis. A lack of response may be due to marked nasal obstruction, and a limited course of vasoconstrictor drops for four or five days to open up the nasal passages used in

conjunction with topical steroids may be helpful. Cases resistant to topical steroids may respond to the topical application of the atropine-like substance ipratropium bromide which reduces mucus secretions.

Symptoms of perennial rhinitis are often attributed to enlarged adenoids and large numbers of children have had their adenoids removed for this condition with no benefit. In doubtful cases a trial of topical steroid therapy and investigation with nasal cytology is indicated before considering referral for adenoidectomy.

Seasonal rhinitis

Seasonal rhinitis, or hay fever, is most often seen in older children and teenagers. Seasonal rhinitis is due to an IgE-mediated reaction to pollen antigens and evidence of specific IgE antibodies can be found by either a skin-prick test or a RAST test. Symptoms occur in spring and summer when the plants are in flower. Plants of major importance are those that rely on wind pollination and include grasses, weeds and some trees. Air-borne pollen grains can travel for many miles from the site of release. There are immunological cross-reactions between pollen allergens from different plants particularly between species of the one genus.

The diagnosis is suggested by a history of seasonal exacerbations of symptoms of nasal itchiness, nasal wateriness and obstruction and sneezing. In addition, ocular conjunctival inflammation and itchiness may be present due to the allergic reaction in the conjunctivae. On examination the child may have conjunctival inflammation, obstruction of the nasal airways, swelling of the nasal mucosa and a watery nasal discharge.

Investigation. A selection of allergens for the demonstration of specific IgE is dependent on a knowledge of the plants in the local environment. Children with seasonal rhinitis will have a positive skin-prick or RAST test to the pollens provoking the symptoms. Nasal cytology in an active case of allergic rhinitis will often show increased numbers of eosinophils.

Management. Topical treatment with steroid sprays or sodium cromoglycate can alleviate symptoms. In the more troublesome cases treatment should be commenced at the start of the pollen season and continued throughout the season. Antihistamines may be helpful in relieving symptoms of itchiness and discharge but do not help nasal obstruction. Non-sedating long-acting antihistamines such as terfenadine and astemizole may be of particular benefit where daily therapy is required. In general, it is preferable to use topical therapy first and add antihistamine if control is not adequate.

Immunotherapy is only indicated in a clear case of

seasonal rhinitis where the appropriate allergen can be definitely identified, an appropriate allergen extract is available for desensitization, and topical treatments have failed adequately to control the symptoms. The expense and the time associated with this form of treatment should also be considered. In view of these problems immunotherapy is not usually indicated in children.

Allergic conjunctivitis

Allergic conjunctivitis represents a spectrum of conditions ranging from acute seasonal conjunctivitis in association with hay fever, seasonal vernal keratoconjunctivitis and persistent vernal keratoconjunctivitis. These conditions are due to an immediate hypersensitivity reaction in the conjunctivae. The allergic reactions are characterized by erythema and oedema of the conjunctivae and papillary hypertrophy, particularly of the upper lid conjunctivae. Oedema and hyperaemia of the limbus may be observed. The papillary hypertrophy of vernal conjunctivitis produces a cobblestone appearance which is seen on the inner aspect of the upper eye lid.

Usually, acute allergic conjunctivitis occurs in association with seasonal rhinitis as part of a more generalized immediate hypersensitivity reaction. A more chronic form may be associated with atopic eczema. Symptoms include itchiness of the eyes, redness of the eyes, a watery discharge, and photophobia. On examination, conjunctival injection and oedema may be noted, particularly in the lower bulbar conjunctivae. Treatment is with antihistamine or sodium cromoglycate eye drops. Steroid eye drops may occasionally be used in the more severe cases.

Vernal keratoconjunctivitis is a more severe form of conjunctivitis which leads to papillary hypertrophy, particularly on the upper eye lids. Involvement of the limbus is also common. This condition has a male preponderance and often starts under ten years of age. Usually there is a history of atopic disease such as asthma or eczema. IgE antigens against environmental allergens can be demonstrated in the tears. The symptoms are often seasonal in nature, being worse in the spring and summer time, but in the more severe cases the symptoms are present all the year round. Treatment is by topical sodium cromoglycate eye drops, four to six times daily. In the more severe cases, or those not responding to cromoglycate, steroid eye drops are used.

Secretory otitis media

Allergic reactions have been suggested to contribute to otitis media with effusion and the incidence of atopy is increased about three-fold in secretory otitis media. However, it is not proven that allergic reactions in the upper respiratory tract can result in a degree of Eustachian tube obstruction and middle ear secretion necessary to produce this condition. In view of the uncertainty about allergic factors, investigation of allergen sensitization and allergen avoidance measures are not indicated in the routine management. An associated allergic rhinitis should be treated.

Spasmodic croup

Some children develop recurrent episodes of laryngeal obstruction in the absence of any obvious infective aetiology. They awake at night with a croupy cough and stridor. The symptoms are transient and usually settle within several hours. This is termed spasmodic croup and should be distinguished from acute laryngotracheobronchitis which is due to a viral infection of larynx, trachea and bronchi. The transient nature of the symptoms, in contrast with the longer course of laryngotracheobronchitis, suggests the possibility of acute laryngeal oedema as a result of an allergic reaction. Approximately 50% of the children have evidence of other atopic features such as eczema, rhinitis, asthma or positive skin prick tests. In addition, both the upper and lower airways are hyper-reactive to histamine. Despite the possible role of mast cells in this condition there is no evidence that measures such as antihistamine, steroids or allergen avoidance are beneficial and the management is symptomatic with warm humidified air.

Occasionally laryngeal oedema with symptoms of croup can occur in association with an immediate hypersensitivity food reaction. In these cases the precipitating food substance is usually apparent and the management is avoidance of these foods.

Asthma

As asthma has been dealt with elsewhere, this section will concentrate on the manifestations of asthma in the atopic child and the possible role of allergens in the provocation of symptoms. Symptoms of recurrent cough and/or wheezing are one of the commonest presenting features in atopic children. Usually, the diagnosis is simple when there is a clear history of recurrent attacks of wheezing in association with other atopic manifestations, but may be more difficult when there is cough alone. Often there is considerable difficulty distinguishing between a cough on the basis of bronchial hyper-activity in asthma and one due to a recurrent infective bronchitis. In fact, there may be no clear distinguishing line, but a continuum between bronchial hyper-reactivity and atopy at one end of the spectrum and infection with excessive mucus production at the other. The presence of recurrent cough, particularly at night or precipitated by exercise or laughing, in a child with other atopic manifestations would suggest an asthmatic cough as the likely basis.

Despite the widespread belief that inhaled allergens are a common provoking cause of attacks of asthma it has been difficult to prove this association. The provocation of asthma attacks by stimuli such as cold air and exercise indicate that an allergen-antibody reaction is not essential to the development of an asthma attack. The most commonly identifiable precipitating cause of asthma attacks is respiratory tract viral infections. Allergens implicated, but rarely proven to provoke asthma attacks in childhood under conditions of natural exposure, include house dust mite antigens, grass pollens and food allergens. A number of children notice attacks of wheezing when exposed to animal danders, particularly cats. A problem with the proposition that inhaled allergens commonly provoke asthma is the finding that particles of the size of pollen grains and house dust mite antigens (10-14 microns) are not inhaled into the lower respiratory tract. Smaller allergen fragments have been demonstrated and can be inhaled into the lower respiratory tract.

A reason for identifying possible provoking allergens is that allergen avoidance may result in a reduction of symptoms. Pollen allergen can travel many miles in the air from the site of release and thus avoidance is extremely difficult. There have been a number of trials of house dust mite avoidance measures which have produced conflicting results. Dust mite avoidance measures used in successful trials include enclosing pillows and mattresses in impermeable covers, removal of clothes, toys, books and carpets from the bedroom and the washing of curtains and blankets every two weeks. It would seem that anything less than the fastidious observance of these measures is unlikely to result in a reduction of house dust mite allergens in the bedroom. Ingested allergens are not a common cause of asthma attacks. Occasionally, there are children who develop wheezing in association with an immediate hypersensitivity reaction to food, usually milk. In these cases there are other generalized manifestations such as urticaria and angioedema. Wheezing alone due to food ingestion in the absence of other immediate hypersensitivity symptoms is most uncommon. There is no evidence to indicate that infantile wheezing is usually caused by immediate hypersensitivity reactions to milk proteins. There have been no trials to demonstrate improvement after the use of a cow's milk substitute.

Wheezing in infancy is not closely associated with the development of food-specific IgE antibodies. Chemicals and preservatives in food, in particular sodium metabisulphite, can promote acute attacks of wheezing by a direct irritant effect rather than by an IgE-mast cell reaction. Sodium metabisulphite is used as a preservative in dried fruits, sausages, pickled onions and packaged fruit juices. Asthma attacks precipitated by metabisulphite occur within minutes of exposure and are often associated with an itchy feeling in the throat.

Investigation

Demonstration of specific IgE antibodies by skin-prick or RAST tests is not usually necessary in management of cases of childhood asthma. On occasions demonstration of sensitization may be helpful in characterizing a child as atopic, particularly when asthma presents as a cough without a clear history of wheeze and there are no other obvious clinical manifestations of atopy. The measurement of a total IgE level is not helpful.

Management

If there is a clear history of asthma attacks on exposure to pets these should be removed from the child's indoor environment and should not sleep in the child's bedroom. Where there is wheezing in association with immediate food reactions or ingestion of metabisulphite-containing foods these should be avoided. The role of house dust mite avoidance is not well defined. There is no role for this measure in episodic asthma in which symptoms have been predominantly triggered by viral respiratory tract infections. House dust mite avoidance should only be considered in chronic asthmatics in whom the symptoms are not adequately controlled by standard treatment regimes and in whom house dust mite-specific IgE can be demonstrated.

Immunotherapy remains an experimental mode of therapy and is not recommended in the routine management of childhood asthma.

Atopic dermatitis

Atopic dermatitis is characterized by itching with an erythematous papulovesicular inflammation on the extensor surfaces in infancy and a dry lichenified dermatitis in the flexural areas in later childhood. In the more severe cases the entire skin surface is involved. The condition tends to improve with time, although a small proportion of cases (about 5%) persists in adult life. Atopic dermatitis is one of the most characteristic manifestations of atopic state and is associated with high level of total IgE in the circulation and specific IgE to a variety of inhaled and ingested allergens. The inflammation in the skin is not simply the result of an immediate hypersensitivity IgE-mast cell reaction. Other immunological mechanisms, such as immune complex deposition and delayed hypersensitivity reactions, may contribute to the inflammation. In addition, the following number of other abnormalities noted in the skin may also be important in contributing to the development of the disorder:

• Blanching after stroking
• Decreased skin surface lipids
• Increased mast cell number
• Increased sweat gland response to acetylcholine.

Atopic dermatitis should not be regarded as having solely an allergic basis.

It is most appropriate to regard ingested allergens as a possible provoking factor rather than a primary cause of the disorder. Food allergens commonly implicated in provoking exacerbations of atopic dermatitis are eggs, milk and peanut products. A number of subjects with atopic dermatitis will demonstrate immediate hypersensitivity food reactions mediated by IgE-mast cell release with symptoms of urticaria and angioedema. In these subjects this immediate reaction will be associated with itching and subsequent worsening of the associated dermatitis. Other cases may demonstrate the delayed onset of erythema and itchiness one or two days after food ingestion. It is possible that these delayed reactions are associated with other immunological mechanisms.

Investigation

Although children with atopic dermatitis usually show a marked increase in total serum IgE levels, this information is of little therapeutic help. Similarly, specific IgE antibodies are usually detected to a range of inhaled and ingested allergens. It should be realized that the presence of specific IgE antibodies to an allergen does not necessarily indicate that that allergen is provoking symptoms. The demonstration of specific IgE antibodies can provide confirmatory evidence where there is a history of a typical immediate food hypersensitivity reaction.

Management

Foods provoking immediate hypersensitivity food reactions should be avoided. A clinical clue to these reactions is attacks of flushing and erythema which occur within one hour of food ingestion. If there is doubt on the history, confirmatory food challenge should be performed under medical observation before advising elimination. More extensive dietary manipulation is not indicated in all subjects but should be restricted to those children with extensive disease in whom standard dermatological treatment is not adequately controlling the symptoms. Such measures are required in less than 10% of children with atopic dermatitis. In these cases the most appropriate measure is a strict elimination diet which is prescribed for a limited period of time (2–4 weeks) with a close follow-up to determine any effect on the dermatitis. This should only be instituted after the topical treatment has been standardized. These diets eliminate foods containing preservatives, yeast, food colourings and dairy products and consist of a restricted range of foods such as lamb, beef, lettuce, carrots, pears and rice. In bottle-fed infants soya milk or a formula containing hydrolysed proteins are substituted for cow's milk. If there is no clear improvement detected after dietary elimination it may be concluded that foods are not a major provoking factor. If the dermatitis is improved after two to four weeks of dietary elimination foods are then reintroduced at the rate of one or two new food groups (e.g. milk, wheat) per week and any exacerbation of dermatitis on at least two occasions should be avoided. Children should not be prescribed strict elimination diets for prolonged periods of time without adequate dietary supervision. It should be emphasized that a total cure is not obtained and despite an apparent improvement on an elimination diet it is often difficult to identify any particular exacerbating food. Dietary elimination should not be prescribed solely on the basis of a positive skin-prick or RAST test.

Food hypersensitivity reactions

Allergic reactions to food in children can be divided into two classes. Immediate, occurring within 1–2 hours of food ingestion, and delayed, which occurs within 24–48 hours (Table 23.3).

True immediate hypersensitivity food reactions are quite common (approximately 1% of the population) and occur particularly in infancy. Delayed reactions are

Table 23.3 Food hypersensitivity reaction

Criteria	Time	
	Immediate (<2 hours)	Delayed (up to 48 hours)
IgE mediated	Yes	?
Diagnosis on history	Yes	Difficult
Frequency	Common	Rare >3 years

less common, and rarely occur in children over three years of age. Egg, milk, and peanut products are the most commonly implicated foods in both reactions.

Common symptoms of immediate food reactions are erythema, either where the food has touched the lips and skin, or more generalized, swelling of the lips and around the eyes, non-specific rashes and urticaria. Vomiting immediately after ingestion of food and irritability may be observed. These symptoms usually occur within 30 minutes of food ingestion and subside after 1–2 hours. Rhinorrhoea and wheezing are occasionally observed. More severe reactions with collapse due to generalized anaphylaxis can occur in the most sensitive individuals. Immediate food reactions may present in fully breast-fed babies on their first exposure to food. This suggests sensitization has occurred via the breast milk. Specific IgE antibodies to the relevant food can be demonstrated in all cases by means of a skin-prick or RAST test.

Delayed reactions are uncommon in older children but more frequent in infancy. They usually present with gastrointestinal symptoms such as vomiting and diarrhoea and occasionally exacerbation of a pre-existing atopic dermatitis. An inflammatory colitis with bloody diarrhoea may occur in infancy. Cow's milk is by far the most common provoking food. The immunological mechanism is unknown but it is not simply an IgE-mast cell reaction.

Investigation

The diagnosis of an immediate food reaction can generally be made on the clinical history. The clinical impression can be confirmed by detection of specific IgE antibodies. Contrary to popular belief, skin-prick tests can be readily performed in infants. A positive skin-prick test or RAST test to a food in the absence of a suggestive history does not establish the diagnosis of a food reaction. There are no immunological tests for delayed reactions.

Management

Management of food hypersensitivity reactions is outlined as follows:

- Immediate reaction with a clear history or specific IgE antibodies – avoidance of relevant food
- Immediate reaction with unclear history or specific IgE antibodies not demonstrated – food challenge
- Delayed reaction – food challenge.

In infancy, where the history is clear and the presence of IgE antibodies confirmed, it is reasonable to advise avoidance of the relevant foods until the child is 18 months to 2 years of age when a rechallenge is usually indicated. A considerable proportion of immediate food reactions will improve with time. If the history is confused or specific IgE cannot be demonstrated, confirmation by an open challenge under medical observation is indicated before advising dietary elimination. When the offending substance is cow's milk protein a soya milk substitute should be used.

The only way to confirm a delayed food reaction is by observing remission of symptoms on withdrawal of the food and relapse after a food challenge. Confirmation is often difficult and may, on occasions, require double blind challenge. In cow's milk enteropathy in infancy, the diagnosis is confirmed by observing remission of gastrointestinal symptoms after withdrawal of cow's milk from the diet and exacerbation after a formal milk challenge with a lactose-free milk. Lactose-free milk should be used on rechallenge to exclude confusion with lactose intolerance. If failure to thrive is present, a small bowel biopsy is essential to exclude other causes. In cow's milk enteropathy the biopsy is characterized by partial villous atrophy and lymphocytic infiltration of the mucosa. In views of the mucosal damage, the risk of subsequent sensitization to soya proteins may be increased and one of the hypoallergenic formulae in which proteins have been hydrolyzed should be used as a substitute food.

Urticaria and angioedema

Urticaria consists of raised areas of erythema and oedema involving the superficial portions of the dermis whilst angioedema consists of a similar reaction in the subcutaneous tissue. Urticaria is usually itchy, in contrast to angioedema. Angioedema commonly involves areas of low tissue tension such as the periorbital area, lip and scrotum. Urticaria and angioedema can occur together.

The lesions may be classified as acute or chronic, meaning a duration of greater than six weeks. The aetiology of the acute lesions, which often last only a few days, is usually unknown although some are associated with a viral or streptococcal infection. Obvious precipitating factors, such as drug ingestion (especially aspirin) and immediate hypersensitivity food reactions, should be identified by the history. Chronic urticaria and angioedema is less common in childhood. In the majority of cases no precipitating factor is identified. Physical urticarias, particularly cold, heat and dermatographism should be excluded. The finding of an IgE-mediated mast cell reaction to ingested allergens as a cause of chronic urticaria is rare (less than 5% of all cases). Other possible precipitating factors to be considered are artificial colouring and preservatives which act independently of IgE. The frequency of these reactions in children is not known.

Hereditary angioedema is an autosomal dominant condition associated with a deficiency of C1 esterase inhibitor protein and can be diagnosed by measuring the level and function of C1 esterase inhibitor. As C4 complement protein is almost invariably low, the measurement of C4 is a useful screening test. In most cases of periorbital or scrotal oedema which present in childhood no cause is found.

Investigation and management

The management of an acute urticarial episode is symptomatic with an antihistamine plus elimination of any obvious precipitating factor. In chronic urticaria the most useful approach is the trial of a strict elimination diet similar to that described above in the management of atopic dermatitis. All episodes should be recorded for two weeks before the institution of the diet and any remission of symptoms observed whilst on the diet. If the symptoms do not remit it is unlikely there is a dietary cause for the urticaria. If the symptoms do remit a series of challenge tests with salicylates, preservatives and food colouring are performed in an attempt to identify the provoking cause. Foods are then added back sequentially and occasionally exacerbation of symptoms may be noted on the addition of a specific food. The use of RAST or skin-prick testing is not a satisfactory way to identify provoking foods. Chemicals which promote chronic urticaria appear to do so by a direct effect on mast cells and specific IgE antibodies are not demonstrated. Despite these measures a considerable proportion of chronic urticarias do not have a cause identified. In these cases the management is symptomatic with antihistamines. If the lesions are causing severe discomfort a short course of oral steroids may be tried. A single dose of antihistamine at night, to minimize the sedative effect during the day, may be sufficient to control the lesions and should be tried before the more frequent use of antihistamines. Where the urticaria is unresponsive to one of the standard antihistamines, the antihistamine hydroxyzine may be effective.

FURTHER READING

Allan-Smith M R, Ross R N 1988 Ocular allergy. Clinical Allergy 18: 1–13
Atherton D J 1988 Diet and atopic eczema. Clinical Allergy 18: 215–228
Block S A 1984 Food sensitivity – a critical review and practical approach. American Journal of Diseases of Childhood 134: 973–982
Kemp A S 1984 The role of allergens in atopic disease in childhood. Australian Paediatric Journal 20: 161–168
Matthews K P 1983 Urticaria and angioedema. Journal of Allergy and Clinical Immunology 72: 1–14
Matthews K P 1982 Respiratory atopic disease. Journal of the American Medical Association 248: 2587–2610
Meltzer E O, Zeiger R S, Schatz M, Jalowdyski A A 1983 Chronic rhinitis in infants and children. Etiologic, diagnostic and therapeutic consideration. The Paediatric Clinics of North America 30: 847–871

Neonatal problems

Mental problems

24. Prematurity and low birthweight

Victor Y. H. Yu

Preterm infants are those born before 37 completed weeks from the first day of the mother's last menstrual period. Low birthweight (LBW) infants are those who weigh 2500 g or less at birth. About two-thirds of LBW infants are also preterm. Small-for-gestation age (SGA) infants are commonly defined as those whose birthweight is below the 10th centile of birthweight for the gestational age at which they are born (Fig. 24.1).

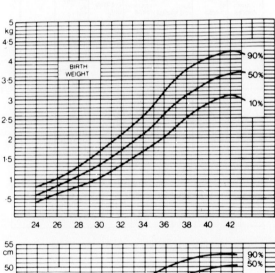

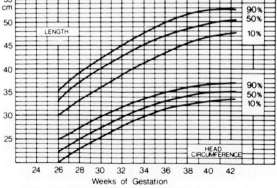

Fig. 24.1 Intrauterine growth percentiles from an Australian population.

It is possible for a LBW infant to be both preterm and SGA. This chapter first describes the problems of the preterm infant and then describes those of the SGA infant.

THE PRETERM INFANT

Incidence

Preterm and LBW infants both comprise about 6% of all live births, yet about 70% of neonatal deaths are LBW. Only 0.8% of live births weigh less than 1500 g but about 40% of neonatal deaths occur in this very low birthweight (VLBW) group. Therefore, LBW and especially VLBW infants assume an importance in neonatal mortality which is disproportional to their overall incidence amongst live births.

Aetiology

The cause of preterm birth is unknown in about 25–50% of cases. Preterm birth is of multiple aetiology. The many separate factors involved are so interdependent that the significance of each factor is uncertain. The associations which have been reported with preterm birth are listed in Example 24.1 but it is uncertain whether such factors are directly causal or purely indicative of a certain type of person. Preterm labour is like other adverse outcomes of pregnancy which occur more commonly in those who have experienced the same complication in past pregnancies; the risk of recurrence in women with one and two previous preterm labours are 40% and 70%, respectively.

Gestational age assessment

A careful history of the date of the last menstrual period gives the best estimation of gestation in about 80% of cases. Ultrasound measurement of fetal size in the first trimester provides reliable confirmation because, at this

Example 24.1 Factors associated with preterm births

Low socioeconomic status
Low prepregnant weight
Extremes of maternal age
Smoking
Alcohol consumption
Previous termination of pregnancy
History of infertility
High gravidity
Multiple pregnancy
First trimester threatened abortion
Abruptio placentae
Placenta praevia
Pre-eclamptic toxaemia
Polyhydramnios
Pyelonephritis
Developmental anomalies of the uterus
Cervical incompetence
Premature rupture of membranes
Chorioamnionitis
Induced labour and delivery
Negative attitudes to pregnancy

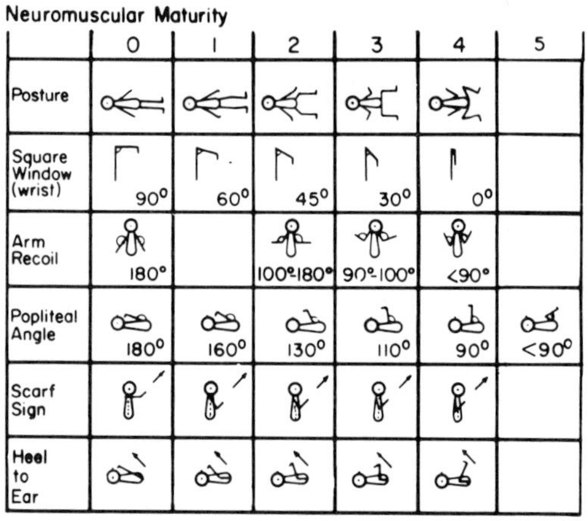

Neuromuscular Maturity

Physical Maturity

MATURITY RATING

Score	5	10	15	20	25	30	35	40	45	50
Wks.	26	28	30	32	34	36	38	40	42	44

Fig. 24.2 Simplified score for gestational assessment (from Ballard et al 1979).

early age, intrauterine growth retardation is negligible. Postnatal assessment of gestation should also be carried out in all LBW infants to confirm the obstetric estimations, as it is essential to differentiate a preterm infant whose weight is appropriate-for-gestational age (AGA) from one who is SGA. Most methods are based on the careful recording of neuromuscular development and external physical characteristics which are known to alter with increasing gestation. A reliable scoring system devised by Dubowitz & Dubowitz (1977) is commonly used but a simplified and rapid method has been formulated by Ballard et al 1979 (Fig. 24.2). The optimal age for testing is on the second day after birth and it is applicable to all infants, including those who are ill. Certain intrauterine and neonatal disorders may render individual criteria within the score less reliable but they do not significantly lessen the reliability of the total assessment.

Complications

Perinatal asphyxia

The preterm infant's condition at birth is the most important perinatal factor influencing survival. Perinatal asphyxia is more common in preterm infants than those delivered at term. Therefore, it is likely that prevention, or prompt detection and appropriate management of perinatal asphyxia would result in improved survival. Personnel competent in neonatal resuscitation should always be present at preterm deliveries.

Hypothermia

Thermal regulation is inadequate in preterm infants because of excessive heat loss (large surface area to volume ratio, reduced amounts of subcutaneous fat) and diminished heat production (reduced amounts of brown fat, decreased muscular activity, inability to shiver). Cold stress increases mortality rate, reduces growth rate and can lead to cold injury. Therefore, the preterm infant should be nursed in a thermoneutral environment (Fig. 24.3).

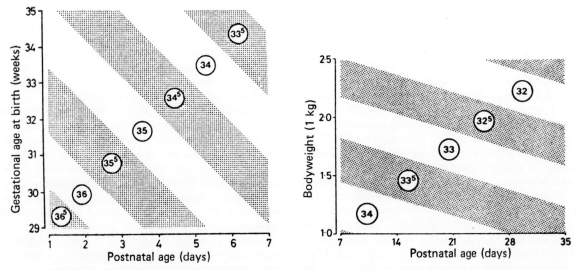

Fig. 24.3   Recommended ambient temperatures (°C) for preterm infants.

Respiratory problems

Immaturity of the lungs and surfactant deficiency cause hyaline membrane disease (HMD) (see Ch. 25). Antenatal steroid therapy and avoidance of perinatal asphyxia are effective in reducing the incidence and severity of respiratory failure from HMD. All preterm infants should be observed closely during the first four hours after birth for signs of respiratory distress in order that the severity of HMD can be determined and the appropriate oxygen and ventilatory therapy given.

Periodic breathing (periods of breathing for about 20 seconds) and recurrent apnoea (attacks lasting longer than 20–30 seconds) are consequences of inadequate development of the neurological control of breathing and the respiratory apparatus. However, before accepting prematurity as a case of recurrent apnoea, predisposing factors such as infection, periventricular haemorrhage or metabolic disorders must be excluded. Continuous electronic monitoring of the heart and breathing rate, with alarms set for bradycardia and apnoea, are required in preterm infants with recurrent apnoea. Aminophylline or theophylline therapy, nursing on an oscillating water bed and assisted ventilation are effective treatments for recurrent apnoea which, potentially, is an important cause of death or major disability from spastic diplegia and mental retardation if inadequately managed.

Cardiovascular problems

In many preterm infants, the ductus arteriosus remains patent after birth and closes spontaneously only as term approaches. Patent ductus arteriosus (PDA) presents in these infants with a hyperdynamic precordium and bounding pulses accompanied by a systolic or continuous murmur. Pulmonary congestion from left-to-right shunting through the PDA results in tachycardia, triple rhythm, crepitations on auscultation, hepatomegaly and recurrent apnoea. Echocardiography provides a non-invasive and quantitative assessment of PDA and has an important role in clinical management. A PDA which results in congestive cardiac failure, respiratory distress or ventilator dependence despite medical management requires pharmacological closure with indomethacin therapy or surgical ligation. Otherwise, the persistence of PDA prolongs oxygen and ventilatory therapy, reduces weight gain, increases the risk of developing bronchopulmonary dysplasia (BPD) and necrotizing enterocolitis (NEC), increases mortality and prolongs hospital treatment.

Neurological problems

With improved management of respiratory failure, periventricular haemorrhage (PVH) is becoming the most common cause of death in preterm infants. The non-invasive method of imaging the neonatal brain with ultrasonography has shown that its incidence is inversely proportional to gestational age, and that the majority are asymptomatic and occur in the first four days after birth. The haemorrhage takes place in the rich capillary matrix of the germinal layer found in preterm infants overlying the caudate nucleus (germinal layer haemorrhage) and this may rupture into the ventricles (intraventricular haemorrhage). For severe cases, there is extension of the haemorrhage into the cerebral white matter (intracerebral haemorrhage). PVH results from the effects of a loss of autoregulation of cerebral blood flow (due to hypoxaemia, hypercapnia and acidosis for which preterm infants with respiratory distress are particularly susceptible) on the prominent germinal layer also found in the same infants. Mild degrees of PVH do not adversely affect outcome. Severe haemorrhages often present as a catastrophic collapse with shock, apnoea and convulsions, leading to death or neurodevelopmental disabilities and hydrocephalus in those who survive. Hypoxic-ischaemic damage to the preterm brain also results in periventricular leukomalacia which can be diagnosed with ultrasonography as cystic degeneration in the white matter several weeks after the primary insult. Survivors of periventricular leukomalacia also have an increased risk of neurodevelopmental disability.

Gastrointestinal problems

Adequate nutrition in the preterm infant is considered to be important for survival and optimal growth and development. However, a poor or unsustained suck reflex, an unco-ordinated swallowing mechanism, delayed gastric emptying and poor intestinal transit make it extremely difficult to estabish milk feeding. Feed intolerance is associated with abdominal distension, cardiorespiratory disturbances, regurgitation of feeds and aspiration pneumonia.

NEC is a more serious complication which is associated with signs of systemic illness (apnoea, lethargy, pallor, temperature instability, metabolic acidosis) and symptoms attributable to gastrointestinal dysfunction (abdominal distension, blood in the stools, bile-stained gastric aspirate and diarrhoea). It is postulated that NEC results from hypoxic-ischaemic insult to the intestinal mucosa aggravated by excessive milk feeding and invasive bacterial proliferation. Often the condition recovers with medical treatment consisting of gastric aspiration, intravenous fluids and antibiotics. Perforation, peritonitis and stricture will require laparotomy and bowel resection.

Hepatic problems

Inadequate glycogen stores in the liver increase the tendency for hypoglycaemia in the preterm infant. Symptoms include lethargy, jitteriness, apnoea and convulsions. However, even asymptomatic hypoglycaemia should be avoided. Prevention is by routine monitoring of blood glucose 4–6 hourly after birth until normal levels are maintained. There is also a tendency for hyperglycaemia during glucose infusion in preterm infants. This is due to persistent endogenous hepatic glucose production and decreased peripheral glucose utilization. Therefore, monitoring of blood glucose is also required during intravenous therapy to avoid complications of glycosuria, osmotic diuresis and dehydration.

Indirect hyperbilirubinaemia is much more common in preterm infants due primarily to the immature liver functions of bilirubin uptake, conjugation and excretion. All preterm infants should be checked daily for clinical jaundice and serum bilirubin levels estimated if the jaundice is more than mild. Bilirubin encephalopathy or kernicterus (lethargy, convulsions, and death or survival with athetoid cerebral palsy, mental retardation and high-tone deafness) is liable to develop at lower levels of serum bilirubin in preterm infants. Successful management involves an adequate fluid and caloric intake, phototherapy and exchange transfusion. Often phototherapy is commenced in preterm infants at a serum bilirubin level of 150 μmol/l, or earlier if excessive bruising or haemolytic disease was present. Exchange transfusion is recommended when the bilirubin level increases to 200–300 μmol/l depending on co-existing factors such as hypoxia or acidosis which increase the risk of kernicterus.

Hypoprothrombinaemia contributes to haemorrhagic disease to which preterm infants are susceptible. Therefore, vitamin K should always be given at birth but if liver dysfunction or other complications are responsible for the coagulopathy, treatment by replacement of clotting factors will be necessary.

Renal problems

Preterm infants are prone to develop fluid imbalance. Compared with infants born at term, their renal concentration and diluting mechanisms are limited. Their larger surface area in relationship to weight and the higher insensible water loss through the skin also contribute to their poor adaptability to inadequate or excessive fluid intake. They are also at risk of sodium imbalance: hypernatraemia from dehydration and hyponatraemia because of excessive urinary losses from immature renal tubular function. An inability of the immature kidneys to conserve bicarbonate is also thought to result in late metabolic acidosis. This is associated with failure to thrive despite adequate nutritional intake.

Haematological problems

Preterm infants commonly develop an early normochromic and late hypochromic anaemia. The exaggerated postnatal fall in haemoglobin is due primarily to a shorter red cell life span and a sluggish response of erythropoiesis; therefore, it is non-responsive to iron therapy. If there is coexisting cardiorespiratory distress, small 'top-up' transfusions are required. Iron supplements are usually commenced at 6–8 weeks of age in preterm infants to lessen the late anaemia which is a result of rapid postnatal growth relative to available iron stores. Late macrocytic anaemia from folate deficiency can also occur in the preterm infant, but this is less common.

Immunological problems

Preterm infants do not have the full benefit of maternally transferred immunoglobulin. Their own ability to produce antibodies is also poorly developed, as are cellular immunity responses. As a result, preterm infants are very susceptible to infections. Clinical features of infection are non-specific and difficult to recognize. These include lethargy, irritability, refusal of feeds, poor weight gain, vomiting, diarrhoea, apnoea, jaundice, temperature instability and pallor. Vigilance by nursery staff is required and, when an infection is suspected, it is best to obtain cultures of blood, urine, nose, throat, umbilicus, or cerebrospinal fluid and then start antibiotics. Routine prophylactic antibiotic therapy in preterm infants is undesirable. Effective prevention requires scrupulous attention to hand-washing techniques in the nursery.

Miscellaneous late problems

Normal skeletal mineralization is dependent mainly on the availability of calcium and phosphorus and the interaction of hormones such as vitamin D and parathormone. Deficiencies of calcium and phosphorus are important in the aetiology of osteopenia and rickets in preterm infants. Breast milk and formulas do not supply enough calcium and phosphorus to match calculated in utero accretion rates. This deficiency is aggravated by the poor oral absorption of calcium by preterm infants. Frank rickets and pathological fractures of ribs and long bones develop especially in those who are extremely preterm. Treatment is by oral calcium and phosphorus supplementation.

Oxygen therapy for preterm infants remains a balanced risk: death or brain damage from hypoxaemia and retinopathy of prematurity (ROP) from hyperoxaemia. Arterial oxygen tensions should be kept between 50–80 mmHg, but with currently available technology even the most impeccable monitoring of arterial oxygen tension does not guarantee against ROP. In the acute stage, there are dilatation of retinal vessels, abnormal formation of new capillaries and haemorrhages. These abnormalities resolve spontaneously in the majority of cases, but fibrous scarring and retinal detachment may occur in severe cases with resultant myopia or blindness. All preterm infants who require oxygen therapy should have their eyes examined by indirect ophthalmoscopy after they recover from their acute illness.

BPD is a condition which results in chronic respiratory distress often of several months' duration and associated with cystic changes in the chest radiograph. It occurs in preterm infants with severe respiratory disorders treated with prolonged endotracheal intubation, mechanical ventilation and a high inspired oxygen concentration. Barotrauma, oxygen toxicity and secondary chest infection probably all contribute to the lung damage. Most infants with resulting BPD have periodic wheezing usually with infection in the first two years of life, but the long-term outlook is generally favourable.

Also, persistent respiratory distress is seen in preterm infants from one week of age without preceding HMD or mechanical ventilation. This conditon is often called Wilson-Mikity syndrome if there are cystic changes in the chest radiograph, or chronic pulmonary insufficiency of prematurity (CPIP) if the chest radiograph shows diffuse atelactasis. Their clinical courses are similar to that of BPD.

Psychosocial problems

The imposed postpartum separation of the parents from their preterm infant is only one factor which increases the risk of parent-infant interactive disturbances. The psychological stress following preterm birth, the abnormal behavioural characteristics of a preterm infant and the unfavourable environment of a special care nursery contribute to the problem in attachment. Open visiting policies and encouragement for early parent-infant contact and participation in care-taking activities must be supported by active parental counselling. This approach aids the development of comprehensive psychosocial management for the preterm infant and the family, both in hospital and during the important months after discharge. Preterm infants in the past were considered to be at particular risk for later child abuse or neglect. This problem can be largely prevented now if the psychosocial needs of the parents are recognized and effectively met.

Prognosis

Studies in preterm children born before 1950 generally showed that those with serious neonatal problems usually died. The few who survived were the ones who had to contend with the least complications and their long-term prognosis was often good. Reports in the 1960s drew rather depressing conclusions because although survival rates had improved, impairments such as cerebral palsy, blindness, deafness and mental retardation were common, for example, 30–80% of VLBW survivors were affected. This was partly because the importance of prevention of hypoxaemia, acidosis, hypothermia, hyperbilirubinaemia, hypoglycaemia and malnutrition was not appreciated and iatrogenic handicap was very much in evidence.

With better understanding of the pathophysiology of preterm postnatal adaptation and advanced technological methods of treatment, more recent years have been associated with an improvement in both mortality and late morbidity rates for all preterm infants, even in those who are less than 100 g birthweight (Table 24.1) or below 29 weeks gestation (Table 24.2). Here the term 'major disability' has been defined as an impairment which would cause a significant interference with what is considered to be a normal lifestyle. As the incidence of major disabilities falls, more 'minor' problems such as learning and behaviour disorders are emerging. Therefore, regular and long- term physical, developmental and psychological assessment, extremely preterm

survivors, should be routinely carried out to detect both major and minor problems, in order that intervention therapy can be initiated to improve the preterm infants' chances of reaching their maximum potential.

THE SGA INFANT

Incidence

SGA infants are those whose intrauterine growth has been abnormally slow and whose birthweight is, therefore, low for the gestation at which they are born. In order that such infants are classified accurately, a growth percentile chart for the population to which the infant belongs is required.

One commonly used definition for SGA is a birthweight below the 10th centile for gestation. This implies that 10% of newborn infants are regarded as SGA. The advantage of this arbitrary dividing line between AGA (appropriate for gestational age) and SGA is that it will include most infants at risk for the special problems associated with intrauterine growth failure. When percentile charts derived from one country are used on infants from a different population, the incidence of SGA may range from 3–30% due essentially to racial and socioeconomic influences.

Aetiology

SGA infants form a heterogeneous group of varied aetiology (see Example 24.2). There are two main categories of SGA infants; either the fetus has an altered growth potential or the intrauterine environment has resulted in diminished support for growth of an other-

Table 24.1 Two-year outcome of singleton inborn ELBW livebirths

Birthweight (g)	No. of infants	No.of survivors	No. of survivors with impairment	No. of survivors with major disability
500–599	30	3 (10%)	1 (33%)	1 (33%)
600–699	38	13 (34%)	3 (23%)	2 (15%)
700–799	36	20 (56%)	4 (20%)	2 (10%)
800–899	49	35 (71%)	6 (17%)	4 (11%)
900–999	53	37 (70%)	8 (22%)	4 (11%)
Total	206	108 (52%)	22 (20%)	13 (12%)

Table 24.2 Two-year outcome of singleton inborn extremely preterm livebirths

Gestation (weeks)	No. of infants	No. of survivors	No. of survivors with impairment	No. of survivors with major disability
23	19	2 (11%)	1 (50%)	1 (50%)
24	35	13 (37%)	2 (15%)	1 (8%)
25	24	10 (42%)	4 (40%)	2 (20%)
26	54	33 (61%)	8 (24%)	5 (15%)
27	68	53 (78%)	4 (8%)	3 (6%)
28	76	57 (75%)	6 (11%)	4 (7%)
Total	276	168 (61%)	25 (15%)	16 (10%)

Example 24.2 Factors associated with SGA births

Altered growth potential
Chromosomal disorders: trisomy 13–15, trisomy 16–18, cri-du-chat syndrome
Intrauterine infections: rubella, cytomegalovirus, toxoplasmosis
Dwarf syndromes: Russell-Silver, Cornelia de Lange
Drugs: antimetabolites, radiation
Genetic: racial, familial

Diminished support for growth
Pre-eclamptic toxaemia
Maternal hypertensive or renal disease
Smoking, alcohol, heroin
Malnutrition or chronic illness
Hypoxaemia: high altitude, cyanotic cardiac or pulmonary disease
Multiple gestations, twin-to-twin transfusion
Circumvallate placenta, infarction, recurrent antepartum haemorrhage

wise normal fetus. The latter is more common and results from a deficiency of growth substrates in the last trimester, as occurs with maternal and placental disorders. This period is a time when weight increases five-fold with a maximum growth velocity between 32 and 36 weeks. This contrasts to a maximum length velocity at 18 to 20 weeks and a much earlier maximum head velocity. Therefore, growth retardation in these infants is mainly for weight, with length and head circumference normal or close to normal.

Complications

General

The SGA infant who is preterm is subjected to the same disadvantages as the AGA preterm infant. However, complications due to functional immaturity of various organ systems are less common in SGA infants compared with AGA infants of similar birthweight but of shorter gestation. These include conditons such as MD, recurrent apnoea, PDA, PVH, feed intolerance, hyperbilirubinaemia and renal dysfunction. Nevertheless, SGA infants are born with special hazards which merit separate description.

Perinatal asphyxia

As gestation advances beyond 34 weeks, the SGA fetus has an increased risk of fetal distress and death in utero. Their ability to withstand the stress of labour and delivery is also impaired. This vulnerability of the SGA fetus to asphyxia is partly related to low stores of liver and cardiac glycogen and impaired placental function. Intensive fetal monitoring is required as decisions on the timing and mode of delivery have to be made, based on the estimated risks of delivery and prematurity versus that of leaving the fetus in utero.

Hypothermia

The larger surface area relative to body weight and diminished subcutaneous fat in SGA infants further narrow their thermoneutral range compared with AGA infants. Therefore, special precautions should be taken to prevent heat loss.

Respiratory problems

Gasping in utero and the passage of meconium into the amniotic fluid are consequences of asphyxia to which the SGA is prone. The infant with meconium aspiration syndrome presents with respiratory distress from birth. Diagnosis is made from the history and confirmed by the chest radiography. The infants should be managed with oxygen, ventilatory and supportive therapy as appropriate, including antibiotics because of the risks of secondary pneumonia.

Massive pulmonary haemorrhage is a much less common condition in SGA infants than it used to be. The usual presentation is on the second to fourth day when blood wells up the trachea and the infant becomes shocked. The pathogenesis is acute left heart failure which results in haemorrhagic pulmonary oedema. Often it is associated with perinatal asphyxia, hypothermia and hypoglycaemia and may be less often seen now because of the success in preventing these disorders.

Hypoglycaemia

Compared with the preterm AGA infant, the SGA infant is at higher risk for hypoglycaemia due to a serious disturbance of carbohydrate metabolism and a greatly deficient store of liver glycogen. Management of the SGA infant includes early feeding, meticulous monitoring of blood glucose and intravenous therapy if hypoglycaemia occurs.

Polycythaemia

An elevated haematocrit and increased red cell volume may be consequent upon acute placental-fetal transfusion during acute fetal hypoxaemia or to an elevation of erythropoetin from chronic fetal hypoxaemia. Hyperviscosity, coagulation disturbances and NEC are further consequences of polycythaemia. The central haematocrit should be measured in plethoric infants and partial exchange transfusion with plasma is recommended for a haematocrit about 65%.

Congenital anomalies

The above hazards apply mainly to the group of SGA infants with diminished growth support in utero. In addition, there is a 10–20 times increase in incidence of congenital anomalies in SGA infants compared with AGA infants. This is due mostly to chromosomal disorders and intrauterine infections. These conditions are the cause rather than the result of intrauterine growth failure. SGA infants should be examined carefully for congenital anomalies and screening for intrauterine infections carried out as appropriate.

Prognosis

The risk of perinatal death is twelve-fold in extremely SGA infants who fall below the 3rd centile for weight.

The most common cause of death in SGA infants is asphyxia either before, during or after birth. Growth and developmental prognosis depends on the cause of intrauterine growth retardation. Those who have a normal growth potential and did not have severe or prolonged growth restriction in utero have a more favourable outcome than those whose growth compromise predated conception or began in early fetal life. Most studies find that SGA infants will ultimately be slimmer and shorter than their gestational for weight peers. Major neurodevelopmental disabilities are infrequent in SGA infants when those with overt anomalies and intrauterine infections are excluded, thus dispelling previously widely held beliefs that SGA infants are doomed before birth. Improved obstetric and neonatal care have been effective in reducing perinatal asphyxia and hypoglycaemia to which the SGA infant is prone.

REFERENCES

Ballard J L, Novak K K, Driver M 1979 A simplified score for assessment of fetal maturation of newly born infants. Journal of Pediatrics 95: 769–774

Dubowitz L M S, Dubowitz V 1977 Gestational age of the newborn. Addison-Wesley, London

FURTHER READING

Kitchen W H, Robinson H P, Dickenson A J 1983 Revised intrauterine growth curves for an Australian hospital population. Australian Paediatric Journal 19: 157–161

Sauer P J J, Dane H J, Visser H K A 1984 New standards for neonatal thermal environment of healthy very low birthweight infants in week one of life. Archives of Disease in Childhood 59: 18–22

Stewart A L, Reynolds E O R, Lipscomb A P 1981 Outcome for infants of very low birth weight: survey of world literature. Lancet i: 1038–1041

Usher R 1987 Extreme prematurity. In: Avery G B (ed) Neonatology: pathophysiology and management of the newborn, 3rd edn. J B Lippincott, Philadelphia, 264–298

Willis S M, Harvey D 1986 Fetal growth, intrauterine growth retardation and small-for-dates babies. In: Roberton N R C (ed) Textbook of neonatology, Churchill Livingstone, London, 199–128

Yu V Y H 1986 Respiratory disorders in the newborn. Churchill Livingstone, London

Yu V Y H, Wood E C (eds) 1987 Prematurity. Churchill Livingstone, London

Yu V Y H, Loke H L, Bajuk B et al 1986 Prognosis for infants born at 23 to 28 weeks' gestation. British Medical Journal 293: 1200–1203

25. The infant with respiratory distress

D. I. Tudehope

At birth major cardiopulmonary changes occur in order to prepare the baby for extrauterine life. In the first instance the fluid-filled fetal lung is replaced by an air-filled lung. Associated with inflation of the lungs and the relative hyperoxia, there is a marked decrease in pulmonary vascular resistance with consequent increased pulmonary blood flow and closure of the fetal shunts, namely, the ductus arteriosus, foramen ovale and ductus venosus. Thus the lungs take over the respiratory function previously carried out by the placenta. This normal sequence of events can be disturbed in a number of ways. Respiratory problems are perhaps the commonest of all disorders in the newborn period. They may present clinically in two different ways:

1. Respiratory distress
2. Upper airways obstruction.

Apnoea and bradycardia may complicate either presentation.

RESPIRATORY DISTRESS

Clinically this is assessed by the presence of tachypnoea (a respiratory rate in excess of 60 per minute), expiratory grunt, chest retraction or recession, flaring of the alae nasae and cyanosis in air. The presence of two or more of the above signs persisting for more than four hours suggests respiratory distress.

There are many causes of respiratory distress in the newborn. Diagnosis will be made by a careful history, physical examination and appropriate investigation. Chest radiographs, anteroposterior and frequently lateral, are essential in the management of any neonate with respiratory distress. Should infection be suspected, bacteriological and virological cultures of blood, urine, CSF and gastric aspirate and full blood count will be necessary. The L/S ratio or 'shake test' on gastric and tracheal aspirates or ammniotic fluid may confirm the diagnosis of respiratory distress syndrome (RDS). Chest transillumination, passage of nasogastric catheters and

haematocrit will diagnose pneumothorax, choanal atresia and polycythaemia, respectively. A hyperoxia or nitrogen washout test may be necessary to distinguish cyanotic congenital heart disease from respiratory distress. Respiratory distress may be due to primary pulmonary diseases or secondary to fetal circulation, congenital heart disease, anaemia, polycythaemia, cerebral damage, infection and metabolic disease.

Transient tachypnoea of the newborn (TTN)

This disorder occurs in approximately 1–2% of all newborn infants. Usually it is benign with symptoms rarely persisting beyond 48 hours. Only rarely is the disorder protracted and requiring intensive therapy.

Pathogenesis

Most of the fetal lung fluid is removed during descent in the birth canal and in the first few breaths after birth. It would appear that in transient tachypnoea, the newborn has either an excess of fetal fluid, a disturbance in the clearing mechanisms, or a combination of both.

Predisposing factors include marginal prematurity (34 to 36 weeks), heavy maternal analgesia, birth asphyxia, Caesarean section, breech presentation, male sex and hypoproteinaemia. The outstanding symptom is tachypnoea. The diagnosis is confirmed by chest radiograph which may show cardiomegaly, venous congestion, perihilar cuffing, fluid in the pleural fissures and, occasionally, small pleural effusions (Figs 25.1 and 25.2).

Hyaline membrane disease (HMD)

This is also known as the respiratory distress syndrome (RDS). It is a specific entity occurring in preterm infants and caused by a lack of surfactant (a surface tension lowering agent) in the alveoli. It has a characteristic clinical picture and a specific radiograph which shows changes of hypoaeration, a diffuse

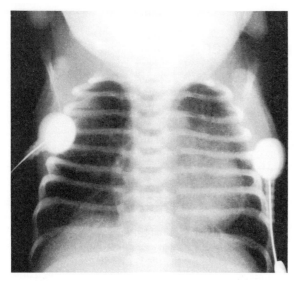

Fig. 25.1   Chest radiograph of transient tachypnoea of the newborn showing cardiomegaly, perihilar cuffing, fluid in horizontal fissure and coarse streaking in lungs.

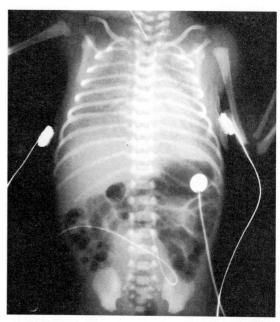

Fig. 25.3   Chest radiograph of RDS with hypoaeration, air bronchograms and diffuse granuloreticular pattern – almost a 'white out'.

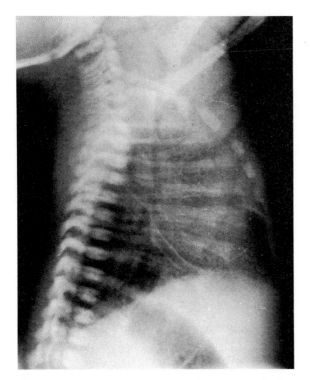

Fig. 25.2   Lateral chest radiograph of TTN showing fluid in oblique and horizontal fissures; generalized lung opacification.

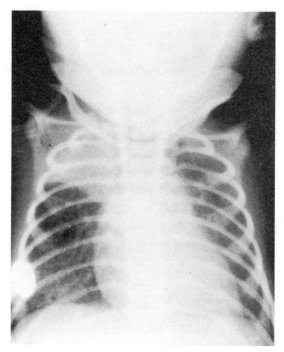

Fig. 25.4   Right upper lobe collapse following extubation after a course of mechanical ventilation in an infant with RDS.

granuloreticular pattern, air bronchograms (Fig. 25.3) and, in its most severe form, a diffuse 'white out'. Frequently lobar collapse occurs secondary to mucus plugging particularly after extubation (Fig. 25.4).

Incidence

This is a common condition and occurs in 1% of all newborns. In spite of recent advances in the management of premature delivery, the incidence has remained markedly static. The incidence of RDS is related to the degree of prematurity (Fig 25.5). The predisposing factors for RDS include prematurity, maternal diabetes mellitus, antepartum haemorrhage, second twin, hypoxia, acidosis, shock, male sex and, possibly, Caesarean section. In an individual case it is not uncommon for a number of these factors to be present simultaneously.

Pathogenesis

Lack of surfactant results in alveoli remaining unexpanded (atelectatic) and impairment of gaseous exchange. Surfactant is a phospholipid secreted by the type 2 alveolar cells in the lung. Its major active component is lecithin but other phospholipids and protein must be present for full activity. These surface active agents, which are released into the alveoli, reduce surface tension thus helping to keep the alveoli open. In HMD some alveoli are widely patent and others atelectatic causing maldistribution of ventilation. This results in biochemical disturbances of acidosis and hypoxia with a consequent perfusion imbalance. Therefore, HMD is characterized by a ventilation-perfusion (V/Q) imbalance. When the lungs of an infant who has survived

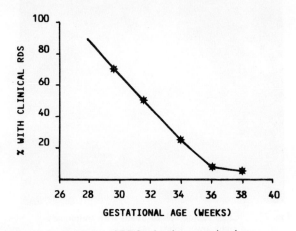

Fig. 25.5 Incidence of RDS related to gestational age.

for several hours after birth are examined at autopsy, hyaline membranes may be demonstrated lining the respiratory bronchioles and alveolar ducts.

Clinical features

The signs of respiratory distress – tachypnoea, chest retraction, expiratory grunting, flaring of the alae nasae and cyanosis may start immediately after birth, or in the first 6 hours of life. These symptoms tend to increase and reach a peak at between 48 and 72 hours, although maximum severity may occur in infants less than 12 hours old. In the early stages, the infant lies in a 'frog-like' position and has difficulty with copious pharyngeal secretions which need constant clearing. With progression of the disease, oxygen will be necessary to abolish cyanosis, the expiratory grunt will diminish and prolonged apnoeic spells may occur. At this stage, breath sounds are decreased and the blood pressure may fall. Initially the infant is oliguric and develops peripheral oedema. At about 48 hours, a diuresis frequently occurs with concomitant clinical improvement.

Prognosis of hyaline membrane disease

With appropriate treatment the long-term outlook is excellent.

Early complications. These include patent ductus arteriosus with congestive heart failure, pulmonary air leaks, such as pneumothorax and pulmonary interstitial emphysema, lobar and segmental collapse and cerebroventricular haemorrhage, the latter being present in 70% of infants who die with HMD.

Late complications. The long-term sequelae from oxygen toxicity are chronic lung disease (bronchopulmonary dysplasia) which may be associated with recurrent wheezing in the first year of life and retrolental fibroplasia which may result in myopia, strabismus and early blindness in its most severe form. Neurological complications are divided into major neurological handicaps, such as spastic diplegia, quadriplegia, post haemorrhagic hydrocephalus, microcephaly and mental retardation which usually manifest in the first year of life whilst the minor neurological handicaps such as ataxia, inco-ordination, specific learning difficulties and minimal cerebral dysfunction may not be recognized for years. The survival of infants with respiratory distress syndrome relating to birthweights in one major neonatal unit (Mater Misericordiae Hospital, Brisbane) from 1985 to 1987 was:

less than 1000 g – 61%
1000 to 1499 g – 93%
1500 to 1999 g – 99%
2000 to 2499 g – 99%

Pneumonia

In the newborn pneumonia is relatively common and is usually bacterial. Particular oganisms involved are Gram- negative bacilli (e.g. *Escherichia coli*, *Klebsiella*, *Pseudomonas*), Group B *Streptococcus* and *Staphylococcus* species. Rarer bacterial pathogens include *Listeria monocytogenes* and anaerobic bacilli. Non-bacterial pathogens include *Chlamydia trachomatis*, *Mycoplasma pneumoniae*, *Candida albicans*, cytomegalovirus and *Pneumocystis carinii*. Pneumonia may be contracted in utero and be present at birth (congenital) or acquired after birth (nosocomial). Congenital pneumonia may be due to ascending infection with prolonged rupture of membranes, or less frequently due to a transplacental infection. The early clinical signs and symptoms are often not specific and may include lethargy, apnoea, bradycardia, temperature instability and intolerance to feeds. At birth it may be very difficult to decide whether a baby is or is not infected. Features of respiratory distress may be present in other cases. It is important that the predisposing factors for infection at birth are evaluated when arriving at a diagnosis of neonatal pneumonia.

On examination of the chest, diminished air entry over areas of consolidation or effusion may be noted. Fine crepitations may be heard on inspiration, but signs may be difficult to elicit. Although radiography is essential for diagnosis, the appearances are often non-specific and the patchy opacities or more confluent areas of radiodensity cannot be distinguished from aspiration syndrome (Fig. 25.6) or transient tachypnoea of newborn (Fig. 25.7).

Pulmonary air leaks

These are common in newborn infants. A variety of types are described e.g. pneumothorax, pulmonary interstitial emphysema (air in the interstitial lung spaces) and pneumomediastinum.

Pneumomediastinum may precede or occur in association with pneumothorax. The air associated with pulmonary interstitial emphysema may loculate to form a pulmonary pseudocyst and occasionally is unilateral resulting in tension to the opposite lung. Rarer, but more severe, pulmonary air leaks include pneumopericardium, pneumoperitoneum and air embolus (air entering the blood stream via pulmonary veins).

Spontaneous pneumothorax occurs in approximately 1% of vaginal and 1.5% of Caesarean section deliveries.

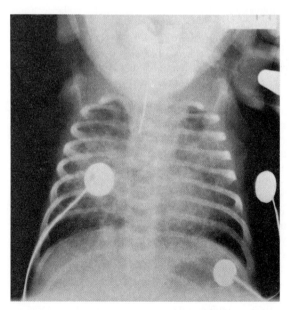

Fig. 25.6 Chest radiograph of group B *Streptococcus* pneumonia.

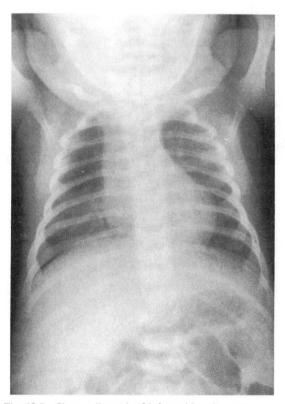

Fig. 25.7 Chest radiograph of infant with pulmonary infiltrate in right lower lobe.

Most of these are asymptomatic and found quite by accident. However, resuscitation with positive pressure markedly increases the incidence of pneumothorax. Pathological conditions in the lung predisposing to the occurrence of pneumothorax include hyaline membrane disease, hyperinflated lungs, and hypoplastic lungs.

The clinical features of infants with pulmonary air leaks comprise the non-specific signs of respiratory distress, but there may be specific signs of mediastinal shift to the opposite side, asymmetrical chest expansion and weak peripheral pulses; a prominent sternum may suggest a pneumomediastinum. Frequently, a pulmonary air leak occurs in a baby who already has respiratory distress so that there may be sudden deterioration with cyanosis, poor peripheral perfusion and bradycardia.

A diagnosis rests on an AP and lateral radiograph of the chest (Fig. 25.8). Chest transillumination is a useful technique to establish the diagnosis in critically ill infants with tension pneumothorax. And occasionally the emergency insertion of a small needle may be a life saving procedure when a delay is anticipated in obtaining a radiograph in a critically ill infant.

Meconium aspiration syndrome

Meconium aspiration results in plugging of airways with consequent atelectasis. This may also cause a ball valve obstruction with hyperinflation of lungs and a high risk of pulmonary air leaks. Meconium is extremely irritating to airways and produces a chemical pneumonitis which may predispose to secondary bacterial infection (Fig. 25.9).

Meconium aspiration is a preventable cause of respiratory distress in the newborn. Meconium staining of amniotic fluid is common, occurring in 9% of deliveries and may be a sign of fetal distress, of postmaturity, or occur normally with a breech presentation. The possibility of aspiration of meconium into the lungs during labour, or at the outset of respiration should always be anticipated.

The clinical features range from severe birth asphyxia, the early onset of respiratory distress to a vigorous baby with no major problems. Typically the infant is born covered in meconium liquor with meconium staining of the umbilical cord, skin and nails. The chest appears to be hyperinflated with a prominent sternum. Infants with meconium aspiration may be irritable and have a slow heart rate, often in the region of 80–90 per minute.

Complications of meconium aspiration include pulmonary air leaks, persistent pulmonary hypertension, hypoglycaemia and hypoxic-ischaemic encephalopathy.

The treatment of meconium aspiration is largely prevention. Thus, with the appearance of the head at birth, the pharynx is suctioned via the mouth and nose. The umbilical cord should be rapidly clamped and the pharynx suctioned under direct laryngoscopic vision. If

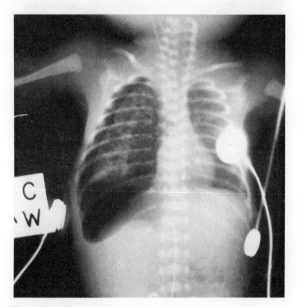

Fig. 25.8 Chest radiograph showing right tension pneumothorax with underlying pulmonary interstitial emphysema.

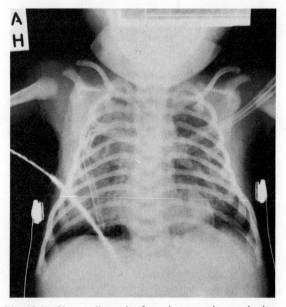

Fig. 25.9 Chest radiograph of massive meconium aspiration showing diffuse coarse opacification with collapse and lung hyperinflation.

meconium is seen at or below the vocal cords the trachea is intubated and aspirated with a 6 French gauge catheter. Instillation of 0.25 ml of normal saline may be necessary to liquify meconium and aid suctioning. As baby is extubated direct suctioning of endotracheal tube is practised. If large amounts of meconium are aspirated the procedure needs to be repeated. The stomach is aspirated and lavaged with normal saline. The infant is transferred to the nursery for further treatment with humidified air (ultrasonic mist) or oxygen, active chest physiotherapy and drainage.

Pulmonary hypoplasia

A sufficient volume of amniotic fluid is necessary for adequate fetal lung development so that with marked oligohydramnios the lungs do not form normally. Many infants with pulmonary hypoplasia have associated facial abnormalities and limb contractures. Also, hypoplastic lungs predispose to the development of pneumothorax. Oligohydramnios may be due to prolonged rupture of membranes or to a renal abnormality. The fetal side of the placenta should be examined for the presence of amnion nodosum which is suggestive of severe oligohydramnios, especially Potter's syndrome.

Infants develop severe respiratory distress from birth with marked hypoxia, hypercarbia and metabolic acidosis. The lungs are very stiff and there is little chest movement even with mechanical ventilation. Severe lung hypoplasia is incompatible with life.

Massive pulmonary haemorrhage

This presents in newborn infants with signs of cardiovascular collapse associated with outpouring of blood-stained fluid from the trachea and mouth. It occurs in about 1 per 1000 births and is usually fatal. Massive pulmonary haemorrhage has been described in association with severe birth asphyxia, hypothermia, small-for-gestational age infants, coagulation disturbances and congenital heart disease. Haemorrhagic pulmonary oedema has been suggested as a possible aetiology.

Treatment

Treatment is for respiratory distress, but particular emphasis must be given to volume expansion with agents such as SPPS, blood and sodium bicarbonate. In the presence of pulmonary oedema, digitalis, frusemide and perhaps morphine are indicated. Coagulation disturbances must be corrected and, should mechanical ventilation be required, high positive expiratory pressures may minimize bleeding.

Congenital diaphragmatic hernia

Usually this is a postero-lateral hernia (Bochdalek type) with 80% being left sided. The defect is due to a persistent pleuro-peritoneal canal with failure of development of muscular components. Herniation of abdominal contents into the thorax results in lung hypoplasia or compression of the lung on the side of the hernia with displacement of mediastinum to the contralateral side. Babies with large diaphragmatic hernias have severe birth asphyxia with persistent cyanosis. Less acute cases may present in the nursery with respiratory distress, or on routine examination when a 'dextrocardia' or scaphoid abdomen will be appreciated. On auscultation of the lungs, bowel sounds may be heard on the side of the lesion if gas has entered the gastrointestinal tract. The diagnosis of diaphragmatic hernia is confirmed by chest radiograph which shows bowel loops in the thorax (Fig. 25.10). However, if the radiograph is taken shortly after birth, there may be some difficulty in determining whether the bowel is in the chest, especially if there is little air in the gastrointestinal tract. The radiograph should be taken with a radio-opaque catheter in the stomach and should

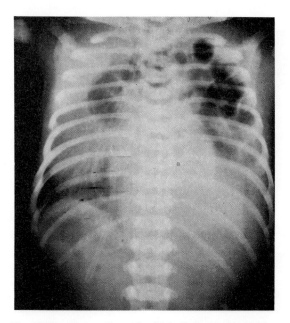

Fig. 25.10 Chest radiograph of left diaphragmatic hernia with mediastinal shift to the right and gas pattern within the thorax.

include the abdomen in order to show a paucity of abdominal gas pattern.

Treatment

If a congenital diaphragmatic hernia is suspected, an orogastric tube should be inserted and the abdominal contents within the chest aspirated of gas and secretions. If the baby requires assisted ventilation, it should be via an endotracheal tube and never by bag and mask because of increasing the bowel distension within the chest. Great care must be taken to prevent rupture of the contralateral lung, as the infant is almost exclusively dependent on this lung for gaseous exchange. After the initial diagnosis and stabilization the baby should be referred to a paediatric surgeon; surgery involves reduction of the abdominal contents, closure of the diaphragmatic defect and correction of any bowel malrotation.

Oesophageal atresia and tracheo-oesophageal fistula

Oesophageal atresia is a congenital anomaly in which there is usually complete interruption of the lumen resulting in a blind upper pouch. This is generally associated with a tracheo-oesophageal fistula. The accompanying diagram shows the various anatomical types (Fig. 25.11).

Clinical features

Maternal hydramnios occurs in 60% of cases and is largely responsible for the high frequency of premature births. Oesophageal atresia is associated with excessive saliva and mucus production and consequently a high incidence of aspiration pneumonia. This is accentuated if the infant is fed, when milk may accumulate in the upper pouch and spill over into the trachea. Aspiration of gastric contents and bile into the bronchial tree via the fistula results in pulmonary complications of collapse and pneumonia. Abdominal distension is due to air passing down the fistula into the stomach. Coexistent congenital anomalies may be present; these include major cardiac disease, intestinal atresias, imperforate anus, skeletal anomalies and renal anomalies. The most important aspect of oesophageal atresia is that it should be recognized as soon as possible after birth; preferably before the first feed, so that pulmonary complications do not occur.

Diagnosis

All babies should have a size 5 nasogastric tube passed sequentially down each nostril and into the stomach shortly after birth. In this way oesophageal atresia and choanal atresia should be diagnosed before feeding. If this is not practised, oesophageal atresia will be recognized by excessive secretions, or because of cyanosis and coughing with feeds. Definitive diagnosis is made by the ability to pass a firm rubber catheter (size 10) into the stomach. If the catheter cannot be passed a radiograph of the neck should be taken to confirm that the catheter has become obstructed. The abdominal radiograph should be inspected for gas in the stomach and the chest radiograph assessed for areas of collapse. Radio-opaque contrast material must not be used because of the danger of aspiration of this material into the bronchial tree. An H-shaped traceho-oesophageal fistula (type E) presents later in infancy with a history of recurrent chest infections; a cine barium swallow will be necessary to confirm this diagnosis.

Treatment

A baby with oesophageal atresia and tracheo-oesophageal fistula should be nursed supine and

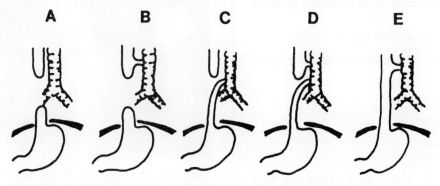

Fig. 25.11 Anatomical types of oesophageal atresia. 85% of all cases are type C.

propped up to 60 degrees. Rehydration and correction of any electrolyte imbalance or hypoglycaemia is necessary before surgery. Antibiotics will be required if there has been significant aspiration pneumonia. The outlook for oesophageal atresia is good but complications and sequelae from surgery are frequent. They include a brassy cough associated with coexistent tracheomalacia, oesophageal stricture, breakdown of anastomosis, recurrence of the tracheo-oesophageal fistula and gastro-oesophageal reflux.

Lobar emphysema

Congenital lobar emphysema is a rare anomaly due to a cartilaginous deficiency of the lobar bronchus. Most commonly this involves an upper lobe or right middle lobe. The onset of respiratory distress is often insidious usually taking two to three weeks to develop and caused by lung collapse around the hyperinflated lobe. The mediastinum becomes displaced and the chest wall is prominent over the affected area. The diagnosis is confirmed radiologically. Once a definitive diagnosis is made, lobectomy is often required. Acquired lobar emphysema may be secondary to an extrinsic or intrinsic bronchial obstruction, such as a mucus plug; this type should be treated conservatively with physiotherapy and postural drainage.

Chronic lung disease

Chronic lung disease in infancy used to be rare, but with the increased survival rate of extremely preterm infants it is becoming more frequent. It is defined as the need for increased ambient O_2 for more than 30 continuous days after birth. Classification of the various types of chronic neonatal lung disease is confusing (see Example 25.1) and only the two classical varieties bronchopul-

---

Example 25.1 Classification of chronic neonatal lung disease

Bronchopulmonary dysplasia (BPD)
Wilson-Mikity syndrome
Chronic pulmonary insufficiency of prematurity (CPIP)
Recurrent aspiration
    pharyngeal inco-ordination
    gastro-oesophageal reflux
    tracheo-oesophageal fistula
Interstitial pneumonitis
    cytomegalovirus
    Candida albicans
    Chlamydia trachomatis
    Pneumocystis carinii
Chronic pulmonary oedema due to a left to right shunt
Rickets of prematurity

---

monary dysplasia (BPD) and Wilson-Mikity syndrome will be described in this chapter.

Bronchopulmonary dysplasia (BPD)

This is usually associated with the healing phase of severe RDS, but occasionally complicates aspiration of meconium, pulmonary haemorrhage, severe neonatal pneumonia or even recurrent apnoea.

Aetiology

Aetiological factors in the development of BPD are multifactorial, but relate to the severity of RDS and degree of prematurity. BPD has only been described with positive pressure ventilation and probably relates to the mean airway pressure. Inspired O_2 tensions in excess of 60% for prolonged periods of time appear to be necessary for its development. Other probable associations are pulmonary interstitial emphysema and pulmonary oedema.

Clinical features

Infants who develop BPD have persistent chest retraction, crepitations and rhonchi on chest auscultation, gross hyperinflation of the lungs and an increased antero-posterior diameter of the chest (Fig. 25.12). In addition, most of these infants have a patent ductus arteriosus and after a period of time may develop right heart failure (cor pulmonale).

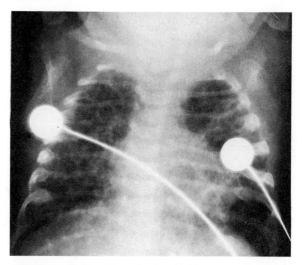

Fig. 25.12 Chest radiograph of stage 4 bronchopulmonary dysplasia showing gross hyperinflation, large cysts and bullae and fractured ribs.

Prognosis

Mortality figures vary from 0–75% depending on when the diagnosis is made. If severe BPD is diagnosed whilst the baby is still requiring mechanical ventilation, the chance of 'weaning' the baby off the ventilator is unlikely. Most infants with resolving BPD have episodes of wheezing often associated with a viral infection in the early years of life. The healing stage is associated with lung growth and may take 2–3 years. The majority of surviving infants are asymptomatic by 2 years and chest radiographs are normal by 2–3 years.

Management

Prevention of BPD requires careful management of infants receiving mechanical ventilation. Avoidance of pulmonary interstitial emphysema, pulmonary oedema from PDA and overhydration decreases the incidence. Early closure of a PDA which is producing congestive heart failure, either medically with indomethacin, or surgically, is desirable. Established BPD is often associated with congestive heart failure when fluid restriction, diuretics and digitalis are indicated. Episodic wheezing is often life-threatening and often resistant to sympathomimetic and xanthine drugs. Steroids may be used, but often take 24 hours to become effective so that the mainstay of treatment for severe bronchospasm is paralysis and mechanical ventilation.

Wilson-Mikity syndrome (or pulmonary dysmaturity)

This condition occurs in preterm infants less than 32 weeks' gestation who did not have RDS. The onset is insidious, usually in the second or third week, and progressing with increasing dyspnoea, chest retraction, apnoea and oxygen requirements. Initially, the chest radiograph is normal, but bilateral course streaky infiltrates with small cysts begin to appear during the second or third week. These cysts enlarge and the lungs become overflated. Osteopenia and at times rib fractures are seen radiologically.

Aetiology

The aetiology of this condition in preterm infants is unknown, but there is an increasingly abnormal air distribution with a ventilation/perfusion imbalance. The incidence of this disease has declined over the last decade while the incidence of BPD has increased.

Prognosis

One-quarter die during the acute phase of the disease.

The signs and symptoms slowly improve over 6 months to 2 years in the survivors. They, like the infants with BPD, are prone to recurrent wheezing episodes often associated with viral infections in the first 2 years of life.

TREATMENT OF RESPIRATORY DISTRESS

Supportive care

The supportive care of the infant with respiratory distress is similar regardless of aetiology. Infants with mild respiratory distress require frequent observations of respiratory and heart rates, temperature, blood pressure and signs of respiratory distress, whilst infants with more severe respiratory distress require continuous monitoring of these parameters with appropriate alarm signals. Accurate fluid balance charts are essential. Adequate thermoregulation may be obtained in a closed incubator or from an open, radiant heat source incubator.

Oxygen

Oxygen is a useful and life-saving therapeutic agent, but potentially dangerous, particularly in the preterm baby when it may damage the eyes (retrolental fibroplasia) and the lungs (bronchopulmonary dysplasia). When administered it should be adequately warmed to 34–36°C and 90% humidified.

Fluids

Infants with respiratory distress should not be breast- or bottle-fed. With mild respiratory distress gavage feeding may be adequate, but with severe respiratory distress fluids via the intravenous or arterial routes will be required. Usually a 10% dextrose solution is used and other electrolytes added after 24 hours, depending on serum levels.

Acid-base studies

With moderate or severe respiratory distress, assessment of acid-base status from arterial blood using samples from intra-arterial catheter, or intermittent puncture of radial or brachial artery is necessary. Continuous transcutaneous monitoring of pO_2 and pCO_2 decreases the requirement of blood sampling and enables rapid detection of fluctuation in clinical status. If respiratory acidosis is severe (pH less than 7.20 with pCO_2 greater than 60 mmHg) assisted ventilation may be necessary. For a severe metabolic acidosis, an infusion of sodium bicarbonate may be indicated. Arterial catheterization is indicated when there is a need for frequent sampling of arterial blood for gas analysis.

Antibiotics

A combination of a penicillin (penicillin G or amoxycillin or ticarcillin) and an aminoglycoside (gentamicin or tobramycin) is used in infants with severe respiratory distress, especially where infection is suspected or when arterial catheterization and mechanical ventilation are being undertaken. Adequate bacteriological investigation, which includes cultures of blood, tracheal and gastric aspirate, is essential.

Prevention of infection involves meticulous hand-washing for all procedures, the use of gloves for tracheal toilets and routine bacteriological surveillance and swabbing of all infants in intensive care nurseries. Active chest physiotherapy may be required for pneumonia, collapsed segments of lungs, aspiration syndromes and following extubation. However, all infants with respiratory distress require correct positioning with frequent changes to facilitate ventilation and lung drainage, and active physiotherapy.

Specific treatment

A tension pneumothorax will need to be released by an intercostal catheter. The rare pleural effusion or chylous effusion in the newborn may require thoracentesis or an indwelling pleural drain. Surgery is required for specific conditions such as diaphragmatic hernia, oesophageal atresia, lobar emphysema, choanal atresia, lung cysts and occasionally the Pierre-Robin syndrome. Dilution exchange tranfusion may be necessary for symptomatic polycythaemia or when the venous haematocrit is greater than 66%.

Support to parents

It is important that the parents are aware of the procedures being carried out. The apparatus used for treating infants in modern special care units is frightening and awesome so that full explanations of the machines and supporting equipment being used can do much to allay the fears of the parents. The special care unit should be a welcoming place, with parents feeling encouraged to participate by handling their infant and being involved in the care as circumstances permit. A satisfactory bonding between parent and the sick infant cannot be overemphasized.

UPPER AIRWAY OBSTRUCTION

Frequently upper airway obstruction presents in the delivery room or nursery due to foreign material in the airway. This can be readily relieved by suction to the airway. Upper airway obstruction not relieved by suction is unusual and may be mild, only occurring at times of stress or during feeds or may be life threatening, presenting in the labour ward.

Clinical features

The cardinal signs of upper airway obstruction are:

1. Stridor (inspiratory if obstruction is extra-thoracic or expiratory if obstruction is intrathoracic)
2. Suprasternal retractions
3. A croupy cough
4. A hoarse cry.

With severe increasing upper airway obstruction the infants may develop cyanosis followed by a secondary apnoea and bradycardia.

Aetiology

The causes of upper airway obstruction may be classified according to the site of obstruction:

1. Intraluminal obstruction from foreign material, such as mucus, blood, meconium or milk, may be relieved by suction. Vocal cord paralysis is a rare complication of traumatic birth. Intramural obstruction in the larynx may be due to subglottic stenosis, laryngeal oedema, a laryngeal web, diaphragm, papilloma or haemangioma.
2. Extramural obstruction may occur with a goitre, vascular ring of cystic hygroma. Nasal obstruction may be due to choanal atresia, or nasal congestion.

Infants with Pierre-Robin anomalad (micrognathia, cleft palate and glossoptosis) are prone to severe upper airway obstruction, especially when asleep, and require careful nursing in the prone position. Stridor due to an infantile larynx (laryngomalacia) usually improves after 6 months of age but requires careful medical supervision with respiratory tract infections.

Diagnosis and investigation

A full physical examination must be undertaken, particularly looking for evidence of cutaneous haemangiomas, cardiovascular system disease and palpation for lingual and pharyngeal cysts. Lateral and antero-posterior radiographs of the neck may demonstrate soft tissue swellings and airway narrowing. Some infants will tolerate laryngeal examination with a neonatal laryngoscope without general anaesthetic. More severe forms of upper airway obstruction will require direct laryngoscopy or bronchocopy under general anaesthesia. A cine barium swallow is necessary to identify a vascular ring. Special investigations, such as tomography, angiography and xerography, may be necessary on occasions.

Treatment

Urgent tracheostomy or intubation may be necessary for neonatal emergencies. Rarely, insertion of an intravenous cannula between the 1st and 2nd tracheal rings may be life saving. Mucosal damage and oedema, especially after prolonged or difficult intubation may be transient, but its resolution may be influenced by the use of corticosteroids. The use of ultrasonic mist and avoidance of further trauma by suction will also assist resolution of oedema. Treatment of the underlying cause may be necessary after consultation between the paediatric respiratory physician and an ENT surgeon.

FURTHER READING

Avery M E, Fletcher B D (eds) 1980 The lung and its disorders in the newborn infant, 4th edn. Saunders, Philadelphia

Avery G B (ed) 1987 Neonatology: pathophysiology and management of the newborn, 3rd edn. Lippincott, Philadelphia

Grasfield J L, Balantine T B N 1978 Oesophageal atresia and tracheosophageal fistula: effect of delayed thoracotomy on survival. Surgery 84: 394–402

Levene M I, Tudehope D, Thearle J (eds) 1987 Essentials of neonatal medicine. Blackwell Scientific Publications, Oxford

Northway W H, Rosan R C, Parker D Y 1967 Pulmonary disease following respiratory therapy of hyaline membrane disease in bronchopulmonary dysplasia. New England Journal of Medicine 276: 357–368

Roberton N R C (ed) 1986 Textbook of neonatology. Churchill Livingstone, Edinburgh

Yu V Y H (ed) 1986 Respiratory disorders in the newborn. Churchill Livingstone, London

26. The jaundiced infant

Ross Haslam

Jaundice in the newborn is clinically apparent in 50% of term babies and more than 80% of prematures. Compared to normal adult values, the serum bilirubin is raised in 100%. Thus icterus is common and, indeed, mostly physiological and benign. However, in a minority of babies it is a frequent general sign of serious underlying disease and should never be ignored. To understand jaundice, a basic knowledge of bilirubin metabolism is essential.

BILIRUBIN METABOLISM (TABLE 26.1)

The vast majority of bilirubin comes from haem protein (haemoglobin) which is oxidized within the reticuloendothelial system to biliverdin and then water soluble bilirubin; 1 gm of haemoglobin produces 600 μmol of bilirubin. A small amount also comes from non-haem proteins such as cytochrome and myoglobin. The newborn has a much larger pool of haem per unit weight compared to the adult. This is a result of an increased red blood cell mass, decreased red cell survival, an increased hepatic haem turnover and ineffective erythropoiesis resulting in increased breakdown of red cell precursors.

Bilirubin is transported firmly bound to albumin. Under normal clinical conditions the albumin binding capacity is rarely exceeded although for some reason the bilirubin bond is not as efficient in the newborn. It improves with postnatal age, but is weakened by illness generally and immaturity. Some drugs (e.g. sulphonamides, salicylates) and perhaps free fatty acids inhibit or compete with bilirubin for the same albumin binding sites.

Albumin transports the bilirubin to the hepatocytes which probably have a specific receptor site. Little is known about carriage across the cell membrane, but once inside the cell a separate transport mechanism aided by ligandins (Y and Z protein) attaches the

Table 26.1 Bilirubin metabolism

Process	Site	Substrate	Catalyst/agent
Oxidation	RES	Haem ↓	Haem oxygenase
Transport	Blood	Bilirubin ↓	Albumin
Uptake	Liver	Albumin=bilirubin ↓	Hepatocyte receptor
Transport	Hepatocyte	Bilirubin ↓	Y and Z protein
Conjugation	Hepatocyte	Bilirubin ↓	UDPGT
Excretion	Bile ducts	BDG (BMG) ↓	Carrier mechanism
Deconjugation	Bowel	BDG (BMG) ↓	β glucuronidase
Excretion	Bowel	BDG (BMG) ↓ Stercobilinogen	Gut flora

Abbreviations: RES = reticuloendothelial system; UDPGT = uridyl diphosphate glucuronyl transferase; BDG = bilirubin diglucuronide; BMG = bilirubin monoglucuronide.

bilirubin to the endoplasmic reticulum. The concentration of these ligandins is low at birth but within 5 to 10 days reaches adult levels.

A conjugation process occurs next, catalyzed by uridyl diphosphate glucuronyl transferase (UDPGT). UDPGT is yet another enzyme whose activity is decreased in the newborn but improves over 2 to 5 days. Bilirubin mono- and di-glucuronide is formed which is then excreted into the bile.

Excretion occurs via a carrier mechanism against a concentration gradient. In all ages, it is the rate-limiting step of bilirubin metabolism being even slower to mature than conjugation. Hence the possibility of raised conjugated bilirubin levels in those conditions causing jaundice by increasing bilirubin production (e.g. haemolysis).

Bilirubin in the bowel is generally metabolized to stercobilinogen by the bacterial flora and excreted. However, some is unconjugated by mucosal beta glucuronidases permitting bilirubin reabsorption in what is called the enterohepatic circulation. This is enhanced in the infant as a result of decreased gut flora and mobility plus increased bilirubin reserves in meconium. Breast-feeding seems to promote this step possibly by aiding deconjugation.

Bilirubin encephalopathy

Unconjugated bilirubin is a neurological poison and as serum levels increase causes first an encephalopathy, which can be transient, but ultimately irreversible brain damage called kernicterus. The transient toxicity presents as irritability or lethargy and poor feeding. Brain stem auditory evoked responses have been found to be abnormal suggesting neuronal dysfunction. Higher and more prolonged levels of free unconjugated bilirubin cause the kernicteric syndrome of opisthotonos, hypertonia, high-pitched cry, fever and convulsions. This occurs when the bilirubin damages the cells of selected subcortical nuclei, particularly in the basal ganglia and hippocampus. Death commonly results, but in those that survive a classic clinical picture of choreo-athetoid cerebral palsy, high-frequency nerve deafness, paralysis of upward gaze, mental retardation, and teeth staining emerges.

Unfortunately, the level of bilirubin which causes these disastrous consequences is totally unpredictable. The same level can be harmless to some babies and life threatening to others and tests of albumin binding capacity and free bilirubin are singularly unhelpful. Toxicity seems to be more likely in haemolytic diseases and it is from retrospective information gained in Rhesus incompatibility that so-called 'safe' levels of

bilirubin have been drawn. A serum unconjugated bilirubin of 340 μmol/l is the level of concern for term babies with Rh disease. Obviously, factors other than the serum bilirubin and albumin binding are important, such as the integrity of the blood-brain barrier which in turn are affected by maturity, hypoxia, acidosis and drugs.

Physiological jaundice (Table 26.2)

Many reasons for the normal jaundice of infants can be found from an analysis of their bilirubin metabolism. This involves an increased bilirubin production, immaturity of several liver enzymes and reabsorption from an active enterohepatic circulation. In a term infant, the serum bilirubin, which in utero is cleared from the blood of the fetus by the placenta, rises quickly after birth to reach a maximum by day 3–5 (phase I), and declines rather rapidly over the next 2–3 days (phase II) before more slowly fading for the next 1–2 weeks (phase III) (Fig. 26.1).

Phase I is due to the high load of bilirubin presented to the liver coupled with a slow hepatocyte uptake and decreased conjugation. Phase II is probably related to the maturation of the intracellular carrier proteins and phase III the more gradual improvement of excretion and reduction of the enterohepatic circulation. This pattern varies with prematurity, when all phases are prolonged, and ethnicity (Asian and Greek races) where phase I is accentuated resulting in a higher peak. From time to time other factors also operate such as polycythaemia, growth retardation, drug effects, delayed feeding, as well as the type of feeding (breast or artificial milk).

Table 26.2 Physiological jaundice

Factor	Cause
Increased bilirubin load	Large red cell mass Sequestered blood Decreased red cell survival Increased hepatic haem turnover Ineffective erythropoiesis
Decreased serum binding	Relative hypoalbuminaemia Deficient albumin-bilirubin bonding
Immature hepatic function	Deficient ligandins (Y and Z protein) Deficient conjugation Delayed excretion
Increased enterohepatic circulation	Meconium bilirubin load Gut immobility Absent gut flora

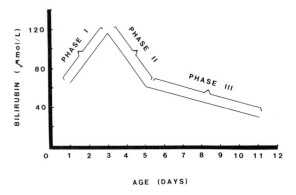

Fig. 26.1 The 3 phases of physiological jaundice in normal term infants.

Whilst accepting that jaundice in the newborn is common and normal, it must also be realized that physiological jaundice is a diagnosis of exclusion. Pathological causes must be actively sought if:

1. Jaundice clinically appears in the first 24 hours
2. Serum bilirubin rises greater than 85 μmol/l/day
3. Total serum bilirubin is greater than 225 μmol/l in the full-term or 250 μmol/l in the premature infant.
4. Direct (conjugated) bilirubin is greater than 35 μmol/l, or there is bilirubinuria
5. Jaundice is clinically apparent after 1 week in the full-term or 2 weeks in the premature infant.
6. Direct Coombs' test is positive
7. Any jaundice in a sick infant.

Pathological jaundice

Pathological causes of jaundice are most readily divided into primarily conjugated or unconjugated varieties. Unconjugated hyperbilirubinaemia is by far the more common. Often difficulties are encountered in coming to an exact diagnosis and even in separating it from physiological jaundice. Most commonly, several adverse factors acting together rather than one single problem result in jaundice outside the physiological range.

Unconjugated hyperbilirubinaemia (Table 26.3)

Increased bilirubin load

1. Polycythaemia results in increased bilirubin levels simply by the high red cell mass producing more haem. The commonest causes are intrauterine growth retardation, maternal diabetes, delayed cord clamping and transfusions (maternofetal and twin-to-twin).

Table 26.3 Pathological jaundice – unconjugated

Pathology	Factor	Disease
Increased bilirubin load	Polycythaemia	Intrauterine growth retardation Maternal diabetes Delayed cord clamping Twin-to-twin transfusion Maternofetal transfusion
	Haemolysis	Blood group incompatibilities Red cell membrane disorders Red cell enzyme deficiencies Infections
	Sequestered Blood	Birth trauma Coagulopathy Swallowed blood
Decreased hepatic function	Conjugation Defects	Crigler-Najjar syndrome Lucy-Driscoll syndrome Gilbert's syndrome Pyloric stenosis
	Multifactorial	Breast milk Hypothyroidism Drugs
Increased enterohepatic circulation	Mechanical obstruction	Gut atresias Meconium plugs
	Neurological	Hirschprung's disease
	Paralytic ileus	Biochemical disorders

2. Haemolysis usually causes the most significant hyperbilirubinaemia. Maternofetal blood group incompatabilities are the more potent causes particularly those involving the Rhesus system, but sometimes the ABO groups. During pregnancy, variable amounts of fetal blood enter the maternal circulation. Where the fetus has a different blood group antigen, the mother then produces antibodies to this antigen which in turn pass back into the fetal circulation and haemolyse the fetal red cells. Some antibodies are naturally occurring (e.g. anti-A and anti-B) and may pre-exist in the mother, whereas others (e.g. anti Rhesus D) are not.

Of the Rhesus antigens, D historically has been the most important, but anti-D gammaglobulin administered after birth to Rh negative mothers who have born Rh positive babies quite effectively (although not completely) absorbs any fetal red cells and prevents maternal sensitization. Since the introduction of anti-D, other Rhesus antigens, especially C and E, have become more common causes of incompatibility.

Haemolysis can also occur as a result of abnormalities of red cell membranes (e.g. spherocytosis) or enzyme deficiencies (e.g. glucose-6 phosphate dehydrogenase deficiency (G6PD), pyruvate kinase deficiency).

Sepsis (e.g. *Escherichia coli* or Group B *Streptococcus*) to which the newborn is far more prone, may cause excessive red cell breakdown as well as hepatocellular damage and hence jaundice.

3. Sequestered blood, such as occurs with cephalhaematomata, swallowed maternal blood and bruising from birth trauma or coagulation defects, may lead to an elevated bilirubin.

Decreased uptake, conjugation and excretion

1. Inherited conjugation defects. UDPGT is the most commonly affected enzyme. It is seldom totally absent such as in Crigler-Najjar syndrome Type I, or only deficient such as in the Type II variety and oddly also in pyloric stenosis. Far more commonly it is delayed or inhibited in so-called transient familial neonatal hyperbilirubinaemia (Lucy-Driscoll syndrome) which becomes a popular diagnosis of exclusion. Gilbert's syndrome is a variably common cause of prolonged mild unconjugated jaundice in which deficient glucuronyl transferase activity plays a part.

2. Breast milk jaundice is best considered as a problem of conjugation whilst also involving excretion delays. However, the precise cause of the well recognized higher and more prolonged hyperbilirubinaemia occurring in about 5% of breast-fed babies is controversial. Conjugation seems to be inhibited (possibly by a steroid or fatty-acids) as well as reabsorption of bilirubin enhanced.

3. Other causes. These include sepsis mentioned above with its generalized effects on hepatocellular function. Hypothyroidism is associated with prolonged unconjugated jaundice and is thought to be a metabolic effect. Some drugs delay metabolism but in this era are minor influences.

Increased enterohepatic circulation

This may occur from intestinal obstruction of any cause or delay which results in more time for bilirubin deconjugation and then reabsorption. Any of the congenital mechanical or neurological obstructions can be implicated as well as intraluminal blockages – the most common of the latter is meconium plug syndrome. Meconium ileus can occur in cystic fibrosis or as an iso-

lated phenomenon. Paralytic ileus occurs in biochemical disturbances, postoperatively and in generally ill babies. The bilirubin concentration in meconium is high and slow clearance from delayed feeding enhances physiological jaundice.

Conjugated hyperbilirubinaemia (Table 26.4)

This is a far less common type of jaundice in the infant and results from abnormalities or illnesses having effects at several points on the bilirubin metabolic pathway. Usually there is a combined unconjugated and conjugated hyperbilirubinaemia with the latter being predominant. There are three main clinico-pathological entities.

Table 26.4 Pathological jaundice – conjugated

Pathology	Disease
Hepatocellular dysfunction	Infective hepatitis, e.g. STORCH infections Metabolic hepatitis e.g. galactosaemia Parenteral nutrition
Biliary atresia	Intrahepatic Extrahepatic
Obstructions	Inspissated bile syndrome Choledochal cyst

Hepatocellular disease

This can be further subdivided into infective and metabolic.

1. Infective problems are perhaps the most common. Generalized neonatal sepsis has already been mentioned, but in particular congenital chronic infections of the STORCH type are included in this group (syphilis, toxoplasmosis, others, rubella, cytomegalovirus and herpes) (see Ch. 63). Often unconjugated bilirubin is more prominent early in these diseases, but later the jaundice becomes almost totally conjugated.

2. Metabolic diseases constitute the other main group. These include cystic fibrosis, galactosaemia and alpha-1 antitrypsin deficiency. Also damage can occur with prolonged parenteral nutrition.

Biliary atresia

This may be either intra- or extrahepatic. Extrahepatic atresia is more common and if diagnosed early (before 6–8 weeks) surgical correction has a high success rate. However, the delayed onset (about 4 weeks) of conjugated hyperbilirubinaemia decreases the chances of early detection and so jeopardizes prognosis. Fortunately intrahepatic biliary atresia is fortunately less common as the prognosis is uniformly bad. Recently, liver transplantation has produced encouraging results for biliary atresia of both types.

Other obstructions

These include plugging of the bile ducts with thickened bile occurring as an isolated phenomenon, after severe illness or due to extraluminal blockage e.g. a choledochal cyst.

CLINICAL APPROACH

History

Family

A history of jaundice or anaemia in parents or siblings may suggest hereditary disorders of red cells or enzyme defects as well as maternofetal blood group incompatibilities.

Obstetric

The mother's health during pregnancy gives important clues. Viral illnesses of the STORCH type must be sought and general diseases like diabetes and hypertension may be influential. The type of delivery gives an idea of the likelihood of trauma, drugs and asphyxia playing a role.

Infant

The baby's behaviour gives an indication not only to the possible causes but also to the likely significance of the bilirubin level. The pattern of jaundice is important, in particular the time of onset, peak and duration.

Examination

General

A general assessment is essential to decide whether the baby is sick or not. An ill infant has either a primary serious underlying disease or, rarely nowadays, toxic hyperbilirubinaemia. A relatively well baby probably has physiological jaundice which has simply become complicated. Maturity and intrauterine growth should be determined.

Nutrition

The baby's feeding must be analysed to determine its hydration and nutritional status. Physiological jaundice is often complicated by poor and/or delayed feeding with breast milk sometimes also a factor.

Haematological

This includes an assessment of the colour looking for pallor, plethora, and cyanosis as well as the intensity of the jaundice. Evidence of excessive bruising or bleeding should be sought as well as hepatosplenomegaly. The colour of the stool and urine is also helpful particularly in conjugated hyperbilirubinaemia.

Neurological

A CNS examination separate to the general assessment is important. Head size and cataracts give clues to STORCH infections. Behaviour and development are affected by bilirubin toxicity.

Investigations

If jaundice is considered clinically significant and treatment of any kind contemplated, then the following number of initial investigations is mandatory:

- Serum bilirubin (total and fractionated)
- Blood grouping of mother and baby
- Direct Coombs' test on cord blood
- Complete blood picture
- Urinalysis for bilirubin, sugar and protein.

Depending on the result of these and the clinical examination, further investigations may be warranted. These will include:

- A search for sepsis
- STORCH serology
- Indirect Coombs' test and antibody titres
- Red cell enzymes (G6PD, and pyruvate kinase)
- Liver enzymes, alpha-1 antitrypsin, etc.
- Thyroid function studies
- Liver ultrasound
- Liver biopsy.

The clinical approach to significant jaundice in the neonatal period is summarized in Table 26.5.

TREATMENT

Prevention

1. Early and adequate feeding prevents dehydration

Table 26.5 Clinical approach – all babies considered significantly jaundiced should have the minimal mandatory tests

Timing	History	Examination	Specific investigations	Diagnosis
Day 1	Previous affected infant Mismatched transfusion	Pale and yellow Hepatosplenomegaly	Blood groups Coombs' test	Haemolysis from incompatability
	Nil, or antenatal illness	Dark jaundice, bruising, petechiae hepatosplenomegaly	STORCH serology	Hepatitis
Day 2–5	Prematurity Feeding delays Poor feeding	Immature Sequestered blood 'Ill'	Nil Nil Cultures	Physiological jaundice Physiological jaundice Sepsis
Day 5–10	Poor feeding Constipated Breast-feeding Mediterranean	'Ill' Lethargic 'Well' Pale	Cultures, glycosuria Thyroid function Nil G6PD analysis	Sepsis, galactosaemia Hypothyroidism Breast milk jaundice Transient familial jaundice, G6PD deficiency
Day 10+	Failure to thrive	Wasted	Liver function Alpha-1 antitrypsin Sweat test	Neonatal hepatitis Biliary atresia Cystic fibrosis

and enhances bowel motility and colonization thus minimizing the enterohepatic circulation.

2. Care at delivery can reduce birth trauma and so decrease the bilirubin load from sequestered blood.

3. Polycythaemia can be prevented by earlier cord clamping and not allowing the baby to become dependent at delivery. In diabetic mothers, improved control helps reduce the likelihood of this complication. When polycythaemia is present (PCV > 60–55) a dilutional exchange transfusion is indicated to minimize complications. These will include excessive jaundice.

4. G6PD deficiency can be detected in susceptible races so that exposure to certain drugs (e.g. sulphonamides) and chemicals (e.g. naphthalene) is avoided.

5. Anti-D gammaglobulin to Rh negative mothers after obstetric procedures and delivery of Rh positive babies has drastically reduced this most severe form of neonatal hyperbilirubinaemia and the prime cause of kernicterus.

General medical care

Attention to detail can significantly reduce the extent and dangers of hyperbilirubinaemia in the baby with established jaundice. Increasing enteral nutrition is important for reasons already mentioned. Careful maintenance of albumin levels, control of acidosis and prevention of hypoxia particularly reduces the risks of kernicterus. Care in the use of drugs which adversely affect albumin-bilirubin binding is essential. In jaundice secondary to other problems, treatment of the primary disease is obviously important (e.g. antibiotics for sepsis and thyroxine for hypothyroidism).

Phototherapy

Bilirubin is a yellow substance which absorbs light in the blue region. In so doing it is oxidized and photoisomerized to non-toxic metabolites. It is an easily administered and, therefore, a widely used therapy. However, therein lies the reason for its common misuse. It is important that its use be limited to specific indications and that users be aware of the complications. These include:

- Temperature instability
- Dehydration – from both insensible water loss and increased bowel transit time
- Retinal damage – which is only theoretical
- Bronze babe syndrome – seen when infants with conjugated bilirubin have phototherapy
- Mother-infant separation – perhaps the most important problem.

Pharmacological

Drugs such as phenobarbitone are enzyme inducing agents which increase Y and Z proteins and UDPGT. It is of most value when given antenatally rather than after birth and is used generally in susceptible racial groups. Where there is a history in a previous child with transient familial hyperbilirubinaemia, it is also worth considering.

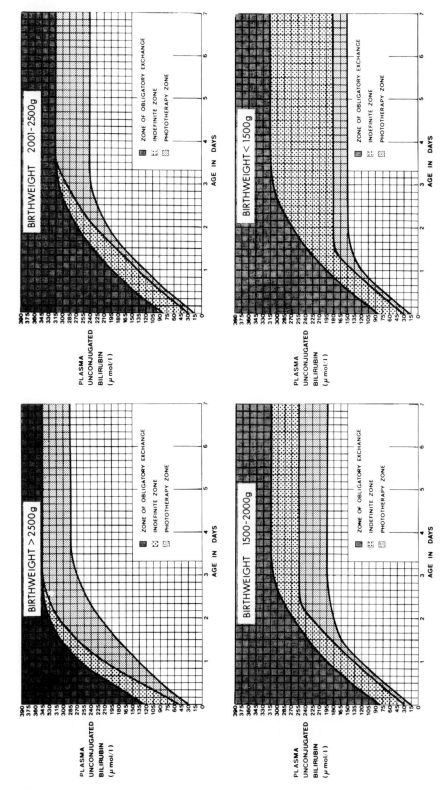

Fig. 26.2 Suggested use of phototherapy or exchange transfusion for different birthweight groups (Cockington 1979, with permission).

Exchange transfusion

This is the ultimate form of therapy and the only means of rapidly reducing bilirubin levels. However, it is a risky procedure and thus is only instituted when kernicterus is a real risk. As the precise level at which bilirubin damages the brain is not known, its indications (like phototherapy) are arbitrary. The graphs of Cockington (1979) (Fig. 26.2) are as good a guide as any. Additional attention should be paid to those factors which specifically increase the risk of encephalotoxicity such as asphyxia, maturity and serious ill health.

Anticoagulated donor blood (Rh negative and cross-matched against both the mother and baby) is exchanged for the baby's blood. An isovolumetric technique can be used with donor blood being infused through a venous line at the same rate as the baby's blood is removed from an arterial line. Alternatively a push-pull method through the umbilical vein is effective. An exchange transfusion accomplishes several things:

● Unconjugated bilirubin is removed
● Immune antibody is removed
● Any anaemia is corrected
● Extra albumin is provided.

It should only ever be performed in a properly equipped nursery as the complications are considerable:

● Fluid overload or hypovolaemia
● Infection
● Thromboembolism (air or blood clot)
● Severe electrolyte enterocolitis
● Hypoglycaemia
● Haemorrhage
● Cardiac arrest.

FURTHER READING

Cashore W J, Stern L 1984 The management of hyperbilirubinaemia. In: Zipursky A (ed) Perinatal hematology. Clinics in Perinatology. W B Saunders, Philadelphia, pp 339–357

Cockington R A 1979 A guide to the use of phototherapy in the management of neonatal hyperbilirubinaemia. Journal of Pediatrics 95(2): 281–285

Odell G B 1980 Neonatal hyperbilirubinaemia. Nomographs in neonatology. Grune & Stratton, New York

Roberton N R C 19 Textbook of neonatology. Churchill Livingstone, Edinburgh

27. Congenital and perinatal infections

G. L. Gilbert

GENERAL CONSIDERATIONS

There are a number of defence mechanisms which protect the fetus and newborn from infection. The placenta separates maternal and fetal circulations and the chorioamniotic membranes and cervical mucous plug prevent upwards spread of vaginal organisms. From about 20 weeks' gestation antimicrobial substances appear in the amniotic fluid and maternal IgG begins to cross the placenta reaching adult levels in the fetus by term. Fetal cellular and humoral immunity can respond to infection from about 16 to 18 weeks' gestation. Breast milk contains concentrated IgA, lymphocytes, macrophages and non-specific antimicrobial substances.

Microorganisms cause infection because of their intrinsic virulence, defects in maternal or neonatal defences or both. They can reach the fetus by crossing the placenta, usually after establishing placental infection, by ascent from the maternal genital tract across intact membranes, or after the membranes have ruptured prematurely. Infection may also arise from maternal genital secretion or maternal blood during delivery. After delivery the newborn may be infected by breast milk or other close contact. Some pathogens can infect the fetus or neonate by more than one route.

The outcome of intrauterine or neonatal infection depends on the stage of development at which it occurs. Only a minority of infants exposed are infected and very few are damaged significantly. Many infections which can damage the fetus are mild or asymptomatic in the mother and can only be detected by routine testing during pregnancy. Whether this is cost-effective depends on the frequency and severity of fetal or neonatal disease and whether effective intervention is possible.

RUBELLA

The ability of rubella virus to cause fetal damage was first recognized in 1941 by an Australian ophthalmologist, Norman Gregg, who described a syndrome of cataracts, deafness and congenital heart disease in infants whose mothers had been infected during pregnancy. Rubella virus slows cellular growth and causes endothelial damage and vascular insufficiency in affected tissues. This results in fetal growth retardation, decreased organ weight and, if it occurs during crucial stages of organogenesis, structural abnormalities e.g. in the heart.

Clinical features

The risk of fetal infection is greatest during the first 8 weeks of pregnancy and rare after 16 weeks' gestation. It can cause spontaneous abortion or fetal death. In infants born alive the clinical manifestations range from none, in the majority, to severe multisystem disease. Manifestations include growth retardation, pulmonary artery hypoplasia, patent ductus arteriosus, cataract, retinopathy, deafness, microcephaly, hepatosplenomegaly, pneumonitis, osteitis and thrombocytopenia. It is important to realize that infected infants who are apparently normal at birth can later develop deafness, psychomotor and intellectual retardation, abnormalities of teeth, bones, genitourinary tract and diabetes mellitus.

Diagnosis

Congenital rubella is confirmed by isolation of virus from saliva, tears, urine, CSF or tissue (such as an excised lens, biopsy or autopsy specimens) during the first three months of life, demonstration of specific IgM in the infant's serum, or persistence of IgG beyond six months. Infected infants excrete virus for many months and are a potential source of infection in others. They should be cared for only by personnel who are known to be immune to rubella. Follow-up is important to detect the development of neurological damage or deafness.

Prevention

The introduction of a live attenuated rubella vaccine during the early 1970s has reduced the incidence but has not eliminated congenital rubella. A combination of universal immunization in young children, supplemented by selective immunization of adolescent girls and susceptible women of child bearing age, would be optimal for prevention of congenital rubella.

The appropriate management of proven rubella (diagnosed by virus isolation, seroconversion or specific IgM) during pregnancy depends on when it occurs. Therapeutic abortion is usually recommended after proven infection during the first trimester.

SYPHILIS

Syphilis is a sexually transmitted infection caused by the fastidious anaerobic spirochaete, *Treponema pallidum*. Congenital syphilis is preventable and routine antenatal screening for syphilis is cost-effective even when the prevalence is low. Transmission of *T. pallidum* to the fetus can occur at any stage of pregnancy and results from intermittent bacteraemia occurring during primary, secondary or early latent maternal syphilis. However, immune-mediated fetal damage does not occur before 18–20 weeks' gestation. If infection is detected and treated early, irreversible fetal damage can be prevented. Later treatment of the mother can cure the fetal infection but cannot reverse tissue damage.

Diagnosis

Maternal syphilis is usually clinically unsuspected and the diagnosis is made by routine antenatal screening for non-specific reaginic antibodies by the Venereal Disease Research Laboratory (VDRL) test or equivalent. A positive result must be confirmed by a specific test for *T. pallidum* antibody.

Clinical features

The fetal outcome of untreated maternal syphilis depends on the stage of the disease. Primary or secondary maternal syphilis causes premature delivery or perinatal death in about 50% of cases and congenital syphilis in most of the remainder. If the mother has latent syphilis of indeterminate duration, about 50% of infants will be normal, 20–40% will have congenital syphilis and there is an increased risk of perinatal death and prematurity. Many infants with congenital syphilis are asymptomatic at birth and develop clinical manifestations weeks, months or years later. Congenital syphilis

is referred to as late when the diagnosis is made after the age of two years. Congenital syphilis is difficult to diagnose in an apparently normal infant whose mother has inadequately treated or untreated syphilis. Under these circumstances serology reflects that of the mother and FTA-IgM is unreliable. The infant should be treated unless the mother has completed a full course of treatment at least four weeks before delivery, clinical and serological follow-up is essential.

Many of the clinical manifestations of congenital syphilis are non-specific. An abnormally large placenta is a useful clue and the diagnosis can often be confirmed rapidly by histological examination. Non-specific features include hydrops fetalis, hepatosplenomegaly, anaemia, lymphadenopathy, jaundice, failure to thrive and radiological changes of osteochondritis. Manifestations typical of early congenital syphilis are: arthropathy or pseudoparalysis; persistent nasal discharge; vesiculobullous rash involving palms and soles, followed by desquamation (Fig. 27.1), and condylomata lata. The diagnosis is made by serology and/or detection of motile spirochaetes in vesicular fluid or nasal discharge by dark ground microscopy. Neurosyphilis is diagnosed by CSF pleocytosis, raised protein level and a positive VDRL.

The clinical manifestations of late congenital syphilis include: dental and skeletal deformities, interstitial keratitis, chorioretinitis and neural deafness.

Treatment

Infants with congenital syphilis should be treated with

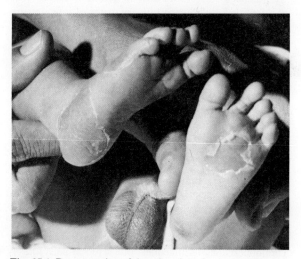

Fig. 27.1 Desquamation of the soles of the feet in a newborn with congenital syphilis.

penicillin. A single intramuscular dose of benzathine penicillin is all that is necessary for asymptomatic infection with normal CSF and normal serum IgM. A full ten days' course is required for infants with clinical or laboratory findings consistent with congenital syphilis. Follow-up should include repeated VDRL testing until negative and clinical examination for evidence of neurological or ophthalmological abnormality or deafness.

CYTOMEGALOVIRUS (CMV) INFECTION

CMV is a member of the herpes family of viruses. Acquired infection is usually asymptomatic or causes a mild febrile illness with atypical lymphocytes. After the initial (primary) infection the virus enters a latent stage and is reactivated from time to time with asymptomatic excretion of virus in urine, saliva or genital secretions. Intrauterine CMV infection can result either from primary maternal infection or from reactivation of maternal infection during pregnancy. Differentiation between these modes of infection requires demonstration of seroconversion or specific IgM in maternal serum during pregnancy. This is rarely possible. In developed countries, 40–60% of women of child bearing age are seropositive. About 1% of seronegative women seroconvert during pregnancy. In developing countries and lower socioeconomic groups, primary infection occurs at a younger age, few adult women are seronegative and primary infection during pregnancy is less common. Infection occurs in about 40% of fetuses of women who have primary infection during pregnancy, but severe fetal damage only occurs early in gestation. About 10% of infants infected during primary maternal infection are abnormal at birth; the remainder are symptomatic but 10–15% subsequently develop deafness or intellectual handicap.

Reactivation of latent infection occurs during pregnancy in 20–30% of seropositive women and 2–5% of their infants are infected in utero. Fortunately, they are asymptomatic and not at risk from long-term sequelae.

Clinical manifestations

The clinical manifestations of severe intrauterine CMV infection include intrauterine growth retardation, hepatosplenomegaly, hepatitis, anaemia, thrombocytopenia, pneumonitis, microcephaly, encephalitis, cerebral calcification and chorioretinitis. Deafness is the commonest long-term sequela but cerebral palsy, intellectual handicap, epilepsy and visual impairment can occur.

Diagnosis

The diagnosis of congenital CMV infection is made by isolation of virus from the urine or saliva during the first two weeks of life. Virus is present in large amounts and usually can be detected within a few days or less using rapid techniques. Serology is unreliable since specific IgM is detectable in the serum of only 60–70% of congenitally infected infants. A positive viral culture after the first two weeks of life cannot distinguish intrauterine from early postnatal infection. This occurs in approximately 15% of infants of seropositive mothers from exposure to virus in maternal genital secretions or milk.

No vaccine or antiviral therapy is available for prevention or treatment of congenital CMV infection. Normal hygienic measures, especially handwashing after contact with urine, are generally adequate to prevent transmission of infection to seronegative individuals caring for infected infants.

TOXOPLASMOSIS

The protozoan *Toxoplasma gondii* infects many types of animal including humans. Sexual reproduction occurs only in the intestines of members of the cat family. Oocytes shed in cat faeces are widely distributed in soil. Infection occurs by ingestion of mature oocytes. Trophozoites are released in the gut, penetrate the epithelium, multiply and spread throughout the body. In the immunocompetent host multiplication is limited but viable organisms persist in tissue pseudocysts. The alternative route of infection is by ingestion of tissue trophozoites; human infection can occur from eating raw or undercooked meat.

Human toxoplasmosis is usually asymptomatic or causes a milk illness with lymphadenopathy, fever, and atypical lymphocytosis. Antibodies are detectable in 20–80% of adults. Infection during pregnancy involves the placenta and fetus in about 50% of cases. The risk of fetal infection increases but fetal damage is less likely with advancing gestation (in contrast to rubella). The estimated incidence of congenital toxoplasmosis in Australia is approximately 1:1000 births.

Clinical manifestations

Severe congenital toxoplasmosis is rare. Clinical manifestations include anaemia, hepatosplenomegaly, jaundice, lymphadenopathy, chorioretinitis and central nervous system damage (intracranial calcification, hydrocephalus and microcephaly). The mortality is high and most survivors have neurological and/or visual impairment. Most infected infants are asymptomatic at birth but repeated examination of the optic fundus eventually reveals chorioretinitis in 80%, about half of whom have permanent or intermittent visual impairment. A smaller proportion (10%) develop neurological sequelae and/or hearing deficit.

Diagnosis and treatment

The diagnosis of toxoplasmosis during pregnancy requires demonstration of seroconversion or specific IgM and is rarely made. Treatment with spiramycin or a combination of pyrimethamine and sulphadoxine can reduce the rate of fetal infection by about 50%. During the first trimester, when the risk of severe fetal damage is high, therapeutic abortion can be justified. Specific IgM in the infant's serum or persistence of IgG in high titre beyond the first few months of life indicate congenital toxoplasmosis; *T. gondii* sometimes can be isolated, in cell culture or by mouse innoculation, from CSF or tissue. Mild or moderately severe congenital toxoplasmosis should be treated, preferably with spiramycin, because damage can progress after birth. Treatment is not appropriate for a severely damaged infant who is otherwise unlikely to survive.

HERPES SIMPLEX VIRUS (HSV) INFECTION

Newborn infants are susceptible to potentially serious infection with HSV type 1 or 2. The possible sources of infection are the maternal genital tract during delivery (usually HSV 2), maternal viraemia during primary infection (HSV 1 or 2) or contact after birth with cold sores, infected saliva or hands (usually HSV 1). Often the source of neonatal infection is unknown.

Primary maternal genital herpes (first infection with either serotype) can cause spontaneous abortion or, seldom, transplacental intrauterine infection. Usually, pregnancy continues without complication but virus excretion can persist after the lesions heal and is likely to involve the cervix. Primary maternal infection in the third trimester can cause premature labour. The risk of the infant being infected from primary maternal genital herpes during vaginal delivery is about 40%. The infant should be delivered by Caesarean section and if maternal infection is severe she should be treated with acyclovir. The risk of infection of the infant during vaginal delivery in the presence of recurrent genital herpes is 5% or less but Caesarean section is indicated if lesions are present when labour begins.

Clinical features

Neonatal herpes occurs in 1:10 000 infants. It may start with skin or mucocutaneous lesions and become disseminated or remain localized. Disseminated neonatal herpes can occur without obvious lesions and is clinically similar to septicaemia with fever, disseminated intravascular coagulation, shock and involvement of the liver, lungs and brain. If untreated, the mortality is about 80% with a high incidence of sequelae in survivors.

Localized infection includes encephalitis due to either HSV 1 or 2. This is unlike HSV encephalitis in older individuals which is due to HSV 1. The mortality from untreated encephalitis is about 50% with a high incidence of severe neurological sequaelae in survivors. Infants with apparently localized mucocutaneous HSV infection may have neurological sequelae from unrecognized encephalitis.

Diagnosis and treatment

Neonatal HSV infection is diagnosed by isolation of virus from skin lesions, unclotted blood, CSF, saliva, urine or tissue biopsy. It can also be made by rapid detection of HSV antigen by immunofluorescence (IF) or demonstration of specific IgM in the serum or CSF. Early treatment of neonatal HSV infection with acyclovir can reduce the mortality and morbidity and should be given to neonates with proven HSV infection, even if symptoms are mild and, after collection of appropriate specimens, when there is reasonable suspicion of HSV infection.

VARICELLA

Fewer than 5% of individuals escape varicella during childhood so it is uncommon during pregnancy. If it occurs, fetal infection is usually uncomplicated but the infant may develop herpes zoster within the first few months of life. During the first half of pregnancy varicella rarely causes the fetal varicella zoster syndrome. This is characterized by growth retardation, skin scarring over a dermatomal distribution, ipsilateral limb or other skeletal hypoplasia, encephalopathy and abnormalities of various organs.

If maternal varicella occurs within 5 days of labour or in the immediate postpartum period, potentially serious infection will occur in about 50% of infants at 5–10 days of age with a risk of dissemination – pneumonia, hepatitis, encephalitis – and a high mortality. When maternal infection occurs more than 5 days before delivery, infection in the infant is usually mild, presumably because of protection by maternal antibody. Infants exposed to varicella after the first few days of life usually have mild disease.

Prophylaxis

Gammaglobulin containing a high level of varicella antibody (zoster immune globulin – ZIG) can prevent or modify the course of disease if given within 4 days of exposure. ZIG is in limited supply and is reserved for use in high risk individuals. These include pregnant women with no past history of varicella who have close contact with varicella, and the newborn infant whose mother develops varicella within 5 days before or 48 hours of delivery. If an infant develops severe varicella, treatment with acyclovir is indicated.

CHLAMYDIAL AND GONOCOCCAL INFECTION

Neisseria gonorrhoeae and *Chlamydia trachomatis* are sexually transmitted organisms which cause cervicitis in women and can be transmitted to their infants during delivery. Generally gonorrhoea is more severe and easier to diagnose than chlamydial infection and, until recently, was more widely recognized. However, in most Western countries the incidence of gonorrhoea has fallen and the relatively high incidence of chlamydial infection and its importance as a cause of infertility has been recognized.

Chlamydial infection

In Western countries, the prevalence of chlamydial infection among women is about 5% overall, but is higher in younger women not in a stable monogamous relationship. Most infants of infected women are normal at delivery but about 60% become infected and half of them develop symptoms. The incidence is much higher in developing countries.

Clinical features

The clinical manifestations of neonatal chlamydial infection are conjunctivitis and pneumonia, each of which occurs in 15–20% of infants exposed. *C. trachomatis* causes up to 30% of cases of conjunctivitis in infants less than one month of age. The incubation period of conjunctivitis ranges from a few days to about two weeks. Symptoms are often persistent but eventually self-limited and blindness does not occur. The diagnosis is confirmed by detection of *C. trachomatis* in conjunctival scrapings by culture, IF or enzyme immunoassay. Chlamydial pneumonia usually begins at 2–6 weeks of age with a subacute onset and an insidious progressive course characterized by pertussis-like paroxysms of coughing, vomiting, weight loss, nasal stuffiness and middle ear abnormalities. Systemic symptoms are minimal and fever absent. Affected infants often have a history of conjunctivitis. Chest radiograph shows hyperinflation, diffuse interstitial changes and areas of atelectasis. The diagnosis is confirmed by detection of *C. trachomatis* in a nasopharyngeal aspirate of chlamydial IgM in serum. Infants often require hospitalization because of apnoea, severe respiratory distress or failure to thrive. Untreated, chlamydial pneumonia runs a prolonged but eventually self-limited course. It is associated with an increased risk of chronic respiratory symptoms and abnormal respiratory function later on in life.

Prophylaxis

Neonatal chlamydial infection can be prevented by diagnosis and treatment (with erythromycin) of maternal infection during pregnancy. Chlamydial pneumonia can be prevented by appropriate treatment of conjunctivitis. Infection in an infant indicates maternal infection which, if untreated, can cause postpartum salpingitis with a risk of secondary infertility. Thus, it is important for both mother and infant that a specific diagnosis is made, even if mild conjunctivitis is the only symptom.

Treatment

Infants with chlamydial conjunctivitis should be treated with oral erythromycin for two weeks. Topical therapy with tetracycline or erythromycin eye preparations does not eradicate *C. trachomatis* from the nasopharynx or prevent pneumonia. A three-week course of erythromycin is recommended for infants with pneumonia. The mother and her sexual partner(s) should be treated for chlamydial infection.

Gonorrhoea during pregnancy is comparatively rare (approximately 1–2 per 1000 in Western communities). About 50% of infants or infected mothers develop conjunctivitis after an incubation period of 3–7 days. Usually, it is mild but a small minority have copious purulent exudate, corneal ulceration and potential blindness. Rarely, neonatal gonococcal infection causes meningitis or septic arthritis.

All cases of neonatal conjunctivitis should be investigated for both gonococcal and chlamydial infection. The diagnosis of gonorrhoea can usually be made rapidly by Gram stain of a conjunctival smear but culture is essential for confirmation and antibiotic susceptibility testing. Treatment is with intravenous benzylpenicillin for seven days or a third generation cephalosporin if the isolate is penicillin resistant. Frequent eye irrigation with sterile saline or chloramphenicol eye drops are also indicated.

HEPATITIS B VIRUS INFECTION

Hepatitis B virus (HBV) can be transmitted to the infant from a mother who is a chronic carrier, i.e. has detectable hepatitis B surface antigen (HBsAG) in serum for six months or longer, or who has acute hepatitis B late in pregnancy. The risk of transmission and the outcome depend on the amount of live virus in maternal serum. A relatively high level of infectivity is indicated by the presence in serum of the hepatitis B e antigen (HBeAg) or DNA polymerase, both of which are associated with active viral replication.

Almost all infants (approximately 95%) of women who are HBeAg-positive carriers or have acute hepatitis B during the third trimester will be infected during delivery and become carriers themselves. They will be at risk from chronic liver disease, cirrhosis and hepatocellular carcinoma, usually in early adult life but occasionally in childhood. Children who are HBsAg carriers are a potential source of horizontal transmission of HBV to other young children.

Infants of HBsAg carrier mothers with antibody to HBeAg (indicating lower infectivity) are less likely to become carriers (approximately 5%) but can develop acute HBV infection. This is usually asymptomatic and provides immunity against HBV but occasionally severe or even fatal hepatitis occurs.

Prophylaxis

HBV infection in infancy can be prevented by routine antenatal screening and immunization of infants of women infected with HBV. They should be given hepatitis B immune globulin within 48 hours of birth and a course of hepatitis B vaccine starting in the first week, with second and third doses at 4–6 weeks and 6 months of age, respectively. This prevents HBV infection in more than 95% of infants at risk. Infants belonging to high risk ethnic groups or to a household in which there is a carrier should be given hepatitis B vaccine even if the mother is not a carrier.

HUMAN IMMUNODEFICIENCY VIRUS (HIV) INFECTION

Women infected with HIV (the cause of the acquired immune deficiency syndrome (AIDS)) can transmit virus to their infants in utero, at delivery or after birth through breast milk. It is a serious problem in populations with a high or increasing incidence of HIV infection in heterosexuals e.g. among intravenous drug users and in countries where HIV infection occurs equally in both sexes. The risk of transmission is about 50% but unpredictable in individual cases. Women known to be infected with HIV should be counselled to avoid pregnancy because of the risk of infection of the infant and of accelerated development or progression of AIDS in the woman herself.

Diagnosis

Diagnosis of HIV infection in the infant depends on demonstrating persistence or reappearance of HIV IgG after maternal IgG has disappeared or isolation of HIV from the infant's blood (which is difficult and expensive). No test for HIV IgM is available. The development of AIDS in infected infants is unpredictable; some develop non-specific symptoms or opportunistic infection within the first few months of life, others remain well for several years. It is assumed that the cumulative risks of AIDS is similar to that in adults i.e. approximately 5–10% per year. HIV infection and AIDS in children are discussed in Chapter 22.

NEONATAL SEPSIS

Aetiology

The bacterial pathogens in neonatal sepsis are different from those of older children. *Streptococcus agalactiae* (Group B *Streptococcus*, GBS) and *Escherichia coli* serotype K1 are the commonest. Pregnant women and neonates are particularly susceptible to infection with *Listeria* monocytogenes although it is relatively uncommon. Numerous other organisms including other Gram-negative bacilli, other streptococci, anaerobes, *Staphylococcus aureus* and genital mycoplasmas are less commonly involved.

Sepsis is more common in premature neonates because they are more susceptible and because intrauterine infection can cause premature delivery. However, sepsis can also occur in apparently normal full-term infants.

Source

The mother is the usual source of infection occurring in the first week of life but infants remain susceptible to 'neonatal' pathogens for several weeks. Infection can occur in utero – by transmission of the pathogen across the placenta or from the maternal genital tract – or after colonization during delivery. After birth, infection can be acquired from other adults or indirectly from other infants within the nursery. Nosocomial infection is more likely in premature neonates who need prolonged intensive care.

Clinical manifestations

It is emphasized that the clinical manifestations of perinatal sepsis are non-specific. Intrauterine infection can cause premature labour or fetal distress. Early postnatal signs include respiratory distress, apnoea, temperature instability, irritability, feeding difficulty, vomiting, diarrhoea and jaundice. Typical haematological changes are neutrophilia or neutropenia, and increase in the proportion of immature neutrophils, thrombocytopenia and coagulopathy.

Pneumonia with tachypnoea, apnoea and cyanosis is a common manifestation of neonatal sepsis and is difficult to distinguish from other respiratory distress syndromes. Meningitis can occur as part of generalized infection or as the only manifestation, especially when the onset of symptoms is some time after birth. Irritability, convulsions, disturbance of conscious state are common but non-specific features. Localized infection of the urinary tract, bones, soft tissues, middle ear and viscera also often cause only non-specific symptoms.

Diagnosis

Sepsis must be considered in any sick neonate. Typical haematological changes and an increase in acute phase reactants such as ESR and C reactive protein may help to distinguish bacterial sepsis from other causes of similar symptoms in neonates. Meningitis is diagnosed by CSF examination. Typical findings are pleocytosis, with a predominance of polymorphonuclear leucocytes, a raised protein and decreased glucose level. Unless the Gram stain is positive or specific bacterial antigens are detected, interpretation of CSF abnormalities in neonates can be difficult. Pleocytosis (up to 25×10^6) white blood cells/l) and an increased protein concentration can occur in neonates in the absence of CNS disease and viral meningoencephalitis (e.g. due to enteroviruses) can cause marked changes similar to those in bacterial meningitis.

The specific bacteriological diagnosis is confirmed by isolation of the causative organism from sites which are normally sterile i.e. blood, CSF or urine collected by suprapubic bladder aspiration.

Gram stain and culture of gastric contents or meconium immediately after delivery, and tracheal aspirate at the time of intubation are helpful, especially if there is no growth from other specimens. In addition to Gram stain, tests for antigens of common pathogens (GBS and *E. coli* K1) in CSF or urine can often provide a rapid presumptive diagnosis.

Specific pathogens

GBS is the commonest cause of neonatal sepsis. It can be isolated from the vaginal flora of 10–20% of healthy women but only 1–2% of their infants are infected. The risk of perinatal infection is determined by a lack of maternal (and hence fetal) serotype-specific IgG antibody against GBS. Apparently up to 50% of infections begin in utero, and are associated with chorioamnionitis and premature labour.

GBS infection can present as fulminating sepsis, pneumonia, meningitis or other localized infection. The mortality is high even when antibiotic therapy is started as soon as the diagnosis is suspected. Various strategies for prevention have been proposed but none is particularly satisfactory. Screening for vaginal carriage during pregnancy and administration of penicillin to the mother during labour and to the infant at birth (single dose) reduces the risk and severity of infection in the infant.

E. coli causes neonatal meningitis with a similar frequency to GBS. Serotype K1 is highly resistant to phagocytosis and most likely to be involved in meningitis. Other Gram-negative bacilli e.g. *Proteus*, *Klebsiella* and *Salmonella* spp. cause neonatal meningitis less commonly. The prognosis in Gram-negative meningitis is generally worse than that in GBS disease, partly because antibiotic therapy is less satisfactory. Therapy has been simplified by availability of newer cephalosporins which cross the blood-brain barrier better than amoxycillin or aminoglycosides and have greater bactericidal activity than chloramphenicol. The effect on long-term sequaelae has not been assessed.

Neonatal listeriosis is relatively uncommon but clusters of cases occur from time to time. *L. monocytogenes* is an animal pathogen and human colonization is probably from contaminated food or water. Human disease is rare except in pregnant women, neonates and the immunocompromised. Maternal infection may be asymptomatic or associated with a subacute febrile, bacteraemic illness. Infection of the infant is transplacental or by contamination during delivery.

Intrauterine infection can cause spontaneous abortion, stillbirth or premature delivery with fetal distress, often associated with meconium staining of liquor. Meningitis is more likely when symptoms occur more than 48 hours after birth. Listeriosis is characterized by generalized granulomatosis affecting many organs including the liver, brain and skin.

Treatment

Usually, antibiotic therapy for neonatal sepsis is started as soon as the diagnosis is suspected and appropriate specimens have been collected for diagnosis. The choice depends on the site of infection and the most likely pathogen. In the absence of meningitis, penicillin or amoxycillin and gentamicin are commonly used. The usual initial therapy for meningitis is penicillin plus a newer cephalosporin such as cefotaxime (which is active against GBS, *E. coli* and most other Gram-negative bacilli but not *L.* monocytogenes).

Even when the pathogen is susceptible to penicillin or amoxycillin, an aminoglycoside (e.g. gentamicin) is usually continued in severe infection because of its synergistic activity. The duration of therapy depends on the severity and site of infection. It is usually 1–2 weeks for non-meningitic disease and 2–4 weeks for menin-gitis. There is a risk of relapse of neonatal meningitis – probably about 5% – even after apparently adequate therapy.

In fulminating infection various other treatment modalities have been used because of the high mortality, despite the use of antibiotic to which the pathogen is susceptible. These include pooled human gam-maglobulin and irradiated leucocyte transfusion. Both can reduce the mortality if used soon after the onset of infection.

REFERENCE

Gregg N M 1941 Congenital cataract following German measles in mother. Transactions of the Opthalmological Society of Australia 3: 35–46

FURTHER READING

Best J M 1987 Congenital cytomegalovirus infection. British Medical Journal 294: 1440–1441
Gilbert G L 1986 Chlamydial infection in infancy. Australian Paediatric Journal 22: 13–17
International Symposium on Prevention of Congenital Rubella Infection 1985 Reviews of Infectious Diseases, Vol 7: (Supp) 1

Leading article. Prevention of perinatally transmitted hepatitis B infection 1984 Lancet i: 939–941
McCabe R, Remington J S 1988 Toxoplasmosis: the time has come. New England Journal of Medicine 318: 313–315
Plotkin S A, Starr S E (eds) 1981 Symposium on perinatal infections. Clinics in Perinatology, Vol 8, No 3
Remington J S, Klein J O (eds) 1983 Infectious diseases of the fetus and newborn infant, 2nd edn. Saunders, Philadelphia
Stagno S, Whitley R J 1985 Herpesvirus infection of pregnancy. New England Journal of Medicine 313: 1270–1273, 1327–1330
Wilson C B 1986 Immunologic basis for increased susceptibility of the neonate to infection. Journal of Paediatrics 108: 1–11

28. Inborn errors of metabolism

A. A. Haan

Inborn errors of metabolism are rare individually, but together they constitute groups of disorders which need to be considered quite frequently in paediatrics and increasingly in adult medicine. Thus, doctors need to be aware of the range of clinical effects of these diseases and to have a general approach to their diagnosis and management.

Diagnosis is important for several reasons. For the child, it may lead to specific treatment and an increased chance of survival. The earlier the diagnosis is made, the greater is the chance that infants and children capable of survival will do so with the least neurological sequelae, and that the lives of infants with lethal diseases will not be prolonged unnecessarily. For the parents and relatives, diagnosis leads to accurate genetic counselling. The birth of another affected child may thereby be prevented through contraception, carrier detection studies and intrauterine diagnosis as appropriate to each disease and each family. Diagnosis needs to be established during life, since postmortem diagnosis is usually impossible unless substantial progress towards a diagnosis has been made before death.

In this chapter the inborn errors of metabolism will be discussed from a general clinical viewpoint. Only a few of the most important conditions will be described in any detail. Further information about particular diseases can be obtained by referring to the books in the reading list.

PRESENTATION

An abnormal family history

An inborn error of metabolism may be anticipated in infants with a family history of a specific metabolic disease and in those with a family history of poorly explained neonatal or infantile deaths. The family history may involve the infant's siblings in the case of recessively inherited diseases or male relatives in the maternal line for X-linked recessive disorders. The

chance of a recessively inherited inborn error of metabolism is increased if the parents of the child who died are consanguineous. These situations allow advanced planning for transfer of the potentially affected infant soon after birth to a centre where rapid diagnosis can occur and appropriate management be instituted.

Mass screening of the newborn population

The principles governing mass screening are discussed in Chapter 3.

The malformed baby

Maternal phenylketonuria is an example of a metabolic disease in a mother which can cause malformations (microcephaly, congenital heart disease) in a developing child, but it is uncommon for inborn errors of metabolism in the baby to be associated with malformations. Recently, exceptions to this concept have been described, e.g. glutaric acidaemia type II and some types of congenital lactic acidosis. Glutaric acidaemia type II has been associated with polycystic kidneys, a dysmorphic facies, external genital anomalies and abdominal wall defects. Some babies with lactic acidosis resulting from pyruvate dehydrogenase deficiency have had agenesis of the corpus callosum, microcephaly and even hydranencephaly. It is presumed that in these conditions either the abnormal metabolites produced and/or the severe effect on cellular energy metabolism are responsible for the errors in development.

The very ill neonate

The newborn baby has a limited number of responses to illness and there is considerable overlap of clinical features between the inborn errors of metabolism and several more common neonatal problems such as sepsis, cardiorespiratory disease, necrotizing enterocolitis and intracranial haemorrhage. It should be remembered that both an inborn error and sepsis may be present, e.g. galactosaemia predisposes to septicaemia. Thus, cot-side diagnosis can be difficult or impossible; making the correct diagnosis rests on the clinician's ability to consider the possibility of a metabolic disease (see Example 28.1).

The child with an inborn error of metabolism is typically delivered at or near term in good clinical condition and with normal birthweight, and remains well in the earliest days of life. The early asymptomatic period is the result of several factors. Firstly, the fetus is growing rapidly before birth and amino acids are being used for protein synthesis rather than being fed into the amino acid degradative pathways and urea cycle. Secondly, the placenta effectively haemodialyses the fetus and removes toxic metabolites which might accumulate in the blood. Thirdly, the fetus is not yet in contact with substances in the diet which could be toxic, e.g. fructose in hereditary fructose intolerance. If the mother eats these substances she generally metabolizes them and they do not reach the fetus.

Exceptions to the general rule of intrauterine protection from inborn errors of metabolism are discussed later.

There are two factors which lead to the start of clinical illness after an initial period of well-being: they are the massive protein breakdown which characterizes the first days of life producing large amounts of amino acids, and feeding the infant with milk. A block in any of the amino acid degradative pathways or the urea cycle

is likely to become manifest at this time. Also, the initial feedings may represent the infant's first exposure to significant quantities of sugars, such as fructose and galactose, and to fats.

It follows that a history of recent feed change is an important indication to an inborn error of metabolism. It may be only later in the newborn period that the child is stressed with protein, e.g. by a change from breast to formula feeding, or exposed to a sugar that it cannot metabolize, e.g. by a change from a lactose-based to a sucrose-based formula. Detailed information regarding all feedings and medications since birth may be very important in diagnosis. For example, one bottle of a sucrose-containing formula given to a breast-fed baby in the middle of the night may be crucial to the diagnosis of hereditary fructose intolerance. Sugared medication can also lead to symptoms in this condition. Other catabolic stresses which may precipitate symptoms include infection, surgery, tissue necrosis and prolonged fasting.

Mild variants of inborn errors of metabolism may present later in the neonatal period, or have only mild symptoms which resolve spontaneously as an anabolic state is established.

A further indication to the presence of an inborn error of metabolism comes from the infant's response to non-specific therapy. Sick babies are treated frequently by intravenous glucose fluids and not fed. Improvement in the infant's clinical condition on intravenous glucose fluids, oral glucose fluids or half-strength feeds, with recurrence of symptoms on reintroduction of full milk feeding should suggest the possibility of an inborn error of metabolism.

Example 28.1 Clinical features and simple test abnormalities suggesting metabolic disease.

1. Persistent vomiting or intermittent vomiting especially when associated with feed changes.
2. Poor feeding and failure to thrive.
3. Neurological abnormalities including depression of conscious state, convulsions, abnormalities in muscle tone or breathing patterns and absence or early loss of functions normally expected in a newborn baby, e.g. ability to suck.
4. Liver function abnormalities including acute liver failure.
5. Acidosis.
6. Abnormal smell, e.g. of sweaty feet in isovaleric acidaemia or of maple syrup in maple syrup urine disease.
7. Hypoglycaemia.
8. Neutropenia and/or thrombocytopenia, e.g. in propionic acidaemia and methylmalonic acidaemia.
9. Hyponatraemic dehydration with or without ambiguous genitalia in the adrenogenital syndrome due to 21-hydroxylase deficiency.
10. Less common features; diarrhoea, hypothermia, abnormal hair, cardiomegaly and cardiac failure, cataracts.

The infant who is abnormal at birth

In some inborn errors of metabolism the fetus is not protected in utero and symptoms can be present at birth. This situation can result when a toxic metabolite is sequestered in a body compartment, thus being relatively inaccessible to placental dialysis. This phenomenon is exemplified by non-ketotic hyperglycinaemia in which disorder there is a defect in breakdown of the amino acid glycine resulting in high levels of glycine in the blood and even greater relative increases in glycine levels in the cerebrospinal fluid; glycine is an important inhibitory neurotransmitter in the spinal cord and brain stem. The placenta is unable to lower glycine levels adequately in the brain's extracellular fluid and often profound neurological abnormalities are present in the baby at birth.

Also, effects on the fetus may occur where metabolites are produced within cells, do not enter the circulation for removal by the placenta and cause toxic effects locally. For example, cataracts may be present in newborn galactosaemics, and girls with this condition may have lost sufficient of their oocytes by birth as to be infertile later in life. In the lysosomal storage disease macromolecules accumulate within cells and do not reach the circulation.

In the peroxisomal disorder Zellweger syndrome, at least some of the clinical features at birth are the result of failure to synthesize complex lipids needed for cell membrane formation, especially in the brain.

Inborn errors of metabolism which involve essential steps in cellular energy production, e.g. glutaric acidaemia type II, or where metabolites accumulate rapidly as a result of the hypoxia associated with birth, e.g. lactic acidoses, may also present immediately after birth.

Important questions to ask when metabolic disease is suspected in newborns are listed in Example 28.2 and tests for the diagnosis of metabolic disease in Example 28.3.

Once an inborn error of metabolism is suspected and the patient severely ill, it is important to discuss the situation with a physician specializing in the diagnosis and management of metabolic disease. By doing so, all necessary investigations can be planned, transfer of the baby to a centre with facilities for the diagnosis and management of metabolic disease can be discussed and preliminary treatment suggestions made. Also, it provides an opportunity to discuss what to do if the child's death becomes inevitable. In this situation it is vital that tissues and body fluids be taken and properly stored so that retrospective diagnosis can be attempted.

Example 28.2 Important questions to ask when a metabolic disease is suspected

1. Is there a family history of neonatal death or consanguinity?
2. Was the baby normal for a period after birth?
3. What type of feeding was given initially?
4. Has there been a change in the feeding with respect to its protein, sugar or fat content?
5. Has anything occurred to the baby which might precipitate metabolic disease, e.g. infection, prolonged fasting or surgery?
6. Has the baby improved on intravenous or oral glucose fluids and relapsed after recommencement of milk feeds?
7. Should I at this stage discuss the case with a physician specializing in the diagnosis and management of children with inborn errors of metabolism?

Example 28.3 Tests which are performed when a metabolic disease is suspected

1. Simple spot tests for urine pH, ketones, ketoacids, non-glucose reducing substances using Clinistix and Clinitest, and for a wide range of compounds which react with ferric chloride using Phenistix.
2. Blood glucose, acid-base, sodium, potassium, chloride, calcium, magnesium, bilirubin, transaminases, albumin, urea, creatinine and a full blood examination.
3. Amino acid profile of urine (e.g. high voltage electrophoresis of amino acid analyser).
4. Carboxylic acid profile of urine (gas-liquid chromatography). A positive result is most likely in the presence of acidosis or abnormal smell.
5. Gas chromatography – mass spectrometry. Used to confirm the identity of compounds detected in the carboxylic acid profile and to identify unknown compounds.
6. Screening test (galactoscreen) for galactosaemia.
7. Plasma ammonia. A positive result is most likely in the presence of marked neurological depression.
8. Other tests which prove useful in particular cases include amino acid profile of plasma, measurement of plasma ketone bodies, short-chain fatty acid profile of urine, e.g. where propionic acidaemia is a possibility, blood and cerebrospinal fluid lactate and pyruvate, cerebrospinal fluid glycine level, where non-ketonic hyperglycinaemia is a possiblity, and plasma 17-hydroxyprogesterone in the presence of hyponatraemic dehydration.

Treatment

The treatment of a child with metabolic disease depends very much on the precise metabolic defect present. Descriptions of the treatment of specific diseases can be found in the books listed in the reading list. However, some general principles should be stated.

1. The major component of treatment of the sick newborn is general supportive care. This may include correction of acidosis, hypoglycaemia and hypocalcaemia, reversal of hypotension, exchange transfusion for marked jaundice or liver failure, vitamin K if there is bleeding, antibiotics, anticonvulsants and assisted respiration.

2. Feeds should be ceased and intravenous glucose fluids commenced. This removes from the child's nutrition those components of food that cannot be metabolized, e.g. galactose in galactosaemia, protein in a urea cycle defect. 10% dextrose is the fluid most often used except when lactic acidosis is suspected. Some forms of lactic acidosis are aggravated by a high carbohydrate intake.

3. Toxic metabolites are removed by exchange transfusion or peritoneal dialysis depending on the

metabolite(s) in question, e.g. ammonia is cleared most effectively by peritoneal dialysis. Indirect ways of removing toxic metabolites may also be possible. For example, in the urea cycle defect citrullinaemia, excess nitrogen atoms can be excreted as hippuric acid and citrulline by giving the patient benzoate and arginine, respectively. Large doses of vitamins are used where the blocked enzyme step has a vitamin as a cofactor, e.g. vitamin B_{12} in methylmalonic acidaemia and thiamine in maple syrup urine disease.

With these forms of therapy it is often, but not always, possible to control the level of toxic metabolites and then gradually to introduce appropriate feedings. Survival is possible if the metabolic disease can be controlled on a diet which allows normal growth.

It should be stressed that, although control of a metabolic disorder may be extremely difficult at the outset, the child who survives may do so with normal intelligence and neurological status and be controlled long term by relatively simple dietary measures.

THE NEWBORN PERIOD

Phenylketonuria

Phenylketonuria has a frequency of 1 in 10 000 births, autosomal recessive inheritance and is caused by phenylalanine hydroxylase deficiency (rare variants involve other enzymes). Symptoms do not occur in the newborn period but neonatal treatment is required to prevent mental retardation. All newborn babies are screened for an elevated serum phenylalanine level, generally by the Guthrie test. A low phenylalanine diet allows normal development. Diet has in the past been ceased between 6 and 10 years of age but some recent evidence suggests that it may be necessary to continue the diet long term if full intellectual potential is to be maintained.

Women with phenylketonuria have a high risk of producing babies with mental retardation, microcephaly and heart malformations. Dietary control of the serum phenylalanine level before conception and throughout the pregnancy appears to prevent this.

Galactosaemia

Galactosaemia has a frequency of about 1 in 60 000 births, autosomal recessive inheritance and is caused by galactose-1-phosphate uridyl transferase deficiency. Neonatal features include vomiting, jaundice, acidosis, hypoglycaemia, hepatomegaly, acute liver failure, cataracts, failure to thrive and developmental delay.

Death or permanent brain damage may result. The condition mimics the picture of septicaemia in the newborn and, in fact, is often complicated by septicaemia so that a high index of suspicion must be maintained.

Galactosuria is suspected when the urine contains a reducing substance (Clinitest positive) which is not glucose (Clinistix negative) and there may be generalized aminoaciduria. The diagnosis can be confirmed rapidly by a screening test on red blood cells, the galactoscreen. Treatment with a galactose-free diet leads to near normal intelligence and normal liver function, and cataracts may regress. The diet needs to be continued for life. A galactose-free diet during the mother's subsequent pregnancies may be useful because galactose crosses the placenta, reaches the fetus and may aggravate the intrauterine effects of the disorder.

Hereditary fructose intolerance

This is a rare condition of autosomal recessive inheritance caused by frutose-l-phosphate aldolase deficiency. These children are well until exposed to fructose in their diet or in medications. Neonatal features include vomiting, hypoglycaemia, acidosis, jaundice, hepatomegaly, acute liver failure and failure to thrive. Older children may have recurrent episodes of vomiting. Affected children usually learn to select a diet free of fructose because nausea, vomiting and abdominal discomfort occur within minutes of eating fructose.

Fructosuria occurs frequently and is suspected when the urine contains a reducing substance (Clinitest positive) which is not glucose (Clinistix negative); there may be generalized aminoaciduria. The diagnosis is confirmed by enzyme assay in biopsied liver. The fructose load test may cause serious symptoms and is now rarely used.

Treatment consists of a frustose-free diet for life. This means omitting such foods as fruit, honey and table sugar from the diet. Children treated in this way are usually of normal intelligence and liver function returns to normal.

Urea cycle defects (the hyperammonaemias)

Urea cycle defects are rare. Argininosuccinic aciduria is the commonest and occurs in about 1 in 75 000 births. All defects are inherited in an autosomal recessive fashion except ornithine transcarbamylase deficiency which is inherited as an X-linked recessive.

Presentation is usually in the newborn period with vomiting, seizures, hypotonia, tachypnoea and coma. Older infants with milder variants of the enzyme deficiencies may present with vomiting, failure to thrive, seizures and developmental delay. Female carriers of ornithine transcarbamylase deficiency may develop symptomatic hyperammonaemia.

Diagnosis of a urea cycle defect rests on the presence of a high plasma ammonia level. Also, orotic aciduria is present in all except carbamyl phosphate synthetase deficiency. Clues to the particular enzyme defect involved come from the pattern of metabolites in urine. The particular enzyme deficiency present is confirmed by enzyme assay in appropriate tissues.

Treatment of the acutely ill child and management in the long term is highly specialized and will not be considered here.

Long-term survival in carbamyl phosphate synthetase deficiency and of males with ornithine transcarbamylase deficiency is unusual, but children with other urea cycle defects may develop and grow normally. Such children are at risk of hyperammonaemic episodes at times of intercurrent illnesses, surgery and prolonged fasting.

The organic acidoses

These comprise a group of rare conditions which cause acidosis. They include the following inborn errors, which are all inherited as autosomal recessives:

Amino acid breakdown, e.g. maple syrup urine disease, methylmalonic acidaemia, propionic acidaemia and isovaleric acidaemia.
Fatty acid metabolism, e.g. medium chain fatty acyl CoA dehydrogenase deficiency.
Glucose metabolism, e.g. the lactic acidoses such as pyruvate dehydrogenase deficiency and pyruvate carboxylase deficiency.

Early features include acidosis, depressed conscious state, vomiting, hypoglycaemia, abnormal smell and failure to thrive. Older children with mild variants may present with episodes of acidosis, ataxia, vomiting and abnormal conscious state.

Presumptive diagnosis is based on the pattern of metabolites in urine (amino acids and organic acids). The particular enzyme deficiency is confirmed by enzyme assay in culture fibroblasts.

Treatment of the acutely ill baby is complex. Often, children who survive the acute illness can be controlled with relatively simple diets and will grow and develop normally. Episodes of metabolic instability may occur at times of intercurrent infection, surgery or prolonged fasting. Diet is continued for life.

Pyridoxine responsive convulsions

This is a condition which produces intractable convul-

sions usually beginning in the first hours of life although presentation can be delayed for several months in some children. It is rare and inherited as an autosomal recessive. It is important because early diagnosis and treatment can prevent much of the mental retardation which follows otherwise.

The diagnosis is made by the clinical response to pyridoxine. Most affected infants will stop fitting within minutes of an intravenous dose (50 mg) of pyridoxine, although the response may be a little delayed.

Pyridoxine needs to be continued for life and most early diagnosed children will have normal or near-normal intelligence.

THE OLDER INFANT AND CHILD

It is more common for inborn errors to present with episodic or chronic symptoms in this age group. The range of symptoms and signs that may accompany these diseases is extremely broad and may involve almost any organ of the body.

In Example 28.4 are set out major modes of presentation of inborn errors in children after the neonatal period. Some result from mild variants of the inborn errors which can present with overwhelming illness in the newborn period. Others result from inborn errors which only rarely are detected in neonates, e.g. many lysosomal storage disorders and neurodegenerative disorders.

The lysosomal storage disorders

They include the mucopolysaccharidoses, GM_1 and GM_3 gangliosidosis, I-cell disease, fucocidosis and mannosidosis. These affect a very wide range of organs. Characteristics include coarse features, stiff joints, thickened skin, corneal clouding, thickened gums, hepatosplenomegaly, umbilical or inguinal herniae and distinctive radiographic changes in most bones of the skeleton (dysostosis multiplex).

Also, often material is stored in brain cells and this leads to intellectual deterioration. In the San Filippo syndrome storage of mucopolysaccharide in brain produces a very characteristic period lasting several years during which the child is difficult to manage because of extreme hyperactivity. Not all patients with a mucopolysaccharidosis are mentally retarded and normal intelligence can coexist with severe physical handicaps, e.g. 'mild' variants of Hunter syndrome or Morquio syndrome.

Rarely, lysosomal disorders can present in the newborn period, with hydrops, ascites, hepatosplenomegaly and early death, e.g. I-cell disease, GM_1 gangliosidosis. Subacute presentations with hepatosplenomegaly,

Example 28.4 Presentations of inborn errors of metabolism in the older infant and child

Mode of presentation	Examples
Episodic symptoms	
(episodes may last from hours to days)	
Vomiting	Hereditary fructose intolerance, urea cycle defects
Altered conscious state	Urea cycle defects
Ataxia	Urea cycle defects, maple syrup disease, lactic acidosis
Acidosis	Organic acidoses
Reye's syndrome-like illness	Systemic carnitine deficiency, dicarboxylic acidurias
Chronic symptoms	
Failure to thrive ± acidosis	Galactosaemia, organic acidoses, Wolman's disease
Mental retardation	Argininosuccinic aciduria, galactosaemia, mild variants of the lactic acidoses, Menkes' disease, homocystinuria
Cardiac failure	Glycogen storage disease type II, systemic carnitine deficiency
Hypotonia	Glycogen storage disease type II, systemic carnitine deficiency, Lesch-Nyhan syndrome
Coarse features, hepatosplenomegaly, stiff joints, corneal clouding, herniae, bone abnormalities on radiograph	Mucopolysaccharide storage: Hunter, Hurler and San Filippo syndromes Mucolipid storage: I-cell disease Lipid storage: GM_1 and GM_3 gangliosidosis, Niemann-Pick and Gaucher's disease Glycoprotein storage: fucosidosis, mannosidosis
Hepatomegaly $+/-$ hypoglycaemia	Glycogen storage disease
Neurodegenerative disorder Loss of previously acquired abilities or failure to progress. May be accompanied by specific neurological signs, e.g. seizures spasticity, visual loss, dystonia, choreoathetosis.	Krabbe's disease, Tay-Sach's disease, neuronal ceroid lipofuscinosis, Menkes' disease, glutaric acidaemia type I
Loss of vision and/or hearing	Gyrate atrophy of retina, Refsum's disease, lactic acidosis
Anaemia	Pyruvate kinase and glucose-6-phosphate dehydrogenase deficiencies causing haemolytic anaemia or orotic aciduria causing megaloblastic anaemia
Chronic or recurrent infection	Adenosine deaminase deficiency leading to severe combined immunoodeficiency

lethargy and failure to thrive are also seen, for example, in Niemann-Pick and Gaucher's diseases.

Initial diagnostic tests include screening the urine for mucopolysaccharides, microscopy of peripheral blood leucocytes and bone marrow cells for inclusions and skeletal radiography. Specific enzyme assays on a variety of tissues will be necessary for definitive diagnosis. This will involve a physician with expertise in metabolic disorders and appropriate laboratory back-up.

ADULT LIFE

Many inborn errors of metabolism present during adult life rather than in childhood, e.g. gout and porphyria.

However, it is less well appreciated that milder variants of the classical inborn errors of metabolism can present during adulthood and sometimes in unexpected ways. For example, hexosaminidase A deficiency, which is usually associated with Tay-Sach's disease, can manifest as a spinal muscular atrophy resembling amyotrophic lateral sclerosis. Similarly, the older female carrier of ornithine transcarbamylase deficiency may suffer only mild ataxia and nausea and have hepatomegaly with fatty change and piece-meal hepatic necrosis on biopsy.

In recent years there has also been an increase in the number of adult disorders whose biochemical basis has been elucidated. The recently described olivo-ponto-cerebellar atrophy due to glutamate dehydrogenase deficiency is an example of this phenomenon which has made it necessary for clinicians caring for adults to think more often about inborn errors of metabolism.

FURTHER READING

Ampola M G 1982 Metabolic disease in pediatric practice. Little, Brown, Boston

Bickel H, Guthrie R, Hammerson G (eds) 1980 Neonatal screening for inborn errors of metabolism. Springer-Verlag, New York

Emery A E H, Rimoin D L (eds) 1983 Principles and practice of medical genetics, Vol. 2, pp 1241–1388. Churchill Livingstone, Edinburgh

Galjaard H 1980 Genetic metabolic disease. Early diagnosis and prenatal analysis. Elsevier/North Holland, Amsterdam

Stanbury J B, Wyngaarden J B, Frederickson D S (eds) 1983 The metabolic basis of inherited disease, 5th edn. McGraw-Hill, New York

Wapnir R A 1985 Congenital metabolic diseases. Diagnosis and treatment. Marcel Dekker, New York

Infection in childhood

29. Infectious diseases of childhood

M. J. Robinson, G. L. Gilbert

MEASLES (RUBEOLA)

Measles is a highly contagious disease, caused by a paramyxovirus. It is characterized by a typical prodrome followed by a generalized maculopapular eruption. The disease has a global distribution and in unimmunized populations it occurs almost exclusively in children, although the very young infant is protected by maternal antibodies. In the healthy, well-nourished child, the disease runs a relatively benign course, but it may have disastrous effects in children who are immunologically deficient, on immunosuppressive therapy or malnourished. Man is the only natural host but monkeys can be infected with measles virus. Transmission to susceptible persons occurs by direct contact with infected droplets. Communicability is greatest during the prodromal stage when cough and coryza are at their peak and continues until 2 days after the onset of the rash.

It is one of the most readily communicable infectious diseases with close to 100% attack rate in susceptible household contacts. Unlike many other infectious diseases it is rarely subclinical but mild infection can occur in individuals with some immunity, e.g. young infants with residual maternal antibody or in those who have had prophylactic immunoglobulin.

Clinical features

The incubation period lasts 10–14 days, but between the seventh and ninth day after contact a transient low grade fever may be noted. The prodromal symptoms and signs are highly characteristic and consist of fever, coryza and cough, conjunctivitis and an exanthem. Occasionally a convulsion occurs at the outset. In the uncomplicated case the fever continues until 2–3 days after the appearance of the rash, when it settles by lysis. Rhinorrhoea, sneezing and a dry incessant hacking cough are such constant features that a diagnosis of measles should not be entertained in their absence. In addition, there is usually intense conjunctival infection, lacrimation and photophobia.

The pathognomonic sign of early measles is the presence of Koplik's spots – tiny white spots with a reddish areola found opposite the molar teeth (the exanthem). They appear on the second or third day of the clinical illness and begin to fade as the cutaneous rash appears.

The exanthem of measles consistently appears on the third or fourth day after the onset of fever, often with aggravation of the prodromal symptoms. The eruption begins as discrete erythematous maculopapules over the mastoid region and the posterior hairline. Within a few hours, a similar rash appears on the neck and face. Later it spreads downwards and by 48 hours, the upper limbs, trunk, lower limbs and even the palms and soles may be covered with exanthem. In a small proportion of children the rash becomes confluent, haemorrhagic and darkens to a red and subsequently violaceous hue. After 2 or 3 days, the eruption begins to fade in the areas where it first appeared. Desquamation invariably follows and may be extensive in the severe case.

Complications

During the clinical course of measles all patients show evidence of viral respiratory tract involvement. Middle ear infection is the most frequent bacterial complication, particularly in children who have had previous otitis media. Bacterial laryngitis, tracheo-bronchitis and pneumonia are also well recognized complications. The offending organisms are usually *Streptococcus pneumoniae*, *Haemophilus influenzae* or *Staphylococcus aureus*.

An uncommon, but well-documented pulmonary complication is giant cell pneumonia. This is a progressive fatal pneumonia observed in children with immune deficiency. In these children the exanthem of measles rarely appears because the rash is a manifestation of cell-mediated immune response. Measles virus persists for long periods in the lung parenchyma without provoking a significant antibody response. Giant cell pneumonia can also occur after measles immunization in children with cell-mediated immune deficiency.

In about 1 in 1000 cases, measles is complicated by clinical evidence of encephalitis. The onset is usually on the fourth to seventh day after the appearance of the rash and hence the term postinfective encephalitis has been used to describe this syndrome. However, encephalitis may occasionally precede the exanthem. There does not seem to be any relationship between the severity of measles, the age of the patient, and the incidence of acute neurological involvement. The symptoms of measles encephalitis vary according to the degree and site of neural tissue involved. There is invariably disturbance of consciousness, ranging from agitation, drowsiness, stupor to coma, in association with one or more of the following – speech and visual disturbance, convulsions, pyramidal signs, cerebellar signs, involuntary movements and cranial nerve palsies. Death occurs in about 10% of cases and neurological and psychological sequelae are present in about 30–40% of the survivors. However, it is very difficult to predict the prognosis during the acute state of the illness as even deeply comatosed children may eventually recover completely.

A subacute form of degenerative brain disease subacute sclerosing panencaphalitis (SSPE) may occur months or years after the measles infection especially in children in whom the initial episode has occurred before the age of two years. The onset is insidious with gradual deterioration of intellect accompanied by motor disturbance, myoclonic jerks and visual loss. The clinical diagnosis is supported by finding high titre measles antibodies in the serum and cerebrospinal fluid together with a typical EEG pattern (Fig. 29.1). The outlook in subacute sclerosing panencephalitis is for death to occur after a protracted illness in almost all cases. Measles

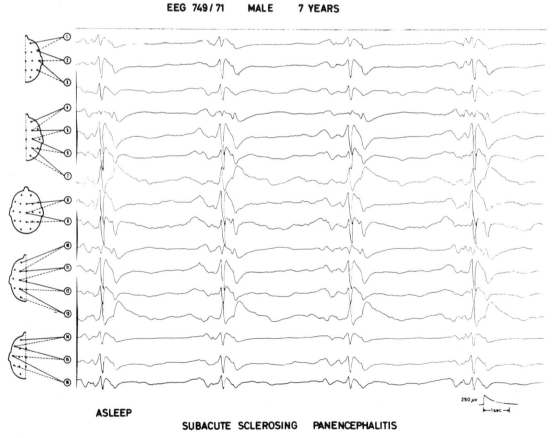

EEG 749 / 71   MALE   7 YEARS

ASLEEP

SUBACUTE SCLEROSING   PANENCEPHALITIS

Fig. 29.1   The EEG in subacute sclerosing panencephalitis. Note the characteristic low voltage activity in all leads and the periodic intervals of brief high voltage slow wave complexes.

virus has been demonstrated in brain tissue in some patients. The incidence of SSPE has declined significantly since the introduction of measles vaccine.

It is well recognized that measles infection regularly produces a transient cutaneous anergy, particularly to tuberculin, but the potential risks of reactivation or aggravation of tuberculous lesions by measles infection have probably been overestimated.

Diagnosis

The diagnosis of measles is usually quite clear from the clinical features described. Other diseases which occasionally cause confusion include rubella, scarlet fever, roseola infantum, rashes associated with Coxsackie and echovirus infection, Kawasaki disease and those due to drugs, including Stevens-Johnson syndrome. Definitive diagnosis of measles depends on detection of virus antigen in exfoliated respiratory epithelial cells by immunofluorescence, culture of the virus or serology (most commonly haemagglutination inhibition or enzyme immunoassay). Serological diagnosis depends on demonstrating seroconversion in paired sera or specific IgM in a single specimen of serum. Usually, these tests are reserved for epidemiological surveys or in an unusual case where the diagnosis is in doubt. The immunity following measles is life-long and second 'attacks' are due to other causes.

Treatment

In uncomplicated measles symptomatic treatment is all that is required. This involves an adequate fluid intake, adequate rest, the use of antipyretics, and mild sedation as necessary. There is no evidence to suggest that antibiotics reduce the incidence of complications and thus should not be prescribed routinely. However, in the presence of definite secondary infection, particularly of the ear and respiratory tract, penicillin is the initial drug of choice. The neurologically affected child needs good nursing care and adequate nutrition. There is no proven pharmacological agent that at present alters the course of measles encephalitis.

Prevention

All children, with rare exceptions mentioned below should be immunized against measles. The severity of the illness, the complications such as middle ear disease, bronchitis and bronchopneumonia, together with the significant incidence of encephalitis, are cogent reasons for making this recommendation. This is particularly important in developing countries where measles is often much more severe because of chronic malnutrition which in turn is aggravated by measles and the mortality is very high.

Children having cytotoxic agents for malignant disease, or a child with immunodeficiency should not be given vaccine. If such a person comes into contact with measles pooled human gammaglobulin in a dose of 0.2 ml/kg intramuscularly should be given within 5 days of exposure. After the sixth day a higher dose is recommended, but the resultant attenuation of the clinical illness is variable.

RUBELLA (GERMAN MEASLES)

The rubella virus, rubivirus, is a member of the Togaviridae family. It can be detected in both blood and in nasopharynx from 10 days before and until 2 weeks after the onset of rash. Regular epidemics of rubella occur usually in the spring. Rubella occurs most commonly in children aged 5–10 years. It is much less contagious than measles, and in unimmunized populations 15–20% of adults are not immune (of 2% for measles). Most rubella infections are subclinical.

Clinical features

The incubation period of rubella is approximately 10–24 days. In children the first symptom is the development of a rash over the face. However, in adolescents and adults fever, malaise and headache are often early complaints. The rash spreads rapidly to involve the neck, trunk and extremities, so that by the end of the first day of the illness the entire body may be covered with discrete, pink, red macules. At times the macules coalesce on the trunk, but not on the limbs. They fade rapidly so that in the typical case, the rash has disappeared by the end of the third day. Sometimes desquamation occurs. Generalized lymphadenopathy is a feature of rubella, although on rare occasions, it may be absent. The nodes particularly involved are the suboccipital, post-auricular and cervical. Fever is usually of mild degree, rarely rising above 38°C in children and rarely lasting longer than one day. Complications in childhood are rare, but especially in adolescent girls and women polyarthritis or arthralgia lasting one to several weeks not infrequently appears on the third day. Encephalitis and thrombocytopenic purpura are extremely rare complications.

Diagnosis

This is suggested from the clinical pattern, but it may be readily confused with the rash of a number of other viral illnesses and with drug eruptions. Because of this and the common occurrence of asymptomatic infection, a history of 'rubella' or 'German measles' correlates poorly with immunity. Confirmation of a suspected case is essential in a pregnant woman or her contacts. Virus can often be isolated from the pharynx for up to 15 days, but the virus grows slowly and the result may not be available for several weeks. Haemagglutination inhibition test and enzyme immunoassay are the most commonly used serological tests. The second specimen is taken 2–4 weeks later. A four-fold or greater rise in titre indicates a recent infection. A more rapid diagnosis can be made by detection of specific IgM in a single specimen of serum, by ELISA.

Prevention

Although postnatal rubella is very mild its effect on the fetus, if it occurs during pregnancy, can be devastating (see Ch. 27). A live attenuated vaccine is available. This can be given, at the same time as measles vaccine, to all children in order to prevent rubella epidemics (the practice in the USA) or to adolescent girls to protect them during childbearing years (the practice in Australia). Each approach has advantages and disadvantages.

ROSEOLA INFANTUM (EXANTHEMA SUBITUM)

This benign disorder of infancy is probably due to infection with a virus closely related to human herpes virus 6 (HHV-6). Roseola infantum affects infants between 6 and 18 months but is rare thereafter; adults are not affected. The onset is with fever up to 40°C, but there are relatively few and mild constitutional symptoms. Occasionally a convulsion occurs with the fever. Other features include irritability, anorexia and a runny nose. After 2–3 days the temperature falls, the constitutional symptoms disappear and a macular or maculo-papular rash appears. The appearance of the rash at the time the fever subsides is characteristic of roseola and helps to distinguish it from rubella and measles. The rash largely involves the trunk, sparing the face and limbs. It disappears within two days without desquamation or pigmentation. A mild lymphadenopathy, particularly involving the nodes of the neck is common. Complications almost never occur and recovery is complete.

ERYTHEMA INFECTIOSUM

This is also known as the 'slapped cheeks' syndrome or fifth disease. It tends to occur in young school-aged children and is due to infection with human parvovirus,

frequently occurring in epidemics. The clinical features consist of a mild constitutional disturbance with fever, enlarged lymph nodes, particularly cervical lymph nodes and at times arthralgia. The facial rash has the characteristics of slapped cheeks, but, in addition, there is a variable reticular rash particularly distributed on the limbs. Characteristically, the rash recrudesces in response to heat or exercise for quite long periods after recovery.

The virus infects red cell precursors in the bone marrow causing transient anaemia. This is usually unnoticed in otherwise normal individuals but causes aplastic crisis, usually without rash, in individuals with chronic haemolytic anaemia such as sickle-cell disease and hereditary spherocytosis. During pregnancy human parvovirus infection (with or without the typical rash illness) can cause fetal death due to severe anaemia and hydrops fetalis.

VARICELLA (CHICKEN POX)

Varicella is a highly infectious but usually benign disorder due to the varicella zoster virus, which is one of the herpes viruses. Children aged between 2 and 8 years are most commonly affected, but varicella may also occur in early infancy despite a past history of varicella in the mother. Also, intrauterine infection has been documented but it is rare (see Ch. 27).

The virus spreads by direct contact with early vesicles, which contain large amounts of virus during the first few days of illness, or by aerosol. It is very contagious and few adults are susceptible to primary infection. After recovery the virus remains in latent form, presumably in dorsal root ganglia. Reactivation causes localized lesions in the distribution of a dermatome (see below).

Clinical features

The varicella eruption appears after an incubation period of 9–21 days. In children the accompanying constitutional upset is mild and consists of a low grade fever and malaise. The initial skin lesion is a small macule but within 6–7 hours it progresses to become a papule and then a vesicle. Crusting of the vesicle occurs almost immediately. Vesicles measure about 2–3 mm in diameter and are surrounded by an area of erythema. Lesions appear in crops involving the trunk, scalp, face and extremities. The mucous membranes of the palate, pharynx, conjunctivae, larynx, trachea and vagina may also be involved. It is characteristic of varicella that lesions in all stages of development may be seen in any area of the body (Fig. 29.2). All lesions crust, scabs

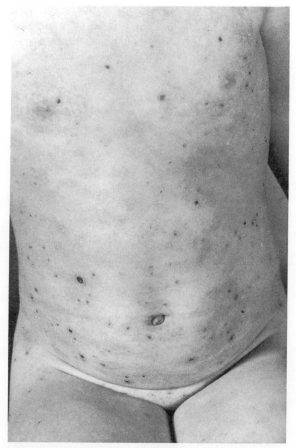

Fig. 29.2 The rash of varicella. Note lesions in varying stages of development.

form and these fall off within 5–20 days. The severity of the rash varies from the mild case with a single crop of scattered lesions to one in which multiple crops appear and the whole body is literally covered. The lesions are characteristically itchy and in the severe case pruritis may be quite distressing.

In children, varicella is almost invariably benign with complete recovery occurring within 3 weeks when all scabs will have disappeared. However, scratching may lead to secondary infection and subsequent scarring. In adults the disorder tends to be more severe and is occasionally followed by varicella pneumonia which may be fatal. Varicella can also be extremely severe, with atypical lesions, visceral involvement and a high mortality in children who are immunologically compromised either because of receiving steroids and immunosuppressants therapy, or in children suffering from primary immunodeficiency syndromes.

In approximately 1 case per 1000 encephalitis complicates varicella, when headache, vomiting, neck stiffness and ataxia occur. Occasionally, there will be convulsions and focal neurological signs. The encephalitis complicating varicella tends to present between the fifth and eighth day of the illness and may complicate either the mild or severe disease. Undoubtedly, cerebellar signs are the most characteristic feature of varicella encephalitis. Most cases resolve completely. An attack of varicella confers lifelong immunity, but the virus may remain latent and reappear years later as herpes zoster.

Diagnosis

Varicella is readily diagnosed on clinical grounds although the virus may be isolated from fluid within the vesicles. The diagnosis can also be established serologically. Varicella has to be differentiated from impetigo, insect bites and papular urticaria.

Treatment

Usually no specific therapy is required for varicella. Paracetamol may be required if fever is high and calamine or some other antipruritic lotion if itching is severe. Fingernails should be cut short to reduce secondary infection from scratching. The management of varicella encephalitis follows the same principles as the management of any other form of viral encephalitis. Zoster immune globulin (ZIG) should be given to children with malignant disease, neonates and others with compromised immune systems and who are varicella contacts. Once clinical signs of infection occur in an immunocompromised patient or when disease is particularly severe (e.g. in adults with varicella pneumonia) it should be treated with acyclovir. An attenuated live virus vaccine is available in some countries but its universal use would not appear to be indicated in developed countries at this time.

HERPES ZOSTER (SHINGLES)

Herpes zoster is due to a reactivation of a latent varicella virus infection. Herpes zoster occurs at all ages; the frequency increases with advancing age. It can occur in children, including infants who have been exposed to varicella in utero. It occurs more often in patients who are immunocompromised especially with malignant disease when it may become disseminated and potentially fatal. Recurrences are uncommon except in compromised patients; when they occur in otherwise normal people herpes simplex infection should be considered.

Clinical herpes zoster is characterized by groups of

vesicles on an erythematous base sited over the distribution of the infected spinal or cranial sensory nerve. Nerve root pain may precede, accompany or occur after the appearance of the vesicles. Lesions may appear on the mucous membrane of the mouth and conjunctivae when the corresponding dermatome is involved. The colour of the vesicular fluid changes from clear to yellow over a day or so, then rupture, crusting and later scarring may occur.

The diagnosis of herpes zoster is suspected from examination of vesicle fluid for giant cells and intranuclear inclusions and confirmed by culture. Analgesics are often required for symptomatic relief. The antiviral agent acyclovir has been shown to be effective in reducing the duration and severity of lesions, especially in the elderly.

MUMPS

Mumps is an acute infectious disease caused by a paramyxovirus. It is predominantly a disorder of childhood, almost 90% of cases presenting before adolescence. However, the infection is rare in infancy presumably the result of persisting maternal antibodies. Transmission of infection usually occurs through direct contact with infected droplet nuclei or fomites contaminated with infected saliva and possibly urine. Intrauterine infection has also been documented following mumps in early pregnancy.

Clinical features

In about one-third of individuals exposed to the infection there is no apparent clinical illness despite a positive serological response. More typically, the disease is heralded by a rapid onset of parotitis which appears two or three weeks after contact. The prodromal symptoms consist of fever, malaise, myalgia and headache, but these are not commonly encountered in childhood infection. The older child may complain of pain and tenderness over the parotid gland before actual swelling becomes evident. Over the next 1–3 days the parotid gland reaches its maximum size and may displace the ear lobe upwards and outwards and obliterate the space between the mandible and the sternomastoid muscle. Pain and swelling are further aggravated by chewing and tasting bitter fluids. In the majority of cases the opposite parotid gland becomes involved 1–5 days later. Other salivary glands, namely the submandibular and sublingual, may also become inflamed but in 10% of cases these glands are involved in isolation. The skin over the parotid gland may become oedematous, red and warm and within the buccal mucosa the orifices of Stensen's

and Wharton's ducts may be erythematous and pouting. Subcutaneous oedema sometimes extends down the neck and anterior chest wall over the manubrium sterni, probably the result of lymphatic obstruction. Constitutional symptoms, such as fever, headache and malaise, are usually severe during this stage of the disease and like the parotid swellings, gradually subside within 3–7 days.

Extra salivary gland manifestations of mumps occur much more frequently in adults than in children. Usually these appear 3–7 days after the onset of glandular swelling, but may precede it or even occur in the absence of parotid gland involvement.

Complications

Meningoencephalitis is the most frequent complication in children. In fact, asymptomatic pleocytosis of the cerebrospinal fluid has been reported in over 60% of cases in which the cerebrospinal fluid was routinely examined. Symptomatic viral meningitis occurs in approximately 10% of cases of mumps. The clinical manifestations relate to increased intracranial pressure and meningeal irritation and are no different from those of any other viral meningitis. Encephalitis due to either direct viral involvement or postinfection demyelination is much less common (less than 1:1000). It is associated with disturbance of conscious state, convulsions and focal neurological signs including poliomyelitis-like illness with transient weakness of the neck, trunk and limb mucles. CSF findings are similar in uncomplicated meningitis and encephalitis, for example, moderate pleocystosis (up to $2000/mm^3$, usually lymphocytes but sometimes polymorphonuclear leucocytes predominate early), moderately raised protein and occasionally low glucose levels. Orchitis, with or without epididymitis, is uncommon in prepubertal males. One or both testes may become painfully inflamed and enlarged to three or four times their original size. Constitutional symptoms frequently accompany testicular involvement and as the gonadal swelling subsides, the affected testis may undergo atrophy, although rarely to a degree to result in absolute infertility. Oophoritis has been estimated to occur in 7% of female patients.

Mumps pancreatitis is rare in childhood. Epigastric pain and tenderness, particularly when accompanied by fever and vomiting in association with an elevated serum amylase level, suggest this complication. Other reported complications of mumps include episcleritis, uveitis, optic neuritis, sensory deafness, arthritis, myocarditis, thyroiditis and nephritis. Spontaneous abortion has been reported to occur more commonly than expected if mumps occurs during the first trimester of pregnancy.

However, there is no increase in the incidence of fetal death or congenital abnormalities resulting from infection later in pregnancy. If the mother is infected near term the infant may also be infected and pneumonia can occur in these circumstances.

Diagnosis

This is readily made during epidemics on clinical grounds, particularly if there is a history of exposure in the preceding 3 weeks. In sporadic cases, other causes of parotid enlargement must be excluded. Parotitis may result from Coxsackie A infection. The parotid and other salivary glands may be enlarged occasionally which is the result of infiltration by neoplasms of the reticuloendothelial system. It is exceptional for mumps virus to cause recurrent parotitis as a single attack confers permanent immunity. However, recurrent parotitis is not rare in children and is usually either the result of salivary calculi or associated with sialectasis. In the absence of parotitis, a painful testicular swelling is the result of torsion unless proven otherwise. A serum amylase level is a useful diagnostic aid as it is elevated in salivary adenitis alone or in association with pancreatitis. The definitive diagnosis of mumps depends on virus isolation e.g. from saliva or CSF and on serology. These tests are rarely required except in the atypical case, or in situations where possible clinical complications of mumps occur in isolation.

Treatment

This is entirely symptomatic. Paracetamol is useful for controlling pain and fever. A fluid or bland diet is probably best tolerated in the presence of a large parotid swelling. Bed rest has not been shown to influence the development of complications and should be guided by the patient's needs. Corticosteroids may provide some relief of pain in mumps parotitis but have no effect on the sequelae and in general are not recommended.

A live attenuated mumps vaccine is highly effective in preventing the natural infection in susceptible individuals. The period of protection is not known at present, but appears to be long lasting. Live mumps vaccine is now available in combination with live measles and live rubella vaccine. It appears very likely that this triple combination will be recommended as routine for all infants, probably at the age of about 15 months.

SCARLET FEVER

Scarlet fever is essentially acute beta haemolytic strep-

tococcal tonsillitis with a rash – the latter being due to a specific erythrogenic toxin produced by this organism. In the pre-antibiotic days scarlet fever had a high morbidity and a not insignificant mortality. In this era scarlet fever is uncommon as are streptococcal infections in general. The importance of scarlet fever related to acute rheumatic fever and glomerulonephritis which were well recognized complications.

Scarlet fever commences abruptly with fever, headache, malaise, vomiting and a sore throat. Some 12 to 24 hours after the onset of these symptoms a skin rash appears. The rash tends to cover the entire body and limbs and is described as a punctuate erythema which blanches on pressure. The skin itself feels rather like sandpaper to the touch. The rash of scarlet fever is more marked over the skinfolds where transverse lines containing tiny petechiae are seen. It is absent around the mouth where an area of circumoral pallor is characteristic. The rash lasts some 2 to 3 days after which desquamation occurs, this being particularly obvious on the palms and the soles of the feet. The pharynx is diffusely reddened as are the tonsils which are swollen and usually covered with a white exudate. The tongue is initially furred and with the enlarged papillae it has the appearance of a 'white strawberry'. Two to three days later this furry superficial layer desquamates giving the tongue a red appearance with enlarged papillae – the strawberry tongue. Regional lymph nodes are regularly enlarged.

The diagnosis of scarlet fever is usually clear from the clinical appearances of the rash and the throat, but difficulties occasionally are encountered in differentiating from enteroviral infections and occasionally from a drug eruption. The diagnosis is usually readily confirmed by culture of throat swabs.

In treatment penicillin is the drug of choice with the symptoms rapidly resolving in 24 hours or so. Local complications such as middle ear disease and pneumonia are now rarely seen as are acute rheumatic fever and post-streptococcal glomerulonephritis.

GLANDULAR FEVER (INFECTIOUS MONONUCLEOSIS)

Glandular fever is now usually caused by the Epstein-Barr (EB) virus. Similar clinical presentation can occur with other infections e.g. cytomegalovirus, viral hepatitis and toroplasma. It is seen most frequently in adolescents and young adults. EB virus infection is not at all uncommon in young children but is often asymptomatic or atypical. It appears to be largely transmitted by infected saliva, thus close contact is essential for its transmission.

Clinical features

The incubation period is probably of 2–6 weeks' duration, but this is not accurately known. Early symptoms consist of anorexia, fever, tiredness and malaise and are accompanied by a sore throat and enlarged lymph nodes, particularly those of the neck. Enlargement of liver and spleen of mild degree are usually present as well. The tonsils may be covered with a whitish exudate and there may be petechial haemorrhage covering the soft palate – features suggestive of diptheria. It is not uncommon for a fine macular rash to be present and for reasons that are not altogether clear, this rash appears particularly if the patient is given ampicillin early in the illness. Complications include hepatitis with clinical jaundice and occasionally aseptic meningitis or encephalitis.

The course of the illness is variable but in most cases symptoms subside within 2–4 weeks. Occasionally, however, tiredness, anorexia and malaise may last for weeks or even months.

The diagnosis is confirmed by finding IgM specific antibodies to the EB virus in serum. Patients with infectious mononucleosis have heterophil antibodies in their sera which are detected by sheep red cell agglutination (the Paul-Bunnell test) or by the Monospot test which uses horse red blood cells. Isolation of EB virus is difficult and is not routinely performed for diagnosis in most laboratories.

Treatment

No specific treatment is available. The reason why some children remain unwell for many weeks is not totally understood.

HERPES SIMPLEX VIRUS

Herpes simplex virus (HSV) is a DNA containing virus which is readily cultured in the laboratory; there are two antigenically distinct serotypes:

- HSV 1, which commonly affects the lips, oral mucous membranes and conjunctivae.
- HSV 2 which usually affects the genitalia and occurs most commonly in adolescents and young adults.

Infection with HSV 1 is very common, especially in the lower socioeconomic groups. Most infections, however, are subclinical.

Infection may be classified as:

1. Primary, representing an individual's first experience with the virus.

2. Recurrent when the lesions are the result of reactivation of a latent infection in an immune host with circulating antibodies.

Primary HSV infection during the neonatal period is often disseminated and/or associated with a high mortality (see Ch. 27).

Primary infection with HSV 1 is most commonly recognized clinically in the age group 1–3 years, but is also seen in early infancy. The child presents with fever and refusal to feed. On physical examination the gums are swollen, bleed readily and are associated with shallow ulcers on the gums, tongue and palate. Regional lymph nodes are readily palpable. Because of fever and refusal to feed, dehydration, particularly in the summer months, may occur. Vesicular lesions may also be seen on the face and involve the conjunctivae producing both conjunctivitis or keratoconjunctivitis with ulceration.

The natural history of primary HSV 1 gingivostomatitis is for symptoms to resolve gradually over a period of 7–10 days. During this period feeding results in pain and bleeding so that careful nursing, attention to hydration and prevention of secondary infection in the mouth by careful mouth toilets is important.

Primary herpes infection is severe in children with generalized eczema. Under these circumstances widespread herpetic lesions occur over the affected skin – eczema herpeticum. In the management, scrupulous care of the skin is essential as is attention to fluid and electrolyte losses.

Occasionally herpes virus may affect the central nervous system in otherwise healthy children. Encephalitis so produced is frequently severe and the mortality high. The encephalitis not infrequently produces focal neurological signs which may be confirmed by EEG and CT scanning (see Ch. 31).

The antiviral drug acyclovir is effective against HSV and is indicated in severe primary infections, especially in neonates, in eczema herpeticum and HSV encephalitis.

Recurrent herpes is manifest by the appearance of vesicular lesions at the oral mucocutaneous junction. These are the result of reactivation of a latent infection which has followed the primary herpes infection in infancy. Recurrent herpes tends to occur at the time of physical illness, but may also be the result of exposure to sunlight, physical exhaustion and probably also emotional stress.

ENTEROVIRUSES

The enteroviruses, a subgroup of the picornoviruses, comprise the Coxsackieviruses, the echoviruses and the polioviruses. They are grouped together because of their similar biological and epidemiological characteristics. A very large number of serotypes exist which are identified by neutralization techniques. Spread of these viruses is via the faecal oral or oral-oral routes. Swimming and wading pools may be important vectors for spread in the summer time. Children are the major sufferers from enterovirus infection probably because of their less hygienic habits. Unrecognized or sub-clinical infections greatly outnumber clinical infections with this group of viruses. However, the younger the patient the less likely is the enteroviral infection to be asymptomatic. Poliomyelitis is described in Chapter 40 and will not be further discussed here.

Pathogenesis

These viruses initially multiply in the mucosa and lymphoid tissue (tonsils and Payer's patches) of the pharynx and gastrointestinal tract (ileum) where they spread to lymph nodes and then to blood, causing a transient (minor) viraemia. In a minority of infected individuals, secondary replication occurs in lymphoid tissue (lymph nodes, liver, spleen, bone marrow) and leads to a more sustained secondary (major) viraemia which may be followed by localization in the central nervous system, heart or skin. The initial febrile illness is associated with the 'major' viraemia.

Clinical manifestations of non-polio enteroviruses

It will be clear from the pathogenesis that Coxsackie- or echovirus rarely produce specific disease patterns – rather a variety of common disease patterns. Virtually any system may be involved.

The commonest manifestation is pharyngitis, the presentation being with fever and sore throat and exudate may be present on the tonsils.

Ulcers on the soft palate which follow small vesicles surrounded by a red blush are characteristic of herpangina – usually due to Coxsackievirus A. Headache, vomiting, myalgia and at times diarrhoea usually accompany the pharyngitis. The illness is short lived with recovery occurring in 4–5 days.

Enteroviruses may at times attack the respiratory system producing croup, bronchitis or pneumonia. Although it can mimic pleurisy or peritonitis, epidemic pleurodynia or Bornholm disease is due to myositis. It is characterized by fever, spasmodic pain and tenderness in the chest and upper abdomen which is accentuated by movement, cough, sneeze and deep breathing. Episodes of pain characteristically last for several hours and can be very severe while they last. Coxsackie B3

and B5 are most often associated with Bornholm disease but other enteroviruses may also be responsible.

The gastrointestinal manifestations of the enteroviruses consist of vomiting and diarrhoea, but their role in infantile gastroenteritis is not clear because of the frequent carrier rate.

Myocarditis and pericarditis are well recognized manifestations of enterovirus infection with Coxsackie B group most often causative, especially in neonates in whom there is a high mortality.

Aseptic meningitis either isolated or epidemic in association with fever, pharyngitis, and perhaps a skin rash is another common manifestation of enterovirus infection. The symptomatology is no different from other forms of viral meningitis. Epidemics of enterovirus meningitis are frequent in the summer months.

The skin lesions of these virus infections vary widely. Most commonly the rash is macular or maculopapular, but at times it may be vesicular or petechial. In hand-foot and mouth disease, vesicles are noted on the pads of the fingers and toes, in the mouth and on the buttocks. Coxsackie A is most frequently the cause of this syndrome, but other Coxsackie types and enterovirus 71 can also produce a similar syndrome.

Enteroviral infections, although very common in paediatrics, are rarely severe except in the neonate in whom myocarditis, hepatitis or encephalitis may be fatal. Treatment of enteroviral infections is symptomatic.

TYPHOID FEVER

Typhoid fever is due to infection of *Salmonella typhi* and is confined to humans. The source of infection is either an active case of typhoid fever or a chronic carrier excreting the organisms in urine or stools. Typhoid fever occurs where standards of hygiene are unsatisfactory, especially where a pure, clean water supply is not available. Faecal or urinary contamination of food or drink is the source of infection. Sporadic cases or small outbreaks in Western communities often result from inadvertent contamination of food during preparation by an unrecognized carrier, often a migrant from an endemic area. Chronic carriage usually lasts for many years. Excretion of *S. typhi* in stools may be intermittent but increases with age.

Clinical features

The initial presentation is usually as a vague illness with malaise, anorexia, muscle aches, cough and particularly headache. Reduced mental alertness is very common. The temperature is almost always raised. Occasionally, patients present with the clinical features of acute gastroenteritis which settles after a few days, but leaves the patient with relapsing fever and headache. However, abdominal pain and constipation probably occur even more commonly.

Occasionally cases are identified through contact with a known case. Sometimes these children are not unwell, but are excreting the organism in the stool. In Western societies, it is unusual for the patient with typhoid fever to develop the severe gastrointestinal complications seen in underdeveloped countries and so vividly recorded in textbooks of tropical medicine. Fever and disorientation with few or no physical signs prompts immediate investigation so that blood cultures are performed early and the diagnosis established rapidly.

Diagnosis

The diagnosis of typhoid fever is established by isolating the organism *S. typhi* from one or more blood cultures. Cultures will usually be positive during the bacteraemic phase of the illness, i.e. during the first week. Isolation of the organisms from stool or urine (usually positive during the second week of the illness) is helpful additional evidence, but not conclusive; for example, it would not prove whether the patient has typhoid fever or is merely a chronic carrier of the disease with a concurrent pyrexial illness. Further evidence can be obtained from the Widal agglutination titres. An initial titre of 'H' or 'O' antibodies in excess of 1:40 in a patient from a non-endemic area who has not had typhoid vaccination is very suggestive of typhoid fever. An initial high 'O' titre and low 'H' titre suggests acute infection; a low 'O' titre and a high 'H' titre suggests previous infection or vaccination.

Treatment

Patients with typhoid fever should be isolated and barrier nursed. Excreta need to be carefully disposed of and scrupulous attention given to hand-washing by medical staff and other attendants. Chloramphenicol is the drug of choice in the treatment of typhoid fever. Ideally it should be given orally, but in a confused and ill patient it will be given intravenously. With chloramphenicol the temperature usually settles over 2(5 days although occasionally it may be 7 days before a response is obtained. The course of treatment should last 14 days. Both ampicillin and co-trimoxazole have also been used with some success in the treatment of typhoid fever.

Relapse

A reservoir of *S. typhi* bacilli in the reticuloendothelial system provides the source for relapse which presents clinically in the same way as the original infection. The incidence of relapse is probably about 5–10%, but higher if shorter courses of chloramphenicol are given.

Carriers

Patients excreting *S. typhi* in stools or urine for a year or more after an acute infection are regarded as carriers. Approximately 3% of all patients become carriers.

MALARIA

Malaria is being seen with increased frequency in Australia. The reasons for this include:

1. Migration, particularly involving refugees from South East Asia.
2. Frequent air travel to tropical countries.
3. The emergence of drug resistant strains of *Plasmodium falciparum*.
4. Failure to comply with recommended protocol for malarial chemoprophylaxis.

A proper understanding of the pathogenesis of malaria involves a knowledge of the life cycle of plasmodium and its transmission. Such aspects are beyond the scope of this work, but the information is readily available in the many excellent texts of tropical paediatrics. In Western societies malaria almost invariably presents as a pyrexia of unknown origin. The clues that malaria is likely to be responsible for the fever are usually apparent from the clinical history which may indicate:

1. The child has recently arrived from an area where malaria is endemic.
2. The child has lived in such an area and has had malaria previously.
3. The child has recently returned from an overseas trip, having travelled through an area where malaria is endemic.

Malaria does not always present with high fever, chills, sweats, headache, vomiting and protraction each second or third day; this classical mode of presentation of tertian or quartan fever is by no means the rule. All types of malaria in the early stage may fail to show the expected asymptomatic intervals; synchronization of the parasitic cycle may be established only after many days, or indeed not at all during the primary episode. Physical examination of a child with malaria often reveals no abnormality although some 30–40% of patients have an enlarged spleen and in about a quarter the liver is also enlarged.

Examination of thick and thin blood films enables the parasites to be identified in the red cells. Frequently there is an associated mild anaemia but the blood examination is otherwise unremarkable. Other investigations do not help with the diagnosis.

The therapy of malaria will not be dealt with in any detail. However, it is important to recognize the following:

1. Resistant strains of falciparum are now very frequent particularly in South East Asia.

2. Apart from *P. falciparum*, the other plasmodial species have persisting exoerythrocytic tissue forms which act as a reservoir for subsequent clinical relapses.

Treatment

Chloroquine resistant strains of *P. falciparum* are now widely distributed throughout the world. Chloroquine phosphate is the drug of choice for *Plasmodium vivax* and *Plasmodium ovale* and for *P. falciparum* in areas where chloroquine resistance is not a problem. In these circumstances the response to oral chloroquine is rapid and cure is complete. *P. vivax* and *P. ovale* have persisting exoerythrocytic tissue forms which act as a reservoir for subsequent clinical relapses. To achieve radical cure in these forms of malaria, primaquine phosphate is administered after clinical cure is obtained with chloroquine. Although primaquine is not required in *P. falciparum* infections, it should be remembered that *P. falciparum* and *P. vivax* infections may occur together in the same patient. Therefore, it is good practice to give all patients with malaria a course of primaquine.

The treatment of choice of chloroquine resistant *P. falciparum* is quinine phosphate and Fansidar (pyrimethamine plus sulphadoxine).

Malarial prophylaxis

With the emergence of insecticide resistance and increasing difficulty in vector control, eradication programmes for malaria will rely at present on mass chemotherapy. It is very important, however, for those travelling to areas where malaria is endemic to realize that the mosquito vector feeds at dusk and in the evening. At these times clothing must cover as much of the body as possible and a mosquito repellant spray should be used. Mosquito netting to windows and beds should also be installed. These measures are at least as important as chemoprophylaxis. Chloroquine phosphate given once weekly commencing two weeks before visiting a malarious area and continuing for 6 weeks after returning home is recommended. In areas where chloroquine resistant *P. falciparum* is endemic, prophylaxis may combine chloroquine and Fansidar (pyrimethamine and sulphadoxine) or chloroquine plus Maloprim (pyrimethamine and dapsone).

Steady progress is being made in the production of a malaria vaccine but almost certainly it will be several years before one is available.

FURTHER READING

Black R H 1982 Malaria in Australia 1981. Tropical medicine technical paper No. 8 Australian Government Publishing Service, Canberra

Christie A B 1981 Infectious diseases, 3rd edn. Churchill Livingstone, Edinburgh

Cirose C 1985 The many faces of infectious mononucleosis: the spectrum of Epstein-Barr virus infection in children. Pediatrics in Review 7: 35–44

Evans A S 1978 Infectious mononucleosis and related syndromes. American Journal of Medical Science 276: 325–339

Fergin R O, Cherry J D 1987 Textbook of pediatric infectious diseases. Vols I and II, W B Saunders, Philadelphia

Krugman S, Ward R, Katz S L 1977 Infectious diseases of children. Mosby, St Louis

Lambert H P, Farrar W E 1982 (eds) Infectious diseases illustrated. Pergamon Press, Oxford

Straus S E, Ostrone M, Inchauspe G et al 1988 Varicella-Zoster infections. Biology, natural history, treatment and prevention. Annual International Medicine 108: 221–237

30. Infections of bone and joint

W. G. Cole

Microbiology

Bacterial bone and joint infections are usually the result of bacteraemia or septicaemia. At all ages *Staphylococcus aureus* is the most common organism cultured from either blood or pus. *Haemophilus influenzae* type B is a rare cause of osteomyelitis but a common cause of joint infection in children from about 4 months to 5 years of age. Group A beta-haemolytic streptococci are cultured from blood and pus in a small percentage of cases. Group B beta-haemolytic streptococci are frequently cultured from neonates.

Many other organisms have been isolated from blood and pus. *Staphylococcus albus* and diptheroids are usually only isolated from blood cultures and may, therefore, represent skin contaminants. Pseudomonas infections of vertebrae and pelvis occur in adolescent drug addicts. Pseudomonas osteomyelitis of the calcaneum also occurs from penetrating injuries of the heel. Salmonella osteomyelitis is frequently associated with sickle-cell haemoglobinopathies. Unusual organisms such as *Candida* sp. and *Aspergillus* sp. occur in patients with severely depressed host-defense mechanisms, or in patients receiving prolonged intravenous therapy or parenteral nutrition. In such patients, bone and joint infections are often multifocal. Osteomyelitis rarely occurs from anaerobic organisms. Polymicrobial infections are usually confined to patients with chronic infections and are more common following compound injuries.

Pathology

Haematogenous osteomyelitis is predominantly a disorder of the metaphyses of long bones in children. Bacteria lodge in the metaphyses because of relative sludging of blood in the sinusoidal metaphyseal vessels. Trauma may also play a role as the lower limb bones are involved more often than other sites.

Without treatment, bacteria in the medullary vessels produce necrosis of metaphyseal bone. Spread of infec-tion involves bone resorption with spread of pus through the thin cortex adjoining the growth plate giving rise to a subperiosteal abscess. In addition, bacteria may extend across the growth plate, via transphyseal vessels to the epiphysis and into the adjacent joint. The hip and shoulder joints are commonly involved in this manner.

Bacterial infections of joints may arise from two mechanisms. The first consists of the spread of bacteria from the adjoining epiphysis or metaphysis; a pattern usually observed in infants and neonates. The second mechanism involves the spread of bacteria from the blood to the synovial membrane. Synovitis results with the production of purulent joint fluid which may become thick and loculated. Polymorphonuclear leucocytes and bacteria produce enzymes which are capable of degrading the articular cartilage.

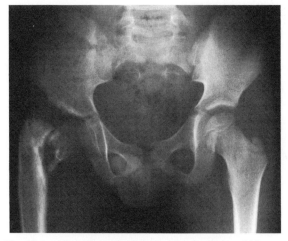

Fig. 30.1 AP radiograph of the pelvis of a 6-year-old boy who had staphylococcal osteomyelitis of the femur and suppurative arthritis of the hip shortly after birth. The bone has healed but growth plate and epiphyseal growth is retarded.

Late treatment of bone and joint infections frequently results in sequestration of bone and chronic osteomyelitis, avascular necrosis, permanent damage to or even total destruction of epiphyses, growth plates and articular cartilage (see Fig. 30.1). In contrast, early treatment is usually curative without any permanent effects.

CLINICAL FEATURES OF OSTEOMYELITIS

The clinical presentation of children with haematogenous osteomyelitis varies due to differences in the duration of the disease, the apparent resistance of the host and virulence of the organism, the age of the patient, and site of the disease. As a result, it is helpful to classify osteomyelitis as acute (early and late forms), subacute (aggressive and non-aggressive forms) or chronic.

Early acute osteomyelitis

This is the most common form of osteomyelitis. Children present with an acute febrile illness of 24 to 48 hours' duration. In addition to the generalized signs of an acute infection, they have localizing signs of acute osteomyelitis. The signs include failure to use the limb normally, and tenderness and swelling over the metaphysis of a long bone such as the distal femur or proximal tibia. At this stage of the illness there is no clinical evidence of an abscess nor any radiological changes in the bone. Alternative diagnoses are suppurative arthritis and cellulitis. Joint signs rather than metaphyseal signs are present in children with suppurative arthritis. Cellulitis is associated with redness of the skin and a spreading edge, while redness and induration only occur with acute osteomyelitis. The signs include failure to use the limb normally, and tenderness and swelling over the metaphysis of a long bone such as the distal femur or proximal tibia. At this stage of the illness there is no clinical evidence of an abscess nor any radiological changes in the bone. The alternative diagnoses are suppurative arthritis and cellulitis. Joint signs rather than metaphyseal signs are present in children with suppurative arthritis. Cellulitis is associated with redness of the skin and a spreading edge, while redness and induration only occur with acute osteomyelitis at a more advanced stage. The white cell count and erythrocyte sedimentation rate are raised in both. A bone scan may distinguish cellulitis from osteomyelitis but it is simpler to repeat the radiographs after 10 to 14 days as the appearance of subperiosteal new bone will confirm the diagnosis of osteomyelitis.

Late acute osteomyelitis

Late onset osteomyelitis is a less common form of osteomyelitis. It is associated with clinical features of an abscess and may be associated with radiological abnormalities of the bone. Although late acute osteomyelitis is seen at all ages, it is more common in neonates, infants and in late childhood.

Neonates and infants

Late acute osteomyelitis is the most common form of osteomyelitis in neonates and infants. The advanced nature of the disease appears to be due to delayed diagnosis. There are two categories of cases:

1. Septicaemic neonates and infants. Septicaemia, which is often due to Group B beta-haemolytic streptococci acquired from the mothers genital tract, usually commences soon after birth. These babies are extremely ill, and as such babies are immobile it may not be apparent that they have osteomyelitis until a mass appears or until lack of spontaneous movement is observed following their recovery from the septicaemia. Multifocal osteomyelitis is common here and osteomyelitis of the proximal humerus and femur is often overlooked. At the time of diagnosis there is commonly a large subperiosteal abscess and suppurative arthritis with the risk of permanent joint and growth plate damage.

2. Relatively well neonates and infants. Most of these babies have returned home and have been feeding and gaining weight in a normal manner. There is often a history of furunculosis while in the neonatal nursery. Subsequently the mother observes a lump or painful movement of a limb (see Fig. 30.2). Osteomyelitis involves most commonly the femur with formation of a huge abscess, when the leg is held in the frog position. Radiographs may show subperiosteal new bone and bone destruction as well as a huge soft tissue mass. The white cell count is elevated with a shift to the left. The erythrocyte sedimentation rate is grossly elevated.

Older children and adolescents

Delayed diagnosis of acute osteomyelitis in children over ten years of age is common. The white cell count and erythrocyte sedimentation count are raised and radiographs taken ten or more days after the onset of the illness show extensive bone destruction and subperiosteal new bone.

Acute osteomyelitis at various sites

The features already described for acute osteomyelitis are those most commonly seen at the metaphysis of a

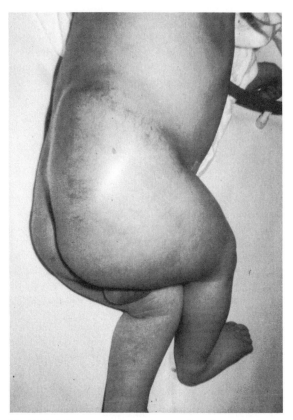

Fig. 30.2 Neonate with huge abscess of the buttocks due to late acute osteomyelitis of the ileum.

long bone but they are less obvious at other sites. The proximal femur and humerus, pelvis and spine are difficult sites to examine and late diagnosis of infections is common.

Discitis and osteomyelitis of the spine

Infection of the spine varies in its severity. When the systemic features are mild it is referred to as discitis and when severe it is referred to as osteomyelitis. The spine is rigid and tender and the children refuse to stand or walk. The white cell count and the erythrocyte sedimentation rate are high. Radiographs are initially normal except for loss of lumbar lordosis and a mild scoliosis. Bone scans may show increased activity on either side of the involved disc. Such changes confirm the clinical diagnosis of discitis or osteomyelitis so avoiding the necessity for additional investigations to exclude intraspinal tumour, neuroblastoma or urinary tract anomalies.

Subacute osteomyelitis

Children with subacute osteomyelitis have minimal systemic reaction to their infection. The white cell count and erythrocyte sedimentation rate may be normal. The radiographs are always abnormal with features of either an aggressive (malignant) or non-aggressive (non-malignant) lesion.

Aggressive form

The radiographic features are those of a malignant bone tumour with destruction of bone, soft tissue mass and the onion skin or sunburst type of subperiosteal new bone formation.

Non-aggressive form

This form consists of a well defined cavity in the metaphysis which may extend across the growth plate into the epiphysis (Fig. 30.3). In young children the cavity may be limited to the epiphysis. These lesions are

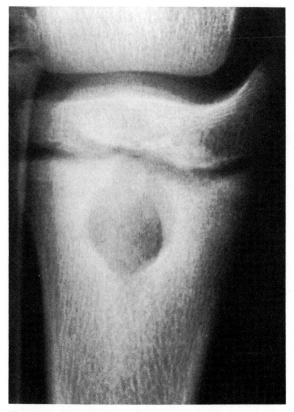

Fig. 30.3 AP radiograph of the proximal tibia showing a lytic area due to subacute osteomyelitis.

frequently referred to as Brodie's abscess but usually they contain granulation tissue rather than pus.

Chronic osteomyelitis

Chronic osteomyelitis is heterogeneous. It is less common in Australia than acute and subacute forms and usually presents as a chronic illness without any preceding acute phase. Chronic osteomyelitis may result from *Mycobacterium tuberculosis* and various fungi but more commonly the cultures are negative or *S. aureus* is cultured. The disease may be unifocal or multifocal (Fig. 30.4). Bone scans are helpful in revealing asymptomatic sites of chronic osteomyelitis.

TREATMENT OF OSTEOMYELITIS

The treatment of osteomyelitis includes the use of antibiotics, surgery and immobilization. Before commencing therapy, swabs of any superficial septic foci and blood are collected for culture. Cultures are also obtained from patients having drainage of pus or bone biopsies. Relevant radiographs and estimations of haemoglobin, white cell count and erythrocyte sedimentation rate are made. Bone scans can also be obtained but should be ordered selectively.

The clinical diagnosis of early acute osteomyelitis is supported by a positive bone scan but is not excluded by a negative scan. As a result, bone scans are of little practical value in the management of early acute osteomyelitis of long bones in which the physical signs are easily observed. In such cases treatment should be commenced immediately and the radiographic features of osteomyelitis sought several weeks later. Bone scans are more useful in confirming early acute osteomyelitis of the pelvis or spine as clinical and plain radiographic assessment are more difficult than in the peripheral skeleton. However, in such cases treatment should also be commenced immediately and the scan undertaken several days later when the child has improved.

Bone scans are also of little value in children with late acute osteomyelitis as the clinical signs of an abscess are obvious and radiographic bones changes are often present. However, they are particularly useful in detecting multiple sites of acute infection in neonates and infants and in detecting asymptomatic sites of subacute and chronic osteomyelitis.

It is helpful to consider treatment in relation to the different types of osteomyelitis.

Early acute osteomyelitis

This form of osteomyelitis can be successfully treated by intravenous antibiotics given over a few days, followed by oral antibiotics and immobilization for a total period of three weeks. Children in this group usually respond rapidly and can be expected to be cured with a single course of treatment without the need for operation. These results indicate the importance of early diagnosis within the first 24 to 48 hours, before a clinical abscess appears.

Blood cultures are positive in about 50% of patients.

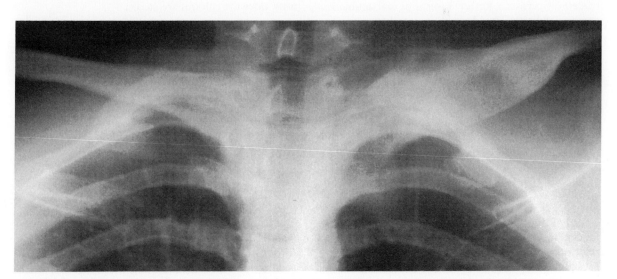

Fig. 30.4 AP radiograph of the clavicles of a 12-year-old girl. The left clavicle is sclerotic and enlarged due to chronic multifocal osteomyelitis.

The positive culture rate can be increased to about 75% by also culturing aspirates from the involved metaphysis. However, aspiration of the infected site, particularly in younger children, requires a general anaesthetic, and is not warranted in children without clinical evidence of an abscess as *S. aureus* is still the most common organism cultured under these circumstances.

The choice of antibiotic is based on the observation that *S. aureus* and Group A and Group B beta-haemolytic streptococci are the most common organisms. Flucloxacillin and benzylpenicillin are given intravenously. If the child is known to be allergic to penicillin, a cephalosporin is given instead. As soon as the antibiotic sensitivities of the pathogen are available, a single antibiotic is selected such as flucloxacillin for *S. aureus* and benzylpenicillin for beta-haemolytic streptococci. If bacteria are not isolated, the antibiotics used initially are continued. Intravenous antibiotics are continued until the child is clinically well, with a normal temperature and a decrease in the local signs. The equivalent oral antibiotics are then commenced and the child returns home 2 days later provided the antibiotics are tolerated and the general condition is satisfactory. Review at the completion of the 3-week course of treatment is essential.

Almost all children are cured by the 3-week course of treatment but the erythrocyte sedimentation rate may not have returned to normal. The radiographs show subperiosteal new bone but may also show cavities. In the absence of tenderness these cavities heal spontaneously over the following 12 to 18 months. If local tenderness persists a further 3 weeks of oral antibiotics and immobilization is indicated.

Late acute osteomyelitis

Treatment of late acute osteomyelitis includes drainage of subperiosteal pus, drainage of pus from adjoining joints as well as antibiotics and immobilization. Subperiosteal abscesses are drained with an incision over the point of maximum tenderness.

In late acute osteomyelitis antibiotics are given intravenously for at least 5 days and oral therapy, initially in hospital and then at home, is continued for a total period of 6 weeks. Serum bactericidal titres and antibiotic blood levels are useful in children who are severely ill or responding poorly to treatment. Immobilization is also continued for 6 weeks. Treatment is stopped at the 6-week review if there is no local tenderness. In neonates and infants the infection is usually resolved by one course of treatment. Necrotic bone is resorbed and replaced, but the outcome depends on

whether there has been permanent damage of the growth plate, articular cartilage or epiphysis. In contrast, bone healing is less effective in older children and adolescents when persistent cavities and sequestra are common and further surgery is often required before cure is achieved.

Subacute osteomyelitis

A biopsy is required in all children with radiological features of an aggressive lesion of bone as the clinical, radiological and haematological features are identical to those of primary malignant tumours such as Ewing's sarcoma. If the pathologist is able, at the time of biopsy, to confirm the diagnosis of osteomyelitis, then the cavity is curetted and treatment with intravenous antibiotics is commenced. Such treatment is usually curative.

Metaphyseal and epiphyseal cavities, with typical features of subacute osteomyelitis, can be successfully treated with a short course of intravenous flucloxacillin followed by oral flucloxacillin and immobilization for a total course of 6 weeks. Curettage is required if there is an abscess or failure of improvement with antibiotics.

Chronic osteomyelitis

Biopsy of one of the lesions is recommended in order to confirm the diagnosis and to obtain material for culture. Preoperative consultation with a microbiologist is recommended as cultures for common and unusual organisms should be undertaken. Specific antibiotic therapy is given when organisms are cultured but in many cases the cultures are sterile.

CLINICAL FEATURES OF JOINT INFECTION

The clinical presentation of children with bacterial joint infections is also variable. In most instances the joint infection is part of a systemic illness with a bacteraemia or septicaemia. Bacteria can also enter the joint from a puncture wound resulting from a needle, nail or thorn.

It is helpful to use a similar classification of joint infection to that used for osteomyelitis.

Early acute joint infection

Acute infective arthritis is also called septic arthritis. Most children present within 48 hours of the start of the illness. The systemic features are the same as those of early acute osteomyelitis. The local joint signs consist of swelling, warmth, tenderness and reduced motion. Pain is often severe at rest. In neonates and infants osteomyelitis and suppurative arthritis frequently coexist.

The radiographs show fluid within the joint but no changes in the bone. In doubtful cases an ultrasound examination may be used to confirm a suspected effusion. The white cell count and erythrocyte sedimentation rate are raised. A bone scan is not usually required to confirm the diagnosis but if done it may show increased activity in the joint.

There are several important differential diagnoses.

Transient synovitis of the hip

The aetiology of transient synovitis is unknown although it is likely to be related to viral infection as many children have a concurrent viral illness or a recent history of one. This condition, also called irritable or observation hip, is common. The principle reason for making the distinction from suppurative arthritis is that transient synovitis is treated with rest; this is clearly inappropriate for children with bacterial arthritis of the hip.

Children with transient synovitis usually have a mild illness and fever with little pain at rest. Movement of the joint is painful and the range of movement is reduced. In contrast, children with suppurative arthritis of the hip are sicker, have pain at rest and no or minimal hip rotation. Radiographs may show a joint effusion. The white cell count and erythrocyte sedimentation rate are raised in both conditions although they tend to be higher in children with suppurative arthritis. Nonetheless, the distinction between the diseases is usually made clinically and when doubt exists it is safer to aspirate the hip as described later.

Acute arthritis with negative bacterial cultures

Negative cultures of blood, joint fluid and synovium are obtained in about half the children who have the clinical features of acute bacterial arthritis. The aetiology of the arthritis remains uncertain in many of these children but several specific disease patterns are observed.

Viral infection of the joint may account for some of these cases. Rubella and parvovirus have been associated with acute arthritis. Acute arthritis can also occur as a reactive arthritis several weeks after *H. influenzae* epiglottis or meningitis. In such cases the joint contains purulent fluid but no organisms are cultured. Reactive arthritis may also occur following enteric and genitourinary infections. For example, sterile acute arthritis may follow enteric infections with *Salmonella*, *Shigella*, *Yersinia* or *Campylobacter* species.

Some children with negative bacterial cultures later show the features of juvenile chronic arthritis.

Other forms of acute arthritis

Rheumatic fever and vasculitis syndromes such as Henoch Schönlein purpura and Kawasaki's disease may present with an acute arthritis. Careful clinical assessment and appropriate investigations will enable these diagnoses to be made. Many other diseases also have arthralgia or acute arthritis associated with them but the underlying disease will be apparent. For example, arthritis occurs in children with chronic ulcerative colitis, Crohn's disease and chronic active hepatitis.

Late acute joint infection

This type of infection is equivalent to late acute osteomyelitis. The children present four or more days following the onset of the illness. The joint is usually grossly distended with thick pus and the child is severely toxic. If affected the hip may be dislocated in neonates and infants. The proximal epiphysis of the femur or other epiphyses may be detached and undergoing autolysis as the result of a pathological feature.

Subacute and chronic joint infections

Children who present with a history of a swollen joint for several weeks to a month rarely have a staphylococcal or haemophilus infection. Some will have synovitis resulting from a penetrating injury, such as thorn synovitis. Synovectomy is required to cure this condition as the thorn breaks up into hundreds of fine spicules which become embedded in the synovium.

Tuberculous synovitis always needs to be considered. Careful clinical assessment is required as well as a chest radiograph and Mantoux test. If a synovial biopsy is obtained it is examined for acid fast bacilli and cultured for mycobacteria. Testing for serum antibodies to *Brucella* species is also undertaken in children from areas where brucellosis is endemic.

In practice, most of the children who present with subacute and chronic arthritis have juvenile chronic arthritis or one of its variants.

TREATMENT OF JOINT INFECTION

The treatment of bacterial joint infection includes joint aspiration, arthrotomy, antibiotics and immobilization.

Early acute joint infection

Blood is collected for estimation of haemoglobin, white cell count, erythrocyte sedimentation rate and plain radiographs are taken. Blood is also collected for culture and an intravenous drip is inserted. Under general anaesthesia the joint is aspirated by an experienced surgeon in an operating room which is set up for an arthrotomy. Should the child have a transient synovitis clear fluid will be obtained from the hip joint. If the fluid from the hip is turbid, a small anterior arthrotomy is made to lavage the joint and a biopsy of synovium obtained for histology and culture. Treatment with antibiotics is commenced and skin traction is applied. In contrast to the hip joint, turbid fluid in other joints can usually be adequately aspirated and the joint lavaged with normal saline without arthrotomy being required. Systemic antibiotics are also given and the joint supported by a plaster slab/sling or traction.

The joint fluid obtained is sent to the laboratory for Gram stain and culture. Also, *H. influenzae* antigen can be detected in the joint fluid, blood and urine, usually before the results of the standard cultures are available. Viral cultures can also be undertaken but are generally not routine.

All children with turbid joint fluid are treated with antibiotics as it is difficult to distinguish between bacterial and other forms of arthritis. A positive Gram stain is helpful in identifying children with bacterial arthritis; however, the Gram stain may be negative in some samples from which bacteria are cultured. Analysis of joint fluid for cell number, cell type and chemical composition may be undertaken, but the results rarely enable a patient to be positively identified as not having a bacterial infection.

Flucloxacillin will cover *S. aureus* and ampicillin or chloramphenicol covers *H. influenzae*. The increasing incidence of ampicillin resistant strains of *H. influenzae* necessitate the use of chloramphenicol or newer generation cephalosporins. A single antibiotic is given when the culture and sensitivity results are available. Should the cultures be negative, flucloxacillin and ampicillin are continued. In neonates flucloxacillin and gentamicin are used to cover *S. aureus*, streptococci and Gram negative organisms.

Antibiotics are given intravenously for several days until the child is well, afebrile and with improvement in the local signs. Oral antibiotics are then commenced and if tolerated the child returns home to complete a total of three weeks' treatment. The joint is mobilized as soon as it becomes comfortable and the swelling subsides.

The joint symptoms and signs usually resolve by the third week, but the erythrocyte sedimentation rate may take a little longer to return to normal. It is rare for children with bacterial infections to require any further treatment. With early presentation and early treatment a cure is achieved with return of the joint to normal.

Parents are notified that the diagnosis remains uncertain when the cultures are negative. Some children will present later with features of juvenile chronic arthritis.

Late acute joint infection

The involved joint contains thick pus and an arthrotomy will be required in order to break down loculations, wash out the joint and determine the state of the epiphysis and articular cartilage. If the hip is dislocated it is reduced and a plaster cast used to maintain the reduction postoperatively. Pus and synovium are collected for culture and synovium is sent for histology and the joint is immobilized. Intravenous antibiotics, as used in early acute joint infections, are given for at least 5 days and then orally, initially in hospital and later at home, for a total of 6 weeks. Careful assessment is made during these 6 weeks although the infection is usually cured with a single 6-week course of treatment. All of the complications that follow bacterial joint infections occur in the late acute group of children. The permanent changes consist of total destruction of the joint, avascular necrosis, growth plate arrest and loss of articular cartilage. Premature osteoarthritis may follow. The severity of these sequelae highlights the necessity for early diagnosis and treatment.

Subacute and chronic joint infection

Careful clinical assessment is made for features suggestive of juvenile chronic arthritis, tuberculosis, brucellosis or thorn synovitis. In addition to other appropriate investigations an arthrotomy or arthroscopy may be used to obtain samples of joint fluid and synovium for culture and histology. Specific treatment is determined by the likely diagnosis.

FURTHER READING

Cole W G, Dalziel R, Leitl S 1982 Treatment of acute osteomyelitis in childhood. Journal of Bone Joint Surgery (64-B): 218–223
Nade S 1985 Acute haematogenous osteomyelitis in infancy and childhood. Journal of Bone Joint Surgery (65-B): 109–119
Ross E R S, Cole W G 1985 Treatment of subacute osteomyelitis in childhood. Journal of Bone Joint Surgery (67-B): 443–448

31. Meningitis and encephalitis in infancy and childhood

M. J. Robinson, G. L. Gilbert

MENINGITIS

Incidence

Bacterial meningitis is essentially a disease of childhood. Approximately two-thirds of all cases occur in children below the age of 15 years and, of these, 80% occur in the first 5 years of life. Neonates and children between the ages of 6 and 12 months are at the greatest risk. Although any bacterial organism may theoretically cause meningitis, in practice the common types seen in childhood in order of frequency are *Haemophilus influenzae* type B, *Neisseria meningitidis* and *Streptococcus pneumoniae* (Fig. 31.1). In the neonatal period the infection is mainly due to Group B streptococci and Gram-negative organisms (see Ch. 27).

Most cases of meningitis begin as a septicaemia, the portal of entry usually being the nasopharynx. In the neonate the original focus may be the umbilicus or occasionally the renal tract often in association with a developmental renal anomaly. This septicaemia phase is partly responsible for the nondescript signs and symptoms which precede the characteristic features of meningitis. Occasionally meningitis may result from direct spread of infection from a compound skull fracture, a leaking meningomyelocele, a congenital dural sinus or other congenital fistulae. Otitis media with or without mastoiditis and infection of valves inserted at shunt operations in the management of hydrocephalus are also possible sources. Formerly, meningitis was occasionally the result of rupture of a brain abscess in a child with cyanotic congenital heart disease but this situation is now very rare in centres where cardiac surgery is performed in early childhood.

H. influenzae type B (HIB) meningitis has become

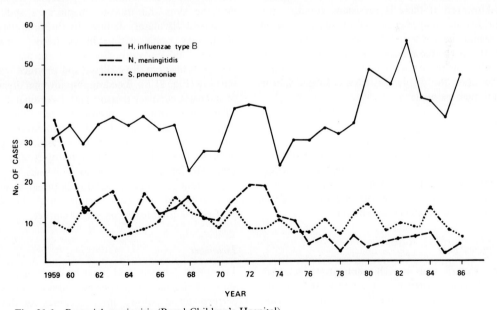

Fig. 31.1 Bacterial meningitis (Royal Children's Hospital).

more common in developed countries over recent years. The reasons for this increase are not clear. A new *H. influenzae* type B (HIB) bacterial vaccine is available which consists of the type b polysaccharide antigen conjugated to protein and is immunogenic in young infants. Preliminary studies indicate that unlike an earlier polysaccharide vaccine it will protect against HIB infections even in children under 2 years of age – an age group in which HIB infections are most common. A pneumococcal vaccine which contains the commonly encountered antigenic strains is also available, but it is not useful under 2 years of age. Pneumococcal vaccine is indicated for older persons at risk from this organism; these groups include postsplenectomy patients and those with asplenia and sickle-cell anaemia.

Clinical presentation

In infancy

Fever, pallor and vomiting in association with alteration in the state of consciousness are the most important clinical features. Some infants are excessively irritable with a high pitched cry, but more commonly the infant is lethargic, refuses to feed and does not appear to recognize the mother. At this age, neck stiffness may be present, but its detection is difficult because so often the infant resents any type of handling. Not infrequently an infant with meningitis will refuse to flex the neck to look down when held above the examiner. Usually the fontanelle tension is increased and sometimes it is actually bulging. However, if there is persistent vomiting the fontanelle tension may be normal or even reduced despite meningitis. Little or no reliance can be placed on spine stiffness or the Kernig's sign in this age group. Occasionally, the presentation of meningitis is with a convulsion when the distinction from a simple febrile convulsion must be made.

In children over the age of 3 years

The signs of meningeal irritation are much more obvious here, the presentation being with headache, fever, vomiting and neck stiffness. Delirium and clouding of consciousness rapidly follows if early symptoms are not recognized and the diagnosis established.

Insidious presentation

This is particularly seen in HIB meningitis which may present with vague symptoms of upper respiratory infection over 1 to 3 days. Antibiotics will often be given with some improvement initially, but quite soon the child becomes ill again and signs of meningeal irritation appear. On the other hand, when antibiotics are given, symptoms may be masked, so there must be a high index of suspicion of meningitis in any child who appears to have a septic illness, but who is not responding to antibiotic therapy.

Neonatal meningitis

Here the initial signs are very vague and the disease must be suspected in any infant who exhibits abnormal behaviour e.g. slight fever, poor feeding, unexplained vomiting. As a rule, by the time the fontanelle bulges there has been wide sutural separation indicating that the disease has been present for some time (see Ch. 27).

Fulminating onset

The presentation may be dramatically sudden with shock, purpura, hypothermia and coma. Almost invariably this indicates meningococcal septicaemia, but occasionally HIB and *Strep. pneumoniae* can cause a similar clinical pattern.

Meningococcaemia

Meningocccaemia is usually followed by meningitis when the clinical features are solely those of meningeal inflammation. Occasionally, the meningococcaemia is overwhelming when the presentation is of a very acute febrile illness associated with petechial haemorrhages into the skin and mucous membranes and signs of peripheral circulatory failure. In the fulminating case, death may occur within hours from overwhelming toxaemia and uncontrollable shock. In such cases the skin petechiae rapidly coalesce and produce widespread purpura (Fig. 31.2). Bleeding into internal organs is due to extensive capillary damage and disseminated intravascular coagulation consequent on the massive septicaemia. Bilateral adrenal haemorrhages are commonly noted at autopsy in fatal cases. All grades of severity exist and the overall mortality is of the order of 25%. Meningococci may be so numerous in the blood stream that they may be seen on a direct blood film or on a smear taken from a purpuric spot. The diagnosis is of course established on blood culture.

Treatment

Treatment is urgent and must be commenced immediately the diagnosis is suspected without even waiting to perform blood culture unless facilities for this are immediately available. Penicillin is the drug of choice and

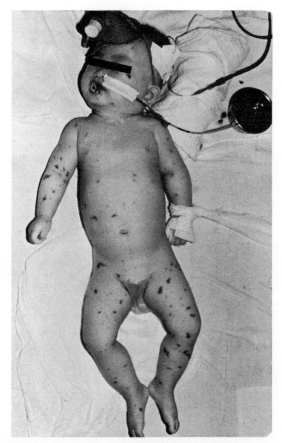

Fig. 31.2 Meningococcaemia – illustrating the characteristic purpuric rash. Circulatory collapse has required resuscitation.

the suggested dosage is 60 mg/kg intravenously every 4 hours. The management of the associated endotoxic shock will involve the use of plasma expanders, e.g. plasma or plasma protein derivative. In persisting shock ionotropic agents, particularly dopamine, will be indicated. The persistence of shock despite volume depletion may indicate myocardial failure and consequently digitilization and oxygen administration. High dosage corticosteroid therapy has been used in the management of severe septic shock, but its efficacy has not been proven. Disseminated intravascular coagulation indicates replacement of coagulation factors and consideration of heparin therapy, but this is unlikely to be successful until the septicaemia has been overcome.

Meningococcaemia occasionally presents as a mild chronic or recurrent febrile illness. An arthritis, usually mono-articular, may be the presenting feature. The presence of petechiae should make the diagnosis of

chronic meningococcaemia suspect and allow for confirmation by blood culture.

Diagnosis of meningitis

This can only be established by spinal puncture which is indicated if the diagnosis is suspect. Occasionally there may be signs of cerebral compression with pinpoint pupils, a very bulging fontanelle and irregular breathing. Under these circumstances spinal puncture may be contraindicated. Such patients will be managed with antibiotic therapy, fluid restriction and appropriate measures to reduce cerebral oedema.

The cerebrospinal fluid in bacterial meningitis is cloudy or opalescent. Microscopic examination will reveal a cell count usually in excess of 1000 polymorphs $\times\ 10^6/l$. Occasionally, the count is within normal limits or only slightly elevated, despite positive culture. Turbidity of the CSF in the absence of a traumatic tap is because of the following:

1. Predominantly polymorphonucleocytes in bacterial meningitis
2. Predominantly lymphocytes in some cases of viral meningitis
3. Large numbers of bacteria and few cells in some cases of fulminating pneumococcal meningitis.

The glucose level of the cerebrospinal fluid is reduced below 2.5 mmol/l and/or to less than 60% of the blood glucose. It may even be undectable in the CSF. The protein level is usually elevated above 1 g/l. Organisms are frequently seen on Gram staining of the CSF when a presumptive diagnosis may be made, but mistakes can occasionally be made on morphological appearances. There are now available simple and sensitive tests for the detection of specific bacterial antigens in CSF and other body fluids, e.g. blood and urine. These are (a) latex agglutination, and (b) co-agglutination. They are available for detection of HIB, *Strep. pneumoniae* and *N. meningitidis*, group B Streptococcus and *Escherichia coli* K1. Falsely positive results are rare, but when testing for urine antigens tests should only be done on sterile specimens because of cross-reactivity between *E. coli*, group B *Streptococcus* and *N. meningitidis*.

The major value of antigen tests is in partly treated meningitis when cultures may be negative. The tests are also useful in fulminating bacterial meningitis with few cells and many organisms visible on Gram staining when the latter may be difficult to identify on morphological grounds.

Occasionally the cerebrospinal fluid examination may be difficult to interpret in cases where antibacterial drugs have been given before spinal puncture. Agglutination tests may also be negative. However, 40% of children with bacterial meningitis have received antibiotics before the diagnosis is made and in most cases the findings are typical. The decision to treat as bacterial meningitis will be a clinical one when the commonly occurring bacteria need to be covered with antibiotic drugs until the CSF is found to be sterile on culture. However, it may be reasonable to observe some children in hospital without chemotherapy if they are not ill. It is also useful to take blood cultures after the spinal puncture. And a total white cell count and differential white cell count may also be helpful.

Treatment of meningitis (between the ages of 3 months and 14 years)

If on spinal puncture the CSF is obviously turbid, crystalline penicillin 60 mg/kg and chloramphenicol 50 mg/kg are given immediately by deep intramuscular injection. If the Gram stain shows pleomorphic Gram-negative bacilli and the test for HIB antigen is positive (and the others negative), use chloramphenicol alone. If the Gram stain shows Gram-positive diplococci and the test for *Strep. pneumoniae* is positive and/or the test for HIB antigen is negative, use penicillin alone. If there is doubt the results should be discussed with the microbiologist, or both chloramphenicol and penicillin used together until the results of cultures are available.

The following antibiotic dosages are recommended in the treatment of meningitis in childhood:

● Chloramphenicol 25 mg/kg 8-hourly intravenously
● Penicillin 30 mg/kg 4-hourly intravenously.

Treatment is continued for a period of 7–14 days, but this will depend upon the clinical course and the type of organism isolated. Occasionally, it may be possible to cease treatment in mild cases of meningococcal meningitis after 5 days, whereas in HIB and *Strep. pneumoniae* meningitis treatment should be continued for 7–10 days at least. Some strains of HIB are resistant to chloramphenicol and alternative agents, which are active against the major causes of meningitis, are available, e.g. cephalosporins, such as ceftriaxone and cefotaxime. These have been shown to compare favourably with chloramphenicol.

Supportive treatment

1. Fluid therapy. Fluid therapy will usually be given intravenously in the first few days because of the risk of vomiting and refusal to take fluid orally. The intravenous route is also convenient for the administration of antibiotic drugs. Fluid intake must be reduced to ap-

proximately 15 mg/kg/day as meningitis in infancy and childhood is frequently accompanied by an inappropriate secretion of antidiuretic hormone (ADH) – see below.

2. Clinical observations. Regular check on the pulse, temperature, respirations and state of consciousness is necessary. The head circumference should be measured daily in any infant with meningitis.

3. Anticonvulsant therapy. This will be indicated in the child who has convulsed or is excessively irritable. Diazepam (valium) intravenously effectively controls most convulsions. If convulsions are frequent and/or prolonged, phenytoin given by intravenous injection is indicated. It should be remembered that when chloramphenicol and phenytoin are used together the usually recommended doses of both drugs should be reduced and blood levels measured daily.

4. Repeated spinal punctures. When the nature of the organism and its sensitivities are known and the clinical progress is satisfactory, repeated lumbar punctures are unnecessary. When chemotherapy is discounted the child may be discharged if the general condition is satisfactory without a follow-up spinal puncture. However, spinal puncture may be repeated under the following circumstances:

1. Persistence of fever
2. Should there be a need to assess progress, e.g. when the diagnosis has been made late or when an organism has not been cultured
3. If a relapse is suspected
4. If an unusual organism is cultured and the prognosis is in doubt.

Problems and complications in meningitis

1. Convulsions. These are common (30% in HIB meningitis, 60% in pneumococcal) and can usually be managed with diazepam. If severe and persistent intravenous phenytoin is indicated.

2. Cerebral oedema. This may occur shortly after the onset, particularly in pneumococcal or HIB meningitis, and is usually a manifestation of the severity of the infection. Thus careful observations for signs of increased intracranial pressure are essential. These include progressive loss of consciousness, stertorous or irregular breathing, pinpoint pupils and finally respiratory arrest. Management of cerebral oedema involves fluid restriction, respiratory and circulatory support, preferably in a paediatric intensive care unit.

In bacterial meningitis in infancy and childhood there is frequently an inappropriate secretion of antidiuretic hormone (ADH). This results in dilution of the extracellular fluid compartment with a consequent water shift into the intracellular compartment. When this involves the brain cerebral oedema occurs. Cerebral oedema in meningitis can usually be avoided by fluid restriction (less than 15 mg/kg/24 hours for the first 2 days or so. The diagnosis of inappropriate ADH secretion is most easily made by measuring the serum sodium concentration. A level of 130 mmol/l is diagnostic of inappropriate secretion of ADH. Treatment involves fluid restriction, but hypertonic saline or hypertonic mannitol may be infused intravenously in an emergency situation.

3. Neurological lesions. These tend to relate to the severity of the infection and the adequacy of treatment; they are frequently reversible. The more common lesions are cranial nerve palsies, particularly third, fourth and sixth. Deafness, monoplegia, hemiplegia, and intellectual impairment may also complicate.

4. Subdural effusions. These are accumulations of high protein, usually sterile fluid in the subdural space. The mechanism of subdural effusions is not well understood. They are often bilateral and are usually situated over the temperoparietal region. The presence of a subdural effusion is suggested from one or more of the following – continuing high fever or recurrence of fever after several days of adequate treatment; persistently positive CSF cultures although this is very rare and likely to indicate resistance of strain to antibiotic; localized or generalized convulsions; persistent vomiting; persistent elevation of CSF protein; increase in skull circumference or fontanelle tension; and sudden appearance of a focal neurological deficit.

The diagnosis of subdural effusion is most readily established by brain CT scanning. In cases where the anterior fontanelle is large, ultrasonography may be useful. Most subdural effusions resolve spontaneously unless large, but a very large effusion may require surgical drainage.

5. Non-specific complications. These include:

- Infection at intravenous sites
- Injection abscesses
- Associated suppurative arthritis
- Skin and other tissue loss due to vasculitis in severe septicaemia.

6. Late complications. These may only be recognized by long-term follow-up. They include:

- Behavioural problems
- Intellectual handicap
- Cerebral palsy
- Deafness
- Blindness
- Epilepsy.

Late complications tend to relate to delay in diagnosis, the severity of infection and the adequacy of treatment. Long-term follow-up is important if some of the more subtle sequelae of meningitis, such as learning or emotional problems, are to be recognized and managed.

Mortality

It should be remembered that meningitis is a serious disorder with a significant mortality. Mortality figures at the Royal Children's Hospital, Melbourne are summarized below:

In HIB meningitis mortality is approximately 3%. There have not been enough cases of pneumococcal and meningococcal meningitis to give accurate figures but it is significantly high in *Strep. pneumoniae* (10–15%). In meningococcal disease death is from fulminating septicaemia and almost never from meningitis per se.

Treatment of contacts

It is important to recognize that there is a significant risk of cross-infection to all close contacts of patients with meningococcal meningitis. There is also a significant risk to cross-infection of close contacts under 4 years of age from patients with HIB. Therefore, there are strict guidelines to the management of contacts.

1. Meningococcal meningitis. Parents need to be warned that should they, their children or other close contacts of the patient feel unwell, medical attention should be sought without delay. In addition, prophylactic chemotherapy using rifampicin should be given to this group as soon as possible. The dosage of rifampicin is 20 mg/kg for 2 days to a maximum of 600 mg/dose. The index case should also be given rifampicin after recovery as therapy does not eradicate this organism from the nasopharynx.

2. HIB meningitis. Parents of children suffering from HIB meningitis should seek medical advice if any of their other siblings, particularly those under the age of 4 years, are unwell. In households where there is another child under 4 years of age all members of the household should be given rifampicin 20 mg/kg (maximum 60 mg/kg daily for 4 days). The index case should also be given rifampicin before discharge from hospital but after completion of chloramphenicol therapy.

Contacts of children with pneumococcal meningitis are not given antibacterial prophylactic treatment. However, parents should be warned that a significant risk to infection of contacts does exist and that medical help should be obtained should a contact become ill over the ensuing week or two.

VIRAL MENINGITIS AND ENCEPHALITIS

A large number of viruses have the capacity to invade the central nervous system and, depending upon the primary site of involvement as judged clinically, the designations meningitis, encephalitis and myelitis are used. Viral or aseptic meningitis implies that the major clinical manifestations are of fever, headache, vomiting, stiffness of the neck, along with other signs of meningeal irritation such as back stiffness and Kernig's sign. Encephalitis implies that the brain has been invaded when the result may be an acute inflammation with neuronal death or damage, or a more delayed demyelination of the white matter. The clinical signs detected in encephalitis will depend upon the site and the extent of the inflammatory process so that the clinical picture will vary enormously. Changes in behaviour and conscious state are most often detected. If signs attributed to involvement of the spinal cord such as paraplegia, neurogenic bladder, are present, the term myelitis is appropriate. Combinations of these syndromes are often encountered.

Even where sophisticated facilities for virus isolation and serology exist, it is common to be unable to define the aetiological agent in aseptic meningitis and encephalitis. Viruses known to be associated with aseptic meningitis and encephalitis are listed in Example 31.1

Epidemic outbreaks of encephalitis in different parts of the world are usually caused by the arthropod-borne viruses. These organisms are closely related and are grouped together as arbovirus group A or B on the basis of their serological reactions. Birds and mammals serve as vertebrate hosts to these viruses and the disease is transmitted to man by the bites of infected mosquitoes

or tics. Enteroviruses are the commonest cause of viral meningitis but some are more likely than others to cause outbreaks of encephalitis. HSV 1 is the commonest cause of sporadic encephalitis.

Clinical features of viral meningitis

The onset may be acute or occur over a day or so. The initial clinical features comprise headache, fever, malaise, vomiting and frequently abdominal pain. Neck and spine stiffness appear quite early in the illness and indicate the need for a spinal puncture. Occasionally a macular rash may accompany viral meningitis and suggest the possibility of an ECHO or Coxsackievirus as the causative agent. Parotid or mandibular swellings will suggest mumps. By definition focal neurological signs do not occur in viral meningitis.

The cerebrospinal fluid cell count is raised and in the initial stages cells are frequently polymorphonuclear leucocytes. Lymphocytes appear in the CSF slightly later. Usually, the spinal protein content is slightly elevated, but the sugar content is normal. Because of the difficulties and time necessary to identify causative viruses in aseptic meningitis, it is of the greatest importance that other disorders, which produce a similar clinical and cerebrospinal picture and require specific therapy, are considered and positively excluded. Such disorders include tuberculous meningitis, cryptococcal meningitis, partly treated bacterial meningitis, cerebral abscess and, rarely, subacute bacterial endocarditis.

Viral meningitis is a benign disease, it requires symptomatic treatment only and complete recovery without sequelae can be expected within a few days.

Clinical features of viral encephalitis and myelitis

The clinical pattern of viral encephalitis varies from a benign illness, almost identical to that seen in viral meningitis, to a most devastating illness which may result in death or recovery with permanent neurological sequelae. The onset of viral encephalitis is usually acute, but may be more gradual over several days. In the encephalitis associated with the exanthematous fevers, e.g. measles, varicella, the onset of neurological symptoms is usually between 2 and 7 days after the appearance of the rash, but may actually precede it. The early symptoms consist of fever, headache, dizziness, vomiting and apathy. Neck stiffness is usually present, but the cardinal feature of encephalitis is an alteration in the state of consciousness and behaviour. In the severely affected child these symptoms are followed by mental confusion, stupor, restlessness and delirium. Focal pareses or paralyses, sensory disturbance, speech difficulties, in-

---

Example 31.1 Common viruses which may cause meningitis and encephalitis

Post-infective encephalitis without direct invasion of CNS
Viruses associated with childhood infections, measles, rubella, varicella, Epstein-Barr virus, *M. pneumonia*
Meningitis and/or encephalitis with viral CNS infection
Mumps – usually meningitis, less often meningoencephalitis
Enteroviruses – ECHO, Coxsackie- and polio viruses these usually cause meningitis but encephalitis can occur.
Arbovirus (arthropod-borne virus) e.g. Australian encephalitis.
Herpes simplex virus type 1 can cause focal (usually temporoparietal) encephalitis. (HSV 1 or 2 can cause encephalitis in neonates)
Progressive encephalitis
E.g. subacute sclerosing panencephalitis due to measles virus infection

voluntary movements and ataxia may occur separately or in combination. Convulsive seizures may occur at any stage and death may occur as the result of brain stem involvement or following seizures.

Spinal cord involvement (transverse myelitis) may occur in association with encephalitis, but is usually the only manifestation of the disease. This has been described in association with mumps, measles, varicella and EBV infection. Acute transverse myelitis is recognized by the rapid appearance of a flaccid paraplegia, loss of tendon reflexes, a neurogenic bladder and a sensory level representing the upper limit of the spinal cord lesion. Any part of the spinal cord may be affected, the commonest site being the mid-thoracic region. Acute cord compression from extradural abscess or some other cause must always be excluded by one of the forms of imaging when a diagnosis of transverse myelitis is made. The outcome of transverse myelitis varies from almost total functional recovery to permanent paralysis of the involved limbs.

Slow virus infection

It is now recognized that viruses can cause a subacute or chronic progressive neurological disease. The term slow virus infection has been applied to these conditions. Examples in childhood are subacute sclerosing panencephalitis and kuru (now virtually non-existent. Subacute sclerosing panencephalitis is a rare late complication of measles (especially when infection occurs very early in life). It is manifest by progressive deterioration of behaviour, personality and intellect and is accompanied by myoclonic seizures and motor disturbances. The onset is usually several years after the attack of measles. The myoclonic spasms classically consist of flexion of the head, trunk and extremities followed by a gradual relaxation phase. These spasms are repetitive occurring at intervals of 10 to 60 seconds and can often be provoked by sensory stimuli. As the disease progresses the motor disturbances become obvious. These consist of spastic paralyses, tremors,

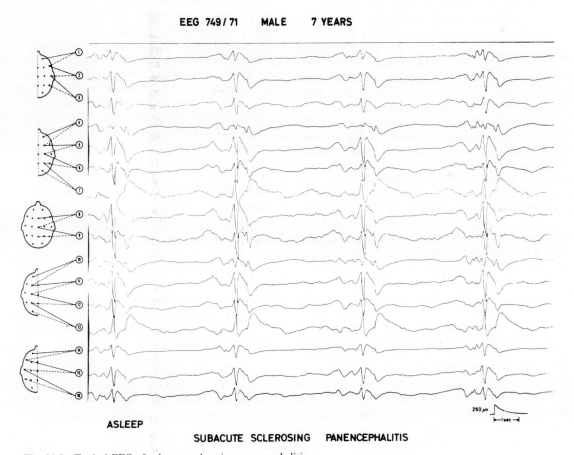

Fig. 31.3 Typical EEG of subacute sclerosing panencephalitis.

athetoid movements and ataxia. The disease runs a variable, but progressive course and is usually fatal within two years. In the early stages of the disease the EEG usually demonstrates a typical 'suppression burst pattern' (see Fig. 31.3). The diagnosis is established by the typical clinical picture and the finding of high titre measles antibody in cerebral spinal fluid.

Diagnosis of encephalitis

Viral encephalitis, presenting during an epidemic or following one of the exanthematous fevers, can confidently be diagnosed on clinical grounds, but in other circumstances the diagnosis is one of exclusion. Other cerebral infections to be excluded include tuberculosis, crytococcal meningitis, partly treated bacterial meningitis and cerebral malaria in areas where it is endemic. Encephalitis may be confused with certain toxic and metabolic disorders such as lead poisoning, salicylate and other drug intoxications. Also to be considered are hypoglycaemia, raised intracranial pressure from a cerebral neoplasm, subdural haematoma or the encephalopathy that accompanies Reye's syndrome.

Herpex simplex encephalitis

This variety of encephalitis specifically mentioned as the causative agent – herpes simplex virus – is amenable to treatment with the antiviral drug acyclovir.

The clinical features of herpes simplex encephalitis (HSVE) are not specific and a laboratory diagnosis may not be possible in the early stages of the illness. Formerly, the diagnosis was established by brain biopsy but, because of the invasive nature of this procedure and because acyclovir is free of serious side effects, many clinicians would prefer to treat on the basis of the clinical history and the CSF findings. The laboratory diagnosis of HSVE is now most commonly established by finding specific antibodies in CSF taken at least 10 to 14 days after the onset of the illness. As HSVE is usually not a primary infection, patients may have IgG antibody in their serum from a previous infection, without IgM. Thus measurement of serum antibodies is often unhelpful. In clinical practice it is now common when a patient presents with fever, convulsions, disturbance of conscious state, with or without localizing signs, together with a mild increase in cells in the CSF and a raised protein to be regarded as possibly having HSVE. As the outcome of this disease depends on early diagnosis and treatment, acyclovir is administered empirically and attempts to establish the diagnosis made by examination of the cerebrospinal fluid after two weeks. This approach appears to have significantly improved the outcome for HSVE. It is recognized that other forms of encephalitis may be treated unnecessarily with acyclovir but, as mentioned previously, the drug is without serious side effects. It is again emphasized that other forms of 'encephalitis' need to be excluded in the first instance before such therapy is commenced.

Reye's syndrome

Reye's syndrome is a disorder characterized by the rapid onset of encephalopathy associated with hepatic dysfunction. Following an upper respiratory infection the child develops seizures and sinks into a coma of varying depth usually within a period of 24 hours. Hepatomegaly due to a fatty liver is common and laboratory tests reveal elevated transaminases, elevated serum ammonia levels, hypoglycaemia and abnormalities of blood coagulation. The serum bilirubin is normal. Apart from the reduced glucose content, the CSF is normal. Reye's syndrome has a high mortality and a significant morbidity, but some patients may recover completely. There is now compelling evidence from epidemiological studies that Reye's syndrome is almost certainly the result of a viral infection (e.g. influenza B or varicella) together with salicylate given for symptomatic relief. In countries where salicylate is no longer used for the febrile child the incidence of Reye's syndrome has been dramatically reduced.

Treatment of encephalitis

The management of encephalitis (other than HSVE) is symptomatic and involves careful clinical observations and maintenance of hydration and nutrition, particularly if the child is unconscious. Sedation will be necessary in the hyperexcitable and convulsing child and diazepam by the intravenous route is probably the best drug. in the presence of hyperpyrexia, tepid sponging, intravenous fluids and chlorpromazine – to prevent shivering – will be indicated. After the acute illness has subsided prolonged physiotherapy and rehabilitation will be necessary for the seriously affected child. Corticosteroids are often used in the treatment of encephalitis, but there is little scientific proof of their efficacy. As already mentioned, acyclovir is indicated should herpes simplex encephalitis be suspected.

FURTHER READING

American Academy of Paediatrics 1988 Committee on infectious disease. Treatment of bacterial meningitis. Pediatrics 6: 904–907

Ho D D, Hirsch M S 1985 Acute viral encephalitis. Medical Clinics of North America 69: 415–429

Klein J O, Feigin R D, McCracken G H 1986 Report of the taskforce on diagnoses and management of meningitis. Pediatrics 78: 959–982

Ratzan K R 1985 Viral meningitis. Medical Clinics of North America 69: 399–413

Sande M A, Schold M, McCracken C H et al 1987 Report of a workshop. Pathophysiology of bacterial meningitis – implications for new management strategies. Pediatric Infectious Diseases 6: 1143–1171

32. Pyrexia of unknown origin (PUO)

M. J. Robinson

Fever in children is usually a transient phenomenon and a manifestation of some intercurrent infection. At least 70% of all infections in children are viral and in most the fever subsides within four to five days. Children have a variable number of infections each year, the number depending upon the age of the child, the position of the child in the family, and the time the child comes into contact with the community. With the recent introduction of day care for young infants the number of infections in this age group has dramatically increased. Before this children stayed at home until about the age of four years when they attended kindergarten so that it was not until this time that the number of infections increased. In the first year or so at school the average child will contract approximately eight separate illnesses per year (see Fig. 20.2). Occasionally there are more so that parents become concerned about the overall health of their child and in particular the child's immune status. Most infections in childhood are minor and fever is usually low grade. However, some of these infections will be more prolonged, but the clinical history, the physical examination and a few simple investigations will establish the cause of the fever in most cases. The investigations performed in this group of children should include a full blood examination, microscopy and culture of urine, radiograph of the chest and Mantoux testing.

Occasionally, a child will present with persisting fever of over one week's duration, the cause of which is not explicable by history, physical examination, nor the tests described above. The clinical picture is often complicated by the previous administration of antibiotics for a presumed respiratory infection, or because of frustration and/or anxiety of the doctor who has been under pressure from anxious parents. The administration of antibiotics under these circumstances compounds the problem, particularly in the interpretation of cultures from blood, urine or cerebrospinal fluid.

The majority of children with a long standing PUO do not as a rule have an overwhelming infection. Severe infections are resolved one way or another within a week and most will require respiratory and circulatory support and broad spectrum antibiotics because of the gravity of the situation. In children with a long standing PUO the child is far from well, with lethargy, anorexia, disinterest, general discomfort and moderate toxaemia. As already mentioned, there is usually substantial anxiety experienced by the parents in large part due to the lack of a positive diagnosis. The doctor must not be unduly influenced by these anxieties and parental pressures, but should approach the problem without undue haste using the skills of history taking and physical examination to determine the most appropriate investigations necessary to establish a diagnosis. Simply requesting a large number of investigations at random and prescribing antibiotics is unscientific, time wasting, expensive and traumatic to the child.

Children who have a fever which persists for over a week or more and who are moderately ill are likely to be admitted to hospital for investigation. When this is done it is important to observe the child carefully while the investigations are being undertaken. Particular note should be made of the height of the fever, whether it is intermittent or sustained and whether there are other signs such as rash, joint pains or swellings, tachycardia or tachypnoea.

PROTOCOL FOR INVESTIGATION OF A CHILD WITH PUO

History

The history of the illness should be taken in the usual way, but there should be a specific enquiry about the following:

1. The health of the immediate family, close relatives and/or neighbours.

2. The occupation of the parents and the place of abode of the child. For example, should the father be a

farmer, disorders such as brucellosis, leptrospirosis and hydatid disease may need to be considered.

3. Pets in the home, for example, pigeons, budgerigars, young puppies or young kittens. This would bring up the possiblity of psittacosis, visceral larva migrans and cat scratch disease.

4. Note should be taken of the presence of any epidemics in the community at the time.

5. The ethnic group of the child. Standards of living are often low in the Aboriginal people and in certain migrant groups – particularly refugees. The incidence of tuberculosis and streptococcal disease is much higher in these groups than in the general community.

6. Have the child and the parents been overseas recently or travelled to areas of endemic disease? If so, enquiries about immunization against typhoid fever and prophylaxis against malaria must be made. It should also be remembered that much of falciparum malaria is now chloroquin resistant worldwide. Despite this, chloroquin is still the most commonly used drug for malaria prophylaxis.

7. Has the child had recent surgery? Under these circumstances one may have to consider a collection of pus as the cause of the PUO. If physical examination does not reveal such a collection it may be necessary to resort to one of the forms of imaging, e.g. CT scanning, radioisotopic scanning, etc.

8. Has there been an insidious onset of weight loss in association with the fever? If so, it is likely that the problem is not a recent one.

9. The past history should always include an enquiry for a congenital malformation, for example, congenital heart disease may predispose the child to endocarditis. Children who have had surgical repair of certain congenital heart lesions are at risk for endocarditis (see Ch. 39). Recurrent urinary tract infections are often due to a congenital renal anomaly.

10. The family history may be contributory, for example, a sibling may have cystic fibrosis or vesicoureteric reflux.

Physical examination

This should be meticulous and complete. The physical examination, while not necessarily allowing one to make a diagnosis, will frequently direct attention to the system involved. It is particularly important to look for subtle signs of CNS involvement, e.g. headache, minor degrees of neck and spine stiffness, subtle neurological signs or deterioration in intellectual performance. The presence of hepatosplenomegaly with or without lymphadenopathy will point to the reticuloendothelial system. Careful palpation of the abdomen may reveal a mass. Palpation of the skeleton and assessment of joint function must also be done. However, a physical examination is by no means always helpful in defining the cause of a prolonged PUO, so that further investigation is often necessary.

The following are three major causes of a prolonged fever:

• Infection
• Connective tissue disease
• Malignant disease.

Infection

The following bacterial infections frequently present as a PUO in a developed society. They are:

– Typhoid fever
– Paratyphoid fever
– Typhus
– Leptospirosis
– Brucellosis
– Subacute septicaemias
– Subacute bacterial endocarditis
– Tuberculosis disease
– Malaria.

In the immunosuppressed child fevers may be the result of infection with a normally non-pathogenic agent, e.g. *Pneumocystis carinii*, *Cryptosporidium*, *Candida albicans* and other fungi. Thus body fluids need to be sent for examination and culture. These will include blood, cerebrospinal fluid, urine and any abnormal collection of fluid, e.g. pleural effusion, pericardial effusion, ascites, joint effusion or abscess. The medical microbiologist should always be consulted in these cases so that anaerobic as well as aerobic cultures are put up. Agglutination tests for typhoid, paratyphoid, *Brucella*, typhus and leptospirosis should also be ordered. Serology and cultures for EB virus, cytomegalovirus and other viruses known to be in the community at present may be indicated. Toxoplasma can produce an illness in children with fever and symptoms similar to infectious mononucleosis. The diagnosis of infectious mononucleosis is now best made by the identification of specific IgM and IgG to the Epstein-Barr virus.

Search for a pyogenic abscess will be indicated in children who have had recent surgery, in children who are febrile with abdominal pain and in those who have the features suggestive of chronic inflammatory bowel disease. Such a search will involve the various forms of imaging including plain radiology, ultrasonography, technetium scanning, CT scanning and perhaps nuclear magnetic resonance imaging if available. Isotope scanning is particularly helpful when low grade osteomyelitis is considered as a possible cause for the continued fever. Osteomyelitis of the pelvis, for example, is a particularly difficult diagnosis to make on clinical grounds.

Tuberculosis as a cause of prolonged fever should be considered particularly in refugee groups and in those where living standards are sub-optimal through crowding and poor sanitation. In disseminated tuberculosis and tuberculous meningitis Mantoux testing may be negative because a state of anergy may develop. Acid fast bacilli may be difficult to identify on the centrifuged deposit of the cerebrospinal fluid and a positive diagnosis may not be made for several weeks until cultures of sputum, CSF, gastric content or urine become positive. It may be necessary when the cerebrospinal fluid findings are compatible with tuberculosis meningitis and not other diagnosis of subacute meningitis is forthcoming, to treat the child as tuberculous until either an alternative diagnosis is made or a positive culture for tuberculosis is obtained. This diagnosis will be facilitated if chest radiology reveals a primary TB complex or a picture consistent with millary disease. Other causes of subacute meningitis include torula, amoebae, cerebral malignancy and rarely cerebral vasculitis as part of a connective tissue disorder. Cytological examination of CSF and appropriate staining techniques, e.g. Indian ink stain for torula will be necessary in these situations.

With few exceptions it should be possible within a week or so to decide from observation and the investigations outlined above whether or not one is dealing with a specific infection. Apart from disseminated tuberculosis, antibiotics should not be given if the patient's general conditon remains stable and cultures and serology are negative. It has been this author's experience that chemotherapy rarely if ever solves the problem of prolonged PUO in the absence of positive bacteriological evidence.

Immune deficiency. This has been covered in Chapter 22. In general, congenital immune deficiency does not present as a PUO but as either overwhelming or recurrent severe infection in comparatively early life. Acquired immune deficiency syndrome (AIDS) is almost certain to become a paediatric problem in this country. It is already a paediatric problem of some magnitude in parts of Africa and the United States. AIDS may present in infancy as failure to thrive, particularly in association with repeated infections. Before the recognition that AIDS could be transmitted from blood transfusions, and other blood products, paediatric AIDS was not frequently acquired by this route; with simple heat treatment to blood AIDS is no longer transmitted in this fashion. Congenital AIDS is almost always ac-

quired in utero from an AIDS positive mother. In older children and adolescents intravenous drug use and homosexuality are the major causes of AIDS. The presentation of AIDS may occur several weeks after the infection was acquired when a febrile illness associated with generalized lymphadenopathy, weight loss, anorexia and skin rash may appear: a clinical pattern that is not dissimilar from that of infectious mononucleosis. Paediatricians and doctors looking after children need to be aware of AIDS and to organize the appropriate serological investigations should an individual with the symptoms described have, in addition, one of the risk factors. Frequently there are no initial signs and the clinical presentation is the fully expressed disease with unusual infections and constitutional symptoms of fever, weight loss and malaise. Infections commonly associated with AIDS include *Pneumocystis carinii* (Fig. 32.1) or other atypical pneumonia, persisting diarrhoea frequently due to cryptosporidium, evidence of a progressive cerebral degenerative disorder and/or unusual skin lesions of Kaposi's sarcoma (Fig. 32.2). Tuberculosis, human or avian, persisting CMV infections and a variety of fungal infections also occur in young people with the fully expressed AIDS complex.

Connective tissue or autoimmune disease

A disorder of this group will need to be seriously considered in cases of prolonged fever where infection appears to have been eliminated. The indications of a connective tissue disorder or an autoimmune process are listed in Example 32.1.

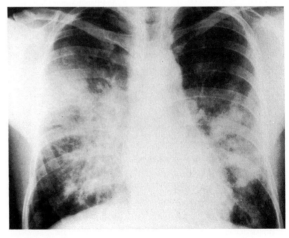

Fig. 32.1 Chest radiograph of a patient with AIDS demonstrating the typical findings of Pneumocystis carinii.

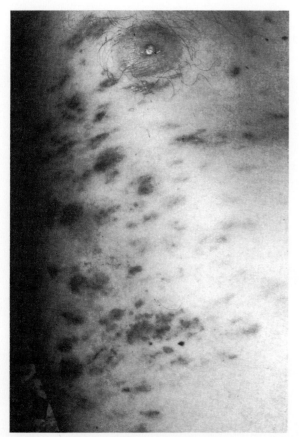

Fig. 32.2 The skin lesions of Kaposi's sarcoma in a young male.

Malignant disease

A number of childhood malignancies present to the doctor with fever as their major cause. In many instances there will be no signs of a mass lesion, hepatosplenomegaly or lymphadenopathy. Radiology of the chest and abdomen may also be non-contributory. The particular malignancies which may present in this fashion include the leukaemias, Hodgkin's disease and other lymphomas, phaeochromocytoma and particularly neuroblastoma. The relevant investigations to exclude malignancy involve repeated examinations of the peripheral blood, bone marrow aspiration and/or trephine, radiological and/or radioisotope bone scanning of the whole skeleton. In children, where there is a

---

Example 32.1 Indications of a connective tissue disorder or an autoimmune process

1. A persistently high erythrocyte sedimentation rate greater than 70 mm in 1 hour)
2. A relatively low leucocyte alkaline phosphatase level
3. Hypergammaglobulinaemia
4. The presence of autoantibodies in serum either to tissue, for example, thyroid, liver, etc. or cell components, for example, a positive antinuclear antibody titre, or a positive Coombs' test.

   The following connective tissue disorders may present purely as a pyrexia of unknown origin with few or no abnormal physical findings: (a) systemic onset juvenile chronic arthritis; (b) systemic lupus erythematosus; (c) mixed connective tissue disease.

Chronic inflammatory bowel disease, namely, ulcerative colitis and Crohn's disease may present similarly as may chronic active hepatitis. Some of the vasculitis syndromes, for example, Kawasaki disease, Stevens-Johnson syndrome, polyarteritis and drug fevers may present with few other symptoms than prolonged fever. The clinical features of these disorders together with the appropriate investigations for their diagnosis are discussed in Chapter 73.

---

progressive downhill course with fever and all other causes of PUO have been eliminated, other forms of imaging such as CT scanning and nuclear magnetic resonance imaging may be required. The type of imaging selected will depend upon the site needing to be imaged and of course the facilities that are locally available. In these circumstances consultation with the radiologist is essential.

Occasionally the fever subsides and no diagnosis is made. Some cases of systemic onset juvenile chronic arthritis (JCA) may resolve with arthritis being little more than minimal. There is a disorder resembling systemic JCA which is self limiting, but responds and resolves with the administration of corticosteroid medication given over a period of 4 to 6 weeks. Treatment with steroids in this situation needs very careful consideration, full investigation to exclude other causes, a significant period of observation and frequently, interdisciplinary consultation. Finally, it should be remembered that fictitious fevers are occasionally reported by parents, nursing staff and other attendants. This was referred to as Muchhausen by proxy and at present is known as Meadow's syndrome. Extreme caution is advised before entertaining this latter diagnosis.

SECTION 8

Paediatric emergencies

33. The collapsed child

Frank Shann

GENERAL PRINCIPLES

Very many conditions may cause a child to collapse; some of the important causes of collapse are listed in Example 33.1. Although the management of a collapsed child depends on the cause of the collapse, some general principles apply regardless of the cause (see Example 33.2).

Cessation of the supply of oxygen to the brain, as in asystole, causes unconsciousness in about 10 seconds. Patients who are unable to breathe take longer to lose consciousness, but this is because they have a reservoir of oxygen in their lungs. The brain is also dependent on a continuous supply of glucose as a source of energy. Glucose and glycogen are used up in about 2 minutes if cerebral flow stops.

Therefore, the first priority in managing a collapsed child is to ensure an adequate supply of oxygen and glucose to the brain. This requires prompt and effective aspiration of the airway, breathing and circulation (ABC), in that order. In the context of a collapsed child, the main purpose of the circulation is to carry oxygen from the lungs to the brain, but there is little point in moving blood from the lungs to the brain if there is no oxygen in the lungs. Valuable time is often lost by feeling the pulse of the collapsed child, when the first priority is to ensure a patent airway and adequate ventilation.

The airway

All unconscious patients should be nursed lying on their side, unless they are intubated, because this improves the size of the airway and reduces the risk of aspiration should vomiting occur. Once the child is lying on the side, the mouth and nasopharynx should be sucked out. It is best to use a large rigid sucker, such as a Yankower sucker, rather than a flexible suction catheter.

It may be necessary to push the child's jaw forward to provide an adequate airway, but often it will be enough just to lie the patient on the side. An oral airway may also be helpful, but it must be the correct size for the child and, even then, an oral airway may actually increase airway obstruction in a small child.

Breathing

After establishing a patent airway, it is important to check that the patient is breathing adequately. Hypoventilation is very dangerous in a collapsed patient. If there is any suspicion of hypoventilation, ventilation

---

Example 33.1 Some causes of collapse in children

Asphyxia	neonatal asphyxia, drowning
Airways obstruction	epiglottitis, croup, asthma
Hypovolaemia	dehydration, haemorrhage
Cardiac failure	congenital heart disease, arryhthmias, cardiomyopathies
Central nervous system	head injury, meningitis, encephalitis, convulsions
Metabolic	hypoglycaemia, hyponatraemia
General	sepsis, 'near-miss' sudden infant death syndrome, drug ingestion, envenomation

---

Example 33.2 Initial management of the collapsed child

1. Lie on the side (or intubate and ventilate if hypoventilating).
2. Suck out the mouth and nasopharynx.
3. Give oxygen at 10 l/min by mask.
4. Pass a large nasogastric tube (0–3 years size 12 FG, 4–10 years size 14 FG).
5. Assess pulse and blood pressure. If hypovolaemic, give 10 ml/kg boluses of blood, SPPS, Haemaccel or saline to restore circulation; start dobutamine 10 μg/kg/min if indicated.
6. Take blood for gases, electrolytes, haemoglobin, glucose cross-match and culture as appropriate.

---

must be assisted by mouth-to-mouth breathing, bag-and-mask ventilation, or by intubation and ventilation. Use 100% oxygen if this is available.

Intubation is by far the most effective way of protecting the airway and ventilating a collapsed child, but it requires considerable experience to intubate a small child. A term neonate should be intubated with a 3.5 mm tube inserted to a depth of 9 cm (measured at the mouth). From one year of age, use a tube size of age/4 + 4 mm (e.g. 6/4 + 4 = 5.5 mm for a 6-year-old child) inserted to a depth equal to age + 9 cm (maximum 20 cm) at the mouth (e.g. 6 + 9 = 15 cm for a 6-year-old child). The amount of ventilation should be judged by watching the child's chest movements. Endotracheal tube and suction catheter sizes are shown in

Table 33.1 Endotracheal tubes and suction catheters (reproduced with permission)

Age	Weight (kg)	Endotracheal tube				Sucker FG
		Int Dia (mm)	Ext dia (mm)	At lip (cm)	At nose (cm)	
Newborn	<1	2.5*	3.4	5.5	7	6
Newborn	1.0	3.0*	4.2	6	7.5	6
Newborn	2.0	3.0*	4.2	7	9	6
Newborn	3.0	3.0*	4.2	8.5	10.5	6
Newborn	3.5	3.5*	4.8	9	11	8
3 month	6.0	3.5	4.8	10	12	8
1 year	10	4.0	5.4	11	14	8
2 year	12	4.5	6.2	12	15	8
3 year	14	4.5	6.2	13	16	8
4 year	16	5.0	6.8	14	17	10
6 year	20	5.5	7.4	15	19	10
8 year	24	6.0	8.2	16	20	10
10 year	30	6.5	8.8	17	21	12
12 year	38	7.0	9.6	18	22	12
14 year	50	7.5	10.2	19	23	12
Adult	60	8.0	11.0	20	24	12
Adult	70	9.0	12.2	21	25	12

* ETT: <1 kg 2.5 mm; 1–3.5 kg 3.0 mm; >3.5 3.5 mm

Table 33.1. Doses of drugs used in resuscitation are shown in Table 33.2.

Circulation

Once it is established that a collapsed patient has a patent airway and is making breathing movements to take oxygen into the lungs, it is important to ensure that there is good circulation to carry oxygen from the lungs to the brain.

Tachycardia and hypotension suggest hypovolaemia. An intravenous catheter must be inserted and 10–20 ml/kg of Haemaccel or SPPS given quickly, and then the circulation reassessed. Another 10–20 ml/kg of fluid may be required in severe hypovolaemia. Note that it is most important to correct hypovolaemia in collapsed patients, but that it is dangerous to give intravenous fluid if the patient is not hypovolaemic.

Patients who have sepsis or who have suffered a severe hypoxic insult (e.g. drowning) may have poor myocardial function. It is very helpful to infuse dobutamine in this situation at 10 μg/kg/min (put 15 mg/kg in 50 ml of fluid and run at 2 ml/hr).

It can be very difficult to insert an intravenous drip in a collapsed child. In an emergency, parenteral fluid can be given through a needle inserted into the bone marrow, which is an intravascular space. This is performed as follows: inject local anaesthetic if the patient is conscious, then take a marrow aspiration needle or a 19 or 21 gauge lumbar puncture needle and hold it perpendicular to the medial surface of the distal tibia at the junction of the medial malleolus and the shaft of the tibia (just above the ankle) (Fig. 33.1). Twist the needle back and forth on its long axis and apply gentle pressure to push the needle through the cortex of bone; you will feel the needle give as the tip enters the marrow. Remove the trocar, and aspirate a little marrow with a syringe to check the needle is in the correct position.

Table 33.2 Doses of drugs used in resuscitation (reproduced with permission)

Age (years)	Birth	1	2	3	4	5	6	7	8	9	10	11	12	13	yr
Weight (kg) kg	3	5	10		15		20		25		30		35		40
Sodium bicarbonate 8.4% 2 ml/kg stat ml	6	10	20		25	30	40		50		60		70		80
Sodium bicarbonate 8.4% 1 ml/kg/10 min arrest time ml	3	5	10		15		20		25		30		35		40

Table 33.2   (cont'd)

Age (years)	Birth	1	2	3	4	5	6	7	8	9	10	11	12	13	yr
Adrenaline 1 in 10 000 0.1 ml/kg. repeat if no response ml	1	1			1.5		2		2.5		3		3.5		4
Calciuim chloride 10% 0.2 ml/kg (maximum 10 ml) ml	1	1	2		3		4		5		6		7		8
Calcium gluconate 10% 0.5 ml/kg (maximum 20 ml)	2	3	5		7		10				15			20	ml
Lignocaine 1% 0.1 ml/kg (1 mg/kg), then 20–40 µg/kg/min ml	0.5	1			1.5		2		2.5		3		3.5		4
Volume expansion. Initially 10 ml/kg, repeat × 2–3 if required ml	30	50	100	125	150		200		250		300		350		400
5Endotracheal tube Internal diameter (mm) mm	3.0	3.5	4.0	4.5	5.0		5.5		.60		6.5		7.0		
Endotracheal tube (oral) Length at lip (cm) cm	8.5	11	12	13	14		15		16		17		18		
Endotracheal tube (nasal) Length at nose (cm) cm	10.5	14	15	16	17		19		20		21		22		
Cardioversion. Atrial arrhythmia 1 joule/kg joule	3	5	10		15		20		25		30		35		40
Cardioversion, Ventricular arrhythmias 5 joule/kg joule	15	50			75		100		125		150		175		200

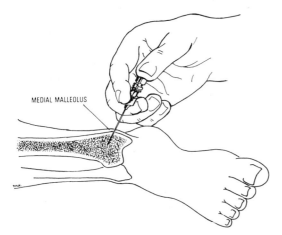

Fig. 33.1 Insertion of a needle into the bone marrow at the distal end of the tibia.

Make a small plaster of Paris splint to hold the needle in position. Fluid can be infused through the needle just as with a normal intravenous drip or it can be syringed in if rapid infusion is required. The distal tibia can be used in children up to 5 years old; in older children use the iliac crest. Do not use the sternum for this purpose in children.

PHYSIOLOGY OF BRAIN INJURY

Many insults injure the brain. These include trauma, prolonged fitting, infection (e.g. bacterial meningitis or viral encephalitis) and hypoxic or ischaemic injury (e.g. neonatal asphyxia or drowning). Nothing can be done to actually cure the brain injury. All that can be done is to provide the brain with the best possible conditions whereby it can heal. It is important to ensure that the

brain is adequately perfused with blood containing oxygen and glucose, and that carbon dioxide is removed from the blood. In order to do this properly, it is necessary to understand the physiology of the injured brain (see Example 33.3).

Cerebral perfusion pressure

The pressure with which blood perfuses the brain is equal to the mean arterial pressure minus the intracranial pressure (Fig. 33.2). Low mean arterial presssure (from hypovolaemia or poor myocardial contractility) is a much more common cause of low cerebral perfusion pressure than is high intracranial pressure.

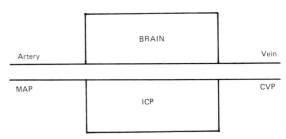

Fig. 33.2 Cerebral perfusion pressure (CPP). (CPP = mean arterial pressure (MAP) − intracranial pressure (ICP).)

Intracranial pressure

Following a traumatic or hypoxic injury, the brain becomes oedematous and swells. This causes raised intracranial pressure, which is dangerous for two reasons. Firstly, a high intracranial pressure may impair the blood supply to the brain and, secondly, very high intracranial pressure may cause fatal coning if the brain stem is squeezed out through the foramen magnum like toothpaste from a tube.

The skull is a rigid box. The pressure inside the box depends on its contents: brain (including brain water, or cerebral oedema), cerebrospinal fluid and blood. It is critical that cerebral blood flow be optimal after a brain injury: too little flow will cause cerebral ischaemia, but too much may cause a dramatic rise in intracranial pressure and coning if cerebral vasodilation occurs when the brain is swollen because of cerebral oedema.

Cerebral blood flow

The relationships between cerebral blood flow (and therefore intracranial pressure) and mean arterial pres-

---

Example 33.3 Physiology of the injured brain

1. The brain needs a continuous supply of oxygen-rich blood. The first priority is to avoid hypoxia and hypotension.
2. Raised intracranial pressure: reduces cerebral blood flow; may cause coning.
3. Intracranial pressure (ICP) depends on the contents of the skull: brain (including oedema), CSF and blood.
4. Cerebral blood flow: too little causes ischaemia; too much increases ICP and may cause coning.
5. Carbon dioxide: high pCO_2 causes cerebral vasodilation and coning; very low pCO_2 may cause cerebral ischaemia (vasoconstriction).
6. Water: too little causes hypovolaemia, hypotension and cerebral ischaemia; too much causes cerebral oedema, coma, fitting and coning.

sure, arterial oxygen tension (pO$_2$) and arterial carbon dioxide tension (pCO$_2$) are shown in Figure 33.3. Cerebral blood flow remains constant over a wide range of blood pressure, although this autoregulation may be lost after brain injury. Therefore, it becomes even more important to maintain a normal blood pressure. Cerebral blood flow is reduced, with the risk of cerebral ischaemia, as the mean arterial blood pressure falls below 60 mmHg (less in very young children). Oxygen tension has no effect on cerebral blood flow if the pO$_2$ is above 50 mmHg, but hypoxia causes marked cerebral vasodilation. This is why hypoxia is so dangerous after a brain injury: not only will each millilitre of blood going to the brain carry less oxygen, but also the cerebral vasodilation will increase intracranial pressure and may cause coning if there is cerebral oedema. Similarly, hypoventilation with retention of carbon dioxide (so that the pCO$_2$ rises above 40 mmHg) will not only cause acidosis, but will also cause cerebral vasodilation with a risk of coning.

On the other hand, the effect of pCO$_2$ on cerebral blood flow provides the most effective treatment for coning. Immediate intubation and hyperventilation will lower pCO$_2$ and cause cerebral vasoconstriction, which will reduce the amount of blood inside the skull; this lowers intracranial pressure in a few seconds. Mannitol

0.25 g/kg should be given intravenously to a patient who is coning, but mannitol takes 20–30 minutes to take effect. Steroids should not be given to reduce brain swelling caused by trauma, infection or hypoxia; they are only effective for the oedema associated with cerebral tumours.

Fluid balance

Very careful attention has to be given to fluid balance in patients with brain injury. Hypovolaemia from blood loss or dehydration is very dangerous because it causes hypotension and cerebral ischaemia. On the other hand, it is important not to overhydrate patients with brain injury, because this may exacerbate cerebral oedema and increase intracranial pressure with a risk of coning or cerebral ischaemia. Although a normal infant is usually given about 150 ml/kg of fluid per day, the full maintenance requirement of an unconscious infant with increased secretion of antidiuretic hormone is only 50 ml/kg/day. Fluid retention implies an intake of less than 50 ml/kg day (even less in older children).

In practice, after correction of hypovolaemia, children with brain injury should be given only 10 ml/kg/day of fluid with careful monitoring of pulse rate, blood pressure and serum sodium. A serum sodium over

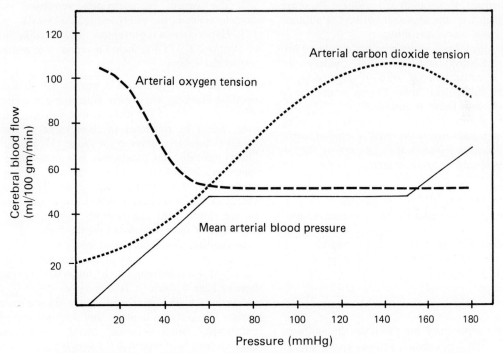

Fig. 33.3 The relationship of cerebral blood flow to mean arterial blood pressure, arterial oxygen tension (pO$_2$) and arterial carbon dioxide tension (pCO$_2$).

150 mmol/l suggests the need for more fluid, a serum sodium of less than 135 mmol/l suggests that too much fluid has been given.

Duration of treatment

After resuscitation from a collapse, children often recover quickly to a semi-comatose state with normal or increased ventilation and good circulation. It is very important that treatment is not stopped at this stage in a child who has had a severe insult, because brain swelling often increases for 24 to 48 hours after the injury. Another collapse (as a secondary insult) can cause irreversible damage in a child who would have made a full recovery if treatment had been continued. *Any child who has needed artificial ventilation or cardiac massage for a collapse should be referred to an intensive care unit for continuing management.*

SOME SPECIFIC CAUSES OF COLLAPSE

Convulsions

A prolonged convulsion causes damage to the brain from the intrinsic effects of fitting on the brain itself. In addition, even a short convulsion can cause irreversible damage in a patient with pre-existing active brain injury because of hypoxia, hypercapnia and acidosis. These are often exacerbated by the depressant effects of anticonvulsants given to control the fitting.

A patient with a brain injury who fits should be immediately intubated and ventilated, unless the convulsion is easily stopped with a single dose of diazepam 0.2 mg/kg (maximum 10 mg) intravenously and the pCO_2 stays below 40 mmHg.

If a child continues to fit after intubation, 1–2 ml/kg 50% dextrose is indicated if the child is hypoglycaemic and the IV diazepam repeated. If fitting persists, the following drugs should be given in turn:

1. Clonazepam 0.25–1 mg IV
2. Phenytoin 20 mg/kg IV over 30 minutes
3. Phenobarbitone 20 mg/kg IV over 30 minutes, and then
4. Thiopentone 3–5 mg/kg/hr slowly IV over 10 minutes (beware hypertension) followed by an infusion of 1–2 mg/kg/hr.

Meningitis

Doctors often concentrate too much on the antibiotic therapy of bacterial meningitis, without giving enough thought to supportive therapy. The commonest mistake is to give too much fluid to children with meningitis.

Such children, given more than 50 ml/kg/day of fluid, often develop hyponatreamia and cerebral oedema, which causes fitting. If the fitting is treated with diazepam, the rise in pCO_2 may cause cerebral vasodilation and coning.

On the other hand, a small proportion of children with meningitis have septic shock with capillary leak and poor myocardial function. They will need large amounts of fluid (20–50 ml/kg IV stat), infusion of an ionotrope (e.g. dobutamine 10 μg/kg/min) and transfer to an intensive care unit for paralysis and ventilation.

A major determinant of the outcome in bacterial meningitis is how soon antibiotics are started. If blood and cerebrospinal fluid cannot be taken for cultures immediately, antibiotics should be started straight away without waiting until cultures can be obtained. A lumbar puncture should not be performed in a comatose child to exclude meningitis; rather, antibiotic therapy should be started immediately and a lumbar puncture performed later when cerebral oedema can be excluded.

Head injury

It is critical that:

1. The airway be preserved – lie the patient on the side, or intubate and ventilate
2. The patient be adequately ventilated – give oxygen, maintain the pCO_2 less than 40 mmHg
3. Hypovolaemia is prevented – give 10 ml/kg boluses of Haemaccel, SPPS or blood if required to restore intravascular volume.

Unexplained hypotension is usually due to intra-abdominal bleeding when early laparotomy is indicated. After restoration of the intravascular volume, fluid intake should be restricted to 10 ml/kg/hr so that the serum sodium level stays in the range 135–150 mmol/l. Unless intubated, the patient who is comatose after head injury should be turned to lie on the side. This applies despite the risk of cervical spine injury. The person in charge of the resuscitation should exert gentle traction on the child's head and carefully turn it to the side, while one or more assistants turn the body.

In children, death from head injury is usually caused by the primary brain injury or cerebral oedema, not intracranial haemorrhage. It is important to exclude haemorrhage because it is a treatable cause of coma and/or focal neurological signs, but it is even more important to prevent hypoxia and hypotension. Skull radiographs rarely provide useful information in children with head injury. A CT scan is needed to define the extent of intracranial haemorrhage and cerebral oedema. A normal cervical spine radiograph does not exclude spinal injury in children, and small children who are unconscious from a head injury should be managed as though they have a fractured spine.

In addition, management must include careful monitoring of the pulse rate, blood pressure, pupil size and response to pain. A rising pulse rate and falling blood pressure suggest hypovolaemia. A falling pulse rate and rising blood pressure suggest raised intracranial pressure. In this situation the child must be intubated, ventilated to a pCO$_2$ of 30 mmHg, the bed tilted head-up, and mannitol 0.25 g/kg IV given stat. Consideration is given to performing a CT scan. The development of focal neurological signs suggests intracranial bleeding. It is very important to record accurately the response to a painful stimulus in the cranial nerve area by exerting pressure on the supra-orbital ridge. The response is noted as normal, semi-purposive, flexor, extensor or absent. Steroids or prophylactic antibiotics are not to be given to children with a head injury.

Ischaemic injury (drowning, 'near-miss' sudden infant death)

Again, the maintenance of the airway, breathing and circulation is the key to management. These children may need to be given very large amounts of SPPS to maintain intravascular volume. This is because the ischaemic damage causes capillary leak with loss of fluid from the intravascular space into the interstitial space. Ionotropes may be needed because of ischaemic damage to the heart. Hypokalaemia is common after drowning.

Very severe asthma

Common mistakes in managing severe asthma are:

1. Not to give 100% oxygen – respiratory depression from oxygen is not a problem in children
2. To give too much water to 'loosen the secretions' – lung water is increased in asthma, so fluid intake should be restricted, and
3. To give submaximal bronchodilator therapy.

In very severe asthma, undiluted 0.5% salbutamol nebulizer solution is given via a mask. Put 5 ml of solution in the nebulizer, and refill it when the level falls below about 2 ml. An oxygen flow of 8 1/min through the nebulizer is required but tape may be needed to stop the tubing disconnecting at this high flow rate). In addition, intravenous salbutamol 5 μg/kg/min, aminophylline 1.1 mg/kg/min and methylprednisolone 1 mg intravenously 4-hourly is administered. The salbutamol and aminophylline must be given through separate drips. Children who are sick enough to require this treatment should be nursed in an intensive care unit. Intubation and mechanical ventilation is dangerous in asthma. The airways' narrowing in asthma results in an inability to get gas *out* of the lungs, whereas a ventilator is a machine which blows gas *into* the lungs. On the other hand, mechanical ventilation should not be withheld until a child becomes so exhausted that breathing ceases. The indication for ventilation is physical exhaustion of the child and this is determined by clinical assessment, not by blood gas results.

Poisoning.

Example 33.4 lists the general principles which are fundamental in the management of poisoning in childhood.

Example 33.4 General principles in management of childhood poisoning

1. Ingestion/envenomation
Any ingestion or envenomation should always be considered as possible causes of an unexplained collapse.
2. Airway, breathing, circulation (ABC)
If the child has collapsed, attend to ABC; that is protect the airway, ensure adequate breathing, and ensure an adequate circulation.
3. Assess the situation
In the event of poisoning identify the suspected agent, find out the probable dose taken and the time of ingestion. It is most important to keep any bottles or containers that contain the poison. Should envenomation be suspected an examination for puncture marks, local swelling and regional lymphadenopathy must be made. It is often necessary to test for venom and drugs in blood and urine.
4. Dilute the poison
If conscious, the child should be given a cupful of milk or water to drink to dilute the poison.
5. Make the child vomit
Vomiting is induced by rubbing the back of the child's throat with a spoon or spatula. If vomiting does not occur, a dose of syrup of Ipecacuanha (15 ml orally) should be given and the back of the throat rubbed again. Attempts to cause vomiting are contraindicated if the poison is: a corrosive acid or alkali; kerosene or other petroleum distillate, or strychnine.

Do not attempt to induce vomiting if the child is unconscious.
6. Activated charcoal
Activated charcoal slows the absorption of poison but can also remove it from the body. A dose of 0.25 g/kg of activated charcoal is given by nasogastric tube every hour. As charcoal often causes constipation, a dose of 50% lactose (1 ml/kg) should be given by nasogastric tube every 6 hours.
7. Get advice early
Special management may be required for poisoned children to prevent absorption of drugs or hasten their removal, or in the case of snake bite to neutralize venom. Consult with a paediatric intensive care unit as soon as poisoning is suspected as the cause for collapse.

Neonatal asphyxia

This form of collapse is often undertreated, with catastrophic consequences. Asphyxiated newborn babies are often extubated soon after they have been resuscitated. They are then sent to the neonatal nursery where they collapse several hours later (as their cerebral oedema worsens), so that they suffer a severe secondary insult. A neonate who takes longer than 5 minutes to start breathing after delivery, and requires cardiac massage, should not be extubated even if appearing to be normal after resuscitation. Such neonates should be transferred to a neonatal or paediatric intensive care unit for mechanical ventilation.

FURTHER READING

Grenvik A, Safar P 1981 Clinics in critical care medicine: brain failure and resuscitation. Vol. 2. Churchill Livingstone, New York
Levin K L, Morris F C, Moore G C 1984 A practical guide to pediatric intensive care, 2nd edn. Mosby, St Louis
Oh T F 1985 Intensive care manual, 2nd edn. Butterworths, Sydney
Rogers M C 1987 Textbook of pediatric intensive care. Williams & Wilkins, Baltimore
Spivey W H 1987 Intravenous infusions. Journal of Pediatrics 111: 639–643

Respiratory disorders

34. The epidemiology of acute respiratory infections

P. D. Phelan

Acute respiratory infections are the most frequent illnesses in infants and young children. It is important that all practising doctors understand the important factors in their epidemiology and details of their clinical manifestations and management.

INCIDENCE

Acute respiratory infections are the most common illnesses in childhood. In 1977–78 a survey was conducted on illnesses in the Australian community; 46 out of every 100 children had an acute episode of some illness in the 2 weeks before the survey – 44% of these illnesses were related to the respiratory tract and most were acute respiratory infections. Put in another way this means that children aged 0–15 years have 1 acute respiratory illness every 5 weeks, or 10 per year.

Many acute respiratory illnesses are not seen by doctors. Nevertheless, acute respiratory illness is the most frequent reason children present for medical attention.

About 95% of all acute respiratory infections involve predominantly the upper respiratory tract and only 5% the lower respiratory tract. As the latter group tend to be the more serious they are disproportionately represented among children presenting for health care.

Acute respiratory infections can begin soon after birth but the actual number a baby has in its first year depends very much on whether there are older siblings in the house, and whether the child is cared for completely at home or in a day care centre. The maximum incidence is between 2 and 5 years of age when the average child has between 10 and 12 infections per year. Within this period there are 2 peaks, one at 18–24 months reflecting the beginnings of socialization by the child. The other is between 4 and 5 years when the child is commencing kindergarten and school. The adult number of 3 to 4 per year is not reached until 11 or 12 years.

Lower respiratory infections are much more frequent in the early years of life. The peak incidence is in the first year when the rate is about 250 infections per 1000 children per year or in other words, 1 child in 4 has a lower respiratory infection during the first year of life.

CLASSIFICATION AND PATTERNS OF ILLNESS

Illnesses are described and classified primarily on an anatomical basis. The limitation of this method is that infection is not restricted by anatomical boundaries. An aetiological classification is not possible as different infecting agents may cause identical illnesses and the same infecting agent may cause various illnesses in different patients. Despite these limitations classification into the following clinical categories provides a useful working basis for diagnosis and management.

Upper respiratory tract infection

This includes four different disorders:

1. Colds
2. Pharyngitis
3. Tonsillitis
4. Otitis media.

Lower respiratory tract infection

This includes the following:

1. Laryngotracheobronchitis
2. Epiglottitis
3. Acute bronchitis
4. Acute bronchiolitis
5. Pneumonia.

These will be described in detail in Chapter 35. The clinical manifestations of illness depends on the part of the respiratory tract involved, the severity of the local inflammatory reaction and the degree of constitutional disturbance. The pattern of illness occurring in any child depends on the interaction of three factors:

1. The infecting agent
2. Host factors
3. Environmental factors.

Infecting agents

Well over 90% of respiratory infections are due to viruses. While bacteria are responsible for some upper and lower respiratory tract infections, their exact role in causing disease is often difficult to determine.

The pathogens responsible for respiratory infection in infancy and childhood are listed in Example 34.1.

Respiratory syncytial virus (RSV). This is the major cause of serious respiratory infection in infancy. It is responsible for almost all bronchiolitis, about 12% of croup, 15% of bronchitis and 30% of pneumonia. About 1 child in 60 will be admitted to hospital with RSV infection during the first 5 years of life. Infants from the lower socioeconomic groups in the community are more likely to be admitted to hospital with it, but the reasons for this are complex and probably include the quality of maternal care, family size, and parental smoking habits. Breast-feeding seems to give some protection against more serious RSV infections.

Example 34.1 Pathogens responsible for respiratory infection in children

Virus
Respiratory syncytial (RSV)
Parainfluenzal types 1,2,3
Influenza types A,B
Rhinovirus
Adenovirus

Bacteria
Beta-haemolytic streptococcus
Streptococcus pneumoniae
Haemophilus influenzae
Mycoplasma pneumoniae

Infection by RSV is usually introduced into the family by an older child. The attack rate in members of the affected families is about 50% and in infants under 1 year 60%. Reinfection occurs and 75% of those exposed to the virus for the second time become infected and 65% of those after a third exposure. With successive exposure there is usually a progressive decrease in the severity of the illness. Occasionally respiratory syncytial viral infection can be fatal – infants with major congenital malformations seem to be at particular risk.

Parainfluenza viruses. These viruses can produce a wide variety of illnesses from mild laryngotracheobronchitis to severe pneumonia and are the major cause of croup. They all cause upper respiratory infection. Reinfection is not infrequent and if it occurs the illness is usually mild.

Rhinoviruses. Rhinoviruses are primarily responsible for the common cold.

Influenza viruses. These viruses play a lesser role in respiratory illness compared with the preceding ones. They commonly cause febrile illnesses with upper respiratory symptoms and can also cause lower respiratory infection. Children do not usually have the systemic symptoms typical of influenza infection commonly seen in adults.

Other viruses. Adenovirus is a cause of pharyngitis, and Coxsackie- and echoviruses also cause upper respiratory infection.

Bacteria. Bacteria play a lesser role in acute respiratory infections and probably are responsible for only about 5% of infections, but these tend to be the more serious ones. However, when previously well children die from acute respiratory infection it is almost invariably from viral infection. Bacterial infection, provided it is recognized promptly and appropriately treated, should rarely be fatal in previously healthy children.

Beta-haemolytic streptococcus is the only cause of bacterial pharyngitis and tonsillitis. It can be difficult to distinguish viral from bacterial pharyngitis and tonsillitis and this is discussed in Chapter 35. *Haemophilus influenzae* type B is the cause of acute epiglottis. *H influenzae* is also an important cause of otitis media and ocassionally causes pneumonia in young children in developed countries. In developing countries both *H. influenzae* type B and non-typeable strains are important causes of pneumonia.

Streptococcus pneumoniae is the major bacterial cause of pneumonia, but, overall, viruses and mycoplasma cause many more episodes of pneumonia than do bacteria. Pneumonia due to *Staphylococcus aureus* is uncommon but it is usually a severe illness.

Mycoplasma pneumoniae. This is an important cause of respiratory infection in children. In younger children it causes coryzal illnesses and pharyngitis and also bronchitis. It is a major cause of pneumonia, particularly in children over the age of 5 years.

Host factors

Host factors are of the greatest importance in determining the pattern of illnesses resulting from infection. Many probably operate immunologically but precise knowledge of the way or ways by which they do so is limited.

Age. The overall incidence of respiratory infection

varies considerably with age. The maximum is between 2 and 5 years.

The most serious respiratory disease occurs in the first 3 years of life, especially the first year. The predominant illnesses are bronchiolitis in the first 6 months of life, pneumonia in the first 2 years and laryngotracheobronchitis between 9 months and 3 years. Most of the deaths and much of the serious morbidity from respiratory disease occur during this period.

Sex. The incidence of upper respiratory tract infection due to viruses and bacteria is the same in boys and girls. Under the age of 6 years boys have a substantially higher incidence of lower respiratory tract infections. This is because RSV infection and infection with the parainfluenza type 1 virus is 1.5–2 times commoner in boys than girls. 60% of children admitted to hospital with either croup or bronchiolitis are boys.

Obesity. Obese infants and children develop more respiratory infection than do normal children for reasons that are unclear.

Atopy. While it has been suggested that children with an atopic background have more respiratory infections than non-atopic children, recent studies have not confirmed the association. Wheezing associated with respiratory infection is significantly more common in children with an atopic background and this is almost certainly asthma.

Immunological factors. There are some children who have an abnormally large number of respiratory infections or alternatively an increased number of the more serious type. In some it is possible to demonstrate an abnormality in immune function which can be deficiencies in immunoglobulin, in the function of phagocytic cells or in lymphocyte function. Often there is an abnormality of more than one mechanism and it has been suggested that immune capacity is best considered as a continuum, extending from gross immune deficiency to excellent immunocompetence. The concept of clear normality and abnormality may be inappropriate. Regrettably, in the present state of knowledge, identification of minor variations in immune function often have little therapeutic implication. Certainly, detailed study of immune function in a child with repeated respiratory infection should only be undertaken if all other host and environmental factors can be excluded.

There is a large group of patients with an abnormal pattern of respiratory infection in whom no specific variation in immune function can be determined. While in some, environmental factors may be important, in many there is no explanation for the abnormal pattern of infection.

Gestational age. While there is an increased frequency of lower respiratory infections in prematurely born infants during their first 12 months of life, this is almost

certainly due to the residual effects of hyaline membrane disease. Babies who survive hyaline membrane disease have about a 20% chance of subsequently being admitted to hospital with bronchiolitis or bronchopneumonia. Other premature infants do not have an increased risk of lower respiratory infections.

Breast-feeding. Babies who are breast-fed have less risk of being admitted to hospital with RSV infection. Why this should be so is unclear and yet it is not simply due to the many social and environmental factors associated with infection and with breast-feeding.

Environmental factors

Quality of maternal care. The quality of maternal care is the most important environmental factor in determining the likelihood of admission of an infant to hospital with RSV infection and probably with other respiratory infections as well. Factors such as maternal attentiveness and affectionate interest, ability to seek appropriate help for an illness, preparation of feeds, clothing, bedding and cleanliness all indicate the quality of maternal care. It is important to recognize that in many situations the mother's social circumstances limit her ability to deliver a high quality of maternal care. Further, our society has been very poor in teaching the skills of mothering, and also, of course, of fathering.

Parental smoking. The incidence of pneumonia and bronchitis in infants during the first year of life is more than doubled if both parents smoke and increased by about 50% where one is a smoker. The risk of developing bronchitis for infants passively exposed to cigarette smoke in the home is about 4 times that for infants from a smoke free environment. Parental smoking is probably the single most important avoidable factor in lower respiratory infections.

Exposure to infection. The incidence of infection in any child is correlated with the closeness and intensity of exposure to infection. The effect, for instance, of having older siblings is quite marked. Babies with older siblings have between 3 and 6 times as many lower respiratory infections in their first year of life as do those who are only children.

Social class. The overall incidence of respiratory infection is not greatly affected by social class. However, there is a very strong correlation of more severe lower respiratory infections with lower socioeconomic groups. This applies particularly to the need for hospital admission with respiratory infections. The reasons for this are complex and are probably largely related to the other environmental factors already discussed – the quality of maternal care, parental smoking habits, breast-feeding and family size.

Atmospheric pollution. The relationship of atmospheric pollution to respiratory infection still remains unclear. There is no evidence that pollution predisposes to a greater incidence of upper respiratory infection. However, it has been shown that there is a significant correlation of recurrent lower respiratory infections with increased air pollution. Many studies that have shown this have not adequately allowed for other social factors and parental smoking. It would seem that atmospheric pollution most probably has a very minor effect.

PREVENTION

Respiratory infections are a major cause of morbidity and a significant cause of mortality in infancy and childhood. They cause considerable anxiety to parents and provide a substantial health cost to the community. Not surprisingly, there have been many attempts at the development of preventive measures but regrettably, so far, these have largely been ineffective.

With the exception of *Bordetella pertussis* and *H. influenzae* type B, effective immunization against the common and more serious respiratory infections does not seem to be a practical possibility within the foreseeable future. The large number of viruses involved and the incomplete understanding of the immunological processes that result from infection with respiratory viruses are the major problems. Modification of environmental factors perhaps gives greater opportunity for prevention, at least in the short term. Parental smoking is a significant factor and one that should be amenable to modification. Improvement of maternal care by health education programmes perhaps also gives some prospect of benefit.

It is unlikely that there will be significant advances of prevention in the near future. Respiratory infection will continue to be a major health problem in infants and children.

35. Clinical patterns of acute respiratory infections

P. D. Phelan

CORYZA OR THE COMMON COLD

This is an illness of short duration in which the main local symptoms are nasal obstruction and discharge. A severe cold may be associated with pyrexia and some constitutional disturbance. Rhinoviruses are the most important causes of coryzal illnesses. Respiratory syncytial virus (RSV), parainfluenza and influenza viruses, Coxsackieviruses, echoviruses and probably *Mycoplasma pneumoniae* can cause an identical illness.

In mild infections respiratory symptoms are usually the early and only manifestation. Some patients notice a mildly sore throat and nasal stuffiness for a day or two before the definite onset. Sneezing, nasal obstruction and nasal discharge are present in the early stages. The nasal discharge varies considerably in appearance and amount. It can be quite thick and yellow without there necessarily being secondary bacterial infection.

In more severe infections, headache, muscular aching, lassitude, malaise and, in young children, irritability and poor feeding, may be prominent symptoms.

The length of the disease is extremely variable. Sneezing and sore throat usually subside early. Nasal discharge may continue for some days and become mucopurulent or purulent. Cough may persist for up to two weeks in a child whose initial symptoms at least were predominantly upper respiratory.

The most important complication is nasal obstruction in young infants, who are normally nose breathers. They may have considerable difficulty sucking while their nose is obstructed.

Spread of infection from the nose to the paranasal sinuses and middle ears is not uncommon. This may be due to the viral infection alone or be the consequence of secondary bacterial infection.

In many colds cough is present, indicating involvement in the inflammatory process of the larynx, trachea or bronchi.

Management of colds

This is symptomatic. Fluid intake should be watched carefully in young babies. Paracetamol can be used for fever if it is very high or causing discomfort. Clearing of the nose with a cotton bud before feeding and administering one or two drops of vasoconstrictor nasal drops can be helpful in a small baby with nasal obstruction.

There is no evidence that antibiotics limit the duration of coryzal symptoms nor reduce the likelihood of secondary bacterial infection. Antihistamines and pseudoephedrine have not been shown to be of benefit.

It is important that parents realize that the symptoms of a common cold may last for as long as two weeks and that pharmacological agents available at present are largely of no benefit.

PHARYNGITIS AND TONSILLITIS

Infection of the tonsils and pharynx are considered together because they are frequently associated, although in many illnesses one or the other is predominantly involved. In pharyngitis there is generalized erythema of the pharynx without localization to the tonsils, whereas in tonsillitis there is local infection of the tonsils, which are red and swollen and often show exudate.

Rhinoviruses, parainfluenza and influenza viruses, RSV, a number of types of adenovirus, Coxsackievirus and echovirus are the common causes of pharyngitis. Pharyngitis associated with coryzal symptoms and bronchitis is a constant feature of the exanthematous phase of measles and pharyngitis with exudate is a common manifestation of infectious mononucleosis.

Group A beta-haemolytic streptococcus is the only significant bacterial cause of tonsillitis and pharyngitis. It is most prevalent in children aged between 4 and 7 years.

In viral pharyngitis, fever and sore throat are the main symptoms. Mild nasal stuffiness and cough are often associated indicating that the infection extends beyond the pharynx to involve the nasal passages and lower respiratory tract. The throat is generally red and the tonsils may become enlarged. Small patches of yellow exudate may be seen on the pharynx or tonsils with adenovirus infection. Extensive exudate on the pharynx and tonsils extending on to the soft palate is typical of infectious mononucleosis.

In bacterial tonsillitis, fever, malaise and sore throat are the prominent symptoms. Enlargement of the tonsils often with exudate is the usual clinical finding. The cervical nodes are often enlarged and tender. Vomiting is commonly associated. Nasal obstruction and cough are unusual in bacterial tonsillitis and strongly suggest viral infection.

It can be difficult on clinical grounds to distinguish viral from bacterial pharyngitis. If the child is under the age of 4 years, streptococcal infection is less likely. In the early school-age child, history of vomiting and fever, a diffusely red throat with oedematous, hyperaemic tonsils and tender cervical nodes are very suggestive of streptococcal infections.

Treatment

Attention to fluid intake, paracetamol for relief of the sore throat and control of the fever, if this is causing discomfort, are the important general aspects of management. The child will probably not eat for some days.

If streptococcal infection is thought likely, oral penicillin for 10 days is the standard recommendation. The major reason for this is to reduce the likelihood of rheumatic fever. In addition, penicillin administration shortens the period of symptoms. Penicillin must be given for a full 10 days if streptococci are to be eradicated. However, many parents will not administer a full 10-day oral course unless the reasons for it are clearly explained. For this reason, a single injection of 'bicillin all purpose' – a mixture of benzathine penicillin, procaine penicillin and benzole penicillin – has often been recommended. However, this injection is painful and has not achieved widespread acceptance. If the streptococcus is not completely eradicated, there is a risk of recurrent infection. Another contributor to recurrent infection is the presence of a carrier in the child's home.

ACUTE LARYNGOTRACHEOBRONCHITIS (CROUP)

Acute laryngotracheobronchitis is the major cause of acute laryngeal obstruction in childhood in temperate climates. It is due to viral infection most commonly with the parainfluenza viruses. RSV, rhinovirus, influenza virus and measles virus are also important causes. It is most frequent in the autumn, winter and spring as indicated by admissions to hospital.

The disease occurs throughout childhood and occasionally also in adults but the peak incidence is in the second year of life — 70% of patients admitted to hospital are males.

Typically the child has coryzal symptoms one or two days before developing evidence of laryngeal inflammation. The first signs of spread to the lower respiratory tract are a harsh, barking or croupy cough and a hoarse voice. With inflammatory narrowing of the subglottic area, an inspiratory stridor rapidly develops. The symptoms most commonly develop during the night when the child awakes with cough. Initially the stridor is inspiratory but with increasing narrowing it is both inspiratory and expiratory.

With moderate to severe obstruction, indrawing of the suprasternal tissues and sternum occurs during inspiration due to a more negative intrapleural pressure. Airways obstruction causes increased respiratory work and in some children may result in physical exhaustion. These children become lethargic and the stridor may in fact decrease in intensity as does retraction. Inexperienced observers may attribute the decrease in stridor and retraction to improvement unless they have observed the rising pulse rate and decreasing breath sounds in the chest.

With severe obstruction there is disturbance of gas exchange. Hypoxia is the major consequence and is manifested by restlessness, rising pulse and respiratory rates and finally cyanosis. When these signs are present the child is at grave risk of cardiorespiratory arrest.

Signs of airways obstruction disappear after one or two days in the majority of children but the dry cough may persist for up to one or two weeks.

Treatment

Children with mild croup can be managed at home. A useful definition of mild croup is absence of sternal or suprasternal retraction at rest. A warm moist atmosphere may help in relieving laryngeal obstruction. This is best obtained by taking the child into the bathroom and turning on the hot taps. No medication favourably alters the course of the illness. In particular, sedatives for restlessness should be avoided as restlessness in a child with laryngeal obstruction is due to hypoxia until proven otherwise.

A child with moderate or severe obstruction as indicated by both an inspiratory and expiratory stridor and sternal and suprasternal retraction at rest should be admitted to hospital. If any signs of hypoxia are present, the child is in serious danger and requires extremely urgent transfer to a hospital with facilities for the treatment of acute laryngeal obstruction in children.

In hospital any measures that may further disturb the child should be avoided. Nursing in a warm humid environment may be helpful but there is no value from particulate water vapour (steam). The pulse rate, the respiratory rate, colour, degree of agitation and of chest wall and soft tissue retraction must be carefully observed if early signs of hypoxia are to be detected. Careful confident nursing is essential. Wherever possible parents should be encouraged to stay with their children. No drugs favourably alter the course of the illness. Antibiotics are not necessary because the disease is viral in aetiology.

Should signs of hypoxia develop, then obstruction must be promptly relieved mechanically. This is done by nasotracheal intubation but tracheostomy is also a satisfactory method.

Recurrent croup

There is a group of children who develop recurrent episodes of acute laryngeal obstruction. The term spasmodic croup is applied to the typical episodes that occur in children with recurrent croup. These episodes are usually of short duration and occur without an obvious respiratory infection. The nature of this illness is obscure but there does seem to be some association with asthma. A child can have a number of episodes of recurrent croup over one or two years and then develop frank episodes of asthma. However, there is no evidence that antiasthma type therapy is at all helpful in this situation.

ACUTE EPIGLOTTITIS

This is a paediatric emergency. Unless children with acute epiglottitis are promptly recognized and admitted to a hospital appropriate for their care, the mortality rate will be high.

It is caused by *Haemophilus influenzae* type B. There is associated septicaemia which is responsible for most of the constitutional features of the condition.

The onset is usually over 3 or 4 hours but there may be a preceding upper respiratory infection. Typically the parents first notice that the child is feverish, lethargic and unwell. If old enough he may complain of a sore throat and will usually refuse to eat or drink. Over some hours he develops difficulty breathing. Cough is usually not a prominent symptom. The voice and cry are muf-

fled rather than hoarse. Most children with epiglottitis look pale, toxic and ill. Temperature is usually above 38.5°C and there is marked tachycardia. Drooling of saliva is common because the throat is too sore to allow swallowing. The affected child generally prefers to sit up and breathes with his mouth open. The stridor is of a lower pitch than in croup and there is usually an expiratory element which resembles a snore.

The diagnosis of acute epiglottitis should be made on the history, general appearance of the child and the quality of the stridor. Direct visualization of the epiglottis is potentially dangerous as it may precipitate an acute obstructive episode.

As the child with acute epiglottitis is at grave risk of laryngeal obstruction, immediate transfer to a hospital with facilities appropriate to the management of acute laryngeal obstruction in children should be arranged. Until decisions on definitive management are made, the child should be propped up with pillows or allowed to lie on his side or stomach. Lying flat on the back may cause complete obstruction.

An antibiotic to which *H. influenzae* type B is sensitive should be given as soon as the diagnosis is suspected. Chloramphenicol is the drug of choice. If the child will be admitted to hospital within 20–30 minutes, then it is probably best to defer the initial dose until the child is in hospital. Sometimes the injection itself will precipitate an acute obstructive episode. The antibiotic needs to be continued for 3 to 4 days.

Almost all children with acute epiglottitis require the insertion of an artificial airway.

ACUTE BRONCHITIS

Mild bronchitis, frequently associated with tracheitis, is a common manifestation of acute viral respiratory tract infection. Cough is usually the only symptom and adventitiae in the chest are uncommon. Cough in association with an upper respiratory infection indicates inflammatory involvement of the larynx, trachea or bronchial tree. It is very unlikely that upper respiratory tract secretions and exudate stimulate the cough receptors in the larynx. Postnasal drip should not be accepted as a cause of cough.

Rhinoviruses, RSV, influenza and parainfluenza viruses, adeno- and Coxsackieviruses and *Mycoplasma pneumoniae* are important causes of bronchitis. Bronchitis is a constant manifestation of measles and whooping cough.

The cough in viral bronchitis is initially dry, but after 2 or 3 days it may become loose and rattling. If it becomes loose, a small amount of mucoid sputum may be expectorated but it is usually swallowed. The sputum may be thick and yellow without there necessarily being secondary bacterial infection. There may be some constitutional disturbance with fever and older children may complain of sternal discomfort. Adventitiae in the chest are absent during the first few days, but subsequently the child may develop a few coarse crackles and low pitched wheezes. Cough usually settles within 1 to 2 weeks. If it persists longer, the possibility of a segmental area of collapse or secondary bacterial infection must be considered. However, there are no data to suggest that secondary bacterial infection is a frequent occurrence. Audible wheezing in association with a viral respiratory infection is almost always a manifestation of asthma. Widespread high-pitched wheezes in the chest of a child with apparent infective bronchitis are also highly suggestive of asthma.

Treatment

No treatment has a beneficial effect on the course of uncomplicated bronchitis. Most cough mixtures are valueless. There is no evidence that the so-called expectorant mixtures, which usually contain either potassium iodide or ammonium chloride, have any pharmacological action. Cough suppressant mixtures such as codeine phosphate and pholcodine are usually contraindicated in any child with a productive cough. Repeated coughing may result in paryngeal irritation and a soothing mixture such as honey and lemon juice in warm water may give symptomatic relief. Proprietary cough mixtures have virtually no place in the management of cough in children.

A major problem is to decide if and when antibiotics are indicated. While there are no scientific data to support their use in acute, presumed viral bronchitis, a reasonable policy may be to prescribe antibiotics if the cough persists after 14 days and is showing no signs of improvement.

PERTUSSIS

Pertussis or whooping cough remains an important cause of bronchitis in infants and children although its overall frequency is less now than 50 years ago. The relative contributions of vaccination programmes and general factors, such as improvement in the standard of living, to the reduction remains unclear but vaccination has been the major influence. *Bordetella pertussis* is the cause of whooping cough. It infects the mucosal lining of the trachea and bronchial tree.

Approximately 70% of unimmunized children will eventually develop pertussis, the majority by their fifth birthday. The source of infection is usually the toddler, school-age child or even young adults, who, as they are often fully immunized, have relatively mild disease.

Immunization does not give total protection, nor is the protection lifelong. Typical pertussis can occur in the fully immunized child and it has been estimated that 95% of immunized subjects are susceptible about 12 years after the initial immunization. Generally, immunized infants and children generally have a milder illness and a high level of herd immunity protects the most at-risk group, infants in the first few months of life.

The illness commonly begins with a nasal discharge. After a few days the child develops a dry cough. This gradually becomes more pronounced and comes in bursts or short paroxysms. During a paroxysm each inspiration is followed by a rapid succession of expiratory hacks. The child goes red in the face and with repeated spasms may become cyanosed, tears stream from the eyes and mucus drools from the mouth. Repeated spasms commonly end in an inspiratory whoop but this may be absent in the fully immunized child. Paroxysms are often followed by vomiting of thick mucus or food. Paroxysms are usually more frequent and severe during the night. Any disturbance such as excitement, anger and feeding may initiate the paroxysms.

Despite the severity of cough there may be little disturbance to general health. Weight loss is uncommon unless there is severe vomiting. Adventitious sounds are not heard in the chest. Between the paroxysms the child is usually perfectly normal and this may obscure the diagnosis unless careful attention is paid to the history.

The history of repeated coughing spasms should suggest the diagnosis of whooping cough. Almost no other acute infectious illness in children causes a cough that lasts 4–8 weeks.

The duration of the illness is variable but paroxysms usually last 4–8 weeks. However, in some children it can last for as long as 3 or 4 months. For weeks or even months after the illness, a fresh respiratory infection is likely to be associated with the return of a cough closely resembling whooping cough. It may be 12 months before the child is permanently free of a distressing cough.

Whooping cough is most dangerous in the first year of life, particularly in infants under the age of 3 months and it is in this group that death is most likely to occur. The major cause of permanent damage and death is hypoxia. This can result from laryngeal spasm at the end of a paroxysm. Alternatively vomiting and inhalation may occur after the paroxysm. At times epistaxis and subconjunctival haemorrhage can result from increased venous pressure. Very rarely cerebral haemorrhage occurs. Bronchopneumonia may result from spread of *B.*

pertussis to the alveoli but can also be due to secondary bacterial infection by *Streptococcus pneumoniae*, *Staphylococcus aureus* or occasionally *H. influenzae*. Bronchiectasis, once thought to be a common complication of whooping cough, is probably a very rare one.

Treatment

No drugs favourably alter the course of whooping cough. Erythromycin estolate but not its other salts may reduce the period of infectivity; however, this is far from certain. Cough mixtures are ineffective. The major aspect of management is good nursing. Infants under the age of 6 months need close observation and this generally means admission to hospital. It is extremely demanding for a mother to care for a small baby with whooping cough. Older children usually manage to cope well and can be satisfactorily nursed at home.

ACUTE VIRAL BRONCHIOLITIS

This is the commonest acute lower respiratory infection in infants. Epidemics occur in communities with temperate winter climates. Almost all cases are attributable to RSV.

Affected infants hospitalized with acute bronchiolitis are usually aged between 1 and 6 months but the disease occurs up to the age of 12 months and very occasionally up to 2 years. 60% of patients are boys and the reasons for this are unclear. Hospitalization is more common in infants from families in the lower socioeconomic groups in the community.

Inflammation typically affects bronchioles of calibre 300 μm down to 75 μm. The bronchiolar epithelium is colonized by the virus which then replicates and produces necrosis of the epithelium. Associated with the bronchiolar inflammation there is a marked increase in airways resistance and lung hyperinflation. The airways obstruction impairs gas exchange with hypoxia and hypercapnia the result of ventilation perfusion mismatch.

The illness typically begins with coryza and over 1 to 2 days the infant develops an irritating cough, distressed, rapid, wheezy breathing and may have difficulty feeding. The infant is usually not toxic and the temperature is rarely higher than 38–38.5°C. Tachypnoea is a feature and is associated with obvious forced expiratory effort and audible wheezing. The chest is barrel-shaped as a result of hyperinflation of the lungs, and there is often retraction of the lower ribs during inspiration.

On auscultation widespread fine crackles are heard towards the end of inspiration, reflecting opening of partially obstructed bronchioles. The fine crackles may be inaudible if the baby is crying and breathing deeply, but will usually be present when he is resting quietly. Widespread wheezes are heard during expiration. The liver is displaced downwards as a result of pulmonary hyperinflation.

As the disease progresses gas exchange may be impaired. Cyanosis in air is common in babies with severe disease and carbon dioxide retention may occur, most often in younger infants and those with the highest respiratory rate. Respiratory failure develops in 1–2% of patients. Physical exhaustion, which results from increased respiratory work is an important contributing factor, especially in weak infants and infants with other diseases such as congenital malformations.

The chest radiograph shows marked hyperinflation of the lungs with depression of the diaphragm (Fig. 35.1). There may be peribronchial thickening, areas of consolidation or segmental or lobar collapse.

Arterial blood gases typically show a low P_aO_2 and a normal or elevated P_aCO_2.

The diagnosis of acute bronchiolitis is usually not difficult as the clinical pattern is a distinctive one. Acute asthma in infancy can produce a similar clinical pattern but fine crackles are less frequent in asthma than in acute viral bronchiolitis. If an infant with features suggestive of acute bronchiolitis has had a previous illness associated with audible wheezing, the diagnosis is more likely to be asthma. Bronchiolitis as such is not a recurrent illness. An infant presenting during summer months or older than 9–12 months is more likely to have an acute episode of asthma precipitated by viral infection. However, to some extent the distinction is arbitrary, as at least 50% of infants who have acute viral bronchiolitis due to RSV have subsequent episodes of audible wheezing which are almost certainly asthma.

Bronchopneumonia is the other disease which may cause confusion. As RSV can cause both, some infants may have features of both diseases. The infant with bronchopneumonia has a higher temperature and more constitutional disturbance. Wheezy breathing is absent and there is rarely hyperinflation of the chest. Alveolar consolidation rather than bronchiolar obstruction is the main pathological change.

It is to be remembered that infants with metabolic acidosis due to renal failure or salicylate poisoning, or infants in cardiac failure can present with tachypnoea.

Treatment

The management of bronchiolitis is essentially conservative. Oxygen is vitally important when there is respiratory distress or hypoxia and there is little evidence that any other therapy is consistently or even occasionally useful. The management depends primarily

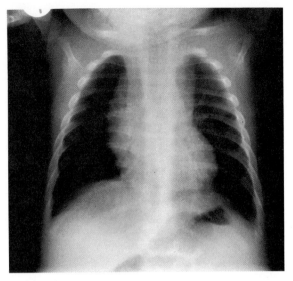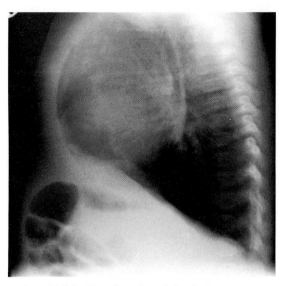

Fig. 35.1   PA (left) and lateral (right) radiographs of the chest in acute bronchiolitis. Note flattening of the diaphragm, bulging of the sternum and hyperexpanded lung anterior to the heart shadow in the lateral view. The thymus shadow is well demonstrated in the PA view.

on good nursing care and avoidance of all unnecessary disturbance. Infants with mild disease can be cared for at home. However, if respiratory distress or difficulty with feeding develops, admission to hospital is indicated.

In hospital, the baby will probably require oxygen and should not be disturbed unnecessarily; careful attention is paid to fluid intake. Babies with respiratory distress are best nursed in a plastic oxygen cot when the initial concentration of oxygen should be about 40%, but this will need to be increased in babies with more severe distress. Measurement of oxygen saturation with a pulse oximeter is the best guide to concentration of inspired oxygen required. The respiratory rate gives a good indication of the P_aO_2, and can be used as a guide to the concentration of oxygen required. If the baby is unable to feed satisfactorily fluid should be given either intravenously or by intragastric tube. The choice will be determined by the skill of the attending medical practitioner in inserting an intravenous needle into a small infant.

As the disease is viral in aetiology antibiotics will not affect the progress of the illness and generally should not be used. Occasionally they may be justified in a very sick infant in whom secondary bacterial infection cannot be confidently excluded.

Prognosis

A mortality rate of less than 1% has been reported. This is due primarily to respiratory failure, not secondary bacterial infection. The majority of infants usually recover within a week or 10 days although a small number may have tachypnoea and cough for up to 3 weeks. As mentioned, at least 50% of babies develop further episodes of wheezing.

PNEUMONIA

Pneumonia is defined pathologically as acute inflammatory consolidation of the alveoli or infiltration of the interstitial tissues with inflammatory cells or a combination of both. Frequently, there is associated inflammatory exudate in the smaller bronchi and bronchioles as the spread of infection is usually from the upper to the lower respiratory tract. Clinically, pneumonia is characterized by acute constitutional symptoms, fever and tachypnoea, and radiologically by lobular, segmental or lobar consolidation. It is a common disease in infants but relatively less frequent in older children. It is still one of the most common causes of death in infants, particularly in those who are weak from any cause such as prematurity, poor nutrition, poor socioeconomic circumstances or congenital malformations.

Most cases of pneumonia in infants and young children are due to viruses, the RSV and parainfluenza type 3 being the most important. *Streptococcus pneumonia* is the major bacterial cause but it is probably only responsible for about 10–20% of pneumoniae.

Mycoplasma pneumoniae is now frequent in all age groups. *S. aureus*, although an uncommon cause, produces a severe pneumonia. *H. influenzae* type B is responsible for about 2% of pneumonia seen in hospital. In developing countries *Strep. pneumoniae* and *H. influenzae*, both type B and non-typeable strains, rather than viruses, are the principal causes of pneumonia in infants and young children.

One of the difficulties with pneumonia is to determine the precise aetiology. If a virus is cultured from the upper respiratory tract and is a known pathogen, then it is reasonable to assume that it is the cause of pneumonia, but mixed viral and bacterial infections occur. However, the culture of bacteria from the upper respiratory tract or sputum is no indication that these organisms are responsible for lower respiratory infection. The only way to be certain that a bacteria is causing pneumonia is to culture it from the blood, in pleural fluid if the latter is present, or by aspirating fluid from the lung. Lung aspiration is a procedure with some complications and should not be undertaken as a routine. Demonstration of *Strep. pneumoniae* or *H. influenzae* type B antigen in the urine in a child with pneumonia is valuable evidence of aetiology.

Causes of pneumonia

Viral pneumonia

Viruses are the major cause of pneumonia in infants and young children in developed countries. They can be responsible for a wide spectrum of illness. At one end the infant may rapidly become dangerously ill with fever, marked constitutional disturbance, respiratory distress, circulatory failure and quite widespread clinical and radiological signs. Death may occur in 1 to 3 days with extensive changes and marked tissue necrosis. At the other extreme is the infant or young child who develops a cough, fever, tachypnoea with mild constitutional disturbance following a coryzal illness. There are few or no clinical signs of lung involvement but a radiograph of the chest shows patchy consolidation.

Mycoplasma pneumonia

Mycoplasma pneumoniae is a frequent cause of pneumonia in children. Often the disease runs in families and the incubation period may be up to three weeks. The onset is usually insidious with constitutional symptoms of malaise, anorexia, headache, fever, nasal discharge and sore throat. A paroxysmal cough develops a few days after the onset of the symptoms. Most patients are not acutely ill and often present some days or even a week or more after the onset of fever and cough. Abnormalities on physical examination of the chest are relatively minor, there being usually no more than a few fine crackles.

The radiological changes can be quite variable and are not diagnostic. Perihilar infiltrate and infiltrates in the lower lobes, while common, are also found in other pneumonias. The diagnosis is confirmed by demonstration of specific IgM by ELISA, by the culture of *Mycoplasma pneumoniae* or by the demonstration of a rise in the level of specific IgG antibody in the serum.

Streptococcal pneumonia

Strep. pneumoniae is the cause of 90% of bacterial pneumonia in developed countries. The incidence in different ages is not known but in childhood the peak incidence is in the second year of life. Commonly there are prodromal symptoms of a mild upper respiratory tract infection for several days. In infants the onset is often with vomiting, refusal to feed, irritability followed by drowsiness and fever. Sometimes convulsions may occur. The infant's breathing becomes rapid and may be grunting in character but often there is little cough. In such infants there may be few or no abnormal physical signs other than a few crackles and radiology will be necessary to confirm the diagnosis. The chest radiograph will usually show a lobular distribution of consolidation.

In the older child, headache, anorexia, restlessness, drowsiness, high fever and an irritating cough are the main general features. The child is usually flushed and has rapid grunting respirations with nasal flaring. Not infrequently he has chest and, at times, abdominal pain which may even simulate appendicitis, the latter usually occurring with lower lobe disease. Upper lobe involvement may produce signs of meningeal irritation. In the early stages of pneumonia reduced movement and diminished breath sounds and a few fine crackles are found over the affected area. Later, with extensive consolidation, the percussion note is dull and the breath sounds may become bronchial in character. The chest radiograph in older children usually shows a typical lobar consolidation (Fig. 35.2).

Staphylococcal pneumonia

Staphylococcal pneumonia is relatively uncommon, but causes a very severe pneumonia. There is frequently an associated septicaemia. The child rapidly becomes ill with marked constitutional disturbance, high fever, and rapid pulse. Clinical signs suggestive of consolidation frequently develop early as lesions are often extensive.

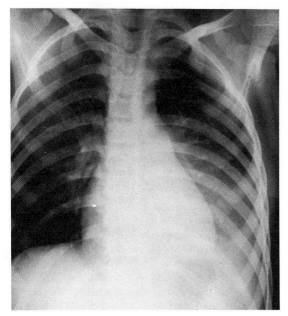

Fig. 35.2   PA radiograph demonstrating consolidation of the left lower lobe. Diagnosis – left lower lobe pneumonia.

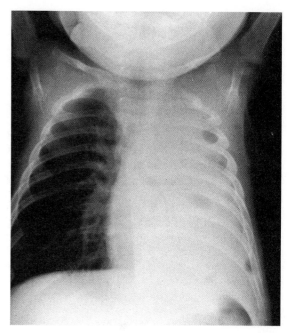

Fig. 35.3   PA radiograph of a chest. The left lung is almost completely opacified. Air and fluid are present in the left pleural cavity and there is a pneumatocoele in the mid zone. Diagnosis – staphylococcal pneumonia.

Pleural complications of empyema and pyopneumothorax are not uncommon as shown in Figure 35.3. The changes may be unilateral. Intrapulmonary air cysts called pneumatoceles often develop after about 1 week.

Pneumonia due to *H. influenzae* is uncommon. There are no characteristic features and the diagnosis is usually made as a result of finding a positive blood culture.

Treatment

Management of pneumonia falls into two sections. The first are general measures to support hydration and oxygenation and require a high standard of nursing care. Most infants under 24 months with pneumonia should be admitted to hospital. Older children who are not constitutionally ill can often be well looked after at home. Physiotherapy is not required in the treatment of acute pneumonia.

While it is now realized that viruses and *Mycoplasma pneumoniae* are the major causes of pneumonia in infants and young children in developed countries, bacterial infection still plays an important part. As there is no simple and rapid method of distinguishing viral from bacterial infection, pneumonia must always be considered potentially bacterial in origin and the patient treated with antibiotics at least until the results of microbiological investigation are available.

Strep. pneumoniae is the major bacterial pathogen in children under the age of 5. In this group penicillin is the initial drug of choice unless the child is so ill constitutionally to suggest the diagnosis of staphylococcal pneumonia. In general practice this means that penicillin is really the only antibiotic that should be considered for the management of pneumonia unless the child is allergic to it. If sufficiently ill to warrant consideration of other therapy, the child should be in hospital under the care of a paediatrician. *H. influenzae* type B pneumonia is uncommon and does not need to be considered at the general practice level. In fact, in hospital practice it is usually treated initially with penicillin and the diagnosis made only after blood culture results become available. Most children with *Haemophilus* pneumonia seem to respond very adequately to the initial penicillin even though the organisms may not be sensitive to this in vitro.

Over the age of 1 year the possibility of *Mycoplasma* pneumonia should always be born in mind. In this age group in general practice, either penicillin or erythromycin should be used. On clinical grounds, if pneumococcal pneumonia is thought probable then penicillin is the drug of choice. However, if the onset of pneumonia is more gradual, then *Mycoplasma* pneumonia is likely and erythromycin is the drug of choice.

All children with complications of pneumonia such as empyema and pyopneumothorax should be in hospital under the care of a team of paediatric thoracic surgeon and paediatric thoracic physician. The management of these complications can be difficult and requires considerable experience.

DIFFUSE LUNG DISEASE IN CHILDREN

Diffuse pulmonary parenchymal disease is much less common than consolidation with a bronchopneumonic distribution in childhood. Diffuse reticulonodular opacities on a chest radiograph imply involvement of all lobes of both lungs. Although the disease is widespread, it need not affect all regions uniformly. For example, the lower lung zones may be involved to a greater or lesser extent than the upper zones, or the central and mid portions of the lungs may be more severely affected than the periphery producing a 'bat's wing' distribution. As a rule, the bases of the lungs appear more involved in diffuse lung diseases due to the greater mass of lung tissue.

The disease process may be interstitial as seen with fibrosing alveolitis or collagen diseases, or may involve the air spaces with air space consolidation due to haemorrhage or oedema.

Other abnormalities such as lymphadenopathy, pleural effusion or cardiac enlargement may be present and may help indicate the likely underlying pathology. In general, all of these conditions present with non-specific symptoms of ill health and tachypnoea. On auscultation, the chest may be clear or there may be diffuse fine inspiratory crackles indicating instability of alveoli or bronchioli.

Conditions that should be considered in a child with non-specific symptoms and a diffuse reticulonodular appearance on chest radiograph (Fig. 35.4) include:

1. Infections. Viruses such as cytomegalovirus, varicella, measles and influenza may produce a pneumonitis during the acute phase of the illness and these occur particularly in children with impaired immunity. Occasionally, staphylococcal infection can result in multiple micro-abscesses throughout the lungs. Similarly, tuberculosis and fungal infections may spread haematogenously and produce a similar appearance. *Pneumocystis carinii* infection in the compromised host produces air space consolidation.

2. Fibrosing alveolitis. A diffuse inflammatory disease of the interstitium may occur without any obvious precipitating factor and present as an idiopathic

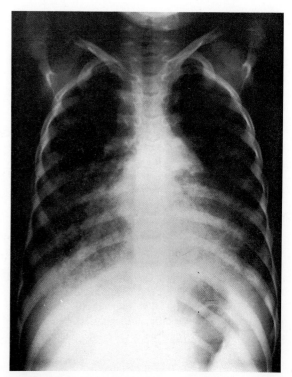

Fig. 35.4 PA radiograph of the chest demonstrating patchy and fluffy bronchopneumonic consolidation involving both lungs. Diagnosis – mycoplasma pneumonia.

pneumonitis. Alternatively, children may produce an immunological response to antigens such as pigeon droppings or fungi and develop an extrinsic fibrosing alveolitis as seen in pigeon fancier's disease or farmer's lung. Pulmonary infiltrates may be associated with a peripheral blood oesinophilia for which no obvious precipitating cause can be found.

3. Collagen diseases. They tend to involve the serosal surfaces but occasionally a diffuse pulmonary parenchymal component may be seen with polyarteritis nodosa, rheumatoid arthritis, systemic lupus erythematosus or dermatomyositis. Pulmonary involvement is a significant component of Wegener's granulomatosis and Goodpasture's disease but these are rare in childhood.

4. Idiopathic pulmonary haemosiderosis. A child with respiratory distress and an iron deficiency anaemia may have idiopathic pulmonary haemosiderosis – a condition in which there is intermittent bleeding into the alveoli producing patchy opacities.

5. Sarcoidosis. Sarcoidosis predominantly presents in older children with lymphadenopathy but may be associated with diffuse parenchymal involvement.

6. *Pulmonary oedema*. Pulmonary oedema can be seen with cardiac failure or circulatory overload and produce diffuse pulmonary opacities. The distribution is generally perihilar and associated with Kerley B-lines and fluid in fissures.

7. *Aspiration*. Aspiration of hydrocarbons can produce a pneumonitis with an appearance similar to that of pulmonary oedema.

8. *Hyaline membrane disease*. The newborn with hyaline membrane disease will have diffuse air space consolidation with an air bronchogram.

9. *Vascular abnormalities*. A diffuse nodular appearance may occur with multiple AV malformations. This radiographic appearance may be acquired with thrombotic emboli deposited in the lung.

10. *Malignancy*. Conditions such as histiocytosis, leukaemia, Hodgkin's disease and metastases from extrapulmonary carcinomas may produce a diffuse lung disease. The lymphomas generally have associated lymphadenopathy. The child being treated for malignancy presenting with this radiographic appearance presents a particularly difficult diagnostic dilemma. The diffuse lung disease may be because of infection in the compromised host with organisms such as *Pneumocystis carinii* or measles. It may be interstitial fibrosis caused by the cytotoxics used (e.g. bleomycin). As well, the diffuse lung disease may be extension of the primary malignancy.

It is often difficult to make a specific diagnosis in many of these conditions. In older children lung function tests will support the presence of diffuse lung disease with evidence of a restrictive defect. Occasionally, investigations such as viral studies, serum antibodies and full blood examination may help. However, one will often need to make a decision as to whether lung biopsy is essential for diagnosis or a therapeutic trial warranted without lung biopsy diagnosis. The relative risks of each need to be considered and these children need the expertise of a paediatric thoracic physician.

FURTHER READING

Phelan P D, Landau L O, Olinsky A 1989 Respiratory illness in children, 3rd edn. Blackwell Scientific Publications, Oxford

36. The child who wheezes

Craig M. Mellis

Noisy breathing is common, particularly in early childhood, and various terms are used to describe the more characteristic sounds (e.g. wheeze, stridor, grunt). These noises signify narrowing or obstruction in a particular anatomical area of the respiratory tract. Wheeze is the commonest, and is typically a high-pitched, musical whistle, more obvious during expiration. Wheeze should not be used interchangeably with bronchospasm nor asthma, as there are many other possible causes. On the other hand, by far the most common cause of wheeze is asthma.

Wheeze arises due to turbulence of airflow in the large airways, although paradoxically, the primary pathology responsible for this is frequently situated in the small or medium sized airways. This paradox is explained diagrammatically in Figures 36.1 and 36.2.

In Fig. 36.1 there is an obvious lesion in the region of the right main bronchus and carina (e.g. an enlarged hilar node due to primary tuberculosis). This results in narrowing of the central airways at this point and an audible wheeze. In Fig. 36.2 there is widespread nar-

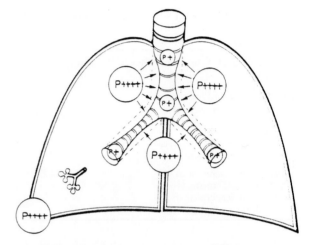

Fig. 36.2 Widespread narrowing of the small bronchioles, e.g. viral bronchiolitis.

rowing of the small bronchioles (e.g. due to acute viral bronchiolitis). In order to transfer gases from the alveoli back to the central airways during expiration, large positive pleural pressures (4+) are required to overcome the obstruction. These pressures are largely dissipated in overcoming the obstruction. Therefore, the intraluminal pressure in the airways is low (1+), yet the pleural pressures and transpulmonary pressures remain high throughout the lung (4+). In small infants, the large central airways are relatively floppy due to the soft cartilaginous rings. Consequently, the central airways undergo dynamic compression, due to the pressure gradient which exists across the central airway wall. The result is widespread narrowing of the central airways, development of turbulent airflow at this point and audible wheeze.

Since wheeze can develop because of narrowing of either the small or large airways, there are many potential causes. In determining the likely cause of wheeze in an individual child, the patient's age has an important

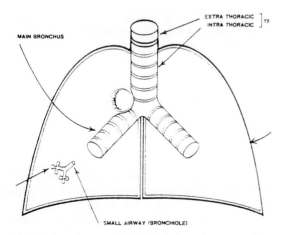

Fig. 36.1 An obstructive lesion in the region of the right main bronchus and carina producing an audible wheeze.

bearing. Accurate diagnosis of the cause of wheeze is important in all age groups, but particularly in infants where there may be a surgical lesion responsible for the wheeze. In other age groups, specific medical therapy (particularly anti-asthma therapy) is the major reason for accurate diagnosis.

For the purposes of this discussion, children are divided into three age groups: infants (0–1 year); toddlers/preschoolers (1–5 years); and school-age/adolescents (5–15 years). Clearly, these groups are arbitrary, and many of the causes will overlap several of these age groupings, especially asthma.

WHEEZE IN INFANTS (0–1 year) (Example 36.1)

Example 36.1 Causes of wheeze in infancy (0–1 yr)

Obstruction of small airways
  Active viral bronchiolitis
  Aspiration
  Asthma
  Bronchopulmonary dysplasia
  Familial bronchiectasis

Obstruction of large airways
  Airway malformations
  Vascular malformations
  Medistinal cysts/tumours

Obstruction of small airways

1. Acute viral bronchiolitis

This is the most common cause of acute wheeze and dyspnoea in infants and is usually due to respiratory syncytial virus (RSV), which is responsible for regular winter epidemics. The clinical features of acute viral bronchiolitis are described in detail in Chapter 35.

2. Aspiration bronchitis/bronchiolitis/bronchopneumonia

This possibility should always be considered in small infants with recurrent or persistent lower respiratory symptoms, including wheeze. Aspiration may be due to gastro-oesophageal reflux, or incoordinate swallowing. In the latter, the aspiration will occur during feeding; in the former, usually 1–2 hours after feeds often in association with vomiting. Incoordinate swallowing is usually secondary to severe central nervous system disease (e.g. cerebral palsy), but some infants simply have delayed maturation of the normal swallowing mechanism. Aspiration may also be due to an anatomical communication, such as laryngeal cleft or tracheo-oesophageal fistula (TOF).

3. Asthma

Although rare in the first months of life, asthma is not uncommon in the second half of infancy. Typically, these infants have persistent low grade wheeze, often without significant breathlessness nor obvious distress. Indeed, they tend to be big, overweight babies and the term, 'fat, happy wheezer' is sometimes used to describe them. There is often co-existent allergic rhinitis and/or atopic eczema. The wheeze is generally resistant to oral or nebulized bronchodilators, steroids, disodium cromoglycate ('Intal') and dietary manipulation (e.g. avoidance of cow's milk).

4. Chronic lung disease of prematurity ('bronchopulmonary dysplasia')

This is becoming an increasingly common cause of persistent cough and wheeze in infancy, and is as a direct consequence of improved survival of the pre-term infant with hyaline membrane disease. The exact cause of the chronic airway and lung pathology is still unclear, but it is thought to result from the interaction of immaturity of the lung, oxygen toxicity, mechanical ventilation and repeated aspiration. Mortality is significant, but in survivors, progressive improvement in respiratory status is usual. However, during the first 12–18 months persistent cough and wheeze plus recurrent lower respiratory tract infection is common.

5. Familial bronchiectasis

Familial bronchiectasis is a rare but important cause of cough and wheeze, as specific antibiotic therapy is necessary and the prognosis is obviously less favourable than most of the other causes of wheeze in infancy. The most common form of familial bronchiectasis is cystic fibrosis, which occurs in 1:2 00 live births in the Caucasian population. Classically, these infants have a combination of both lower respiratory tract symptoms (cough, wheeze and repeated lower respiratory infection), plus gastrointestinal symptoms (steatorrhoea and poor weight gain). The wheeze is due to persistent viral or bacterial bronchiolitis. Treatment entails aggressive use of systemic antibiotics, chest physiotherapy, inhalation therapy plus pancreatic enzyme replacement. Other forms of familial bronchiectasis which may present in infancy with wheeze and cough include primary ciliary dyskinesia, (immotile cilia syndrome or Kartagener's syndrome) and immune deficiency syndrome (e.g. sex-linked hypogammaglobulinaemia or Bruton's disease).

Obstruction of large airways

1. Airway malformations

Tracheomalacia/bronchomalacia. This is due to a primary malformation of either tracheal or bronchial cartilage resulting in excessive floppiness of the central airways. This causes a brassy, 'seal-bark' cough, wheeze and sputum retention. Tracheomalacia may also be complicated by sudden, very severe obstructive episodes, due to transient total apposition of the anterior and posterior tracheal walls.

Congenital lobar emphysema. Usually this results from a congenital deficiency of cartilage in a lobar bronchus. This causes obstruction to the bronchus, overdistension of that lobe and subsequent compression of the adjacent lung and mediastinum. The most common lobe involved is left upper, followed by right middle and right upper lobe. Involvement of the lower lobes is rare. Generally, these infants present in the neonatal period with respiratory distress accompanied by wheeze and over-distension of the chest. Treatment is surgical removal of the affected lobe and the long-term prognosis is excellent.

Subglottic haemangioma. These lesions are absent at birth (as with cavernous haemangioma of the skin), but appear during the first few months of life. Therefore, the symptoms of expiratory wheeze, inspiratory stridor and respiratory distress typically occur between the ages of 2 and 6 months. Approximately half of these infants will also have cutaneous cavernous haemangiomata in the head and neck region. The diagnosis can only be made reliably by bronchoscopy under general anaesthesia. Spontaneous resolution of the haemangioma may take from 1–2 years, and during this time, a permanent tracheostomy is usually necessary.

Tracheal/bronchial stenosis. This can occur anywhere in the central tracheobronchial tree, resulting in varying degrees of obstruction. Normally, these infants will present with breathlessness, expiratory wheeze and/or inspiratory stridor (depending upon the site and extent of the narrowing). Unfortunately, surgical correction of the severe or extensive lesions has proved difficult.

2. Vascular malformations

Vascular ring. The true vascular ring is usually due to a double aortic arch malformation. This results in early onset of wheeze and stridor, cough and recurring lower respiratory tract infection. Diagnosis can be made on barium swallow, which demonstrates an abnormal indentation of the oesophagus posteriorly plus an indentation in the anterior wall of the tracheal air column on lateral views. Diagnosis is confirmed at bronchoscopy and surgical excision of the smaller arch is indicated after delineation of the anatomy by angiography. Other vascular malformations which may cause symptoms include innominate artery compression of the trachea (often associated with localized tracheomalacia), aberrant subclavian artery and rare forms of pulmonary artery sling. Apart from the latter, surgical treatment of these lesions is rarely necessary.

Large left to right cardiac shunt. External compression of the bronchi can occur in the presence of enlarged, hypertensive pulmonary arteries, particularly when there is associated left atrial enlargement. The left atrium lies immediately adjacent to the tracheal bifurcation and infants with this combination seem particularly prone to bronchial compression (e.g. ventricular septal defect; persistent ductus arteriosis). Clinically, this obstruction results in over-distension of one or both lung fields with associated wheeze and breathlessness. The peak incidence of respiratory difficulties in the presence of a large left to right shunt occurs between the ages of 2 and 9 months. Development of this complication necessitates early corrective cardiac surgery.

3. Mediastinal cysts and tumours

Cystic hygroma/lymphangioma. Usually these contain elements of both cystic hygroma (cavernous lymphangioma) and capillary lymphangioma within the same lesion. Although the majority are in the neck, they can involve the mediastinum where they tend to be more cystic and can cause compression of the central airways. In this site surgical removal may be indicated, but because of their size and infiltrative nature, surgery is difficult and multiple operations may be necessary.

Bronchogenic cysts (Figs. 36.3 and 36.4). These are usually located in the region of the lower trachea, carina or main bronchi. Although embryologic in origin, they can present quite late in childhood, or even adulthood. However, if large, they will present with wheeze and breathlessness and an obvious middle mediastinal mass will be noted on chest radiograph. Treatment is surgical excision.

Oesophageal duplication cysts, and neurenteric/gastroenteric cysts. These are usually in the posterior mediastinum and, therefore, less likely to impinge upon the airway. However, duplication cysts

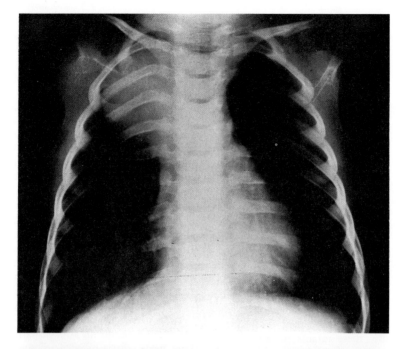

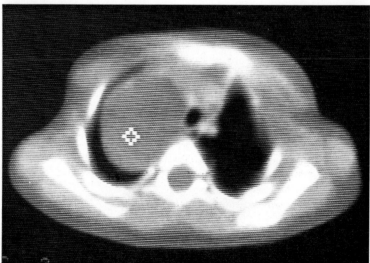

Figs 36.3 and **36.4** Chest X-ray (Fig. 29.3). Showing large opacity in right upper zone pushing trachea to the left and causing persistent wheeze. CT scan (Fig. 36.4). Of same child showing very large fluid-filled cystic lesion which appears to be arising from the mediastinum. Subsequently this was excised and found to be a bronchogenic cyst.

may be in the middle mediastinum and result in wheeze and respiratory difficulty. Treatment is by surgical excision.

Teratoma. These are the most common of the germ-cell tumours and while most are in the sacrococcygeal region, between 10% and 15% are found in the medias-tinum. Usually they are in the anterior mediastinum and frequently cause compression of adjacent structures, particularly trachea or main bronchi. These tumours may be benign (dermoid cysts) or malignant. Malignancy can only be determined after histological evaluation and clearly, excision is mandatory.

Assessment of the infant with wheeze

Obviously, there are a large number of potential causes of wheeze in infancy, some of which are extremely serious and require urgent intervention. In this age group, the diagnosis of asthma can only be made on clinical grounds as there are no specific tests which can confirm the diagnosis. Thus, full evaluation of the infants with recurrent or persistent wheeze may entail chest radiograph, lateral neck radiograph, barium swallow and possibly bronchoscopy/oesophagoscopy by a competent paediatric endoscopist and anaesthetist. Computerized axial tomography (CAT scan) can be particularly helpful in the evaluation of mediastinal masses.

WHEEZE IN CHILDREN (1–5 years) (Example 36.2)

Example 36.2 Causes of wheeze in toddlers/preschool children (1–5 yrs)

Obstruction of small airways
Asthma
Suppurative lung disease/bronchiectasis
Acute viral bronchiolitis

Obstruction of large airways
Inhaled foreign body
Ingested foreign body
Mediastinal masses

Obstruction of small airways

1. Asthma

Asthma is particularly common in this age group and may reach a prevalence of 20%. Most asthmatic children will develop their asthma symptoms during this period. A large percentage will only wheeze in association with intercurrent viral respiratory tract infections. Although terms such as 'wheezy bronchitis', 'allergic bronchitis', 'asthmatic bronchitis', have been used to describe these children, they simply represent the mildest end of the asthma spectrum. Asthmatic children over the age of 12–18 months respond well to bronchodilator drugs, but many in this age group are unable to use the various hand-held aerosol devices (see Ch. 37).

2. Suppurative lung disease/bronchiectasis

In this age group both the familial forms (especially cystic fibrosis) as well as the acquired forms will be seen. Although the predominant symptom is chronic productive cough, wheezing due to diffuse small airways

obstruction is common in young children with suppurative lung disease. The acquired forms of bronchiectasis usually follow major insults to the lungs such as chronic aspiration or severe adenoviral pneumonia. However, in some children there is no underlying abnormality nor previous lung injury to explain the insidious development of their suppurative lung disease.

3. Acute viral bronchiolitis

Although classically acute viral bronchiolitis (due to RSV) occurs in the first year of life, older children can develop this illness as the immunity following RSV infection is transient. Indeed, prospective studies of young children have shown repeated infection with each winter epidemic is to be expected, and clinical bronchiolitis is not uncommon during the second and third bouts of RSV infection. Nevertheless, hospitalization for children with acute RSV bronchiolitis is uncommon beyond infancy. A very severe form of necrotizing bronchiolitis/bronchopneumonia due to adenovirus (especially types 7 and 21) is occasionally seen in this age group. This virus causes gross airway and lung damage with considerable mortality and morbidity. The major long-term complications are bronchiectasis and obliterative bronchiolitis.

Obstruction of large airways

1. Inhaled foreign body

The majority of children presenting with an inhaled foreign body are in this age group. The most common foreign bodies are nuts (especially peanuts), but other food material and small objects (e.g. plastic toys, grass seeds, leaves) can be inhaled into the airways. The most common symptom is acute onset of wheeze, usually accompanied by cough and breathlessness. Unfortunately, many of the children will not have a history of a choking episode, and therefore a high index of suspicion is essential when dealing with children in this age group presenting with acute onset of respiratory symptoms. Chest radiographs may show a ball-valve obstruction, particularly if both inspiratory and expiratory views are taken (Fig. 36.5a and b). If the inhaled foreign body has been retained for a period of time, the child develops symptoms and signs consistent with persisting lower respiratory tract infection (chronic productive cough, fever and wheeze). Chest radiograph in these patients will usually show extensive collapse of the lung distal to the foreign body.

It should be remembered that a child with an inhaled foreign body can have a normal chest radiograph.

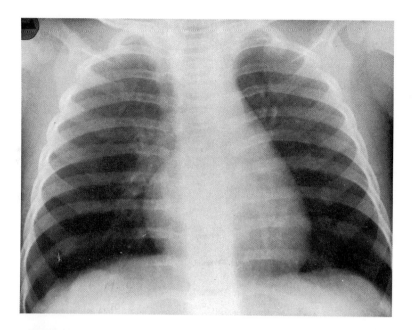

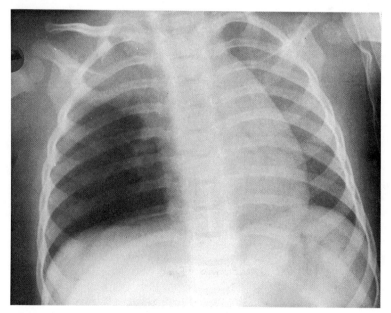

Figs 36.5a and b Radiographs of 3-year-old-child with acute wheeze during inspiration (Fig. 36.5(a) (top) and expiration (Fig. 36.5(b) (bottom). Inspiratory film is normal. Expiratory film shows marked air trapping in the right lower zone, consistent with a ball valve (partial obstruction) in the right main bronchus. At bronchoscopy, a peanut was removed from the right bronchus.

Similarly, although there may be auscultatory signs of diminished breath sounds or localized high-pitched expiratory rhonchi, physical signs may be absent.

In short, if a foreign body is suspected, then bronchoscopy/oesophagoscopy should be performed, despite the absence of physical signs or history of inhalation.

2. Ingested foreign body

Quite large foreign bodies (coins, toys, bones) may be swallowed and fail to pass through the relatively narrow upper oesophagus. If these foreign bodies are large (Fig. 36.6), or irregularly shaped, they may cause significant obstruction to the adjacent extra-thoracic trachea. In most cases, this will produce inspiratory stridor, but expiratory wheeze may also be audible. These children will have difficulty swallowing of recent onset, plus persisting fever and malaise as a consequence of inflammation of the oesophagus from the foreign body. Radio-opaque foreign bodies will be visible on radiography providing the upper portion of the airways is present on the chest film. Management is by removal of the foreign body by oesophagoscopy under general anaesthesia.

3. Mediastinal masses

In this age group, extrinsic compression of the main bronchi is most commonly due to enlarged hilar lymph nodes secondary to primary tuberculosis. Classically these children have recent onset of weight loss, cough and fever, followed by wheeze and breathlessness. The chest radiograph will show hilar lymphadenopathy, narrowing of the adjacent main stem bronchus and frequently a parenchymal lesion, representing the primary complex (Fig. 36.7). The Mantoux test will be positive at this stage of the illness. Should there be increasing respiratory difficulty, bronchoscopic suctioning of the caseous node may be possible, or alternatively, surgical excision by thoractomy. Late development of bronchial stenosis at the site of the compression and erosion is common, but usually asymptomatic. Other causes include lymphomas arising from hilar nodes or thymus gland.

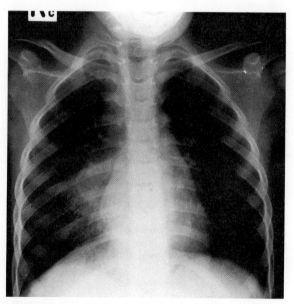

Fig. 36.7 Primary tuberculosis with enlarged hilar lymph nodes on the right, resulting in compression of the right main bronchus and wheeze localized to the right lung.

WHEEZE IN SCHOOL CHILDREN/ ADOLESCENTS (5–15 years) (Example 36.3)

Obstruction of small airways

1. Asthma

This is by far the most common cause of recurrent wheeze in the school-aged child and confirmation of the

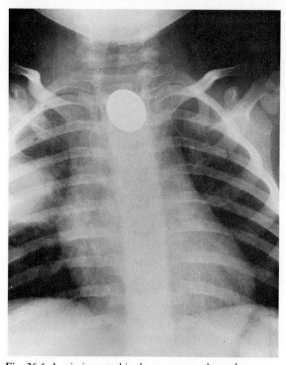

Fig. 36.6 A coin impacted in the upper oesophagus has distorted the adjacent trachea causing wheeze and resulting in consolidation — collapse of the right upper lobe.

Example 36.3 Causes of wheeze in school children/adolescents (5–15 yrs)

Obstruction of small airways
 Asthma
 Mycoplasma pneumoniae infection
 Suppurative lung disease/bronchiectasis

Obstruction of large airways
 Inhaled/ingested foreign bodies
 Mediastinal masses/tumours
 Bronchial adenoma
 Alpha$_1$-antitrypsin deficiency
 Hysterical wheeze/stridor

---

diagnosis by pulmonary function testing is usually possible. A past or present history of co-existent, eczema or perennial allergic rhinitis is usual. Moreover, a history of atopic disease in either the parents or siblings will be present in the majority. Thus, in this age group, the diagnosis of asthma does not usually present major difficulties.

2. Mycoplasma pneumoniae infection

Recent epidemiological studies have underlined the importance of *Mycoplasma pneumoniae* as a cause of wheezing respiratory disease in school-aged children. More commonly, however, school-aged children wheezing with intercurrent respiratory infections are suffering from asthma, and the virus or *Mycoplasma* is simply the trigger for that particular bout of wheeze. Features which would make one suspect *Mycoplasma* bronchitis/bronchiolitis include protracted fever, cough, headache, malaise, extensive chest radiograph changes, diffuse moist crepitations of auscultation and a poor response to penicillin/amoxycillin. There is usually a rapid improvement after administration of erythromycin.

3. Suppurative lung disease

Both the familial and acquired forms of bronchiectasis may present during this age group with a combination of chronic, productive cough and persistent clinical plus chest radiograph abnormalities. Recurrent wheeze is a common accompaniment.

Obstruction of large airways

1. Inhaled/ingested foreign bodies

These are far less common in this age group and in most instances a history of a choking/aspiration episode will be forthcoming.

2. Mediastinal masses/tumours

Lymphomas arising from thymus or other lymphoid tissue in the anterior and middle mediastinum (causing compression of central airways and subsequent wheeze and breathlessness) most commonly occurs in this age group and in young adults. Co-existent inspiratory stridor, recurring fever, malaise and weight loss are characteristic. Also, in this age group, primary tuberculosis with enlarged hilar lymph nodes resulting in compression of central airways is a possible cause.

3. Bronchial adenoma

Although these occur more typically in adults, they can occur in children under the age of 15 years. The clinical manifestations are usually due to the mechanical effects of the tumour, namely, wheeze and breathlessness. Wheeze may be unilateral because of partial obstruction of the bronchus. In addition, persistent irritating cough is common and haemoptysis may occur because of ulceration of the tumour.

4. Alpha$_1$-antitrypsin deficiency

Normally, the patients with this enzyme deficiency develop respiratory symptoms during the third or fourth decade. However, a number have been reported whose symptoms date back to early childhood and adolescence. Classically, the symptoms are progressive breathlessness on exertion associated with episodes of wheeze and cough. Most children and teenagers with alpha$_1$antitrypsin deficiency will have had this disease diagnosed in early infancy as a consequence of neonatal hepatitis or a known family history. Thus, it is sometimes possible to detect respiratory symptoms from this disease at a very early stage.

5. Hysterical wheeze/stridor

Fictitious asthma is occasionally seen in childhood, particularly in adolescent females. The wheezing is self-induced and heard best over the neck, rather than over the lung fields. The wheeze appears to be generated by the vocal cords (which are held in apposition during exhalation), although there may also be a component of dynamic compression of central airways due to the violent expiratory effort.

Further enquiry usually reveals considerable emotional disturbance within the child and family. It is more common to develop hysterical inspiratory stridor than expiratory wheeze, and the different noises may be a consequence of varying degrees of inherent stability of the central airways, as well as paradoxical vocal cord movements.

FURTHER READING

Felman A H 1983 The paediatric chest. Radiological, clinical and pathological observations. Thomas, Illinois
Henderson F W, Clyde W A, Krolier A M, Denny F W 1979 The aetiologic and epidemiologic spectrum of bronchiolitis in paediatric practice. Journal of Paediatrics 95: 183–190

Milner A D 1987 Childhood asthma: diagnosis, treatment and management. Dunitz, London
Phelan P D, Landau L I, Olinsky A 1982 Respiratory illness in children, 2nd edn. Blackwell, London

37. Asthma in childhood

Louis I. Landau

Asthma is a disease characterized by increased responsiveness of the airways to various stimuli and manifested by widespread narrowing of the airways that changes in severity either spontaneously or as a result of therapy. Asthma is the most common chronic illness in childhood.

Definition

Surprisingly, there is no definition that satisfactorily covers the range of clinical and physiological manifestations of asthma. To the clinician, asthma refers to repeated bouts of wheeze, cough and dyspnoea. To the physiologist, asthma is a state of hyperresponsiveness of airways and reversible airflow obstruction. To the pathologist, smooth muscle hypertrophy, mucosal swelling and mucous plugging of small airways characterize the changes seen in severe asthma.

Clinically, recurrent wheeze is the most characteristic feature of asthma. However, asthma may be present in the absence of wheezing and manifest as a persistent cough, exercise induced dyspnoea or recurrent collapse or lung segments seen on chest radiographs. A wheeze is the continuous musical note heard on expiration and although all that wheezes is not asthma, most is (see Ch. 36).

The concept that asthmatic children have a common basic disorder, bronchial hyperresponsiveness, with attacks precipitated by a variety of trigger mechanisms, provides a useful working model. The bronchial hyperresponsiveness can be demonstrated by:

1. Variability in daily peak flow measurements.
2. A change of more than 10% in peak flow rates or forced expiratory volume in one second (FEV^1) following a bronchodilator.
3. Increased bronchial responsiveness with a fall in flow rates of greater than 20% with inhaled chemicals (histamine, methacholine, beta-blockers), inhalation of cold dry air or an exercise challenge.

Asthma may be a primary condition manifested in a predisposed child or it can be associated with underlying lung disease such as cystic fibrosis and bronchopulmonary dysplasia.

Pathophysiology

The predisposition to asthma appears to be inherited and the pattern is most compatible with polygenic or multifactorial determinants. Most children with asthma have coexisting atopic disease which is also inherited. The inheritance of bronchial hyperresponsiveness and atopy is not strictly concordant and all will have various combinations of these two basic pathophysiological disturbances. It is assumed that an individual is born with the predisposition to asthma and the clinical syndrome is then induced by various environmental factors. These inducers include viral infections, allergens and some irritants such as ozone and cigarette smoke (Example 37.1). Although these agents can be shown experimentally to induce bronchial hyperresponsiveness which will last for weeks or months, their specific role in the induction of clinical asthma has yet to be confirmed. Once a state of hyperresponsiveness is established, there are a number of triggers which can precipitate attacks of

---

Example 37.1 Inducers and triggers of asthma

Inducers
  Viral infections
  Allergens, irritants (ozone, cigarette smoke)

Triggers
  Non-allergic:
    Infections: viral, pertussis, mycoplasma
    Exercise, hyperventilation of cold dry air
    Irritants (ozone, SO_2, cigarette smoke)
    Coughing, laughing
    Emotional
  Allergic:
    Inhalant – mite, pollen, animal dander
    Ingested – nuts, milk, eggs

---

asthma (see Example 37.1). The most common factors in children are viral upper respiratory infections, exercise, allergens and irritants. Often, however, the cause of an acute attack of asthma can not be readily identified.

Chemical mediators can induce bronchoconstriction which resolves spontaneously in a few hours. However, most clinical attacks of asthma are more prolonged and it is argued that the initial trigger stimulates airway inflammation which is responsible for ongoing changes. Airway epithelial cells produce metabolites (lipoxygenase-dependent metabolites of arachidonic acid such as leukotriene B^4 and 5-hydroxyicosatetraenoic acid) that affect the activities of nerves, smooth muscle, glands, neutrophils, mast cells and eosinophils. Mast cells release numerous mediators including histamine, prostaglandins, leukotrienes and other chemotactic factors which perpetuate the inflammatory process. The link between inflammation and bronchial hyperresponsiveness is not yet clearly defined.

The pathology of asthma is difficult to define as most of the information is based on postmortem histopathology from children who die with an acute attack. In this situation, the bronchial smooth muscle is thickened as a result of hypertrophy and hyperplasia, the mucosa is oedematous and infiltrated with inflammatory cells, and the bronchial mucus glands are hypertrophied. There are plugs in the lumen consisting of mucus, shed epithelium and eosinophils.

Prevalence

During childhood, it is estimated that 20–30% of children in Australia will show some manifestations of asthma. Most start to wheeze between 6 months and 3 years of age. In 30% the onset is later than 3 years of age. Most children have only a small number of attacks of wheezing in association with intercurrent viral respiratory infections and the majority of this group stops wheezing by 7 to 10 years of age. Approximately 10–15% of children will have repeated bouts of wheezing requiring ongoing treatment. Less than 5% have frequent wheezing episodes and less than 0.5% have chronic asthma with symptoms present most days for a number of years. Chronic asthma is more common in boys than girls, although infrequent wheezing is fairly evenly distributed between boys and girls.

Natural history of asthma

Most children with asthma have fewer symptoms as they grow into adolescence and adult life. Approximately 60% of those with infrequent episodic asthma will cease

to wheeze by early adult life, but only 20% of those with frequent episodes of asthma and less than 5% of those with chronic asthma become wheeze free in adult life. Those who have early onset of troublesome asthma requiring frequent admission to hospital and those with ongoing eczema and chronic abnormalities of lung function are less likely to improve during childhood and adolescence. With increasing age there is an increasing incidence of hayfever. There is convincing evidence that a combination of childhood asthma and smoking leads to persistence of cough and wheeze in early adult life and deterioration of lung function during middle age.

The death rate from asthma between 5 and 20 years of age in Australia runs at between 1 and 2 per 100 000. This does not appear to have altered significantly in the past 30 years. Most of the deaths are unexpected and occur at home or school. There is no evidence that deaths are due to drug toxicity. Most appear to be a result of underestimation of the severity of asthma by either the patients, their families or health provider. Morbidity from asthma can be marked if it is not adequately treated.

Clinical features

There is a spectrum of increasing severity of asthma with progression from those who have a few episodes of wheezing associated with viral infections, to those who have frequent episodes of wheezing precipitated by infections, exercise or allergens, to those who have symptoms most days. These children with chronic asthma will cough with exercise, wake in the night with cough and wheeze, require bronchodilators on wakening first thing in the morning, and have wheezes on auscultation of their chest and physiological evidence of airflow obstruction when apparently free of overt symptoms.

At times, the major component of a response may be mucus secretion with less bronchospasm so that the predominant symptom is a moist cough. This may present as the 'chesty child'. In other children, the major symptom may be a dry nocturnal cough present either on going to bed or on wakening early in the morning. In others, extensive mucous plugging may cause collapsed segments on a chest radiograph. The right middle lobe is particularly liable to collapse. This hypersecretory type of asthma is frequently misdiagnosed as recurrent pneumonia.

In some children, recurrent croup occurs early in infancy which at 3 to 4 years of age changes to typical asthma. Approximately 50% of children with bronchiolitis subsequently wheeze. Some believe this bronchiolitis is the first attack of asthma in a predisposed infant. Others feel the bronchiolitis induces a state of bronchial hyperresponsiveness which is different to classical asthma as it is less severe, equally prevalent in boys and girls and less associated with atopy.

Investigations

The majority of children with asthma, particularly those with infrequent episodes, do not require detailed investigation. In some, however, investigations will help describe the pattern of asthma and possible trigger factors.

1. Diary card recording

Details of cough, wheeze, limitation of activities and medication used can be helpful in documenting the pattern of asthma and response to treatment.

2. Peak flow measurements

Recording peak flow rate with a simple peak flow meter provides the most practical objective assessment of airway obstruction and lability. Children from the age of 4 or 5 years should perform peak flow measurements whenever seen for their asthma. Those with troublesome symptoms should be given a peak flow meter to help at home to document the bronchial lability. Morning and evening peak flow rates, before and after bronchodilator, will objectively define the pattern of asthma and response to therapy.

3. Pulmonary function tests

Some children will need more detailed lung function tests with spirometry and lung volume measurements to characterize their degree of airway obstruction and its responsibility with bronchodilator. If there is a lack of response to bronchodilators, a course of steroids will usually be necessary. Lung function measurements can accurately document return of bronchodilator responsiveness and establishment of optimal lung function.

4. Immunological investigations

These are not necessary in the majority of children with asthma. If there is uncertainty about the presence of atopy, simple skin testing to common allergens such as house dust mite and rye grass pollen may be useful (see Ch. 23).

5. Chest radiograph

A chest radiograph is warranted in any child with chronic asthma. It is necessary where clinical features suggest a possible alternative diagnosis. It is required where a complication such as pneumothorax or lobar collapse is suspected.

Management

The main aims of therapy are outlined in Example 37.2.

Example 37.2 Management of asthma

Education
  natural history
  drugs
  drug usage
  inhaler technique
  lifestyle
  crisis management

Assess severity with objective measurements

Aim for control of symptoms and best lung function

Drugs
  beta-2-sympathomimetics
  theophylline
  anticholinergics
  disodium cromoglycate
  corticosteroids

Control trigger factors if possible

Review regularly

As the pattern of asthma varies from child to child, the treatment must be individualized and will vary from a single drug in those with mild episodic asthma to long-term multiple drugs for those with chronic asthma.

In all cases, counselling the child and family about the basic cause of asthma, trigger factors, drug therapy and crisis management is vital. Careful instruction on the use of aerosols and regular review of technique is essential. Drug therapy is the mainstay of treatment and this is specifically aimed at alleviating symptoms and restoring normal lung function.

Allergen avoidance measurements are used where it is clear that allergens have triggered attacks of asthma and dietary manipulation is sometimes necessary. However, these measures do not alter the natural history of asthma in most children. Hyposensitization injections have little effect, they carry the risk of acute life-threatening anaphylactic reactions and are generally not recommended in the management of childhood asthma. Physiotherapy is rarely needed for asthmatic children unless there is mucous plugging and lobar collapse. All asthmatic children should be encouraged to play sport.

Swimming is frequently used as the warm humidified atmosphere is less likely to induce bronchoconstriction than the cold dry air in free range running. However, with adequate prophylaxis and warm-up exercises, any sport can be undertaken by asthmatic children.

Anti-asthma drugs

There have been advances in the pharmacological management of asthma in the past 25 years. The drugs most commonly used include bronchodilators, and prophylactic agents (see Example 37.2). Antibiotics, antihistamines and cough suppressants do not have a role in specific management of asthma. Antihistamines may be used for the treatment of hayfever and occasionally antibiotics for secondary bacterial infections. However, most episodes of asthma are related to viral infections for which antibiotics do not have a role.

The **beta-2-sympathomimetics** are effective bronchodilators with minimal cardiovascular effects. The major side effects are tremor and hyperactivity. This group of drugs is available as aerosols, nebulizer solutions, injectable and oral preparations. The various preparations, routes of administration and dosages are listed in the addendum at the end of this chapter. The preparation should be used by can aerosol where possible. Most children from 3 or 4 years of age can use the Rotahaler and those from 7 or 8 years a standard metered aerosol. Sometimes, a spacer attachment will allow use of the aerosol in children who cannot co-ordinate the metered aerosol alone. Spacers can also be used to give larger doses of the beta-sympathomimetic agent during an acute attack of asthma. Dry powder aerosols cannot be used with severe airways obstruction. Beta-2-sympathomimetic agents can be nebulized effectively with a compressed air pump or oxygen during an acute attack of asthma and this is the mainstay of treatment in this situation (Fig. 37.1). There is a small number of asthmatic children who cannot use any of the regular forms of aerosol because of their age or who have troublesome chronic asthma. They require long-term treatment with a nebulizer at home. Oral preparations of beta-sympathomimetic agents should rarely be used and are only considered for the treatment of mild asthma in very young children where there is no other practical alternative.

Theophyllines are available as oral, rectal, and intravenous preparations. The absorption of the rectal preparation is erratic and often incomplete and this form should rarely be used. The oral preparations are effective bronchodilators and have significant prophylactic value.

There is considerable variation in the phar-

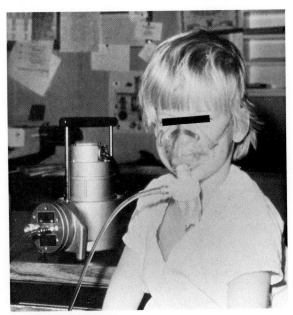

Fig. 37.1   Child receiving nebulizer therapy via face mask.

micokinetics from patient to patient. Theophyllines should only be used in the slow release preparations such as slow release tablets or spinkles. They are generally given in conservative doses as illustrated in the addendum. Side effects from oral theophylline include poor concentration, nausea, behavioural changes, vomiting, haematemesis, headaches, and rarely, arrythmias or convulsions. If used in high dosage for severe asthma, serum measurement of levels is necessary to ensure that satisfactory therapeutic levels are achieved. Intravenous aminophylline is a useful preparation for the treatment of severe acute asthma. An initial loading dose of 5–6 mg/kg is given, provided theophylline has not been recently administered in which case the dose should be reduced. This can be repeated every 6 hours or a constant infusion used.

Ipratropium bromide is an anticholinergic agent available as a metered aerosol or nebulizer solution. It is a moderately good bronchodilator. Its main use is in combination with beta-2-sympathomimetic agents in patients with severe acute asthma.

Disodium cromoglycate is a prophylactic agent reducing the frequency and severity of episodes of asthma in children with frequent episodic or chronic asthma. It can be given via a dry powder inhalation, metered aerosol or nebulizer solution. There are no significant side effects with this drug although some complain of throat irritation following inhalation of the powder. It must be given on a regular basis over a number of weeks or months as it is purely prophylactic. An initial course of 6 to 8 weeks is given and if there is no response to treatment then it is unlikely that the drug will be useful. Sodium cromoglycate should be commenced when airway function is normal or near normal so it is usually used, at least initially, with bronchodilators.

Aerosol corticosteroids are very effective in the prophylaxis of asthma and can be given by metered aerosol or dry powder aerosol but not by nebulization. They are particularly useful in those with frequent episodic or chronic asthma. Although they are important anti-inflammatory agents, one of the main actions is to potentiate the activity of the beta-2-sympathomimetic agents and they are used in combination with them. Side effects such as oral candidiasis are very rare in children.

Oral corticosteroids will be required by a small group of children during their treatment of acute attacks of asthma and for ongoing prophylaxis. Oral prednisolone is the steroid of choice.

Acute asthma

The onset of symptoms is reasonably consistent. A previously well infant or child develops what seems to be a cold with rhinorrhoea. This is followed by irritability, a tight cough, tachypnoea and wheezing; symptoms may progress slowly or extremely rapidly. A sympathomimetic by inhalation using a metered aerosol and spacer, or a nebulizer driven by oxygen or air compressor pump will usually give relief. If not available, subcutaneous administration is an acceptable alternative. If the single dose of inhaled bronchodilator relieves the attack, ongoing bronchodilators should be continued until wheeze-free for 48 hours. The most appropriate medications would be sympathomimetic agents by metered aerosol with a spacer if necessary or rotacaps.

Should a single dose of nebulized bronchodilator not produce relief in 15 to 30 minutes, the dose may be repeated. If this is not adequate, hospitalization is probably indicated. In a hospital setting, the nebulized beta-2-sympathomimetic agents can be used very frequently to ensure maximum benefit. There is increasing evidence that a short course of steroids will be helpful to reduce the morbidity of an acute attack of asthma in those likely to have a prolonged course. They should be used if there is not a rapid response to 2 or 3 doses of beta-2-sympathomimetic given over 60 minutes.

A child who fails to respond to nebulized bronchodilator has severe, acute asthma previously termed 'status asthmaticus'. This refers to an attack of asthma which does not respond to regular bronchodilator therapy. Management is outlined in Example 37.3. This child will have severe airway

---

> **Example 37.3 Management of severe asthma**
>
> Beta-2-sympathomimetic nebulized with oxygen
> Corticosteroids
> IV aminophylline
> Monitor closely
> Assisted ventilation (rarely).

obstruction, gross overinflation of both lungs and will be hypoxic with an arterial oxygen saturation of less than 70 mmHg (Fig. 37.2). If moderately unwell the arterial carbon dioxide tension will be low, but if severely obstructed it will be high. Most patients will have a pulsus paradoxicus of greater than 10 mmHg. Continuous nebulization with a beta-sympathomimetic agent using oxygen is essential. Intravenous steroids and aminophylline will have been commenced. If there is inadequate response to this combination the use of intravenous sympathomimetic agents, and occasionally, ventilatory support will be considered.

Episodic and chronic asthma

Patients who are truly episodic have periods when they are totally symptom free. When reviewing children with asthma it is essential to ask for details about their pattern of asthma. Questions must establish whether they have nocturnal cough, whether there is a need for bronchodilators on waking first thing in the morning, the frequency of use of the metered aerosol, and par-

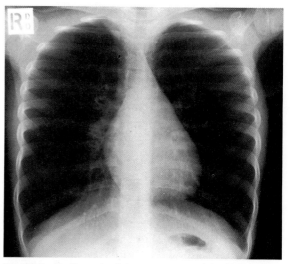

Fig. 37.2 Radiograph of 4-year-old child with severe asthma showing gross overinflation of both lungs, narrow upper mediastinum and flat, depressed diaphragms.

ticipation in sport. If there are truly many weeks where none of these symptoms occur, the pattern is episodic. If there is never more than 1 to 2 weeks free of these symptoms it is chronic. Infrequent episodic asthma can be treated with intermittent courses of bronchodilators as mentioned above. Inhaled sympathomimetic agents will generally be used although slow release theophylline may be helpful for those with nocturnal symptoms.

If the child has frequent episodes with weather change, exercise, allergens and infections which occur for 1 to 2 weeks every month or two, long-term prophylactic therapy is indicated. Sodium cromoglycate in association with intermittent bronchodilators will be the first line of therapy. If this is not adequate a combination of regular sodium cromoglycate and bronchodilators is indicated. Failure to respond, provided there is good compliance and good aerosol technique, warrant the substitution of aerosol corticosteroid for the sodium cromoglycate. Prior to corticosteroids, a short course of oral prednisolone may be necessary to optimize airway function.

Should a child have symptoms most days, a pigeon or barrel chest deformity, a wheeze heard on auscultation when free of overt symptoms and possibly some growth retardation, chronic airways obstruction is highly likely. This needs regular intensive bronchodilator and oral steroid therapy. These children need a clear plan of treatment for failure to respond to regular therapy. They should have advice regarding action to take when their bronchodilator does not last 3 to 4 hours. In some, this may mean an extra dose of oral prednisolone, in others it is important to have a plan for rapid admission to hospital.

Every patient with asthma should have a crisis plan for the occasional situation when a severe episode develops suddenly and does not respond to 1 or 2 doses of inhaled bronchodilator. Such a patient should urgently summon emergency help, usually an ambulance, and continue to take very frequent or continuous bronchodilator until this arrives.

Special problems

Wheezing in infants warrants special consideration as it is a more difficult diagnostic and therapeutic problem. They must be properly evaluated to exclude cystic fibrosis, bronchiolitis or milk inhalation. They are less likely to respond to regular bronchodilator therapy and often require hospitalization for oxygen and intravenous fluids.

Recurrent life-threatening episodes of asthma in children of any age are more frightening and very difficult to treat. Prophylactic therapy in this group is disappointing. Parents should have clear instructions of the approach to take with the first signs or symptoms of asthma. This group of children need a peak flow meter at home to record daily measurements and so recognize early the development of a severe attack.

Most children with asthma will complain of wheeze and tightness in the chest whilst exercising, particularly with vigorous running. Typically the wheeze commences towards the end of the period of exercise, becoming more severe once the child has stopped exercising. With swimming and intermittent sprints, exercise-induced asthma is less likely to occur as it is less likely to involve hyper-ventilation with cold dry air. The child and parents need to be familiar with the problem and have a satisfactory plan of action to prevent this exercise-induced asthma. This may include warm-up exercises and administration of beta-sympathomimetic agent or sodium cromoglycate before exercise. Asthmatic children should be encouraged to participate in sport with adequate control of their asthma.

Conclusion

Asthma is very common in childhood and is usually controllable with safe, effective drug therapy. The natural history of childhood asthma is generally favourable. Management requires co-operation between patient, family, medical and paramedical personnel. With appropriate treatment, the child's asthma can be controlled so that a happy, normal childhood can be lead and adult life reached with no physical or emotional disability. Children with asthma must not smoke otherwise they risk the development of chronic lung disease in adult life.

FURTHER READING

Buchanan N, Van Asperen P 1985 Asthma education for all. Medical Journal of Australia 142: 287–288
Editorial 1986 Acute asthma. Lancet 1: 131–133
Kelly W J W, Hudson I, Phelan P D, Pain M C F, Olinsky A 1987 Childhood asthma in adult life: a further study at 28 years of age. British Medical Journal 294: 1059–1062
Landau L I 1979 Outpatient evaluation and management of asthma. Pediatric Clinics of North America 26: 581–601
Phelan P D, Landau L I, Olinsky A 1989 Respiratory illness in children, 3rd edn. Blackwell, Oxford
Sears M R, Rea H H, Fenwick J et al 1986 Death from asthma in New Zealand. Archives of Diseases in Childhood 61: 6–10
Silverman M 1984 Bronchodilators for wheezy infants? Archives of Diseases in Childhood 59: 84–87
Weinberger M 1988 Corticosteroids for exacerbations of asthma: current status of the controversy. Pediatrics 81: 726

Addendum: Drugs in asthma

Agent		Strength	Recommended dose
(a) Beta-2-sympathomimetics			
Salbutamol (Ventolin)	Metered aerosol	100 μgm/puff	2 puffs up to 3–4 hrly
	Rotahaler	200 μgm/capsule	1 capsule up to 3–4 hrly
	Nebulizer solution	0.5% (5 mg/ml)	0.02–0.03 ml/kg to a maximum of 1 ml up to 3–4 hourly
		or	1 ml diluted in 3 ml saline for 10 min irrespective of age
	Oral syrup	2 ml/5 ml	0.15 mg/kg/dose to a max. of 4 mg every 6 hrs
	Oral tablets	4 mg	1 tablet 6 hrly f > 25 kg
	Injectable	500 μgm/ml	10–20 μgm/kg/dose SC or IM. 5–10 μgm/kg stat IV followed by infusion at 0.1 μgm/kg/min increasing as necessary
Terbutaline (Bricanyl)	Metered aerosol	250 μgm/puff	2 puffs up to 3–4 hrly
	Nebulizer	1% (10 mg/ml)	0.02 ml/kg to max. of 1 ml up to 3–4 hrly
		or	1 ml diluted in 3 ml saline for 10 min irrespective of age
	Oral syrup	0.3 mg/ml	0.075 mg/kg/dose to a max. of 5 mg 6 hrly
	Oral tablets	2.5 mg	1 tablet 6 hrly if > 25 kg.
	Injectable	0.1 mg/ml 0.5 mg/ml	0.005 mg/kg/dose subcutaneously
Fenoterol (Berotec)	Metered aerosol	200 μgm/puff	2 puffs up to 3–4 hrly
	Nebulizer solution	0.1% (1 mg/ml)	0.02 ml/kg dose to a max. of 1 ml 3–4 hrly
		or	1 ml diluted in 3 ml saline for 10 min irrespective of age
	Oral syrup	2.5 mg/5 ml	0.1 mg/kg/dose to a max. of 2.5 mg 6 hrly
	Oral tablets.	2.5 mg	1 tablet 6 hrly if > 25 kg
(b) Theophylline			
Theophylline (Nuelin)	Slow-release tab.	250 mg 500 mg	8–10 mg/kg/12 hrs
	Sprinkles	50 mg 100 mg	8–10 mg/kg/12 hrs
	Syrup	80 mg/15 ml	4–5 mg/kg/6 hrs
Theophylline (Theodur)	Slow release tab.	200 mg 300 mg	8–10 mg/kg/12 hrs
	Sprinkles	125 mg	8–10 mg/kg/12 hrs
Choline theophyllinate (Brondecon)		50 mg/5 ml	7–8 mg/kg/6 hrs
Theophylline (Elixophylline)	80 mg/15 ml	4–5 mg/kg/6 hrs	
Aminophylline (Somophylline)	Oral syrup	105 mg/5 ml	5–6 mg/kg/6 hrs
	Sprinkles	100 mg	8–10 mg/kg/12 hrs
	Injectable	250 mg/5 ml	5–6 mg/kg stat slowly and repeated 6 hrly or constant infusion (0.9 mg/kg/hr)

Addendum: Drugs in asthma (cont'd)

Agent		Strength	Recommended dose
(c) Anticholinergic			
Ipratropium bromide	Metered aerosol	20 µgm/puff	2–4 puffs/dose
(Atrovent)	Nebulizer solution	250 µgm/ml	1 ml in 3 ml saline for 10 min
(d) Disodium cromoglycate			
Intal	Spinhaler	20 mg/capsule	1 capsule 3–4 times/day
	Metered aerosol	1 mg/puff	2–4 puffs 3–4 times/day
	Nebulizer solution	20 mg/2 ml	2 ml 3–4 times daily
(e) Corticosteroids			
Beclomethasone	Metered aerosol	50 µgm/puff	2–6 puffs 2–4 times/puff
(Aldecin, Becotide)		100 µgm/puff	
		250 µgm/puff	
	Rotacaps	100 µgm/capsule	1–2 capsules 2–4 times/day
Prednisolone	Oral tablets	1 mg	Varies
		5 mg	
		25 mg	
Methylprednisolone	Injectable	40 mg/ml	1–2 mg/kg/dose 3–6 hrly
Hydrocortisone	Injectable	100 mg/2 ml	4–5 mg/kg/dose 3–6 hrly
		250 mg/2 ml	

38. The child with a persistent cough

Anthony Olinsky

Cough is a most efficient mechanism for protecting the lungs against the accidental inhalation of particulate and foreign matter and for the removal of excess secretion or exudate. It is the commonest symptom of recurrent and chronic lower respiratory disease in children. The cough reflex is a primitive but very important reflex which developed during the evolution of the lung to protect the respiratory tract from inhalation of food or foreign matter, especially during swallowing. Cilial action is very effective in keeping the airways clean, the mucous sheet being constantly swept up the airways to the glottis and into the pharynx where it is then swallowed. However, if the cilia are injured or destroyed, as frequently occurs in acute and chronic infections of the airways and in asthma or if there is excess secretion, as with infections and asthma then effective coughing becomes very important. Failure to keep the airways clear of secretion or exudate leads to airway obstruction, pulmonary collapse and subsequent infection, with progressive destructive inflammatory changes in the airways and parenchymatous tissue.

Although a cough can be initiated or suppressed voluntarily, it is usually the result of a complex reflex that begins with stimulation of a receptor (afferent component). Impulses from these receptors are conducted to a central area (central co-ordinating cough centre) and then passed down appropriate efferent nervous pathways to the expiratory muscles (efferent component). Coughing consists of an explosive blast or series of blasts of gas expelled at high velocity through the glottis. The normal sequence of events is a deep inspiration followed by a sudden forcible expiration with synchronous closure of the glottis and rapid release of gas by sudden opening of the glottis 0.2 seconds later. An effective cough depends on the integration and normal function of each component of the reflex arc. Sensory neurofibrils, which are situated between the ciliated columnar epithelial cells, occur throughout the airways but are concentrated within the larynx, posterior wall of the trachea and the carinae of the large and medium sized bronchi. They send afferent messages via the vagus to the brain stem and pons. These receptors are sensitive to mechanical stimulation from touch or foreign substances, to irritation from inflammation, to pressure from tumours or glands either within or without the bronchial tree, and to chemical irritation from noxious gases. Cough receptors are not present in alveoli, so that cough may be absent with extensive lobar consolidation.

No specific cough centre has been defined, but a co-ordinating region exists in the upper brain stem and pons. Afferent fibres from the sensitive nerve endings in the larynx and airways are received here and efferent impulses transmitted. Efferent impulses travel via the vagus and spinal nerves from C3 to S2 to the larynx, thoracic muscles, diaphragm, abdominal wall and pelvic floor. During coughing, sudden forcible co-ordinated contraction of these muscles results in rapid elevation of intrathoracic pressure. The larynx is initially closed for 0.2 seconds and then suddenly opens as the pressure in the airways rises. It is important to appreciate that the cough reflex is under voluntary control and may be either inhibited or initiated at will. Voluntary inhibition of coughing may prevent effective clearing of the bronchial tree of excess secretions. Depression of higher centres and of the brain stem, damage to afferent or efferent terminals and weakness of muscles from any cause reduces or abolishes the cough reflex. In any of these situations pulmonary infection occurs and is often persistent.

This chapter is concerned with the approach to diagnosis and management of the child with a persistent cough. Cough of recent onset is discussed in Chapter 35. Not infrequently parents will state that their child has a persistent cough when, in fact, there are significant periods of time when the cough is absent. It is important that this point is clearly established, as the diagnosis, management and prognosis of recurrent cough is different from that of chronic or persistent cough.

APPROACH TO DIAGNOSIS

In diagnosis, the history must establish the fact that the cough is continuous and has been present for weeks at least. In many instances the cough may have been present for months or even years. The type of cough – whether dry or productive must be noted. One can only be certain of this point by hearing the child cough, as parents are not always aware of the distinction. A dry, barking cough is suggestive of pathology in the trachea. Paroxysmal coughing is characteristic of pertussis but is also seen in *Mycoplasma* and *Chlamydia* infections as well as some children with cystic fibrosis. A bizarre, loud, honking cough is usually of psychogenic origin. All children with a persistent loose cough should be postured to see if they can produce sputum. The type and amount of sputum produced must be noted. Clear mucoid sputum is suggestive that allergy is the basis whereas yellow or green sputum containing polymorphonuclear cells on microscopic examination usually indicates infection is present. A history of haemoptysis, although uncommon in childhood, must always be sought. Sputum streaked with blood is sometimes seen in chronic suppurative lung disease. The age of onset of the cough may be helpful in diagnosis; cough commencing early in infancy is suggestive of an underlying congenital lesion, or raises the possibility that the infant may be inhaling milk due to feeding difficulties. All infants who have a persistent cough should be observed feeding. Persistent cough in the toddler age group should suggest the possiblity of an inhaled foreign body, lung collapse or cystic fibrosis. In the young school child asthma is a frequent cause whereas the adolescent who develops a recurrent or persistent cough should be suspected of smoking. A family history of allergy, tuberculosis or cystic fibrosis may be significant and a similar cough in a sibling or close relative may suggest the diagnosis.

On physical examination particular attention must be paid to the growth of the child. Failure of growth in chronic chest disease is related either to chronic suppuration, chronic hypoxia or both. Growth failure is common in bronchiectasis and severe asthma. Finger clubbing in childhood bronchiectasis is uncommon and its presence should alert one to the possibility of cystic fibrosis. Chest deformity, such as barrel chest or a pigeon deformity (pectus carinatum), if present, will also suggest a long-standing lesion as the cause of persistent cough. Examination of the chest will usually enable one to establish whether the disease is generalized or localized. Generalized chest disease, as manifest by the presence of widespread physical signs, is more consistent with a diagnosis of cystic fibrosis, bronchitis or

asthma. Physical signs localized to areas of dependent drainage are suggestive of bronchiectasis or of pulmonary collapse. The presence of wheeze should be noted and although this does not have diagnostic implications, it certainly implies airway obstruction. Stridor in association with persistent cough is much more suggestive of obstruction to the upper airways, usually by a mass lesion.

When a carefully obtained history and physical examination does not lead to a specific diagnosis, supplementary laboratory investigations are then considered. A chest radiograph is almost always indicated in a child with chronic cough. If inhalation of foreign body is suspected, inspiratory and expiratory films are warranted. A barium swallow may be indicated for evidence of inhalation or extrinsic pressure from a mediastinal mass. A lateral neck film may also be useful with a tracheal cough. Sputum examination, although helpful in management, is not of great value in diagnosis except where tuberculosis is suspected. All children with a persistent cough require a Mantoux test. In the child in whom allergy is suspected, examination of the nasal mucus for the presence of eosinophils and mast cells may be helpful.

Pulmonary function tests

Pulmonary function tests are useful in older children to:

1. Provide objective evidence of disease.
2. Provide objective measurement of severity where the clinical history and physical examination do not agree.
3. Document progress in chronic conditions such as cystic fibrosis.
4. Document response to treatment regimens such as steroids in asthma or fibrosing alveolitis.
5. Provide objective measurements with which to compare one's clinical assessment and so improve clinical skills.

For non-variable, chronic conditions such as cystic fibrosis, a single lung function test performed every few months will be a useful measurement of clinical progress. For a variable condition such as asthma, a single test may help indicate severity but daily measurements will more accurately describe the pattern of disease.

The use of lung function tests is limited by the age of the child as forced expiratory manoeuvres cannot be performed accurately under the age of 6–8 years. For lung function tests to be reliable it is essential to have a co-operative child, reliable equipment, adequate instruction to the child and reproducibility of measurements.

Those tests commonly performed include:

1. Peak expiratory flow rate. Peak expiratory flow rate is measured after filling the lungs to maximum capacity and blowing as hard as possible into a peak flow meter. This is a simple, reproducible test requiring inexpensive equipment. It can be performed in a laboratory, in a doctor's surgery, or at home. This test is most useful for conditions such as asthma which require repeated measurements.

2. Spirometry. A spirometer is a more expensive piece of equipment which provides a volume-time plot of a forced expiration. The child takes in a maximum breath and then expires from full inspiration to full expiration. The spirometric trace will indicate whether the underlying condition is obstructive or restrictive, the degree of obstruction and the presence of small airway disease.

The volume from maximum inspiration to maximum expiration is the forced vital capacity (FVC) and the normal range is between 80% and 120% predicted for height and sex. The FVC is reduced in obstructive and restrictive lung disease. In obstructive lung diseases the reduction is because of early airway closure. In restrictive lung diseases the primary pathology causes restriction of lung or chest wall expansion.

Forced expiratory volume in 1 second (FEV_1) is the volume exhaled from maximum inspiration in the first second. The normal value is 80–120% predicted for height and sex. At least 75–80% of the FVC should be exhaled in the first second so that the normal FEV_1/FVC is greater than 75–80%. The FEV_1 is reduced in airway narrowing. FEF_{25-75} is the forced expiratory flow between 25% and 75% of the vital capacity. It is a more sensitive measure of airway obstruction and may be decreased when FEV_1 is normal. It is calculated by drawing a line between 25% and 75% of the vital capacity exhalation trace on the spirometer. The slope of this line is the mean flow in that range. A normal child should have a FEF_{25-75} between 67% and 133% predicted normal for height and sex.

A diagnosis of asthma will require evaluation of a response to bronchodilator if airway obstruction is present. An increase in FEV_1 of 20% is considered significant and evidence of asthma. However, asthma can be episodic and a child may have normal lung function at the time of testing. If the diagnosis is in doubt, increased bronchoreactivity can be demonstrated by seeking a fall in FEV_1 in response to exercise or an inhalation challenge with histamine aerosol, methacholine aerosol or cold dry air.

Blood gas measurements are the most appropriate tests to perform in the acutely ill patient. Arterial pO_2, pH and pCO_2 can be measured in samples taken from the brachial or radial arteries or occasionally the femoral artery. Oximetry and transcutaneous oxygen electrodes can provide a non-invasive measurement of oxygenation. A capillary sample will provide an accurate measurement of pH, bicarbonate and pCO_2 but not pO_2.

Hypoxia is present with a pO_2 below 75 mmHg. The hypoxia may be due to hypoventilation, when it will be accompanied by an elevated pCO_2. The hypoxia may be due to an anatomical shunt and in this situation there will be no increase in pO_2 when breathing 100% oxygen. The most common cause of hypoxia is ventilation-perfusion imbalance.

It is more difficult to use a specific value of pCO_2 as indicative of respiratory failure in children as pCO_2 rises more readily due to the smaller airways, lack of collateral ventilation and weak chest wall. A diagnosis of respiratory failure will be made on a combination of clinical status and blood gas measurement. The level of bicarbonate will help indicate whether the elevated pCO_2 is acute or chronic. With chronic CO_2 retention, the bicarbonate level will be increased in an attempt to compensate for the respiratory acidosis.

Other investigations

The majority of children with a persistent cough can be diagnosed and managed by the techniques described above. Bronchoscopy, bronchography and angiography may be necessary on rare occasions. It should be emphasized that the majority of cases of bronchiectasis can be diagnosed without these techniques. Should asthma be suspected, but the typical signs be absent, lung function studies may be helpful in establishing bronchial hyperreactivity – the basis of asthma. Occasionally skin testing is performed on a child suspected of allergy, but interpretation can be difficult and hence such tests should be viewed with caution.

On occasions persistent cough in association with a chronic chest lesion will remain undiagnosed despite the methods outlined above. Immunological function tests and lung biopsy may be indicated in these children.

CAUSES OF PERSISTENT COUGH

Persistent cough in childhood results from persisting infection, allergy, from a pathological lesion compressing of infiltrating the bronchial tree and as the result of a psychogenic disturbance. Not infrequently a secondary cause is superimposed on the primary cause, for example, infection may be superimposed on either a primary allergic disorder or following airways obstruction from any cause. The more important causes are listed in Example 38.1.

Example 38.1 Causes of persistent or recurrent cough

Bronchitis
   Viral bronchitis – subsequent collapse
   Chemical – milk inhalation, smoking
   Secondary bacterial bronchitis
   Bronchitis in disadvantaged children associated with chronic upper respiratory infection

Asthma

Specific infections
   Pertussis
   Mycoplasma pneumoniae infection
   Tuberculosis

Suppurative lung disease
   Cystic fibrosis
   Bronchiectasis
   Secondary infection of collapsed lobe, cyst or retained foreign body

Focal lesions
   Foreign body
   Mediastinal or pulmonary tumours, cysts, glands
   Tracheomalacia

Nervous or psychogenic cough

Reflex cough

Infection

Primary

Occasionally the nature of the infecting organism is the basis of a persistent cough, for example, pertussis, which may persist for many months; *Mycoplasma* infections may behave similarly. These disorders have been discussed in Chapter 35. Some children suffer a persistent low grade bronchitis of varying but often unknown aetiology. More frequently the pattern is one of recurrent bouts of cough with wheeze and fever; attacks may take weeks to subside but recurrences occur very frequently. In most cases the aetiology is viral often with superimposed secondary bacterial infection. In areas where living standards are poor and medical care suboptimal, a number of these children progress to chronic suppuration and bronchiectasis. Tuberculosis in childhood is rarely associated with persistence of cough unless bronchial compression by enlarged hilar lymph nodes occurs.

Secondary

Persistent pulmonary infection is far more often secondary and the result of pathology within the airways whereby the normal process of drainage is compromised, secretions accumulate, infection flourishes and a persistent cough associated with other features of lung suppuration follows. The pathological process may initially involve the mucosa with consequent impairment of cilial activity, the bronchial lumen may be partially or completely obstructed and ultimately the entire bronchial wall may be involved.

There are a number of disorders in children where persisting infection is the result of some mechanical disturbance to lung drainage. These may be generalized or localized, congenital or acquired.

Congenital lesions

Cystic fibrosis

Cystic fibrosis is the commonest of all inherited disorders with an incidence of 1 in 2500 live births. The modes of presentation (Fig. 38.1) are as follows:

1. In the neonatal period, with intestinal obstruction – meconium ileus. This is due to accumulation of tenacious meconium in the large bowel, the result of pancreatic achylia.

2. With recurrent or persisting cough often associated with wheeze and frequently commencing in early infancy.

3. With manifestations of malabsorption – large, pale, bulky and offensive stools.

4. Because of failure to thrive, the result both of persistent chest infection and malabsorption.

5. Occasionally the mode of presentation is because of rectal prolapse and, rarely, through heat stroke.

6. A number of cases are identified because of disease in a sibling i.e. routine sweat testing of siblings. However, it is now also possible to diagnose cystic fibrosis antenatally by 2 methods in situations where parents have had a previously affected child. One method is by measuring a group of microvillar enzymes in amniotic fluid taken during the second trimester. The second and better method is chorionic villus biopsy. In this test DNA markers to the cystic fibrosis gene are sought. The cystic fibrosis gene has been localized to somewhere on the long arm of chromosome 7. This test can be done in the first trimester of pregnancy but it is important to first test the parents and affected child for these DNA markers.

7. As part of a neonatal screening programme – measurement of immunoreactive trypsin (IRT) in a blood sample.

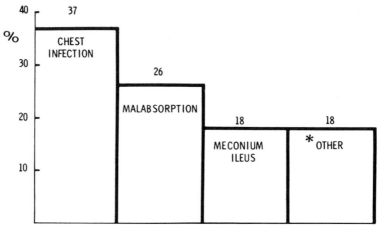

Fig. 38.1 Modes of presentation of patients with cystic fibrosis.

Lower airways obstruction constitutes the pathology of cystic fibrosis. This was formerly attributed to tenacious and sticky mucus, but is now regarded as the result of persisting infection. In addition to the persistent cough, recurrent episodes of acute chest infection occur and general health is poor. The chest is clinically and radiologically overexpanded; other physical and radiological signs will depend on the stage at which the child is seen. (Fig. 38.2a and b). Finger clubbing occurs early.

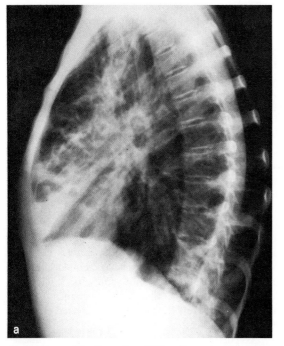
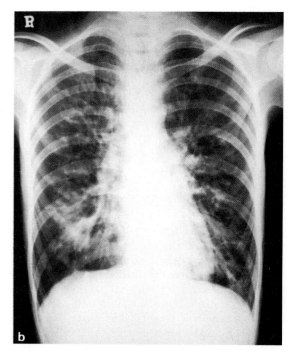

Fig. 38.2 a and **b** Lateral and PA radiographs of the chest of a child with cystic fibrosis. Note gross emphysema and the involvement of both lungs with cystic dilatation of bronchi.

The diagnosis will be delayed unless a high suspicion of cystic fibrosis is present. Should there be any doubt a sweat test should be performed. In cystic fibrosis the sweat chloride level is in excess of 60 mmol/litre. It is important to emphasize that the sweat test should be performed by the technique of pilocarpine iontophoresis and should only be done in centres experienced in the technique. Accuracy is essential; the consequences of an incorrect result should be very obvious.

In management, infections should be treated early and vigorously with appropriate chemotherapy. Most chest infections are the result of *Staphylococcus aureus*, but *Pseudomonas aeruginosa* is now frequently causative. Physiotherapy should be commenced early in life and regularly maintained. Malabsorption will require pancreatic enzyme replacement. At times special dietary therapy is indicated – particularly when growth is unsatisfactory. In the hot weather attention to fluid and salt intake is essential.

Cystic fibrosis is occasionally complicated by diabetes mellitus and liver disease. Men are infertile because of absence of the epididymis and vas deferens. Most females are fertile but pregnancy may be inadvisable for many. Progressive suppurative lung disease, pulmonary fibrosis and right heart failure is the commonest mode of death.

At present it is possible to keep many of these children well and the majority survive into early adult life with little disability. However, the treatment programme is very demanding on both the child and the family. The basic defect in cystic fibrosis remains to be identified. It is not yet possible to detect the carrier state nor is curative therapy possible.

Tracheomalacia

In this disorder the cartilage of the trachea is deficient. The deficiency may be localized or generalized. Most commonly tracheomalacia is associated with oesophageal atresia and tracheo-oesophageal fistula when the lesion is a localized one. These children present with a characteristic barking cough. Localized tracheomalacia may also be the result of external compression from a vascular ring. In tracheomalacia, the trachea collapses when pleural pressure is increased by coughing so that the cough is ineffective in removing secretions and infection is an ever present risk. Should this result in small airways obstruction, pleural pressure will further increase and in the more severe case, episodes of cyanosis occur. The diagnosis of tracheomalacia is established at bronchoscopy when the trachea is found to collapse during expiration.

Bronchial cysts

These are uncommon lesions but if communication with a bronchus is present, infection will inevitably result. Such children will present with a persistent productive cough and signs of chest infection. The diagnosis will be established by bronchography performed because of persistent cough and unresolved chest infection. Treatment involves surgical resection. A number of varieties of bronchial cysts exist.

Sequestrated lung

This is an uncommon developmental anomaly in which an area of lung tissue has no bronchial connection and it is not supplied by a bronchial artery. Ultimately communication with the normal lung via alveoli occurs and infection rapidly ensues resulting in persisting infection; this manifests as an unresolved pneumonia. However, cough may be minimal, the child presenting as fever of unknown cause. Sequestration is suspected should a chest radiograph reveal a persistent cystic lesion, particularly one posterior to the cardiac shadow. The bronchogram will indicate that the lesion is separate from the normal lung and without bronchial connections. Surgical resection is indicated.

Acquired lesions

Bronchiectasis

This disorder should be regarded as an end result of a number of different pathological processes. When fully established, the clinical features consist of persistent cough, purulent sputum, recurrent acute episodes of chest infection and poor general health with growth failure. Finger clubbing is uncommon in childhood bronchiectasis. It appears to be a disorder associated with poor nutrition, poor standards of living and substandard medical care. While this disorder is still prevalent in developing countries, the incidence has greatly diminished in countries where living standards and medical care are high.

Bronchiectasis may occasionally follow a severe chest infection that never completely resolves, e.g. severe bronchopneumonia, pertussis or following severe measles. Most cases, however, arise insidiously and parents are unable to date the onset of the cough. Bronchiectasis may at times be localized, for example, following an unrecognized inhaled foreign body, or as the result of a congenital or acquired bronchial stricture. It is important to recognize this group, as removal of a foreign body may result in reversal of the bronchiectasis.

In all types of bronchiectasis there is a history of a persistent cough often from early infancy. The sputum is yellow or green and may vary in amounts up to a cupful or more per day. Symptomatic bronchiectasis always involves the dependent areas of the lung, namely both lower lobes, the right middle lobe and the lingular segment of the left upper lobe where drainage is against gravity. Because of pooling of secretions, chronic infection with recurrent acute exacerbations of pneumonia is the rule. In the severe and poorly managed case, lung abscess, haemoptyses, empyema and pulmonary fibrosis are frequent complications. On physical examination, in the uncomplicated case physical signs are found over the dependent areas of drainage and consist of fine crepitations (crackles) brought out by coughing. Wheeze is not frequently present; other physical signs will depend on the presence of complications.

The chest radiograph in the early case will show only an accentuation of lung markings over the affected areas. Later, areas of lobular or segmental pulmonary collapse may be noted. The bronchogram in the early stages shows defective bronchial branching, defective filling of peripheral bronchi and poor alveolar filling. Later in the disorder bronchial dilatation will be obvious.

It appears that recurrent viral and bacterial infection of the smaller bronchi is the initial lesion in bronchiectasis. In the dependent lobes drainage is poor so that continued infection with damage to the bronchial wall and ultimate dilatation result.

Most cases of bronchiectasis involve most or all of the dependent lobes. Management consequently involves control of infection with chemotherapy, postural drainage under supervision and attention to general health. Surgery is reserved for cases of localized bronchiectasis, for the child who produces large amounts of foul sputum, or in whom lung abscess, severe haemoptysis, bronchopleural fistula or empyema complicate. Most children with bronchiectasis can be kept in good health and the symptoms controlled with the measures outlined above. Many who are well controlled in childhood become symptomless in adult life despite the persistence of bronchiectasis as demonstrated bronchographically. Very few should develop complications with present-day treatment.

Pulmonary collapse

This is a frequent complication of respiratory infection in childhood and a very common cause of persistent cough. Failure to recognize the presence of a pulmonary collapse may result in progressive suppuration and bronchiectasis in the affected area. The symptoms of pulmonary collapse are persistent cough which rapidly becomes productive and signs of toxaemia – fever, anorexia and weight loss. Physical signs within the chest will depend on the extent of the collapse but unless it is large they will usually only consist of fine crepitations over the affected area brought out by coughing. A chest radiograph will always be necessary to confirm the diagnosis (Fig. 38.3a and b).

Pulmonary collapse may follow the inhalation of a foreign body, from obstruction due to mucus and exudate as in pneumonia and in asthma, or from pressure on a bronchus from any cause. Management involves control of infection with appropriate chemotherapy after sputum culture, suitable postural drainage and physiotherapy, together with an intensive search for the precipitating cause. Bronchoscopy will be indicated if a foreign body is suspected but as a rule it is not helpful, and most cases will re-expand with the measures outlined.

Inhalation

The possibility of inhalation of milk should always be considered in the infant with a persistent cough and wheeze. This situation is particularly likely to occur in the infant with sucking and swallowing difficulties (e.g. due to congenital anomalies of mouth, tongue, pharynx) and in the brain-damaged infant. Inhalation is also seen in association with gastro-oesophageal reflux (Fig. 38.4). This diagnosis will be suspected if, while watching the infant feeding, cough or resistance is noted in addition to the wheeze and persistent cough which characterizes this disorder. The radiological signs depend on the severity and duration of the inhalation. The distribution of the lesions relate to the position in which the child feeds. If the child is fed in recumbancy the upper lobes are involved; if in the upright position the dependent lobes will be involved.

The diagnosis of inhalation is suggested by the finding of fat-laden macrophages in the tracheal aspirate. Their absence does not exclude the diagnosis. Tracheal aspirate is performed at direct laryngoscopy without anaesthesia. The secretions are fixed with formalin and stained with Fetrot when the fat will be readily demonstrated. Management of this conditon in the first instance implies management of the underlying cause. Careful techniques of feeding must be taught and the infant kept in the upright position if gastro-oesophageal reflux is present. Chemotherapy or bronchodilators have no place in the management. In the infant with persistent inhalation from gasto-oesophageal reflux and who fails to thrive, surgery – fundoplication – should be considered.

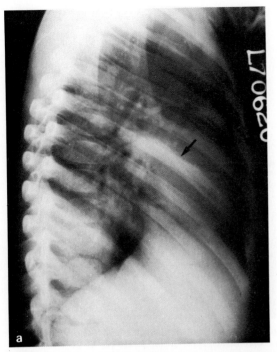 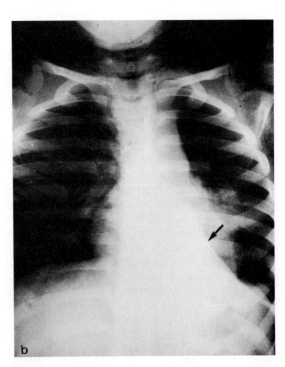

Fig. 38.3 a and **b** Chest radiographs (lateral and PA) demonstrating collapse of the left lower lobe and lingula. Note the opacity over the lower thoracic vertebrae in the lateral view.

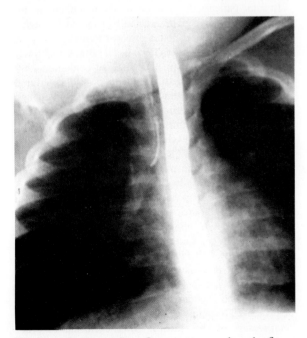

Fig. 38.4 Barium swallow. Gross gastro-oesophageal reflux was demonstrated during screening. Note the fine line of barium adjacent to the oesophagus. This is barium which has been aspirated into the trachea.

Immotile cilia syndrome

This is a rare disorder in which there is a defect in the ultrastructure of the cilia. This results in ineffective clearing of mucus and consequently chest infection. It is recessively inherited and in the fully expressed form the clinical features include (a) situs inversus, (b) chronic chest infection, (c) sinusitis, and constitute the Kartagener triad.

The diagnosis is established by examination of cilia under electron microscopy. Immotile but live spermatozoa are present in the ejaculate.

Immunodeficiency

Recurrent infection in infancy characterizes primary immunodeficiency (see Ch. 22). The immunological status of a child may also be compromised by cytotoxic drugs and steroids. Both groups of children are particularly susceptible to persistent chest infection. No constant pattern of infection exists so that the index of suspicion must be high. A diffuse pulmonary infiltration, seen on the chest radiograph, which responds poorly to treatment, together with a clinical history of recurrent infections of any type are indications for investigation for immunodeficiency. Children receiving immunosuppressive or cytotoxic drugs must be carefully observed should a cough develop. Management is usually very difficult because of the problems associated with the underlying immunodeficiency. However, in sex-linked agammaglobulinaemia, monthly injections of gammaglobulin are usually very helpful.

Asthma as the basis for persistent cough

There is usually no difficulty in establishing the presence of asthma as there will usually be a history of recurrent wheezing, other manifestations of allergy, such as rhinitis or atopic dermatitis, and a positive family history. Occasionally this history is not volunteered and the child presents simply because of a persistent cough. On questioning it will be found that the cough is non-productive, occurs almost entirely when the child is in bed, although it may be brought on by exercise. This cough is usually loud, often described as barking, frequently paroxysmal and at times associated with vomiting. The child is not constitutionally disturbed and physical and radiological examination of the chest is clear. Little relief is obtained from chemotherapy or various cough suppressants. It is inferred that asthma is the basis for this cough, as many, but by no means all of these children later develop wheezing. The wheeze can frequently be brought out by exercise or pulmonary tests that assess airway hyper-activity. Also a number have a definite allergic rhinitis and some past history of atopic dermatitis. In addition, there is frequently a family history of allergy. Radiology of the chest is only occasionally helpful (Fig. 38.5).

Treatment of this cough is difficult. Many of these children are relieved by propping them up in bed at night. Most, but not all gain relief from bronchodilators, e.g. sympathomimetics and/or the methyl xanthine drugs.

Emotional disturbance and persistent cough

Persistent cough is occasionally the mode of presentation of an emotional disorder. There are two main features in children who are brought to the doctor with a so-called nervous or psychogenic cough. Firstly, there is a great deal of either overt or covert anxiety by the parents concerning the child's cough and, secondly, there is no evidence of underlying respiratory disease. It should be remembered that it is the mother who almost always reports, and not infrequently interprets the child's symptoms. It is, therefore, essential to find out what she believes is the cause of the cough and why she has brought the child for consultation.

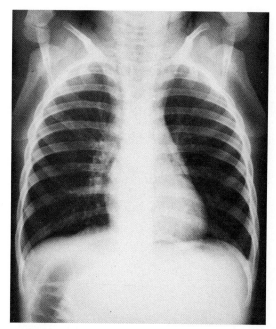

Fig. 38.5   Radiograph of chest. Note chest is hyperinflated, ribs horizontal and diaphragm depressed. There is surgical and mediastinal emphysema present. Diagnosis – asthma.

In some patients the cough is similar to a habit spasm, the child frequently giving a series of short, dry coughs, particularly if his attention is directed to his cough. The cough often develops following an attack of lower respiratory infection, yet long after all evidence of inflammation has subsided, the child is still coughing. Often the child's attention has been drawn to the cough by a repeated comment either during or when he is recovering from the infection, and this often causes a vicious cycle. This cycle will frequently be revealed during consultation. The child may give a little dry cough whereupon the parents will exclaim 'there it is doctor' or 'just listen to that'.

Another type of psychogenic cough is seen in children and adolescents, particularly girls. It is an explosive, foghorn, bark-like, honking cough repeated frequently while the child is awake, but absent during sleep. Clinical and laboratory findings are negative and medications ineffective. It may have started with a respiratory tract infection, but goes on for weeks or months. Psychological stress such as school phobia or family tension may be present. The cough is probably produced by dynamic compression of the trachea. After exclusion of other conditions, the cough is treated by suggestion and reassurance, and assistance in correcting the psychological stress.

Smoking

In the older child and particularly in the adolescent, smoking should always be considered as a possible cause for a persistent cough. This can be obvious at times from the patient's breath or from nicotine staining of the fingers. On the other hand, it may be necessary to inquire directly from the patient in private about smoking habits. The smoker's cough tends to be dry, short and persistent. Smoking, of course, will significantly aggravate all chest disease, but particularly suppurative lung disease. It is, therefore, of the utmost importance that children who have chronic chest disease are adequately informed from an early age of the dangers of smoking. If this advice is frequently reinforced and if the parents do not smoke, children with chronic chest disease avoid smoking.

Miscellaneous causes of persistent cough

A persistent cough is seen in many retarded chidren, particularly those who are debilitated and confined to bed. It is also a feature of certain muscular dystrophies and in poliomyelitis and polyneuritis when the resporatory mucles are involved. In these disorders the cough reflex is disturbed so that, although it is persistent, it is weak and ineffective. It is for this reason that chest infections so frequently prove fatal in those children. Thus the recognition of even a poor and ineffectual cough in these situations is of great importance. Management will of course depend upon the nature of the underlying lesion but it is often very difficult.

Management

Correct treatment of a persistent cough is impossible until its aetiology is determined. The indiscriminate use of antibiotics is to be condemned on a number of grounds. In the first instance infection is by no means always the cause and, even when present, it may not be bacterial.

Treatment of cough depends on determining the underlying cause and initiating specific therapy for that disorder. Cough is usually a protective mechanism for the clearing of excess secretions and only when the cough performs no useful function or its complications represent a significant hazard should symptomatic treatment be considered.

The two main groups of non-specific drugs used are cough suppressants and expectorants and mucolytic agents. Very few well designed and well controlled studies of their value have been reported. The suppression of coughing is clearly contraindicated in the presence of suppurative lung disease or other conditions in which the production of sputum is increased. However, such pharmacological agents may be indicated when the cough is dry and irritative, when it is keeping the child awake at night, or is very distressing, as in older children with pertussis. Most cough suppressants act by depressing the central component of the cough reflex. Therein lies their major disadvantage, since in addition to suppressing the cough centre, they act as general depressants on the central nervous system and may even depress respiration. More importantly, none of the cough suppressants presently available are particularly effective. Narcotics such as codeine are widely used. Pholcodine has a stronger action than codeine in suppressing cough and has less potential for addition and depression of the central nervous system. Non-narcotic cough suppressants are not particularly effective. Many available in combination 'cough preparations' have not been studied objectively. Some mixtures contain a cough suppressant and expectorant, which is quite illogical. Sympathomimetics, when used as bronchodilators in asthma are effective.

Expectorants and mucolytic agents are purported to increase the output and alter the composition of respiratory secretions. With the exception of hydration, there are no expectorants that are effective and free of side effects. Although N-acetyl-cysteine (Mucomyst) and bromhexine (Bisolvon) have been found to alter favourably the rheological properties of sputum in vitro, it has been extremely difficult to show any objective improvement in clinical trials. Sympathomimetic agents (e.g. salbutamol) stimulate mucociliary transport in normal subjects as well as in those individuals with bronchial asthma, chronic bronchitis and cystic fibrosis. However, research is required to see whether these drugs may prove valuable in conditions other than asthma.

In summary, antitussive medications have a very limited place in paediatric practice. Occasionally the use of a cough suppressant such as pholcodine may be of benefit, particularly if the cough is dry and irritative but only after the physician has determined that the cough is serving no useful physiological purpose or if specific therapy is going to take some time to be effective.

PULMONARY TUBERCULOSIS

Tuberculosis has infected mankind for many centuries. In 1882, Robert Koch isolated the tubercle bacillus and demonstrated tuberculosis to be infective. The clinical disease is a manifestation of the interaction between the organism *Mycobacterium tuberculosis*, and the host. Infection occurs when the tubercle bacillus is present without symptoms and is usually recognized as a positive tuberculin test without clinical or radiological features. Tuberculous disease may occur weeks or years after infection, but the risk is greatest in the first one to two years after infection. About 5–15% of those infected will develop tuberculous disease. While the risk for developing tuberculous disease in the newly infected individual is highest in the first one to two years after acquiring infection, an untreated infected person carries the risk for tuberculous disease for a lifetime. Tuberculosis is as much a social disease as an infective disease, as the mortality decreases considerably with improved social conditions.

Tuberculous disease usually starts by inhalation of tubercle bacillus which multiply at the site of infection. This is often sub-pleural and is accompanied by a lymph node response, so producing the primary complex. Four to eight weeks after infection the body is sensitized to tuberculo-protein and a cell-mediated immune response will produce a positive tuberculin skin test. Approximately 1.5% of children in the State of Victoria are positive reactors at 14 years of age. Uncommonly, this sensitization to tuberculo-protein may be associated with fever, erythema nodosum or phlyctenular conjunctivitis.

This primary focus usually heals but occasionally the lesion may progress.

1. Caseation may occur with extensive lung destruction.
2. The lymph nodes may enlarge causing, initially, ball-valve obstruction and then atelectasis.
3. Rupture of the node into the bronchus may cause tuberculous bronchopneumonia. The lung pathology is a combination of infection and an allergic response to the tuberculo-protein.
4. Effusions may occur in the pleura or pericardium.
5. Haematogenous spread may occur producing miliary tuberculosis or tuberculous meningitis.

Tuberculosis is spread by droplets from adults with open tuberculosis. Children with primary tuberculosis are not infectious.

The primary focus is usually asymptomatic. However, enlargement of the nodes may produce cough or wheeze. Tuberculosis should be considered in any child with:

1. Persistent cough
2. Persistent chest radiographic changes (Fig. 38.6).
3. Enlarged mediastinal or hilar lymph nodes
4. Meningitis with a subacute onset
5. Vomiting as a prominent symptom
6. Non-specific illness especially if the child has had recent contact with overseas visitors.

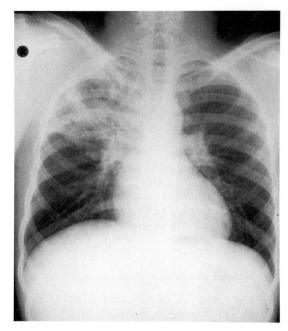

Fig. 38.6 Chest radiograph demonstrating consolidation of the right upper lobe. This child had a strongly positive Mantoux test. Diagnosis – primary pulmonary tuberculosis.

Diagnosis

1. Positive tuberculin skin test. Ten units of purified protein derivative (PPD) in 0.1 ml is injected intradermally, the usual site being the volar aspect of the forearm. The reaction is read 48–72 hours after the injection and is recorded as diameter of induration in mm measured transversely to the long axis of the forearm. Induration of 10 mm or greater is regarded as a positive reaction. Erythema without induration is often difficult to interpret but is not generally considered evidence of tuberculous infection. False negatives occur with advanced disease in malnourished children, in the early weeks of infection, or occasionally in anergic patients.
2. Early morning gastric lavage will provide material for culture of the organism. Tubercle bacilli usually accumulate in the stomach over-night and significant numbers will be available for culture if a secondary lesion is present.
3. Tubercle bacilli may also be seen by smear and culture from pleural fluid of cerebrospinal fluid.

Treatment

Treatment will depend on the extent of the disease. A

positive skin test without any clinical signs or radiological abnormalities is indicative of infection and is treated with chemoprophylaxis using daily isoniazid for 12 months. This treatment will significantly reduce the risk of subsequent disease. The risk of hepatitis from isoniazid is very low in children and peripheral neuropathy is not seen.

Disease with radiographic features of a primary complex is treated with a combination of isoniazid and rifampicin for 6–12 months. Extensive tuberculous disease is treated with triple drug therapy using a combination of isoniazid, rifampicin and pyrazinamide, or ethionamide. Ethambutol is usually not used until the child is old enough to have vision checked. Steroids are sometimes used in children with extensive collapse of the lung and complicated tuberculous meningitis. The Health Department must be notified of all cases in order to commence surveillance to find the source and identify infection in contacts. Once treatment has begun resolution is slow, taking 4–6 months.

Management

The major objective in management should be prevention of tuberculosis. Social factors are of prime importance with this condition and improved social circumstances will lead to reduction in the prevalence of infection and the severity of disease. All immigrants from high endemic areas should be screened for tuberculosis. There is considerable controversy regarding the role of BCG (attenuated strain of the bacillus of Calmette and Guerin). BCG certainly limits the spread on exposure as evidenced by the reduction in tuberculous meningitis in endemic countries. The efficacy has been reported as varying from 0–80%. At present, indications for BCG immunization include all children in communities with high endemic rates of tuberculosis, at-risk groups such as health care workers in any cmmunity, and children exposed to adults with tuberculosis. Following BCG, a 5–10 mm response to tuberculin skin testing is normal. A response of greater than 15 mm should be considered as possible evidence of tuberculous infection.

FURTHER READING

Bramen S S, Corrao W M 1987 Cough: differential diagnosis and treatment. Clinics in Chest Medicine 8: 177–188

Mellis C M 1979 Evaluation and treatment of chronic cough in children. The Pediatric Clinics of North America 26(3): 533–564

Miller F J W 1982 Tuberculosis in children. Churchill Livingstone, Edinburgh

Phelan P D, Landau L I, Olinsky A 1982 Respiratory illness in children, 2nd edn. Blackwell Scientific Publications, Oxford

Cardiac disorders

39. Heart disease in infancy and childhood

A. W. Venables

HEART MURMURS

Physical examination of the cardiovascular system in infancy and childhood does not differ essentially from that in adults, but there are certain aspects that should be highlighted. Auscultation of the heart is of particular importance as the majority of heart disorders in childhood are the result of a structural abnormality, when murmurs are usually present. In most cases of congenital heart disease a heart murmur is heard either on routine examination or in association with symptoms referable to the cardiovascular system.

Murmurs can be graded conveniently in four grades according to their loudness:

Grade 1 – soft
Grade 2 – moderately loud
Grade 3 – loud
Grade 4 – very loud

This is a subjective classification requiring experience for its application. Murmurs are often classified louder than appropriate because of inexperience or because the child is seen when the loudness of the murmur is actually increased by increased cardiac output due to fever.

Ejection murmurs

These are the result of turbulence created by flow out of the heart into the great vessels and are crescendo-decrescendo in character. The length of the murmur varies with the length of the ejection period. Normally ejection murmurs are heard maximally at the base of the heart and radiate cranially. The commonest examples are the murmurs of pulmonary and aortic stenosis. When the stenosis is at valvar level, there will also usually be an early systolic sound known as an ejection sound which helps to identify the nature of the murmur.

Regurgitant murmurs

These are caused by the flow from a high pressure to a low pressure area and are normally pansystolic. They are the murmurs of atrioventricular valve incompetence and of ventricular septal defect. At times it may be difficult to distinguish an ejection murmur from a regurgitant murmur, e.g. in atypical mitral incompetence, subaortic stenosis, infundibular stenosis, and in certain varieties of ventricular septal defect. The site of maximum intensity and radiation are ordinarily helpful in differentiation. Most regurgitant murmurs are heard best away from the base of the heart but this rule does not always apply.

Continuous murmurs

These are the result of turbulence arising from one source and continuing from systole through the second sound into diastole. They are heard in association with a patent ductus, aortopulmonary collateral arteries, arteriovenous fistulae, and in the venous hum.

To and fro murmurs

These are biphasic. There may be a gap between the two elements. The classical to and fro murmur is that of combined aortic stenosis and incompetence.

Diastolic murmurs

These may be short or long. They are usually classified as early or mid diastolic according to their time of onset. The early diastolic murmur (EDM) commences immediately or soon after the relevant component of the second heart sound and is characteristic of aortic and pulmonary incompetence. The mid-diastolic murmur (MDM) commences with opening of the mitral or tricuspid valve and represents flow into the ventricle.

Atrial contraction may produce a late diastolic or presystolic murmur characteristic of mitral stenosis with sinus rhythm.

Innocent murmurs

There are four types of innocent murmur:

1. The short systolic murmur best heard along the left sternal edge and usually maximal at the third to fourth intercostal space, with a characteristic high-pitched rasping, honking or vibratory quality, often called the innocent musical murmur. It is recognized particularly by this quality.

2. A soft murmur maximal at the pulmonary area and appearing to arise in the right ventricular outflow tract. This murmur can be readily confused with that of an atrial septal defect. There must be no signs of right ventricular volume loading. A radiograph and electrocardiogram should always be taken, and if there is any doubt at all, expert opinion should be obtained to ensure that an atrial septal defect is not overlooked.

3. A short, soft systolic murmur, heard over the aortic area with no thrill palpable in the neck, and with no other abnormality, is frequently innocent. In particular there should be no early systolic sound at the apex to suggest an abnormal aortic valve.

4. Venous hum. This is a continuous murmur of variable loudness heard at the base of the heart and in the neck. It is related to body and head position and disappears when the child lies down, so that it is not ordinarily heard when the child is examined in the supine position. If children are not examined in this standard position this murmur may be confused with that of a patent ductus. Compression of neck veins will also cause the venous hum to disappear.

Often, doctors who care for children are faced with the problem of deciding whether a murmur heard during the course of a routine physical examination is a significant one, indicating structural disease, or whether it is innocent. Failure to recognize a significant murmur, on the one hand, may place the child at risk and, on the other hand, failure to reassure the parents and child of the innocent nature of a murmur may create anxiety and lead to unnecessary restrictions on activity.

Ejection sounds

These are early systolic sounds. The ejection sound of aortic valve stenosis is best heard at the mitral area and along the left sternal edge. It does not vary with respiration and gives the impression of a split first heart sound. An early systolic click at the apex with no murmur suggestive of aortic stenosis probably indicates a bicuspid aortic valve. The ejection sound of pulmonary valve stenosis is best heard over the pulmonary area, at the upper left sternal edge. Normally this sound disappears during inspiration. As no first sound is heard with it, it initiates the murmur.

A precordial midsystolic click together with, or even without, a late apical systolic murmur may indicate the presence of mitral valve prolapse.

Splitting of the second sound

Normally the second heart sound is split and the width of the splitting increases in inspiration. Splitting is not heard at the apex because pulmonary valve closure is not heard there. Splitting of the second heart sound is due to asynchronous closure of the two semilunar valves, the aortic closure preceding pulmonary valve closure. In atrial septal defect the second heart sound may be split widely and respiration has little effect on the width of the split.

The pulmonary component of the second heart sound

This sound is accentuated in pulmonary hypertension and reduced or absent in pulmonary stenosis. The pulmonary component of the second sound can often be felt in severe pulmonary hypertension. It is absent in the tetralogy of Fallot.

The pulses

It is important to feel the femoral and brachial pulses. Femoral pulses are absent or reduced in volume in coarctation of the aorta except when a large ductus arteriosus supplies the descending aorta. Generally, pulses may be of small volume in severe aortic stenosis and full in patent ductus arteriosus. With a large patent ductus in an infant the palmar pulses may be palpable, but vasodilation in hot climates may produce a similar effect.

Chest radiograph

The chest radiograph provides the most accurate information about heart size. In a correctly taken PA view, the heart is enlarged when the heart shadow is more than half the maximal internal width of the chest (Fig. 39.1). (The maximal width is usually the distance between the inner borders of the rib cage at the level of the top of the right diaphragm.) In early infancy a cardiothoracic ratio figure of 60% is usually taken to indicate cardiac enlargement.

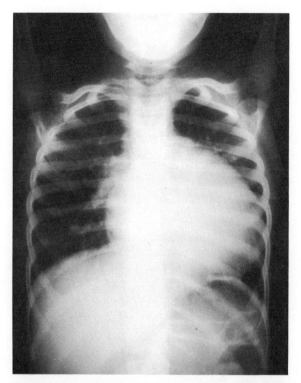

Fig. 39.1 PA radiograph of the chest showing cardiomegaly.

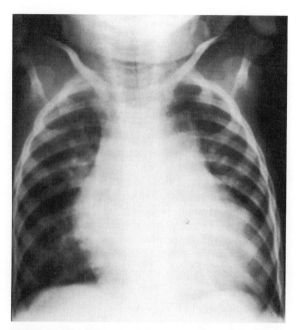

Fig. 39.2 PA radiograph of the chest demonstrating cardiomegaly and increased pulmonary vasculature.

The chest radiograph also provides information about the appearances of the great vessels and the state of the pulmonary vasculature as illustrated by the intrapulmonary shadows. As the hilar shadows are mainly vascular, an increase or decrease in these shadows tends to correlate with the size of the pulmonary vessels and usually with pulmonary flow (see Figs 39.2 and 39.3). Individual cardiac chamber size is usually difficult to assess on plain radiographic films. Such radiographs will of course detect associated intrapulmonary lesions.

Electrocardiography

The surface electrocardiogram represents electrical forces generated by the heart and is displayed along various axes or leads to allow its assessment and interpretation. The leads are standardized and those ordinarily used are:

1. Standard limb leads (bipolar) – I, II, III
2. Unipolar limb leads – aVR, aVL, aVF
3. Chest leads from V4R to V6.

The P wave depicts atrial activity, the QRS ventricular depolarization, and the ST segments repolarization.

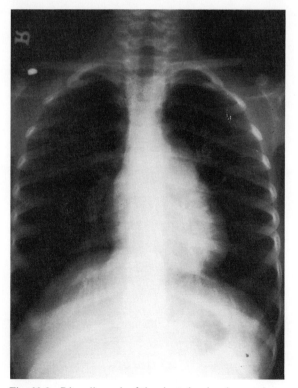

Fig. 39.3 PA radiograph of the chest showing decreased pulmonary vasculature.

Study of the ECG provides information about cardiac rhythm, in particular the site of the pacemaking area, and about transmission of the impulse through the heart, together with the balance of the ventricular forces. Cardiac rhythm abnormalities can be examined as can ventricular hypertrophy or hypoplasia interfering with ventricular balance. ECG 'axis' is deduced from study of the net limb voltages and has some empirical significance, including the recognition of the abnormal vector pattern of atrioventricular septal defect (AV canal).

At birth the right ventricular mass is relatively greater in proportion to the left ventricle than in adult life or older childhood since both ventricles carry systemic loads in utero. Therefore, the normal neonatal ECG pattern shows right ventricular activity similar to right ventricular hypertrophy due to systemic right ventricular loading in later life (see Fig. 39.4). There is

right axis deviation and the R waves are normally dominant in the right chest leads. The T waves are (normally) upright in the right chest leads at birth but become negative by about 48 hours of age. After this time persistently positive T waves in these leads indicate abnormal right ventricular loading.

In the normal infant there is progressive evolution of the ECG towards the adult pattern which is seen from about 7–8 years of age. The R wave of the right chest leads remains equal to or greater than the S wave till about 3–4 years after which it is expected to be smaller than the S wave. T waves become positive again in adolescence. Failure of the neonatal right ventricular pattern to evolve normally also indicates persistent right ventricular loading.

Abnormal dominance of one ventricle in the neonate with congenital heart disease is more likely to be due to hypoplasia of one ventricle disturbing the electrical

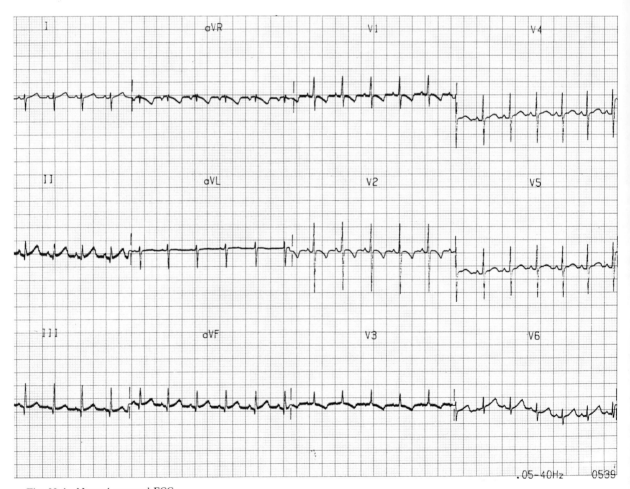

Fig. 39.4 Normal neonatal ECG.

balance than to hypertrophy. Thus, with a hypoplastic right ventricle there will be left ventricular dominance and with a hypoplastic left ventricle abnormal right ventricular dominance.

Volume loading of the right ventricle produces a typical ECG pattern with rsR complexes in the right chest leads and wide S waves in V6 (see Fig. 39.5). This pattern overlaps with normal. There is no similar characteristic pattern of left ventricular volume loading.

Assessment of ventricular hypertrophy is largely conducted along similar lines to adults with reference to voltages of complexes measured on calibrated tracings (see Figs. 39.5 and 39.6).

HEART DISEASE IN INFANCY

This is most commonly the result of a congenital cardiac anomaly. Approximately 1% of all newborn infants have some type of cardiovascular abnormality, but fortunately many are not severe. The majority of infants with congenital heart disease will now reach adult life if appropriate management is provided.

Other causes of heart disease in infancy are rare but include:

Myocarditis

This is most commonly due to Coxsackie- and echoviruses, but almost any virus can be implicated. *Mycoplasma* is also capable of causing myocarditis. Diphtheria is no longer an important cause in countries with effective immunization programmes.

Metabolic and storage diseases

Heart disease may be associated with cardiac

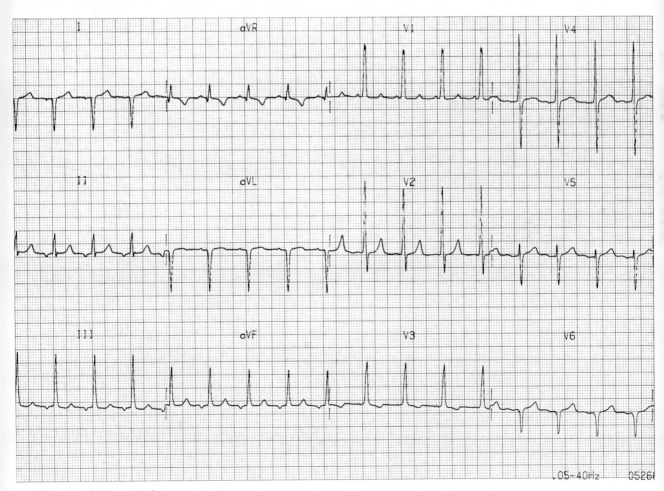

Fig. 39.5 RV hypertrophy.

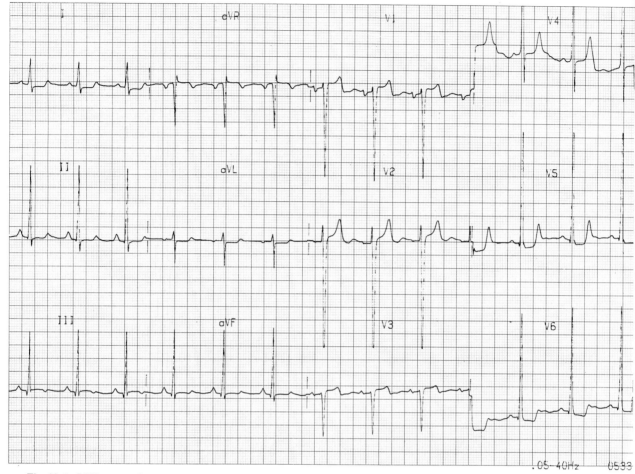

Fig. 39.6   LV hypertrophy.

glycogenosis (Pompe's disease), certain mucopolysac-charidoses, and carnitine deficiency.

Endocardial fibroelastosis

This is a syndrome of unknown aetiology. The endocardium is thickened and is accompanied by myocardial hypertrophy and impaired cardiac function. Heart failure results but the outlook is quite variable. A form of endocardial fibroelastosis may complicate certain congenital structural lesions such as severe aortic stenosis or aortic coarctation.

Cardiomyopathies

This term is given to situations of unexplained heart muscle pathology. A number of varieties are recognized on clinical grounds.

Hypertrophic cardiomyopathy. This may be associated with obstruction to the outflow of blood from the ventricles. There is also a form of hypertrophic cardiomyopathy not associated with obstruction.

Congestive cardiomyopathy. In this variety there is ventricular dilatation usually in association with congestive heart failure.

A *constrictive* form of *cardiomyopathy* is described but is rare. It presents with clinical features simulating constrictive pericarditis.

Signs suggesting the possibility of heart disease in infancy

Arterial desaturation

With experience arterial desaturation may be suspected on the basis of a dusky or leaden complexion and before frank cyanosis is apparent. Cyanosis implies the presence of at least 5 g of reduced haemoglobin per 100 ml of blood in the skin capillaries. Should this be suspected as due to congenital heart disease the hyperoxic test will be helpful. This involves the administration of 100% oxygen by face mask for a few minutes. Usually cyanosis will be relieved if caused by pulmonary disease but in the presence of congenital heart disease the desaturation will be little changed. Objective evidence of this is obtained by measuring arterial oxygen tension. If cyanosis is suspected to be caused by congenital heart disease the infant should be transferred immediately to a paediatric cardiac centre. Failure to take this action promptly may seriously compromise management or even result in the death of the infant before definitive treatment can be instituted.

Transposition of the great arteries is the commonest form of congenital heart disease to cause cyanosis in early neonatal life. Cyanosis may be relatively mild initially, but the normal haemodynamic changes that follow birth, closure of the ductus arteriosus and cessation of flow through the foremen ovale, may lead to rapid increase in cyanosis. The associated severe hypoxia is followed rapidly by the development of metabolic acidosis, which, if not corrected, will cause the death of the infant. In the tetralogy of Fallot, cyanosis may not be apparent early in life, but when it appears the same principles of management apply. Complete atresia of the right ventricular outflow tract will, of course, lead to severe cyanosis and hypoxia when the ductus closes.

Cyanotic heart disease must be differentiated from pulmonary disease, neonatal polycythaemia, facial bruising, and methaemoglobinaemia. If neonatal pulmonary disease is sufficiently severe to produce cyanosis, there is inevitably considerable respiratory distress with marked chest retraction and grunting. Cyanotic congenital heart disease in the absence of metabolic acidosis or accompanying lung disease is usually not associated with tachypnoea. Again the hyperoxic test will help in assessment.

Arterial desaturation may also result from persistence of the fetal circulation. This results from right to left shunting through the ductus arteriosus and at times through the foramen ovale as a result of raised pulmonary resistance. It is important to recognize that these infants do not have congenital heart disease. This can be done by the use of echocardiography and invasive investigations should not be required. Infants with persistent fetal circulation may require ventilatory support for survival.

In neonatal polycythaemia the infant's condition is usually good, there are usually no signs of heart disease, the cyanosis is relieved by oxygen and haemoglobin levels are excessively high. Heart failure is unusual. Facial bruising due to a face presentation is recognized by the distribution of the cyanosis, failure to blanch on pressure, and the presence of many petechiae.

Methaemoglobinaemia is a rare cause of neonatal cyanosis. The diagnosis is usually made after exclusion of other causes. Some help may come from examining the colour of the blood on filter paper but confirmation requires direct measurement of methaemoglobin levels in the blood.

Dyspnoea

This is a not uncommon mode of presentation of congenital heart disease in infancy, particularly when there is a large left to right shunt as for instance with large ventricular septal defect with or without aortic coarctation. In addition to the actual dyspnoea the chest is often overdistended and there may be associated profuse sweating. Dyspnoea may be constant and sufficiently severe to prevent normal feeding so that gavage feeding is required, or it may only occur during feeding. Failure to thrive is common in dyspnoeic babies with congenital heart disease and feeding problems. Dyspnoea may be accompanied by wheeze so that the small infant is mistakenly thought to be suffering from lung disease. Paroxysmal dyspnoea may also occur and may not be recognized as such. Dyspnoea with costal margin retraction indicates decreased lung compliance. This may just be due to stiff lungs from increased flow but also often indicates heart failure.

Heart murmurs

Heart murmurs are not only important signs of possible cardiac abnormality, but they can often be used when an abnormality is present to allow a diagnosis to be made, e.g. patent ductus arteriosus, pulmonary artery stenosis, etc. Some of these murmurs may be quite soft and perhaps be mistaken for innocent murmurs. Any murmur heard immediately after birth, particularly if loud, is likely to be significant and should be evaluated promptly as the severity of the underlying lesion may be very difficult to assess at that time. It is conceded that auscultation may be difficult in small infants because of rapid heart and respiratory rates, particularly when the infant is restless and crying. Auscultation needs to be performed patiently, under good conditions and with a good stethoscope. Absence of an audible heart murmur does definitely not exclude heart disease – in a number of cardiac malformations murmurs may be soft or absent. The murmur of ventricular septal defect is usually delayed in its appearance after birth until a significant shunt is established and may not be recognized for several weeks.

Physical examination

Cardiomegaly

Cardiomegaly always implies significant heart disease although a heart of normal size does not exclude it. Cardiomegaly may be difficult to detect clinically, particularly in the neonate and small infant. The most important sign of cardiomegaly is the presence of ventricular overactivity, assessed by the unusually forceful characteristic of the cardiac impulse, including parasternal heave and obvious epigastric pulsation. Assessment of heart size by percussion is not easy in the neonatal period but should be attempted.

Peripheral pulses

All major peripheral pulses should be assessed, including carotid pulses as well as brachial and femoral pulses when the two latter are poor in volume. This may allow correct identification of such lesions as aortic coarctation and some forms of aortic arch interruption. Variations in calibre of the ductus may lead to variations in femoral pulse volume when the ductus is supplying the descending aorta in a neonate.

Radiology

Chest radiography is the only certain means of establishing heart size in infancy. If heart disease is suspected a radiograph is absolutely essential.

Echocardiography

The development of echocardiography has made available a most important noninvasive method of obtaining information about the heart that can be used to obtain accurate diagnostic material with greater ease and much less risk than previous techniques such as cardiac catheterization.

Echocardiography involves scanning the heart through the available sound 'windows' around the chest with beams of high frequency sound of at least 2 megahertz.

2D echocardiography (sector scanning) provides a series of cross-sectional cuts through the heart displayed in real time that can be synthesized by the observer to provide anatomical structural information. The scanners achieve their cuts with either mechanical devices or electronic means to steer the beam of sound from the transducer. Addition of Doppler interrogation increases the information available about cardiac function. Information is recorded, mainly on videotape, to allow subsequent review.

M mode echocardiography, in which a single beam is used, and which was the original technique used, still provides useful information about chamber size and wall thickness.

2D echocardiography, with its advantages of ease of application and lack of complications, together with the information that it provides, has become the mainstay of diagnostic assessment. It has almost completely done away with the need for cardiac catheterization in infancy, particularly in the newborn period, expediting management and reducing risks. Catheterization still has limited applications in this age group, to fill in gaps in information and to perform relevant therapeutic procedures such as balloon atrial septostomy in transposition of the great vessels. However, it is important that echocardiography be performed by individuals who are experienced in the technique and well trained in cardiac anatomy, and that taped material is constantly reviewed to ensure maximum accuracy in assessment.

HEART FAILURE IN INFANCY

The diagnostic triad of heart failure in infancy is:

1. Dyspnoea
2. Hepatomegaly
3. Cardiomegaly (see Fig. 39.7).

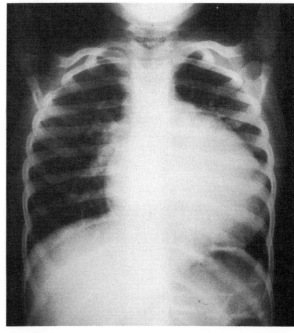

Fig. 39.7 PA radiograph of the chest showing gross cardiomegaly and pulmonary congestion – heart failure.

Other features commonly present are profuse sweating; skin pallor; chest retraction; and tachycardia.

In heart failure tachycardia is almost invariably present and a gallop rhythm may be heard. But the extra sound can be very difficult to time because of the tachycardia. If heart failure is associated with complete heart block the rate will be slow.

It should be remembered that pericardial effusion with compression of the heart (tamponade) mimics heart failure. Echocardiography will exclude this problem.

Treatment

Heart failure in infancy creates an emergency, and when it is suspected the general practitioner should immediately confer with a paediatric cardiologist about referral to a major cardiac centre. The speed and means of transport of such an infant are often critical and at times this is best performed in the company of an expert in resuscitation. It may be in the infant's best interest for certain treatment to commence before being moved. At present, initial management of heart failure in infancy involves often admission to an intensive care unit and respiratory support, with assisted ventilation. Total management is aimed at facilitating diagnostic assessment, using echocardiography, and when indicated, cardiac catheterization, in parallel with any necessary resuscitation, to allow relevant surgery to proceed with least risk and maximum productivity at the most appropriate time. Recent advances mean that a great deal more 'reparative' surgery can be performed in small infants with low mortality rates.

Nevertheless, it is important that the following principles of treatment of heart failure in infancy are understood:

Rest

Infants should be disturbed as little as possible, in a position that prevents the liver splinting the diaphragm and interfering with its movement. Reduction of metabolic activity may be important in a very sick infant. Paralysis and assisted ventilation contribute substantially to this.

Oxygen

Adequate oxygenation should be provided by relevant means. Mechanical ventilation also allows control of CO_2 levels.

Feeding

The infant may require feeding by gavage tube, or to have fluid balance maintained by intravenous infusion. When oral feeding is able to be continued the milk mixtures may best be diluted to provide low solute loads.

Circulatory support

Digoxin is best avoided in acute heart failure in infancy, particularly when surgery may be performed, to avoid the risk of digoxin intoxication precipitated by a metabolic disturbance not uncommon in this situation. Intravenous dopamine is the best inotropic agent in such infants. Should digoxin be indicated the infant must be observed closely for signs of toxicity, including vomiting, irregularity of the heart rhythm or bradycardia. An ECG should optimally be performed before starting therapy and if any disturbance of rhythm occurs. Serum digoxin levels should be monitored.

Diuretics

Frusemide (Lasix) is the diuretic of choice. It may be best given parenterally at first. If diuretics are required for more than a limited period potassium depletion may occur. Potassium supplements should be given or Aldactone combined with the Lasix. Serum electrolytes should be monitored but the development of intracellular potassium depletion may only be revealed by appearance of a metabolic alkalosis.

Treatment of infection

The presence of pulmonary infection in particular should be recognized and treated appropriately. In small infants with left to right shunt associated chest infection may be difficult to exclude. Antibiotic therapy is indicated if there is any doubt.

Correction of acidosis

Combined respiratory and metabolic acidosis often occurs in infants with heart failure. Acidosis rapidly supervenes in infants with cyanotic heart disease with duct closure. Prostaglandin E_1 administration, to maintain duct patency or reopen it, may be indicated even before transport to a cardiac centre. Acidosis may also require correction with sodium bicarbonate. Uncontrollable acidosis increases the need for appropriate intervention.

Surgery

Heart failure provides an urgent indication for assessment and often for relevant surgical treatment, so that such infants should be transferred promptly to a centre where both assessment and surgery are available.

CURRENT TREATMENT POSSIBILITIES

The majority of congenital heart lesions can now be treated surgically, but some residual potential problems remain in most cases. True cure is probably restricted to ligation of isolated patent ductus arteriosus, the treatment of which carries minimal mortality, and for which contraindications rather than indications should be sought. However, special consideration needs to be given to management of patent ductus in low birthweight premature infants, now surviving with ventilatory support.

There are few other lesions that cannot at least be palliated in many cases with a view to later secondary intervention. Procedures have now been devised even for hypoplastic left heart syndrome but their role still needs evaluation.

Closure of atrial septal defects should also carry minimal risk and this procedure is indicated electively in most cases.

Ventricular septal defects carry a substantial prospect of spontaneous decrease in size and even closure, but surgical treatment is indicated in infancy when there is heart failure, failure to thrive because of the defect, or the defect remains large with the threat of development of pulmonary vascular disease. The risks of direct closure in infancy are now small and comparable to those in later childhood. Palliative pulmonary artery banding is now only required in special circumstances for infants with ventricular septal defect.

The tetralogy of Fallot can now also be repaired quite early in life at low risk, but small infants requiring treatment for this condition will still often have an initial shunt procedure and later secondary, elective, repair. Most patients with this condition should reach adult life but the ultimate consequences of postoperative pulmonary incompetence, and the real risks of sudden death from ventricular arrhythmia and its cause are not yet clearly known.

The prognosis of complete transposition of the great arteries has changed greatly. Initial palliation by creation of an atrial septal defect either by balloon septostomy or surgically, followed by more definitive surgery, leads to survival of most affected infants. Repair by inflow diversion, in which venous inflows are switched at atrial level by the techniques of Mustard or Senning has been replaced widely by the arterial switch operation in which the great arteries are restored to their correct positions. This can now be performed in many centres safely in the neonatal period, and does away with the possible problems of the continuing systemic loading of the right ventricle following atrial inflow operations.

The incidence of recurrence of aortic coarctation following repair in infancy has been reduced substantially by present surgical techniques.

Aortic coarctation is a very common cause of heart failure requiring surgery in early infancy, either alone or with other lesions.

Nonsurgical techniques such as balloon valvuloplasty are also becoming applicable to small infants as an alternative to surgery in relevant lesions.

HEART DISEASE IN OLDER CHILDREN

Heart disease in the older child may present with symptoms, or more commonly be identified incidentally during physical examination. Its causes are discussed below.

Congenital

Most cases of congenital heart disease are now detected in infancy because of better surveillance and increased referral in this age group. Occasionally, these conditions will be identified at routine preschool or school physical examinations. The most common such lesions are:

1. Small ventricular septal defects (VSD)
2. Atrial septal defect (ASD)
3. Patent ductus arteriosus (PDA)
4. Aortic and pulmonary stenosis
5. Aortic coarctation.

The clinical features of these conditions are discussed in Chapter 40.

Rheumatic heart disease

This is now rare in developed countries. Its clinical features are described below.

Renal disease

Cardiac disease is a well-established complication of acute poststreptococcal glomerulonephritis and occurs early in the disease. However, this disease is also becoming rare in developed societies and the features of increasing dyspnoea and signs of left ventricular failure that characterize this complication are now not often seen. In chronic renal failure heart disease may be associated with hypertension.

Primary myocardial disease

This is of varied aetiology. Viral infection is perhaps the commonest cause and many viruses may be involved. Many cases of myocardial disease in childhood are unexplained. Rare causes include type 2 glycogen storage disease, Duchenne muscular dystrophy, and some varieties of mucopolysaccharidosis.

Arrhythmias

See below.

Chronic refractory anaemia

Chronic anaemia is occasionally complicated by heart disease. Beta thalassaemia was frequently associated with heart disease, cardiomyopathy or pericardial effusion, before the high transfusion regime and use of desferrioxamine treatment for chelation of iron were instituted. Heart disease now seen in patients with leukaemia and solid tumours is more likely to be due to the drugs used in treatment than to anaemia.

Management of heart disease in childhood

The principles do not differ significantly from those in adult patients. The management of heart failure in infancy has already been discussed. It should be recognized that children resent restriction of activity rather more than adults and great difficulty is often experienced in keeping children at rest after they have recovered from the effects of acute heart disease. Anxious parents will be inclined to restrict children with the result that there are often superadded behavioural problems. A common-sense attitude to rest is called for from those involved in the management of heart disease in children. Children with significant heart disease almost invariably play within the limits of their tolerance. Certain competitive sports may need to be banned, but a satisfactory alternative can usually be found if sufficient thought is given to the problem.

Where surgery is indicated, parents and children must be carefully informed to the level of their understanding of the nature and outcome of the surgery. This will apply particularly when only palliative procedures can be offered.

Children with inoperable congenital heart lesions require follow-up so that their quality of life can be made optimal and problems freely discussed as they arise. Any new developments that become available can also be offered. Children with congenital heart disease and with rheumatic heart disease are at risk for bacterial endocarditis and should have antibiotic prophylaxis whenever they have dental extractions or surgical procedures. Provided that the child is not on prophylactic penicillin, is not allergic to penicillin, and does not have an intravascular prosthesis, an oral penicillin is given to cover the procedure, usually now as oral amoxycillin, on that day.

RHEUMATIC FEVER

Rheumatic fever is probably the result of an abnormal immune response on the part of the host to certain streptococcal antigens, resulting in an autoimmune response against certain host antigens, for example, heart, synovial membrane, etc. Recently, it has been noted that a very high percentage of patients with rheumatic fever have a specific antigen on their B cells (lymphocytes) and that 95% of such patients have one of two specific antibodies in their serum. Thus, it would appear that one can now identify patients susceptible to rheumatic fever through these specific genetic markers. The relationship between them and the pathogenic mechanisms postulated above is still not clear.

Rheumatic fever is now very rare except in developing societies where it continues to be the commonest cause of acquired heart disease.

Clinical manifestations

Rheumatic fever may present in a number of ways, either singly or in combination.

1. Most commonly as a migratory arthritis, mainly affecting larger joints and which ultimately resolves leaving no residual disability.

2. As a carditis manifest by tachycardia, cardiomegaly, heart murmurs, and if severe, congestive heart failure.

3. With jerking movements of one or more limbs, facial grimacing, muscular weakness and emotional instability – Sydenham's chorea.

4. Rarely with skin lesions – erythema marginatum, or with nodules.

In the severe case fever, arthritis, carditis, and skin manifestations may be combined.

The diagnosis of rheumatic fever is a clinical one dependent on the features described above, together with evidence of recent streptococcal infection either from throat culture or from serology. The ESR is always elevated at the onset of the disease.

The course of rheumatic fever is variable, with complete recovery the rule in the absence of carditis. In the presence of carditis, morbidity and mortality are greatly increased both in the short and long term. However, surgery has now improved the outlook for both aortic and mitral valve disease. In between 20% and 50% of those affected the disease will recur if these patients do not receive prophylactic antibiotic therapy against further streptococcal infection. Since approximately one half of all streptococcal infections are asymptomatic, continuous prophylaxis against streptococcal infection is essential in all children who have had rheumatic fever. Oral penicillin is the most satisfactory prophylactic drug and should be taken indefinitely.

Treatment

No specific curative treatment is available. During the acute stages of the illness, and particularly in the presence of fever and arthritis salicylates are specific and should be given in full therapeutic dosage. Careful observations on pulse, respiration, and cardiac status must be made. In the presence of significant carditis, corticosteroids are recommended, although there is no reliable evidence that their administration in the acute stage prevents the development of chronic valvular disease.

INFECTIVE ENDOCARDITIS

In children with cardiovascular lesions, microorganisms from septic foci may enter the bloodstream and become implanted on abnormal endothelium or thickened valves. Rarely virulent organisms may infect normal valves. Vegetations produced allow proliferation of the organisms and further endothelial and valve damage. The vegetations, which largely consist of fibrin may break off and produce peripheral emboli.

Clinical features

In developed societies heart disease is usually identified early in life and generally supervised by persons experienced in heart disease in childhood. Any child with structural heart disease who develops fever, or becomes unwell for no apparent reason, should be considered to have bacterial endocarditis until proven otherwise. This also applies to children who have had cardiac surgery and particularly to those who have had valve replacements, the insertion of prosthetic material to close defects, and to individuals who have had ventriculoatrial shunts inserted for treatment of hydrocephalus. An increasing number of cases of infective endocarditis are now related to intravenous drug abuse and this diagnosis

must be considered in adolescents who are using drugs of addiction intravenously. Under these circumstances the right side of the heart may be involved. Murmurs may be insignificant and symptoms relate to the lungs as a result of infected emboli lodging there.

The features of endocarditis described in older textbooks are related to longstanding, late diagnosed, endocarditis. They include continuing fever, weight loss, anaemia, peripheral emboli, splenomegaly and clubbing. These are now infrequent features because of expected much earlier diagnosis.

Once the diagnosis of endocarditis is suspected at least six blood cultures should be taken over a few hours. Immediate consultation with the microbiologist is essential to ensure appropriate culturing, both aerobic and anaerobic, and earliest possible identification of an organism and its antibiotic sensitivities. Echocardiography may demonstrate vegetations on affected heart valves.

The alpha-haemolytic streptococcus (*Streptococcus viridans*) is responsible for about 75% of cases of infective endocarditis in childhood. Staphylococci (*Staphylococcus aureus* and *Staphylococcus albus*) account for between 10% and 20%. Other causes include species of enterococci, *Escherichia coli*, *Pseudomonas aeruginosa*, *Haemophilus influenzae*, and fungi, of which *Candida albicans* is the commonest. Antibiotics are, of course, the mainstay of treatment and are chosen in collaboration with the microbiologist on a basis of the determined sensitivities of the organism isolated. Bactericidal drugs rather than bacteriostatic drugs should be used and treatment continued for some weeks until the organism is eradicated. In the case of the sensitive *Strep. viridans*, the response may be rapid and intravenous chemotherapy can be suspended after two to three weeks and oral therapy continued for a further period. Initial therapy should always be by the intravenous route. Supportive therapy may include digitalization, diuretics, and anticoagulants, but will always involve careful clinical observations of pulse, temperature and fluid balance. Surgery may need to be considered if there is intractable heart failure, but may also be required for uncontrolled infection, or to prevent dangerous embolization.

CARDIAC ARRHYTHMIAS

The commonest is sinus arrhythmia, which is a normal phenomenon in which the heart rate varies with respiration, slowing in expiration and quickening in inspiration. It is important that it is not confused with a serious arrhythmia.

There are three types of arrhythmia that need particular consideration in childhood.

Paroxysmal atrial tachycardia

This is characterized by rapid atrial beats at 200–300 per minute. Each atrial beat is conducted to the ventricles. The fastest rates occur in small infants. The cause is usually not found but some of those with recurrent re-entrant tachycardia have the ECG abnormalities that typify the Wolff-Parkinson-White syndrome.

Short spells of paroxysmal atrial tachycardia may be symptomless or may be associated with palpitations and chest discomfort. Prolonged atrial tachycardia may cause congestive heart failure, particularly in small infants. Ventricular filling is defective at high rates.

The treatment of paroxysmal atrial tachycardia is aimed firstly at stopping the immediate attack, and secondly at preventing further attacks. Vagal reflex stimulation, including the application of ice packs to the face of an infant, may stop an attack but carotid sinus massage is not often effective in children. When simple measures fail, digoxin is the drug of choice for treatment, but if cardiac output is impaired a DC shock offers a satisfactory method of terminating the attack, particularly in infancy when the use of intravenous verapamil for that purpose is dangerous. DC shock can be given to an infant using adult defibrillator paddles placed 'fore and aft', on front and back, of the chest. Only small amounts of energy of the order of 10 joules are usually required.

Heart block

In most cases heart block is an isolated congenital problem and is complete, but well tolerated. This variety may be recognized in utero. There is an association between this form of congenital heart block and systemic lupus erythematosus in the mother. A small number of cases is associated with cardiac defects, the commonest of which is so-called corrected transposition of the great arteries. Heart block may complicate surgery from damage to the conducting system. It can also result from digoxin toxicity.

Complete heart block is recognized by the presence of constant bradycardia, usually at rates of about 40–50 beats per minute. The congenital form may accelerate, sometimes substantially, with exercise. Although many tolerate the problem well, some children have syncopal attacks (Stokes-Adams attacks), which may lead to death. One such attack is an indication for insertion of an electronic pacemaker. Other indications for pacemakers also exist.

Ventricular arrhythmias

An increasing number of ventricular arrhythmias are being recognized in children, particularly as causes for syncopal attacks. This cause should always be considered as a possible basis for unexplained syncope and appropriate investigation arranged because of the dangers offered by these arrhythmias, which occur mostly in individuals with otherwise apparently normal hearts. The resting ECG may show prolongation of the QT interval, which is an important predisposing factor in some individuals. In some, prolonged monitoring of the ECG, or monitoring during exercise, may confirm the occurrence of episodic ventricular arrhythmia.

40. Common congenital heart lesions

J. Wilkinson

Congenital malformations affecting the heart and/or great vessels occur in approximately 1% of newborn infants and as such comprise the largest single system group of congenital abnormalities.

Eight defects are relatively frequent and together make up approximately 80% of all congenital heart disease (see Table 40.1). The remaining 20% is made up of a large number of defects which are individually uncommon or rare and combinations of abnormalities which may add up to highly complex congenital heart disease.

Table 40.1 Approximate frequency of common congenital heart defects

Defect	Approximate frequency (%)
Ventricular septal defect (VSD)	30
Persistent ductus arteriosus (PDA)	12
Atrial septal defect (ASD)	8
Pulmonary stenosis (PS)	8
Aortic stenosis (AS)	5
Coarctation of the aorta	5
Tetralogy of Fallot	5
Transposition of the great arteries (TGA)	5

Defects may be broadly divided into those which are 'acyanotic' and those which are 'cyanotic'. Acyanotic defects comprise defects associated with an isolated left to right shunt (e.g. VSD, PDA, ASD) and those in which no shunting is present (e.g. obstructive defects – PS, coarctation). Cyanotic defects are those in which a right to left shunt occurs. Such defects are always associated with a septal defect, usually associated with other malformations which equalize or reverse the pressure gradient between the left and right sides of the heart or the difference between the levels of systemic and pulmonary vascular resistance. The common cyanotic defects are tetralogy of Fallot and transposition of the great arteries.

PRESENTING FEATURES

The major presenting features are:

1. The presence of an abnormal murmur
2. Development of symptoms or signs of congestive heart failure
3. Central cyanosis
4. Any combination of above.

Diagnosis

The clinical features of individual defects are frequently sufficiently characteristic to allow for a diagnosis to be made with a relatively high degree of confidence. However, confirmatory investigations are often necessary and these include:

Chest radiograph – to assess heart size and contour and lung vascular markings (which may be increased in the presence of a left to right shunt or diminished if pulmonary blood flow is low (e.g. in Fallots tetralogy).
Electrocardiogram – allows assessment of heart rhythm and presence of ventricular or atrial hypertrophy or hypoplasia.
Echocardiogram – a useful noninvasive tool for examining the heart with ultrasound. Cardiac anatomy and function can be analysed in detail and most defects can be accurately diagnosed (Fig. 40.1).
Cardiac catheterization – an invasive investigation which may produce some morbidity and is associated with a significant risk of complications and occasionally death. It permits measurement of intracardiac pressures directly. Blood samples may be taken for assessment of oxygen content at different sites. Injection of radio-opaque contrast material allows radiological visualization of intracardiac and extracardiac anatomy in detail (angiography).

ACYANOTIC DEFECTS

These comprise approximately 75% of all congenital

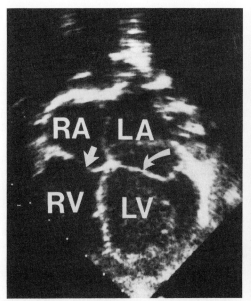
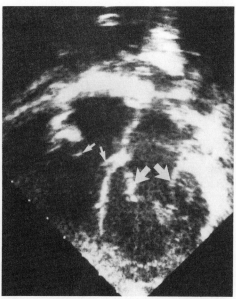

Fig. 40.1 Echocardiograms: 'four chambers view'. (**a**) Shows the four cardiac chambers with the mitral valve (curved arrow) and tricuspid valve (straight arrow) closed during ventricular systole. The ventricular septum separates the left ventricle (LV) and right ventricle (RV) and the atrial septum separates the left atrium (LA) and right atrium (RA). (**b**) Shows the same anatomy during diastole with the four cardiac chambers as in (a) and the mitral valve (large arrows) and tricuspid valve (small arrows) open.

heart defects and can be broadly subdivided into those which are associated with (a) an isolated left to right shunt and (b) those which are not associated with any shunting (in which no septal defect is present).

Defects with a left to right shunt

Ventricular septal defect

Defects in the ventricular septum are common and comprise 30% of all cardiac defects. They vary from tiny defects of pin hole size to huge defects involving most of the ventricular septum. Small defects are more common than large ones and are often asymptomatic. Defects are frequently situated in the region of the membranous part of the ventricular septum immediately below the aortic valve, but VSDs involving the muscular ventricular septum are also very common (see Fig. 40.2).

In the presence of a small VSD the characteristic clinical findings are of a loud harsh high-pitched systolic murmur audible at the left sternal border and frequently associated with a thrill. The heart sounds may be otherwise normal and there are often no other abnormal findings. The murmur is most often 'pansystolic' in timing, but this is not invariably so.

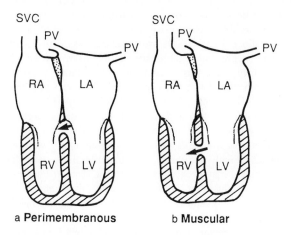

Fig. 40.2 Diagram of sites of VSD. In (**a**) the defect is close to the membranous part of the ventricular septum (perimembranous VSD). In (**b**) the defect is in the middle of the muscular septum (muscular VSD).

With a larger VSD clinical signs of cardiac failure may be present and the cardiac findings may be different. These may include a parasternal heave (evidence of right ventricular dilatation/hypertrophy), displaced apex and atypical ausculatory findings. In some cases the systolic murmur may be considerably softer or an additional diastolic murmur may be heard at the apex. Infants with a large VSD often thrive poorly, suffer dyspnoea with feeds and are prone to recurrent chest infections. Tachypnoea, dyspnoea, sweating and hepatomegaly are frequent findings.

The chest radiograph and electrocardiogram are helpful in assessing the significance of a VSD. With small defects these investigations are frequently normal and this is good evidence that a VSD is of very minor haemodynamic significance. With larger defects the chest radiograph shows cardiomegaly and increased pulmonary vascular markings (pulmonary plethora). The electrocardiogram often shows biventricular hypertrophy.

The natural history of a ventricular septal defect varies depending on its size and haemodynamic significance, and is also related to some degree to its site in the ventricular septum. Small defects frequently undergo a process of progressive reduction in size culminating in spontaneous closure which may occur in 30% or more of cases during early childhood. Some moderate or larger defects may also diminish in size to an extent where the shunt becomes relatively insignificant. Important complicating problems may develop even in the presence of a relatively small defect – such as the development of progressive aortic incompetence or infundibular pulmonary stenosis (see below tetralogy of Fallot). Large VSDs are invariably associated with some degree of pulmonary hypertension which is primarily related to transmission of systemic pressure through the defect into the right ventricle and pulmonary circulation. Such pulmonary hypertension is present from birth and, if the defect remains large, it usually leads to the development of pulmonary vascular obliterative disease. Progression of pulmonary vascular damage, with associated rise in pulmonary vascular resistance, may eventually lead to the disappearance of a left to right shunt and the appearance of a right to left shunt with cyanosis (referred to as Eisenmenger's syndrome).

Surgical repair of ventricular septal defect is indicated if congestive heart failure appears in infancy, or if pulmonary hypertension is present. It is important to establish the diagnosis of pulmonary hypertension at an early stage before pulmonary vascular disease develops as severe pulmonary vascular damage contraindicates surgery. Cardiac catheterization is usually necessary in affected patients who are symptomatic in infancy or if the clinical findings or ECG/chest radiograph suggest a large shunt or pulmonary hypertension. Surgery can be carried out at any age from the newborn period –

though most affected infants with a large VSD do not become symptomatic until the second or third month of life. Therefore, it is unusual for surgery to be indicated in the neonatal period.

Persistent ductus arteriosus

Failure of the ductus arteriosus to close normally in the newborn period may be due to a congenital abnormality of the ductus or to severe prematurity. In the small premature infant delayed closure of the ductus will often occur after a period of weeks or even months, but if the infant is symptomatic treatment may be required.

The clinical findings depend on the size of the ductus. Patients with a small PDA frequently remain asymptomatic and the only abnormal finding may be a loud continuous murmur audible at the upper left sternal border (in or above the pulmonary area). Such murmurs may be present throughout the cardiac cycle (machinery murmur) but sometimes disappear during diastole and may be sufficiently short to be mistaken for a purely systolic murmur.

In the presence of large ductus collapsing pulses are frequently apparent. The apex may be displaced and forceful and an apical mid diastolic murmur may be heard.

Symptoms such as failure to thrive, dyspnoea and recurrent chest infections are similar to those of a large VSD.

The chest radiograph and ECG are useful indicators of the size of the ductal shunt. If they are normal this is almost invariably associated with a small ductus which is not likely to lead to major problems in the short term. The presence of cardiomegaly and pulmonary plethora on the chest radiograph indicates a large shunt and left ventricular hypertrophy will usually be seen on the electrocardiogram if this is present. The diagnosis can be confirmed by echocardiography and cardiac catheterization is not usually necessary.

In symptomatic premature infants specific medical treatment with drugs which inhibit prostaglandin synthesis (e.g indomethacin) may be effective in promoting spontaneous ductal constriction. Unfortunately, drug treatment is not effective in mature infants with a persistent ductus and in such patients surgical ligation is indicated. This should be carried out at an early stage in symptomatic patients (including premature infants if indomethacin is ineffective) but may be delayed until the second year of life or subsequently in asymptomatic patients with a small ductus. In such infants surgery is indicated to eliminate the risk of infective endocarditis rather than to treat cardiac failure or pulmonary hypertension.

Atrial septal defect

Defects of the atrial septum are usually situated in the region of the fossa ovale and are termed 'persistent ostium secundum' or secundum ASD (Fig. 40.3). Unlike small VSDs and PDAs – which are commonly associated with a loud murmur – small atrial septal defects may go completely undetected. With larger defects a significant shunt is present but this is not associated with pulmonary hypertension (with rare exceptions) and seldom leads to symptoms during infancy.

The characteristic findings in children with an isolated ASD are related to the increased blood flow through the right side of the heart which results from the shunt. An ejection systolic murmur due to high pulmonary flow is present in the pulmonary area and a soft mid diastolic murmur may be heard in the tricuspid area. A parasternal heave due to a dilated right ventricle may be palpable. The aortic and pulmonary components of the second heart sound are widely separated and frequently remain equally well separated during both phases of respiration (fixed splitting).

Whilst most children are free of any major symptoms their growth is often mildly impaired compared with siblings and exercise tolerance may be slightly reduced.

Chest radiograph characteristically shows increase in transverse cardiac diameter with pulmonary plethora. The electrocardiogram tends to show features of partial right bundle branch block (due to the right ventricular dilatation). The diagnosis may be confirmed by echocardiography and cardiac catheterization is not usually required.

Treatment is surgical and should be recommended in all cases where there is evidence of a significant shunt. The defect is usually closed by direct suture but may require insertion of a patch.

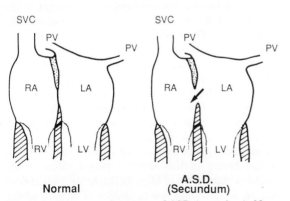

Fig. 40.3 Diagrams of anatomy of ASD (secundum). Note that the defect is in the middle of the atrial septum (fossa ovale) and is well separated from the mitral and tricuspid valves.

Atrioventricular septal defect

This category of defect which accounts for approximately 3% of all congenital cardiac defects includes a group of atrial septal defects low in the atrial septum which abut on the atrioventricular valves and may involve the upper part of the ventricular septum as well. When the ventricular septum is intact (partial atrioventricular septal defect) only an atrial communication is present. This is referred to as an 'ostium primum ASD' and is almost invariably associated with malformations of the mitral and tricuspid valves which are often incompetent (e.g 'cleft mitral valve').

Children with this type of defect may become symptomatic in infancy or early childhood if mitral incompetence is severe. In the absence of significant mitral regurgitation, however, the features resemble those of a secundum ASD.

When a significant ventricular septal defect co-exists (complete atrioventricular spetal defect – common atrioventricular canal) the presentation resembles that of an isolated large VSD and most infants become symptomatic with difficulty feeding and failure to thrive in the early months of life.

The chest radiograph usually shows quite marked cardiomegaly and pulmonary plethora, especially in the complete form of the defect. The electrocardiogram characteristically shows left axis deviation accompanied by partial right bundle branch block. The presence of left axis deviation distinguishes ostium primum ASDs from secundum defects. Echocardiography confirms the diagnosis and will differentiate partial from complete atrioventricular defects. Cardiac catheterization is usually required to document the severity of pulmonary hypertension and the degree of mitral incompetence.

Surgical repair is almost always required. When pulmonary hypertension is present this is generally recommended in the early months of life (e.g. 3–6 months) in order to obviate the risk of pulmonary vascular disease. In patients with an isolated ostium primum ASD, when pulmonary hypertension is absent, surgery may be delayed until the age of around four years. Operation involves placement of a patch to close the ASD and repair of the mitral valve cleft to eliminate mitral incompetence if present.

Defects with no shunt: obstructive lesions

Pulmonary stenosis

Pulmonary stenosis which is usually valvar in site is the commonest of the pure obstructive malformations. The pulmonary valve is abnormal with thickened leaflets and partially fused commissures. In some cases the valve may be bicuspid.

Other sites of pulmonary stenosis occur infrequently. These include muscular subpulmonary obstruction involving the right ventricular outflow tract (infundibular stenosis) and supravalve or branch pulmonary stenosis.

Most patients are asymptomatic in infancy and childhood. An ejection systolic murmur best heard in the pulmonary area and radiating through to the back is the characteristic finding. The murmur may be associated with a thrill. The pulmonary component of the second sound is often abnormally soft or inaudible though in mild cases it may be heard and the degree of splitting is often increased. An early ejection sound (ejection click) is usually audible at the left sternal border with valvar stenosis. Characteristically the click is louder during expiration and fades on inspiration.

The chest radiograph usually demonstrates a normal heart size but the main pulmonary artery is often unusually prominent (post-stenotic dilatation). This produces an abnormal convexity on the upper left heart border just below the aortic knuckle. The electrocardiogram may be normal with mild obstruction but shows right ventricular hypertrophy in more severe cases.

Mild pulmonary stenosis is generally a benign condition and often nonprogressive. More severe pulmonary stenosis leads eventually to effort intolerance, angina on exertion and cardiac failure. Rarely, severe pulmonary stenosis may present in early infancy with cyanosis due to right to left shunting through a normal foramen ovale.

The diagnosis may be confirmed by echocardiography, but cardiac catheterization is usually required to assess the severity more precisely.

Traditionally treatment involved surgical valvotomy but in recent years this has largely been replaced by a catheter technique involving inflation of a balloon in the valve orifice to separate fused commissures (balloon pulmonary valvotomy or valvuloplasty). This procedure is simple and effective in most cases and as it requires only a very short hospital stay and saves the patient an open heart operation it has much to commend it.

Aortic stenosis

Like pulmonary stenosis the valve is abnormal with thickened leaflets and fused commissures. In most cases with aortic stenosis the valve is bicuspid. Subaortic stenosis with a fibrous stricture or with muscular obstruction (hypertrophic subaortic stenosis) also occurs but is in the ascending aorta above the aortic valve (supra-aortic stenosis).

With rare exceptions affected children are symptom free in infancy and early childhood and present with the chance finding of an ejection systolic murmur over the precordium and in the aortic area. Characteristically, with valvar stenosis the murmur is best heard to the right of the sternum and radiates to the carotids. A thrill is commonly present over the carotids and may also be felt in the aortic area. An ejection click is usually heard with valvar stenosis and is often most easily audible at the apex or lower left sternal border. In mild and moderate cases there may be no other abnormal finding. In more severe cases a forceful apical impulse due to left ventricular hypertrophy may be apparent.

The natural history of aortic stenosis is generally one of gradual progression. Symptoms include dizziness and syncope on exertion, angina pectoris, effort intolerance and sudden death. In a small minority of cases severe congestive heart failure may appear in early infancy.

In mild and even moderate aortic stenosis the chest radiograph and ECG may show little abnormal. In more severe cases the electrocardiogram tends to show left ventricular hypertrophy but this is often late in appearing. Echocardiography allows assessment of the site and severity of the obstruction but cardiac catheterization is usually indicated if there is evidence of moderate or severe stenosis.

Treatment is surgical and should be recommended if significant stenosis is confirmed at cardiac catheter – even in the absence of symptoms. Operation involves aortic valvotomy on heart lung bypass. Balloon aortic valvotomy is feasible and has been carried out on some patients but at the present time this is not regarded as the treatment of choice in children with aortic stenosis.

Coarctation of the aorta

In this condition a discrete stricture is present in the distal part of the aortic arch close to the site of the ductus arteriosus. The maximal site of obstruction is usually opposite to or just proximal to the aortic end of the ductus arteriosus or ligamentum arteriosum (Fig. 40.4).

Coarctation of the aorta is often associated with other cardiac defects including aortic stenosis, ventricular septal defect and mitral valve abnormalities. A bicuspid aortic valve is present in 40% of cases even in the absence of other malformations.

Coarctation often leads to the development of severe cardiac failure in the newborn period (often in the second or third week of life). Alternatively, presentation may be delayed until late in childhood or even adolescence or adult life.

The characteristic physical findings are of diminished or absent femoral pulses. Simultaneous palpatation of

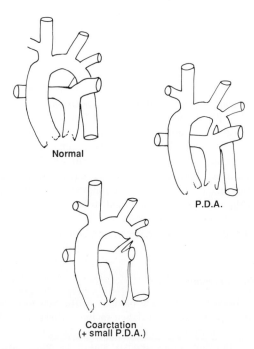

Fig. 40.4 Diagram of the aorta and pulmonary artery to show persistent ductus arteriosus (PDA) and site of coarctation (often associated with small PDA).

the right brachial pulse and the femoral pulse frequently shows quite obvious delay in the appearance of the latter. Upper limb blood pressure is often elevated (sometimes severely so) and there is a marked discrepancy between arm and leg blood pressure (usually greater than 20 mmHg).

The chest radiograph and ECG findings vary according to the age of presentation. In symptomatic infants cardiomegaly and pulmonary congestion are usually seen on the chest radiograph and the ECG shows right ventricular hypertrophy. In later childhood the radiograph may show an abnormal appearance of the aortic knuckle and rib notching due to the presence of enlarged intercostal arteries which act as collateral routes for flow of blood into the lower systemic segment (this is seldom seen before the age of eight years). The electrocardiogram may show left ventricular hypertrophy.

Treatment. In infancy the onset of congestive heart failure is often related to closure of the ductus arteriosus. (Before closure of the ductus the pulmonary artery pressure is usually sufficient to allow adequate flow of blood into the descending aorta via the ductus but after the ductus starts to close the flow of blood in the lower part of the circulation becomes inadequate.)

For this reason infusion of prostaglandin E_1 or E_2 intravenously may ameliorate symptoms (by causing the ductus to reopen). Other medical measures may help to ameliorate heart failure and improve the condition of the infant before operation. Early surgery is always indicated in symptomatic cases (as soon as the diagnosis is established). Patients who remain free of symptoms should be assessed carefully for the development of hypertension and if this is present surgery should be carried out during early childhood. In other patients operation may be deferred until later in childhood. Infants who require relief of coarctation may develop restenosis at the repair site – although this is less common with newer surgical techniques.

Unoperated patients with coarctation (i.e. those who escape detection during childhood) are at a high risk from serious complications or death during adolescence or early adult life. These include left ventricular failure, aortic dissection and subarachnoid haemorrhage due to ruptured berry aneurysm.

Hypoplastic left heart syndrome

A small subgroup of infants with both severe aortic stenosis and coarctation may present with associated gross hypoplasia of the left ventricle. In some cases the aortic valve and/or mitral valve are atretic (Fig. 40.5).

Such infants present with severe cardiac failure or

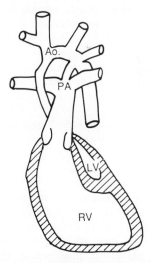

Fig. 40.5 Diagram of hypoplastic left heart syndrome, showing hypoplasia of the left ventricle and ascending aorta. Note that the ductus arteriosus is patent and provides an alternative pathway for blood to enter the systemic circulation via a right to left shunt from the pulmonary artery and right ventricle.

shock in the early days of life. All peripheral pulses are diminished or absent and manifestations of cardiac failure are severe.

The condition is invariably lethal without surgery. Medical treatment including infusion of prostaglandin and other measures may lead to improvement. Surgical procedures for this conditon remain experimental at this stage although a small number of affected infants have survived after drastic reconstructive cardiac surgery.

CYANOTIC CARDIAC DEFECTS

The presence of cyanosis in a child with congenital heart disease indicates that deoxygenated blood from the systemic venous system is being directed back into the systemic circulation without transiting the pulmonary vascular bed.

Cyanotic defects account for approximately 25% of all congenital heart malformations. All such defects are associated with the presence of a septal defect coupled with additional abnormalities which alter the pressure relationship between the two sides of the heart so that, instead of pure left to right shunting, right to left or bidirectional shunting occurs producing cyanosis.

Three major subgroups exist. In the first group (exemplified by tetralogy of Fallot) pulmonary blood flow is reduced due to a combination of obstruction to normal flow into the lung circulation and a septal defect behind the obstruction through which blood may shunt from right to left. In tetralogy of Fallot the shunt is almost completely right to left, whereas in some other defects associated with low pulmonary flow the physiology is more complex with right to left shunting at one level and left to right shunting at another (e.g. tricuspid atresia, pulmonary atresia). In all such defects the net result is low pulmonary flow and cyanosis which is proportional in severity to the reduction in pulmonary flow.

In the second group of cyanotic defects bidirectional shunting is associated with very large communications between the left and right sides of the heart with free mixing of blood (e.g. 'single ventricle', truncus arteriosis). In such defects pulmonary blood flow is usually high and pulmonary hypertension is a feature. Cyanosis is generally very mild and may pass unnoticed.

A third group of cyanotic defects, best exemplified by transposition of the great arteries may be considered as a 'plumbing problem'. In transposition, the aorta and pulmonary artery are connected to the wrong side of the heart and as a result systemic venous blood is directed straight through into the systemic circulation again (see below).

Tetralogy of Fallot

Of the four components which comprise the tetralogy (VSD, pulmonary stenosis, right ventricular hypertrophy, overriding aorta) the important ones are pulmonary stenosis and the VSD (Fig. 40.6). The presence of severe pulmonary stenosis, which is characteristically associated with infundibular muscular obstruction coupled frequently with valvar hypoplasia and commissural fusion, leads to elevation of right ventricular pressure. In most patients the systolic pressure in left and right ventricles is equal but the marked resistance to ejection into the pulmonary circulation due to the stenosis produces right to left shunting into the aorta (the degree of right to left shunting is not influenced much by the overriding aorta).

Clinical features

Cyanosis is not usually obvious in the newborn period but appears later in infancy in most affected children. A systolic murmur is audible along the left sternal edge (due to infundibular stenosis) and in the pulmonary area and radiates through to the back. The second heart

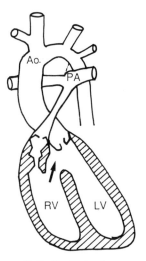

Fallot's Tetralogy

Fig. 40.6 Diagram of the anatomy in tetralogy of Fallot. Note the large subaortic VSD which carries a right to left shunt. Pulmonary stenosis is predominantly infundibular, but also affects the pulmonary valve and is often associated with hypoplasia (narrowing) of the main pulmonary artery and/or pulmonary artery branches. The aortic valve overrides (sits astride the VSD).

sound is often quite loud but single (because the pulmonary closure sound is inaudible).

Cyanosis appears gradually during the early months of life or rarely in later childhood, and is characteristically more obvious on crying or on exertion. A characteristic feature is the development of intermittent episodes of severe hypoxia and cyanosis (hypoxic spells) which may appear spontaneously but are quite commonly precipitated by stress or exercise. Such spells are characterized by marked pallor or cyanosis with dyspnoea and distress. Loss of consciousness may occur. Hypoxic spells are associated with increased right to left shunting and a sharp reduction in pulmonary flow. In the past these have been attributed to infundibular 'spasm' – though in practise the physiology is more complex and 'spasm' does not occur. First aid treatment of spells (which are potentially dangerous) involves soothing and pacifying the distressed infant with a view to trying to induce sleep. In severe cases intramuscular morphine may be helpful.

Older infants and children have reduced exercise tolerance and often adopt a squatting posture at regular intervals during exertion. This manoeuvre, in which the child squats down on to the haunches with knees up to the chest, increases systemic venous return and systemic vascular resistance. The latter reduces right to left shunting and the increased venous return produces a significant transient rise in pulmonary blood flow with improved oxygenation.

Course and prognosis

Cyanosis generally progresses gradually with diminishing exercise tolerance, finger clubbing and in severe cases growth retardation. Development of cardiac failure is unusual but the severe cyanosis leads to extreme compensatory polycythaemia and cerebral thromboembolic complications (e.g. stroke) may occur. Bacterial endocarditis and cerebral abscess are also important complications.

Investigations

The chest radiograph shows the heart size to be normal with an uptilted apex and concave pulmonary segment associated with reduced lung vascularity (oligaemia). In severe cases the cardiac contour may resemble the shape of a wooden clog – 'coeur en Sabot' – (often referred to as 'boot shaped'). The electrocardiogram usually shows right ventricular hypertrophy. Echocardiography is diagnostic but cardiac catheterization is usually required before surgical intervention.

Differential diagnosis

In infancy, before the onset of cyanosis, the murmur is often mistaken for that of a small VSD.

Other cyanotic defects such as tricuspid atresia may be differentiated by the help of ancillary investigations such as ECG, radiograph and echocardiogram.

Treatment

Total correction involving repair of the ventricular septal defect and relief of the infundibular and pulmonary valve stenosis can be carried out even in early infancy if the anatomy is suitable. However, many affected children have quite marked hypoplasia of the branch pulmonary arteries and this may make it desirable to delay repair and to carry out one or more palliative 'shunt' operations first. These involve creating a communication between the aorta and a pulmonary artery to increase pulmonary blood flow (allowing better growth of the branch pulmonary arteries).

Infants who are having significant hypoxic spells can be treated medically in the short term with beta-adrenergic blocking drugs, e.g propanolol, to prevent spells while the child is awaiting surgery.

Transposition of the great arteries

In this condition the aorta and pulmonary arteries arise from the incorrect ventricles. This is described as 'ventriculo-arterial discordance' (Fig. 40.7). Systemic

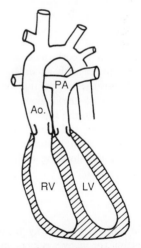

Fig. 40.7 Diagram of transposition of the great arteries. Shows right ventricular origin of the aorta and the pulmonary trunk connected to the left ventricle.

venous blood is directed through the right side of the heart back into the aorta and pulmonary venous blood through the left side of the heart and back into the pulmonary circulation. Survival is dependent on transfer of blood across from each circuit into the other via a foramen ovale, ductus arteriosus or a septal defect. Affected infants generally survive for several days or even weeks due to shunting through the foramen ovale and/or ductus arteriosus, but few live longer than a month without help unless they have a coexisting septal defect (e.g large VSD).

Clinical features

Cyanosis is present from the early hours of life and usually progresses gradually over the next few days. Metabolic acidosis may also develop if the situation persists untreated (due to the tissue hypoxia). Apart from the cyanosis the infant may appear completely normal. Palpation reveals a forceful right ventricular impulse at the left sternal edge, but on auscultation there is frequently no murmur audible.

Investigations

The chest radiograph shows a relatively normal sized heart with a contour which sometimes resembles an 'egg on its side'. Pulmonary vascular markings are usually mildly increased. The electrocardiogram shows normal ventricular complexes but may manifest T wave abnormalities.

The diagnosis may be established rapidly by echocardiography.

Treatment

Cardiac catheterization is performed as an emergency procedure and a catheter with an inflatable balloon at the tip is passed into the left atrium via the foramen ovale. After inflation of the balloon the catheter is withdrawn with force into the right atrium producing a tear in the atrial septum and hence creating an atrial septal defect (balloon atrial septostomy). This allows more effective interatrial shunting with amelioration of the cyanosis and hypoxia.

Surgery

After successful balloon septostomy most infants will manage comfortably for many weeks or months.

Surgical correction can now be performed in the newborn period by transferring the pulmonary artery and the aorta back to their appropriate ventricles. It is also necessary to transfer the tiny coronary arteries across from the aortic root (above the right ventricle) to the new aortic origin from the left ventricle. The operation is technically difficult and needs to be performed in early infancy (usually the first month of life) before the left ventricle has adapted to feeding the low pressure pulmonary circulation.

An alternative approach which has been widely used in the past (and is still used in many centres) involves waiting until the infant is three to six months old or older and then re-routing blood at atrial level by insertion of a complex intra-atrial patch or baffle (Mustard's operation) or by repositioning the patient's own atrial septum and infolding of part of the right atrium (Senning's operation). These operations, although conceptually difficult to understand, are relatively straight forward to perform and carry low surgical mortality. For this reason they have been preferred by many surgeons to the 'arterial switch' procedure described above.

Tricuspid atresia

In this malformation the tricuspid valve is completely blocked and there is no communication between the right atrium and ventricle. Systemic venous blood passes via the foramen ovale or an atrial septal defect into the left side of the heart and at ventricular or arterial level a left to right shunt exists (via a VSD or PDA). This allows blood to perfuse the pulmonary circulation – usually in reduced amounts.

Clinical features

Cyanosis develops early. A systolic murmur is audible along the left sternal border.

Diagnosis

The diagnosis may be suspected on the characteristic ECG pattern of left axis deviation, right atrial hypertrophy, left ventricular hypertrophy, right ventricular hypoplasia. Echocardiography confirms the diagnosis.

Treatment

A palliative shunt operation (see above under tetralogy of Fallot) may be performed in infancy. Later in childhood reconstructive cardiac surgery is usually feasible and involves the creation of a wide anastomosis between the right atrium and the pulmonary arteries allowing systemic venous blood to pass directly into the pulmonary circulation (a Fontan operation).

Pulmonary atresia

In this condition the origin of the pulmonary artery from the right ventricle is completely obstructed or absent. Blood in the right side of the heart passes via an ASD, foramen ovale or VSD into the left ventricle and aorta. The pulmonary circulation depends on collateral flow from the aorta (via a PDA or other collateral channels).

Clinical features

Cyanosis develops early and many infants have an easily audible continuous murmur due to the associated persistent ductus arteriosus or other collaterals feeding the pulmonary circulation from the aorta.

Diagnosis

The diagnosis is usually confirmed by echocardiography though it may be suspected strongly on clinical grounds coupled with ECG and radiographic findings.

Treatment

Early treatment usually involves a systemic-pulmonary shunt procedure. At a later stage which depends on the associated defects, surgical correction may be performed by opening up a way through from the right ventricle into the pulmonary arteries (often by insertion of a 'valved conduit').

Persistent truncus arteriosus

This rare defect is associated with the presence of a single artery which branches shortly after arising from the heart to give rise to the pulmonary artery and aorta. The truncal valve usually sits astride a large ventricular septal defect and receives blood from both right and left ventricles.

Clinical features

Cyanosis is usually mild or absent and congestive heart failure often appears in the newborn period. Both systolic and diastolic murmurs are frequently heard (due to the abnormal truncal valve which is often incompetent).

Diagnosis

The diagnosis can be made by echocardiography. Chest radiograph and ECG findings are usually non-specific.

Treatment

The only effective treatment is surgical correction which needs to be carried out often in early infancy. The pulmonary artery is separated from the truncus and after closure of the VSD leaving the aorta arising from the left ventricle a valved conduit is placed to connect the right ventricle to the pulmonary arteries.

Haematology and oncology

41. The pale child

M. J. Robinson

PALLOR

The colour of the skin is dependent on several factors. The quantity of melanin produced by melanocytes of the basal layer of the epidermis obviously determines the racial differences in skin colour. The pigmentation seen in adrenal insufficiency is also largely the result of excess melanin produced in response to the excessive secretion of melanocyte-stimulating hormone – a feature of this disorder. Skin colour is modified by other abnormal deposits, most obvious in the case of liver disease, particularly obstructive liver disease, when the skin appears almost green. Milder degrees of jaundice may at times simulate pallor. The deposition of iron in skin, characteristic of inadequately treated thalassaemia major, or urates in chronic renal insufficiency and carotene in carotenaemia, are further examples where the skin colour has been modified by pigmentary deposition.

In addition, skin colour is dependent under normal circumstances on the blood flow through the subpapillary venous plexus. Adrenergic nerve fibres to skin vessels modify their calibre and hence the amount and rate of blood flow within them. This, in turn, influences the degree of haemoglobin reduction which will take place within the skin vessels. The adrenergic nerves supplying the skin vessels respond physiologically to temperature, pain and emotion, all of which may be accompanied by skin pallor. Pathologically, cutaneous vasoconstriction is seen in shocked states and in situations where there is pathological hypersecretion of adrenalin, e.g. in hypoglycaemia and in phaeochromocytoma.

Parents frequently complain that their child is pale so it is useful to have a diagnostic approach to this problem. One such approach is shown in Figure 41.1.

Pallor of recent onset associated with fever, but without anaemia

In this situation the child is usually toxic and, although pale, the skin is hot. The pale febrile child often has a serious infection and a careful search must be made to identify the source. Because of the acute nature of the illness, the history may yield little information and when symptoms are mentioned they are frequently nonspecific, e.g. malaise, irritability, anorexia, fever or vague abdominal pain. The physical examination must be very complete and disorders such as meningitis, septicaemia, pyelonephritis and pneumonia must be

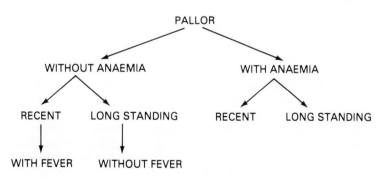

Fig. 41.1 Diagnostic approach to the pale child.

considered. This applies particularly in the neonatal period.

Pallor of recent onset unassociated with fever and anaemia

Despite the absence of fever, infection cannot be excluded particularly in the neonatal period; this is less common in the older infant or child unless there is gross debility.

The most obvious situation here is acute circulatory insufficiency. Here the child is pale, the extremities are cold, clammy or blue, the pulse is rapid, weak, and thready and the blood pressure low. Circulatory failure and hypovolaemia may be because of the following:

1. Acute blood loss
2. Fluid loss from bowel or renal tract
3. Massive toxaemia
4. Renal disease
5. Congestive heart failure.

Acute blood loss

Pallor due to acute blood loss may be obvious, particularly as a result of severe trauma. Initially the haemoglobin is not reduced, but anaemia will be obvious by 24 hours. Internal bleeding, possibly the result of a rupture of the spleen or liver, or from a haemothorax, must always be considered in the pale child who has experienced recent trauma. Acute overt blood loss is not common in children apart from trauma, but may occasionally occur from a bleeding Meckel's diverticulum or from gastric and oesophageal varices. Bleeding from peptic ulceration of the upper gastrointestinal tract is an uncommon cause and haemoptysis is very rare in childhood. Pallor may precede the overt bleeding and this may cause confusion unless the possibility is kept in mind.

Concealed haemorrhage in the neonatal period may also cause problems in diagnosis, particularly if it is not recognized that the normal haemoglobin at birth is 15.9–17.9 g/dl and the haematocrit 55%. Bleeding from an abnormal insertion of the umbilical cord into the placenta, into a twin, or into the mother, may result in a haemoglobin of 11–12 g/dl or less. Such an infant may be pale and shocked, although the neonate may be well compensated if the blood loss has been gradual. Bleeding from the cord, too early clamping of the cord, cephalhaematoma, intracranial bleeding, bleeding from spleen, liver or into muscle, the result of birth injury, may also result in a pale baby whose haemoglobin by standards at other periods of life will seem normal, but

who is in fact grossly anaemic. Any neonate with a haemoglobin value less than 13 g/dl should be considered anaemic.

Hypovolaemia

The pallor associated with hypovolaemia consequent on vomiting and diarrhoea rarely poses a problem in diagnosis. Here signs of dehydration are present and the history and physical findings usually indicate the diagnosis. Gastroenteritis is by far the commonest cause, but other lesions of the gastrointestinal tract should be considered. The dehydration with pallor which may accompany adrenal insufficiency will not cause problems if it is recognized that there have been insufficient losses of fluid from the bowel to explain the degree of dehydration present. This suspicion should be heightened if the genitalia are abnormal. Serum electrolyte values reveal gross lowering of serum sodium and elevation of serum potassium in an adrenal crisis.

Overwhelming infection with severe toxaemia

This may be the cause of pallor in the absence of fever or anaemia. Generally, this would imply septicaemia or an intra-abdominal catastrophe, e.g. rupture of a viscus, intussusception, etc.

Renal disease

This is also very frequently associated with pallor, when anaemia may or may not be present. In infancy renal insufficiency may present as a pale infant with either dehydration or failure to thrive, or a combination of both. Urinary tract infection may coexist, but there may be no overt signs to suggest its presence.

Pallor is a feature of acute poststreptococcal nephritis and of the nephrotic syndrome, even in the absence of anaemia. This often relates to the oedema whereby the overall thickness of the skin is increased.

Congestive heart failure in infancy and childhood

This is frequently accompanied by pallor in the absence of fever or anaemia. The diagnosis will not be missed if it is appreciated that the most important signs of heart failure in infancy are tachypnoea and hepatomegaly. The heart will always be enlarged, but this may be difficult to detect in a small infant without a chest radiograph. Tachycardia or a gallop rhythm are usually present, but the absence of murmurs will in no way exclude a diagnosis of heart failure. It must also be appreciated that peripheral oedema is infrequent in infants with heart failure and the lung fields are frequently clear to auscultation.

Long-standing pallor without anaemia

The physician is not infrequently consulted by parents who complain that their child has been pale for weeks, months or even years. General health may have been good otherwise, but often there are vague associated symptoms such as tiredness, malaise, anorexia or recurrent abdominal pain. Physical examination may reveal little in this group and investigation may be required. The more common causes of pallor in this group are:

1. Psychological
2. Allergic
3. Metabolic

Psychological

Here anxiety is the basis of the symptoms and of the pallor. A carefully taken history should establish, firstly, that there is anxiety, and, secondly, that there are reasons for it.

Allergy

It is common for the allergic child to present purely because the parents are concerned about skin pallor. Physical examination may reveal a dry skin, swollen nasal mucous membrane indicating allergic rhinitis, or signs within the chest may indicate asthma (see Ch. 23).

Metabolic

Certain metabolic disorders may present because of pallor with little or no anaemia. In general those children tend to be in poor health. Because of this, and the absence of specific physical findings, investigations may be indicated. Renal disease should be excluded by urinalysis, microscopy and culture of urine, blood urea and serum creatinine estimations. Rare inborn errors of metabolism, if suspect, will be identified from amino acid chromatography of urine, high voltage electrophoresis and gas liquid chromatography of urine and blood. Hypothyroidism, which may present in this way, should also be considered, but congenital hypothyroidism is less likely in countries where universal neonatal screening is undertaken. Hypothyroid children are generally pale even in the absence of anaemia. The facies, however, is typical and there is physical and mental sluggishness. The diagnosis is confirmed by thyroid function studies. Treatment with thyroxine is curative and the pallor disappears.

Pallor associated with anaemia

Anaemia implies a decrease in the concentration of haemoglobin. It cannot be diagnosed with certainty by simple inspection of the skin and mucous membranes and, in childhood, anaemia is frequently symptomless. Children may tolerate very severe anaemia with few or no symptoms at all if the anaemia is long standing, and the child only presents because of an unrelated acute illness. Some acute haemolytic anaemias may present as an infection with fever, chills and rigors.

The diagnosis of anaemia is made by estimation of the haemoglobin concentration or, more properly, by measuring the haemoglobin concentration and the haematocrit (Hct) or packed cell volume (PCV). Under normal circumstances the haematocrit corresponds to three times the haemoglobin concentration (g/dl).

It is of fundamental importance to appreciate the normal haemoglobin values throughout infancy and childhood. These are illustrated in Figure 42.2 page 345. It therefore follows that levels of haemoglobin, which may be regarded as normal in later infancy and childhood, represent a severe anaemia in the neonatal period. Conversely physiological levels at the age of 2–3 months may be mistakenly regarded as constituting anaemia.

Red cell indices

Red cell count and mean corpuscular volume (MCV) are directly measured by electronic counter. As measured by electronic counter, the MCV is a more accurate index than when it was calculated from the centrifuged haematocrit and the chamber red cell count.

The mean corpuscular haemoglobin (MCH) is usually proportional to the MCV, but is a more complex and less accurate calculation. It is derived from the haemoglobin concentration divided by the product of the MCV and the red cell number.

The MCV confirms the size of red cells inferred from examination of the blood film (normal 78 to 85 femtolitres (fl). The MCH usually follows the same direction as the MCV but can be helpful in distinguishing iron deficiency anaemia from thalassaemia. This is very difficult from the blood film alone. Normal values for MCH – 27 to 31 pg.

MCV between 65 and 75 fl, coupled with an MCH between 20 and 25 pg is far more likely to be due to thalassaemia minor than iron deficiency.

MCV below 65 fl, especially if the MCH is less than 20 pg, is more likely to be due to iron deficiency. It must be remembered that patients with thalassaemia minor can also have iron deficiency.

DIAGNOSIS OF THE CAUSE OF ANAEMIA

Once anaemia has been established the cause must be found. This, in the first instance, involves a full paediatric history and complete physical examination. In diagnosis, the age of the child is particularly relevant; the more important points of history are set out in various age groups.

1. Neonatal period

Period of gestation. Preterm and 'small for dates' infants are at risk for iron deficiency.

Jaundice. A history of neonatal jaundice, particularly if exchange transfusion or simple blood transfusion was necessary, will often be relevant to subsequent anaemia.

Haemorrhagic manifestations. Easy bruising and bleeding, or a single episode of haemorrhage not adequately treated, will be of significance in the diagnosis of anaemia in later infancy.

2. Infancy

Diet. At this time diet is of the greatest importance in the prevention of anaemia. Thus, enquiry must take in the total milk intake, the time that solid foods were introduced and exactly what types of food were offered.

Infection. A recent infection may be relevant to the presence of anaemia; recurrent infections almost certainly will. Bowel habits and the characteristics of stools must be noted as a history of recurrent or chronic diarrhoea will be of importance in diagnosis. The possibility of malaria as a cause of anaemia must always be kept in mind, particularly in migrants from tropical countries.

3. Childhood

In this period it is equally important to enquire into both the quantity and quality of the diet. A history of recurrent infection, particularly bowel infection, will almost certainly be significant in this age group. The history of blood loss is obviously important.

4. At any age

The following details of history will be relevant to establishing the cause for anaemia: jaundice, drug ingestion, abnormal bruising or bleeding and a family history of abnormal bleeding or bruising. The onset and the length of illness should be noted, for example, a long history suggests either a long-standing deficiency or a long-standing haemolytic anaemia. An acute onset, particularly with constitutional symptoms (fever, abdominal pain, vomiting), is suggestive of a haemolytic anaemia. The ethnic group (e.g. Mediterranean or South East Asian) is particularly relevant in regard to G-6-PD deficiency, thalassaemia or sickle-cell anaemia.

Physical examination

This must be complete, but special notice taken of the following:

1. The skin and mucous membranes for pallor, bruising, petechial spots or telangiectases.
2. The conjunctivae for the presence of pallor and jaundice.
3. The liver, spleen and lymph nodes – enlargement of one or all of these will point to the presence of a systemic disease, e.g. leukaemia, reticulosis, connective tissue disorder, or to acute or chronic haemolysis.
4. Growth failure – anaemia alone may be causative, but more usually this will imply the presence of a chronic systemic disorder.

Investigations relevant to anaemia

The type of anaemia present may be determined in most cases from a few simple tests. These include:

1. Haemoglobin, haematocrit and other red cell indices (MCV, MCH)
2. Peripheral blood film (Fig. 41.2)
3. White cell count and differential white cell count
4. Reticulocyte count
5. Urinalysis
6. Serum bilirubin.

Examination of the blood film

Abnormalities in red cell morphology. These include:

Microcytes. These are found particularly in iron deficiency anaemia, but also in the thalassaemias.

Macrocytes. These will be seen in the anaemia of folic acid or vitamin B_{12} deficiency.

Microspherocytes. These are specifically seen in congenital spherocytosis but also in acquired haemolysis, e.g. ABO incompatibility, autoimmune haemolytic anaemia.

Immature red cells. Increased numbers of reticulocytes, normoblasts or polychromatic red cells indicate active regeneration.

Distorted cells. These can take the form of burr cells or other bizarre forms and may be seen in renal disease and in many haemolytic disorders (Fig. 41.3).

Target cells. A large number of these cells indicate the

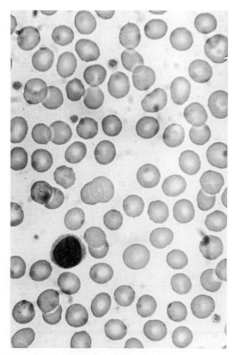

Fig. 41.2 The normal blood film.

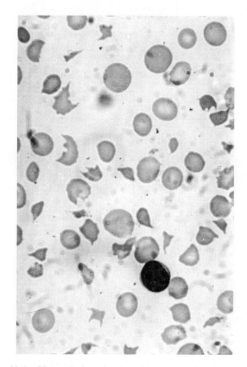

Fig. 41.3 Haemolytic uraemic syndrome.

possibility of iron deficiency, thalassaemia, a structural haemoglobinopathy or liver disease.

Howell-Jolly bodies. These are red cell inclusion bodies and may be seen after splenectomy, in congenital asplenia, after drug-induced haemolysis and in other severe haemolytic anaemias.

Red cell inclusions particularly malarial parasites. Malaria must always be considered as a likely cause of anaemia in tropical countries but must not be forgotten in recent migrants and in overseas travellers.

Examination of the blood film will also detect abnormalities of the white blood cells such as immature leukocytes, hypersegmented neutrophils and gross platelet deficiencies. The reticulocyte count indicates the presence of red cells which have been formed in the past 24–48 hours. Normally this is 0.4–1.6% of the total red cells, provided that the red cell count is normal. Counts in excess of 2–3% are abnormal and imply a hyperactive responding bone marrow but should be correlated to the red cell count to ensure that there is absolute increase of reticulocytes. A decreased reticulocyte count indicates poor red cell production. Thus, the reticulocyte count is a very sensitive index of bone marrow activity at the time of observation and consequently very helpful in diagnosis. Normally a reticulocytosis results in elevation of the haemoglobin levels. If, despite an elevated reticulocyte count, the haemoglobin level does not rise, increased destruction of red cells is implied. A decreased reticulocyte count implies decreased red cell production and is always associated with a fall in haemoglobin level.

CLASSIFICATION OF ANAEMIA

When blood loss is excluded, anaemia is the result of one of two mechanisms:

1. Defective production of red cells
2. Increased destruction of red cells in excess of production.

Anaemias due to the defective production of red cells

These are summarized in Tables 41.1 and 41.2.

Although these disorders may often be diagnosed on the blood film, confirmation is frequently necessary because of the implications for treatment and prognosis. In this group of anaemias the following confirmatory tests may be indicated in Table 41.3.

Aplastic anaemia

This disorder may occur as the result of damage to

Table 41.1 Anaemias due to defective production of red blood cells: dietary

Aetiology	Mechanism	Disease entity
Iron deficiency	Inadequate intake Blood loss	Iron deficiency anaemia Haemorrhage from any site including the bleeding and coagulation disorders
Folic acid deficiency	Inadequate intake Increased utilization	Malnutrition Recurrent infections Chronic haemolysis
Vitamin B_{12} deficiency	Lack of intrinsic factor Defect in absorption	Congenital pernicious anaemia Regional ileitis Ileal resection Abnormality of specific B_{12} transport protein Blind loop syndrome
Vitamin E	Temporary malabsorption	Infantile pyknocytosis
Combined deficiencies	Inadequate intake Malabsorption	Malnutrition Coeliac disease Tropical sprue Certain parasitic infestations

Table 41.2 Anaemias due to defective production of red blood cells: bone marrow

Aetiology	Mechanism	Disease entity
Bone marrow defect (generalized)	Congenital Drug induced Idiopathic	Aplastic anaemia
Bone marrow suppression (generalized)	Bone marrow replacement	Leukaemia Neuroblastoma Any skeleto-endothelial systemic malignancy Lipid 'storage' disease
Localized RBC defect	Congenital Chronic infection Chronic renal disease Pyridoxine deficiency	Blackfan Diamond anaemia Pure red cell hypoplasia

precursor cells so that an adequate quantity of haemopoietic cells cannot be supplied. Damage to the stroma surrounding these precursor cells – the so-called microenvironment – is now regarded as being of equal importance in the genesis of aplastic anaemia. Damage to precursor cells will result in depression of all blood elements – erythroid, myeloid and megakaryocytic. Should the damage occur at a later stage, that is, after differentiation has occurred, pure red cell aplasia, agranulocytosis or thrombocytopenia may occur singly.

Pancytopenia may arise as part of congenital aplastic anaemia (Fanconi's anaemia). This is a genetically determined disorder transmitted in an autosomal recessive fashion. Associated congenital abnormalities include a variety of skeletal abnormalities (especially involving the thumb), short stature, skin pigmentation, microcephaly

and renal abnormalities. The onset of the aplastic anaemia in Fanconi's anaemia is usually between 4 and 7 years in boys and 6 and 10 years in girls, although it may occur at an earlier age.

Aplastic anaemia may also follow the ingestion of a large number of drugs and chemicals, following viral infections, or after irradiation and leukaemia. Whether these agents are directly causative or whether they act as a trigger factor in an individual with a genetic disposition to aplastic anaemia is not clear. Drugs associated with aplastic anaemia include chloramphenicol (the commonest), sulphonamides, including sulphonamides without antibacterial effect. The anti-inflammatory agent phenylbutazone and the anticonvulsants mephenytoin (Mesantoin) and trimethadione (Tridione) are also associated with aplastic

Table 41.3 Investigations for anaemias in childhood

Test	Clinical significance
Serum iron	Low in iron deficiency and in the anaemia of chronic infection. High in chronic haemolysis.
Total iron binding capacity	High in iron deficiency and low in anaemia of chronic infection.
Serum ferritin	Low in iron deficiency, normal or elevated in chronic infection and elevated in thalassaemia.
Serum folic acid	May be low in macrocytic anaemia due either to dietary deficiency, excess needs or malabsorption.
Serum vitamin B_{12}	May be low in certain macrocytic anaemias, e.g. malabsorption, malnutrition and in juvenile pernicious anaemia.
Platelet count	Low in thrombocytopenic purpura and in certain states of excessive platelet consumption.
Bone marrow aspiration	Diagnostic in leukaemias, other types of marrow infiltration and aplastic anaemia.

anaemia. Chemicals implicated in causing aplasia are benzene, organic solvents and insecticides such as benzene hexachloride (Lindane), chlorphenothane (DDT) and chlordane. Gold and penicillamine therapy may also be followed by bone marrow aplasia. Aplastic anaemia may rarely occur after viral hepatitis when it is often fatal.

The onset of aplastic anaemia is usually insidious, with pallor, skin bruises and petechiae. Tiredness and anorexia due to anaemia then appear. As the disease progresses bleeding may occur from almost any site and a sore throat with mouth ulceration consequent on profound leukopenia may occur. Physical examination reveals little except pallor and skin bleeding; the liver, spleen and lymph nodes are usually not enlarged. The diagnosis is established from the blood examination, which shows pancytopenia, together with the bone marrow examination, which indicates hypoplasia or aplasia. An adequate marrow aspiration must be obtained from a number of sites, together with marrow trephines to demonstrate the degree of aplasia. Iron stores in the marrow will be absent but the serum iron is high and the iron binding protein fully saturated.

Patients with profound aplastic anaemia who have a suitable bone marrow donor within their family should proceed to bone marrow transplantation as soon as possible. Repeated blood and platelet transfusions soon result in the patient becoming sensitized and a successful marrow transplant less likely. When a suitable donor is not available the treatment of choice is antithymocyte globulin. There is no scientific evidence that androgens or corticosteroids influence recovery from aplastic anaemia. Blood and platelet transfusions will be required for anaemia and control of bleeding. Chemoprophylaxis will be required in severe leukopenia to control infection.

Transient erythroblastopenic anaemia of childhood

This is a self-limited aregenerative anaemia of childhood of unknown cause. The child may present because of increasing pallor, or a blood examination performed for some other reason may disclose a significant anaemia (normochromic and normocytic). The reticulocyte count is low. Physical examination does not demonstrate any abnormality but a history of a preceding infection is frequently obtained. Investigation reveals an elevated serum iron and a low total iron binding capacity. On bone marrow examination a decreased number of precursor cells will be noted. This disorder resolves after a variable time but one or more blood transfusions may be required before this.

Leukaemia and other marrow infiltrations will not be further discussed here. As causes of anaemia, the diagnosis of these disorders will usually be suspected on physical examination. The peripheral blood film will indicate anaemia (usually of the normochromic type), thrombocytopenia and in most cases, immature or abnormal white blood cells. Bone marrow examination will establish the diagnosis (see Ch. 44).

Anaemia due to increased destruction of red cells

The list of causes of haemolytic anaemia is a very long one and can be readily obtained from any textbook of haematology. The presence of haemolysis can frequently be made on the basis of the peripheral blood film when alterations in red cell morphology as described above will be noted (see Fig. 41.4).

Confirmatory tests for the presence of haemolysis will include:

1. Reticulocyte count.
2. Heinz body preparation.
3. Serum haptoglobin – low or absent in haemolytic states.

4. Detection of free haemoglobin or methaemalbumin in plasma – positive in intravascular haemolysis.

5. Detection of oxyhaemoglobin in urine in intravascular haemolysis.

6. Serological tests to detect antibodies on the red cells or in the serum (Coombs' tests, cold agglutinins, Landsteiner tests, – Ham's acid serum test).

7. Bone marrow examination – will indicate red cell hyperplasia in haemolytic states.

8. Isotopic red cell survival studies.

The following is a simple and practical classification of haemolytic anaemia in childhood.

A. Haemolytic disease in the neonatal period

1. ABO incompatibility
2. Rh incompatibility
3. Minor blood group incompatibilities (Kell, Duffy, Kidd)
4. G-6-PD deficiency, pyruvate-kinase deficiency and other rarer red cell enzyme defects.

Haemolytic disease in the neonatal period is always associated with jaundice and in diagnosis the relevant investigations involve:

1. Haemoglobin, blood group and Rh typing
2. Peripheral blood film
3. Serum bilirubin
4. Coombs' test (direct and indirect)
5. G-6-PD assay.

Microspherocytes in the peripheral blood indicate either ABO, Rh incompatibility or hereditary spherocytosis (Fig. 41.4). Maternal antibody studies will confirm ABO incompatibility. Osmotic fragility tests for autohaemolysis and family studies will be necessary to confirm hereditary spherocytosis.

Management of the haemolytic anaemias in the neonatal period is particularly concerned with the management of the associated hyperbilirubinaemia. It is of the greatest importance in management that blood is taken for investigation before any exchange transfusion is commenced.

B. Intravascular haemolysis

Haemoglobinaemia is the feature of this group. The urine may have a port wine or tea colour and oxyhaemoglobin will be detected spectroscopically. Oxyhaemoglobin must be distinguished from bile and pigments and from haematuria.

The commonest haemolytic anaemias in this group are:

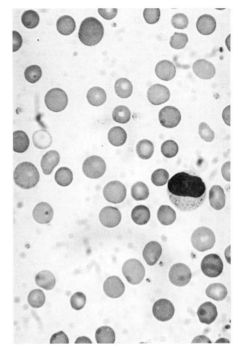

Fig. 41.4   Hereditary spherocytosis.

1. G-6-PD deficiency
2. Autoimmune haemolytic anaemia (see Fig. 41.5).

In G-6-PD deficiency males are usually affected, the precipitating factors being drugs, broad beans and infections. In autoimmune haemolytic anaemia the direct Coombs' test will be positive. Rarer causes of intravascular haemolysis include the haemolytic uraemic syndrome, anaemia of collagen disease, haemoglobin H thalassaemia and malaria.

C. Haemolytic anaemias associated with marked splenomegaly

The common conditions in this group are:

1. Beta thalassaemia major
2. Hereditary spherocytosis.

The diagnosis of thalassaemia is made by haemoglobin electrophoresis (see Ch. 43). Hereditary spherocytosis is confirmed by the demonstration of abnormal osmotic fragility and tests of autohaemolysis.

The management of hereditary spherocytosis involves observations of the haemoglobin level and blood transfusion as necessary. This routine should be continued as long as possible in childhood to avoid splenectomy which carries with it a significant risk of overwhelming infection. It should be noted, however, that many

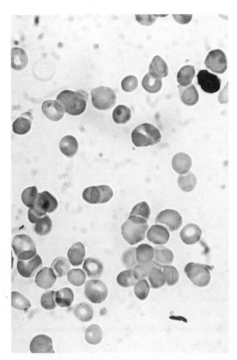

Fig. 41.5 Autoimmune haemolytic anaemia (showing red cell agglutination).

children with congenital spherocytosis are asymptomatic and never require splenectomy. Symptomatic congenital spherocytosis is cured after splenectomy but, of course, the basic red cell anomaly remains. The management of Beta thalassaemia is discussed in Chapter 44.

D. Haemolytic anaemia associated with minor enlargement of the spleen

In this group the anaemia is not severe, the problem is not acute and the disorders may only be suspected when a routine blood film is examined or family studies are being performed. The peripheral blood film shows hypochromia which may be confused with mild iron deficiency.

The two disorders to be considered in this group are:

1. Beta thalassaemia minor
2. Haemoglobin H thalassaemia.

These are diagnosed by haemoglobin electrophoresis and by incubation of whole blood with brilliant cresyl blue, when inclusion bodies are seen in thalassaemia (Ch. 44).

Management of anaemia

Anaemia is a symptom and not a disease in itself. It must, in the first instance, be diagnosed by the methods that have been indicated and be followed by a plan of investigation that will determine the cause. As a general rule a good history and physical examination will provide the best leads which will allow the diagnosis of the type of anaemia to be made with the aid of very few standard haematological tests. Logical treatment will only follow when the nature of the disorder producing the anaemia is known. The widespread use of iron in the treatment of anaemia is to be condemned; it should be reserved for iron deficiency. Iron treatment is, in fact, contraindicated in a number of anaemias, particularly the thalassaemias. The management of the deficiency disease is clear-cut – define the cause and replace the deficiency. Management of anaemia associated with bone marrow defect is complex and depends on the cause, as has already been discussed. With regard to the haemolytic anaemias, a knowledge of the underlying cause is even more essential as therapy for one type of haemolytic anaemia may be completely inappropriate for another.

FURTHER READING

Baehner R L (ed) 1980 Pediatric haematology. The Pediatric Clinics of North America 27: 2
Ekert H (ed) 1982 Clinical paediatric haematology and oncology. Blackwell Scientific Publications, Oxford
Gill G M, Schwarz E 1972 Anaemia in early infancy. The Pediatric Clinics of North America 19(4): 841–854
Willoughby M L N 1977 Paediatric haematology. Churchill Livingstone, Edinburgh

42. Iron deficiency in childhood

Geoffrey P. Tauro

Iron deficiency remains the most common cause of anaemia, affecting hundred of millions of children and adults. While it is most prevalent in the lower socioeconomic groups, especially in the developing world, it is still to be found in more affluent societies.

IRON METABOLISM

Excess iron is very toxic to body tissues. We protect ourselves by limiting our absorption. The daily requirement for iron in an adult is 25 mg, of which 24 mg is obtained from previously used iron which has been returned to the metabolic pool. Intestinal absorption is limited to 1–1.5 mg per day. There appears to be no effective mechanism to excrete excess iron stores in the body.

Before birth the fetus absorbs iron from the mother across the placenta against a concentration gradient. At the time of birth iron stores are 75 mg/kg, bearing a constant relationship to bodyweight. Thus, a small birthweight baby has low iron stores relative to a normal birthweight baby. After birth absorption occurs from the intestine, mainly the duodenum and upper jejunum, with small amounts absorbed from the stomach and distal small bowel.

Dietary iron, mainly ferric iron complexes in the food, is broken down and reduced by gastric hydrochloric acid and absorbed by gut mucosal cells and appears in the plasma bound to the transport protein, transferrin. It is carried to sites of utilization, mainly the bone marrow, for use in the production of haemoglobin, myoglobin and iron containing enzymes. Should body iron stores be high the mucosal cells in the gut retain the absorbed iron, which is lost when the mucosal cell is shed 2 to 3 days later.

Factors which increase the amount of iron absorbed include a negative iron balance, increased iron presented to the gut, and the presence of compounds such as as-corbic acid, citric acid, fructose and amino acids in the diet. Heme, found in meat, appears to be more readily absorbed than elemental iron. Substances such as tannates (in tea), phosphates, EDTA, clay and antacids decrease iron absorption.

Body iron is distributed into two pools. The metabolic pool contains three quarters of the body iron; 70% is in haemoglobin, 4% in myoglobin and 1% in iron containing enzymes. The remainder is held in the storage pool, in two related compounds, ferritin and haemosiderin. These two compounds are distributed evenly between the liver, spleen and the bone marrow, sited in the parenchymal cells and in reticuloendothelial cells. Stores can be visualized by staining the tissues using the Perls' stain (potassium ferrocyanide). Small amounts of ferritin are found in plasma and under normal conditions reflect body iron stores (1 μg/l of ferritin being equivalent to 10 mg of stored iron).

IRON REQUIREMENTS

Iron is an essential requirement for compounds concerned with oxygen transport, electron transfer and for a large number of enzymes. The daily requirement for iron is about 25 mg for adult males, slightly more for menstruating females. Our ability to conserve catabolized iron means that we have only a limited need to absorb iron to replace normal losses by intestinal blood loss, in bile, in mucosal cells and in desquamated skin. Adult males need to absorb about 0.9 mg iron daily, menstruating females 1.4 mg. The pregnant woman needs to absorb 6 mg per day during the last trimester to provide iron for herself and for the developing fetus.

Children need to increase their iron stores from about 260 mg at birth to 2–3.5 g by the time they reach adulthood. During the first year they need to absorb 150–200 mg of iron to provide for the increase in their blood volume, to build stores and fulfil their other iron requirements. The rate of iron acquisition is thus 1.5 mg per day. Low birthweight children need to absorb even larger amounts, to catch up with their low body iron stores and to keep pace with their more rapid rate of growth. The American Academy of Pediatrics has, therefore, recommended that normal birthweight infants should be given supplementary iron at the rate of 1 mg/kg/day of elemental iron (up to a total maximum of 15 mg per day) commencing at 4 months of age at the latest, continuing until 3 years of age.

Additionally, they recommended that low birthweight infants be given 2 mg/kg of elemental iron per day, commencing at 2 months. A second period of rapid body growth occurs during adolescence, a time when iron deficiency once again becomes prevalent.

Food sources of iron vary both in their content and their bioavailability. Breast milk and cow's milk have low amounts of iron (0.5–1.0 mg/l), but breast milk has a very high rate of absorption (50%), while only 10% of cow's milk iron is absorbed. It should be noted that cow's milk may occasionally induce intestinal bleeding in some children due to allergy. Meat and fish contain from 1–3.2 mg of iron per 100 g, with as much as 20% absorption. Dried fortified cereals contain from 32–50 mg of iron per 100 g, but have a low rate of absorption (0.9%) (see Table 42.1).

Table 42.1 Iron content of infant food

Food	Iron
Iron fortified cereal	32–50 mg/100 g
Organ meats (liver, heart)	>5 mg/100 g
Wheat germ, egg yolk	>5 mg/100 g
Dried beans, fruits	>5 mg/100 g
Muscle meat, fish, fowl	1–5 mg/100 g
Green vegetables, cereals	1–5 mg/100 g
Yellow vegetable	<1 mg/100 g
Milk (cows, human)	0.5–1 mg/l

IRON DEFICIENCY

Anaemia is the final manifestation of iron deficiency. During the initial stage of iron deficiency the body's iron stores are progressively depleted and the level of ferritin in the serum falls, followed by a fall in the serum iron and percentage of transferrin saturation. The final stage sees a progressive fall in the haemoglobin, mean cell volume and mean cell haemoglobin. The rate of fall of haemoglobin will affect the production of symptoms, so that a slowly developing anaemia may not produce obvious symptoms until the haemoglobin reaches very low levels.

Aetiology of iron deficiency in infants and children

Causes of iron deficiency can be divided into a number of categories:

1. Increased requirements
2. Inadequate intake
3. Malabsorption
4. Blood loss.

Multiple causes may be present in the one patient.

Increased requirements for iron occur at a number of key times in the life of a child; during the first year of life, during the phase of growth at about 5 years and during adolescence. Neonates do not suffer from iron deficiency, except following blood loss before or at the time of birth, as the result of fetomaternal bleed, a feto-fetal bleed (Fig 42.1), placental bleed or after inadequate blood replacement following exchange transfusion. Low birthweight babies may develop iron deficiency anaemia from 4 months after birth and infants who do not receive adequate iron in their diet begin to develop anaemia from about 9 months. Diets rich in milk and cereals, but poor in meat, vegetables and iron supplementation will result in iron deficiency. The effect of poor eating habits (with current fads for 'junk food') may also lead to iron deficiency in young school age children and adolescents.

Inadequate intake of iron rich food or lack of iron supplementation in young children is probably the most important cause of iron deficiency in paediatrics. This is especially a problem in poor countries and the poorer sections of more affluent societies. Nutritional iron deficiency may be associated with other deficiencies, e.g. folic acid, vitamin and protein deficiencies, and must be sought when assessing the patient's diet.

Malabsorption of iron is uncommon in children, but may be seen associated with chronic diarrhoea or in malabsorption syndromes such as coeliac disease.

Blood loss is a significant, but not the most common cause of iron deficiency in children. The gastrointestinal tract is the most usual site of blood loss, with a large variety of lesions being implicated. These are listed in Example 42.1.

After birth there is a physiological fall in the haemoglobin value, reaching as low as 9.5 g/dl at about 2 months (Fig. 42.2). This is due to a shortened red cell survival in the neonate (about 80 days compared to the normal 120 days), coupled with a decreased red cell

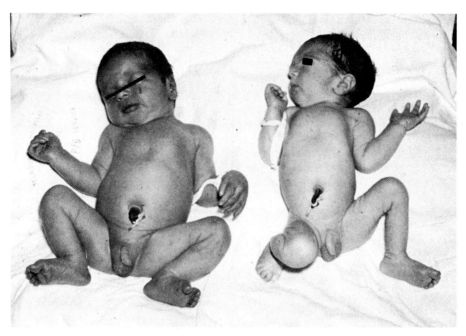

Fig. 42.1 Twin to twin transfusion. One twin is large and plethoric the other pale and small.

Example 42.1 Causes of iron deficiency anaemia

Inadequate supply of iron
Inadequate iron stores following birth:
  1. Low birth weight, prematurity
  2. Blood loss before or at time of birth
Inadequate intake:
Cow's milk diet, delayed addition of iron containing foods to diet, lack of or inadequate iron supplementation

Excessive demands
  1. Prematurity, low birth weight infants, rapid body growth (twins)
  2. Adolescence, menstruation
  3. Chronic intravascular haemolysis (congenital or acquired haemolytic anaemias)

Impaired absorption
  1. Chronic diarrhoea
  2. Malabsorption
  3. Iron deficiency induced malabsorption

  4. Gastrointestinal abnormalities

Blood loss
  1. Perinatal haemorrhage: into mother, twin, placenta, external haemorrhage
  2. Umbilical cord: rupture, haemorrhage, exchange transfusion
  3. Gut: iron deficiency induced bleeding, cow's milk allergy, epistaxis, hiatus hernia, varices, peptic ulceration, duplication of gut, Meckel's diverticulum associated peptic ulceration, colitis, polyps, neoplasia, hereditary telangiectasia, inflammatory bowel disease, haemorrhoids, Henoch-Schönlein purpura
Drug-induced bleeding e.g. aspirin, steroids
Parasites e.g. hookworm
Malabsorption: severe diarrhoea
  4. Lung: pulmonary haemosiderosis, Goodpasture's syndrome
  5. Uterus: menstrual loss
  6. Kidney: neoplasia, trauma, nephrotic syndrome

---

production of new red cells during the first 2 months after delivery. Recovery in red cell production occurs at about 2 months. At about this time factors such as low birthweight followed by rapid weight gain, poor absorption of iron from cow's milk, cow's milk intolerance leading to blood loss, or early clamping of the umbilical cord may lead to the development of iron deficiency.

Clinical features

Clinical presentation

While iron deficiency anaemia in children most frequently occurs between the ages of 6 months and 2 years, it can be found at any age. Early stages may pass undetected by parents and those close to the child, first

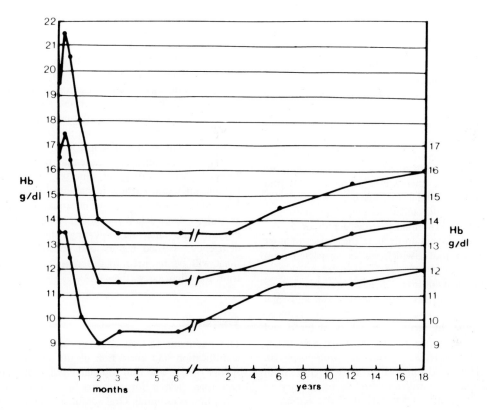

Fig. 42.2   Normal haemoglobin values according to age (± 2 sd).

being observed by casual observers. The children can often tolerate moderate to marked degree of anaemia (4–5 g/dl) before symptoms occur, especially if the anaemia has a gradual onset. Decompensation may only occur after an intercurrent illness, (e.g. viral infection) or after an acute bleed.

Symptoms usually detected are pallor, lethargy, irritability, anorexia and excessive fatigue after physical activity. Abnormal dietary habits may occur, with children chewing on solid objects (pica), or eating dirt or clay (geophagia). The child may have altered attention span, their alertness may be diminished and there may be decreased learning capacity. An increased incidence of infections may be noted.

A history of predisposing factors should be sought. Perinatal events are important in children under the age of one year and a detailed history should be taken. Appraisal of the nutritional adequacy of the diet in meeting iron and other food requirements and the history of iron supplementation and compliance must be made. While an obvious acute bleeding episode will be remembered, the parent will not be aware of chronic or occult blood loss, particularly if it occurs from the intestinal tract.

Physical examination

Pallor is the hallmark of anaemia. It can only be reliably detected once the haemoglobin has fallen below the level of 7 g/dl. It is most readily detected in the creases of the palm, the nail beds and on the mucosal surfaces. The child will have a general pallor, but this may be obscured in children with dark skin pigmentation or accentuated in children with fair complexions. The nails may be fragile and thin, but koilonychia is uncommon in children. The spleen may be enlarged 2–3 below the costal margin in a proportion (10–30%) of cases. In severe anaemia tachycardia, cardiac enlargement and congestive heart failure may be present. The site of the blood loss must be sought, e.g. a bleeding nose, skin or mucosal telangiectasia, the presence of melaena or haemoglobinuria.

Laboratory investigations

The haemoglobin is decreased below the lower limit of normal for the age of the child – usually less than 10 g/dl. The mean cell volume (MCV) is reduced below normal (80–96 fl), values usually being less than 65 fl, and the mean corpuscular haemoglobin (MCH) is reduced (to 20 pg or less). Examination of the blood films show small pale red cells (microcytic hypochromia) and variations in shape (poikilocytosis), with elongated cells, target cells and distorted shape being prominent. Usually, the diagnosis can be confidently made from the blood film, although other causes of these blood film changes should be sought (thalassaemia minor, thalassaemia major, chronic inflammation, lead poisoning sideroblastic anaemia). Bone marrow aspiration is not usually required, except to exclude the causes of poor use of iron listed above, which will be suspected from the history.

Confirmatory tests of iron deficiency anaemia include a serum ferritin, together with a serum iron and total iron binding capacity. The ferritin is reduced (<10 μg/l), while the serum iron will be reduced and the transferrin level raised with the saturation below 16%. Where available, an erythrocyte protoporphyrin level is helpful to distinguish iron deficiency from thalassaemia minor. It will be found to be elevated in iron deficiency anaemia and normal in thalassaemia.

Differential diagnosis

Thalassaemia minor is the main differential diagnosis at higher haemoglobin levels and thalassaemia major at more profound levels of anaemia. Blood film differences separating thalassaemia minor from iron deficiency are often too subtle to be reliable, but the MCV tends to be higher in thalassaemia minor, ranging between 65 and 75 fl. Iron deficiency in association with thalassaemia major is usually readily discernible from severe iron deficiency alone. The finding of a large liver and spleen, together with laboratory tests on the child and the family help to confirm this diagnosis.

Hypochronic microcytic anaemias may be found associated with a variety of illnesses. The anaemia of chronic infection, chronic juvenile arthritis, iron losing haemolytic anaemias and lead poisoning may all present as either iron deficiency anaemia or as microcytic hypochromic anaemia indistinguishable from iron deficiency. A good history and appropriate investigations will be required to differentiate these disorders from iron deficiency (Fig. 42.3).

Treatment

The treatment of iron deficiency should be based on identification and correction of the underlying cause. Advice on diet and iron supplementation play an important role. Search for a source of blood loss and its correction is essential. Oral administration of simple ferrous salts, such as ferrous sulphate, provides inexpensive and satisfactory treatment, but is often poorly tolerated by the patient. Ferrous gluconate mixture is better tolerated and is recommended. The

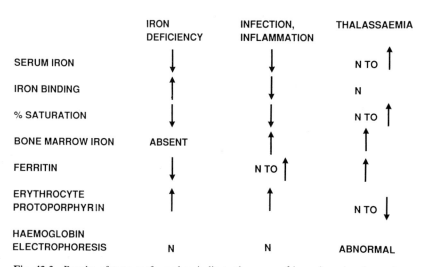

	IRON DEFICIENCY	INFECTION, INFLAMMATION	THALASSAEMIA
SERUM IRON	↓	↓	N TO ↑
IRON BINDING	↑	↓	N
% SATURATION	↓	↓	N TO ↑
BONE MARROW IRON	ABSENT	↑	↑
FERRITIN	↓	N TO ↑	↑
ERYTHROCYTE PROTOPORPHYRIN	↑	↑	N TO ↓
HAEMOGLOBIN ELECTROPHORESIS	N	N	ABNORMAL

Fig. 42.3 Results of tests performed to indicate the cause of hypochromic microcytic anaemia.

therapeutic dose is calculated in terms of elemental iron; ferrous sulphate contains 20% and ferrous gluconate 10–12% of elemental iron by weight. A daily therapeutic dose of 6 mg/kg of elemental iron, given as 3 divided doses, provides the optimal amount of iron for treatment. Better absorption results when iron is given between meals, particularly if ascorbic acid in the form of orange juice is given at the same time.

Parenteral iron is not recommended, but may be indicated under some circumstances, such as:

1. Poor absorption, e.g. idiopathic steatorrhoea or following gut resection
2. Compensation for frequent blood loss when not possible by other means e.g. with hereditary telangiectasia
3. Intolerance to iron by mouth
4. Non-compliance of administration, when it cannot be assured that the medication will be either given or taken.

Intramuscular iron-dextran or iron sorbitol-citric acid complexes are available. Side effects of iron-dextran include local pain, headaches, vomiting, fever, urticaria, angioneurotic oedema, and arthralgia. Rarely, systemic illness with fever, inguinal lymphadenopathy and anaphylaxis have been reported. Only local reactions have been reported with iron sorbitol-citric acid complex.

The dose of parenteral iron should be calculated to raise the child's haemoglobin to 12.5 g/dl. The calculated dose should be increased by a further 20% to restore iron stores. The dose is to be calculated from the following formula:

$$\text{Blood volume} \times \frac{(12.5 - \text{Hb})}{100} \times 3.4 = \text{dose in mg}$$

(Blood volume is assumed to be 80 ml/kg bodyweight.)

The response to parenteral iron is no more rapid or complete than that obtained with correct oral administration of iron. Within 72 hours to 96 hours of iron administration a peripheral reticulocytosis will commence. The height of the response is inversely proportional to the severity of the anaemia, reaching its maximum at about 1 week (see Fig. 42.4). Following the reticulocyte response the haemoglobin level will rise by as much as 0.5 g/100 ml per day in cases of severe anaemia. Oral iron therapy should be continued for 4–6 weeks after haemoglobin values have returned to normal.

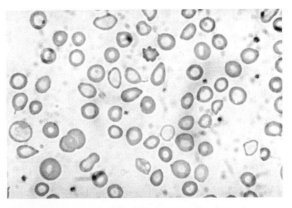

Fig. 42.4 Dimorphic blood film: patient has been commenced on iron therapy. The red cells show a mixture of small cells with greatly reduced amounts of haemoglobin, and normally haemoglobinized red cells indicating response to treatment.

Blood transfusion is only rarely required in patients with iron deficiency anaemia and should only be used in emergency situations, such as in incipient or actual cardiac failure, or when the patient requires correction of a severe anaemia before urgent surgery. The transfusion should be approached with caution, using packed red cells and diuretics when indicated, to avoid cardiac decompensation. Partial transfusion correction of the anaemia may be wise in these situations, with slow administration of 5–10 ml/kg weight of packed red cells sufficient to raise the haemoglobin to a safe level. Exchange tranfusion may be required in some circumstances. Subsequent administration of oral iron is recommended.

Prevention

The recommended oral intake of iron for normal term infants is 1 mg/kg of elemental iron per day, to a maximum of 15 mg/day, commencing at 3 months of age. This is given with a diet of iron fortified cereals and solid foods rich in iron, such as meats and green vegetables. Infants at risk (premature or low birthweight infants, children who have had exchange transfusions or who have had anaemia at birth) require an intake of 2 mg/kg of elemental iron per day.

FURTHER READING

Cook J D 1982 Clinical evaluation of iron deficiency. Seminars in Haematology 14: 6–18

Dallman P R 1982 Manifestations of iron deficiency. Seminars in Haematology 14: 19–30

Finch C A 1982 Erythropoiesis, erythropoietin and iron. Blood 60: 1241–1246

Finch C A, Huebers H 1982 Perspectives in iron metabolism. New England Journal of Medicine 306: 1520–1528

Hallberg L 1982 Iron nutrition and food iron fortification. Seminars in Haematology 14: 31–41

Simes M A, Addiego J E Jr, Dallman P R 1974 Ferritin in serum: diagnosis of iron deficiency and iron overload in infants and children. Blood 43: 581–590

Smith N J, Rios E 1973 Iron metabolism and iron deficiency in infancy and childhood. Advances in Pediatrics 21: 239–280

43. Abnormal bleeding

Henry Ekert

Abnormal bleeding is one of the more dramatic symptoms in childhood and few physicians would not take it seriously. Abnormal bleeding is considered when bruising or petechial spots appear spontaneously or when bleeding persists for an unusually prolonged period following cuts, minor trauma, surgical operations or following dental extractions. There are a very large number of causes of abnormal bleeding and for this reason many physicians have difficulties in approaching the problem of diagnosis in a logical manner. The results tend to be that either a few haphazard tests are ordered or that unnecessarily prolonged investigation is undertaken. As a general rule, it can be stated that most causes of abnormal bleeding will be found by the usual techniques of history taking and physical examination together with a small number of relatively simple laboratory tests.

Abnormal bleeding is basically the result of a disorder of one of the following:

1. The blood vessel or its supporting tissue
2. The platelet
3. The coagulation mechanism.

CLINICAL APPROACH TO DIAGNOSIS

In the approach to the child who bleeds it must never be forgotten that it is the clinical history, with particular reference to the past and family history, that provides the most valuable information. The history should in particular bring out the following points.

The onset of bleeding

Bleeding in the neonatal period may suggest an intrauterine or postnatal infection and bleeding from the gastrointestinal tract in the second to fifth day of life is characteristic of haemorrhagic disease of the newborn, the result of defective functional activity of the prothrombin complex. Prolonged bleeding following circumcision in the neonatal period is suggestive of haemophilia but its absence at this time in no way excludes this diagnosis. A history of prolonged bleeding following cuts or other trauma, tonsillectomy or dental extractions must never be ignored. On the other hand, its absence after these incidents will almost certainly allow one to rule out the possibility of a serious bleeding disorder. Recurrent epistaxes are most commonly due to a local abnormality of blood vessels, but if these can be excluded, Von Willebrand's disease, thrombocytopenia or a platelet dysfunction should be considered. A history of bruising in unusual sites, particularly if associated with skeletal trauma must always alert to the possibility of child abuse.

The family history

Haemophilia and Christmas disease are transmitted in a sex-linked recessive fashion. Von Willebrand's disease and haemorrhagic hereditary telangiectasia are transmitted as Mendelian dominants; platelet function disorders are usually inherited in a recessive manner. Simple enquiry about bleeding within the family is inadequate; a proper family tree must be constructed. Despite this, a negative family history does not rule out these hereditary disorders as fresh mutations of haemophilia A and B account for about one-third and one-fifth of all new cases, respectively. In Von Willebrand's disease symptoms in the affected parent may be so slight as to escape detection.

The past history

A past history of easy bruising, bruising at abnormal sites, prolonged bleeding following trivial trauma, or bleeding following surgery and dental extractions are all absolute indications for investigation.

The site of bleeding

Bleeding into the joints is characteristic of haemophilia

A and B and rare in virtually all other bleeding disorders. The nose is the major site of bleeding in Von Willebrand's disease and disorders of platelet function. In scurvy the abnormal bleeding typically involves the gums, the skin and under the periosteum of the long bones. A retro-orbital haemorrhage in a small child is also suggestive of scurvy.

The diet

Vitamin C is essential to the intercellular matrix and a proper dietary history must always be taken. The maternal intake of vitamin K may be relevant to gastrointestinal bleeding in the neonatal period.

Associated diseases

In the presence of such disorders as systemic lupus erythematosus, liver disease, extrahepatic portal hypertension, gross splenomegaly, giant haemangiomata, reticuloendothelial malignancies and leukaemia, bleeding is anticipated and readily explicable. Bleeding is a feature of a number of less common systemic disorders.

Drug ingestion

Drugs may produce abnormal bleeding through direct irritation (salicylates), depression of clotting factors (anticoagulants, liver toxins), bone marrow depression (chloramphenicol, cytoxic agents, radiation), antigen-antibody reactions with platelet membranes (quinine group of drugs) or by direct inhibition of enzymes in platelets (acetylsalicylic acid). Aspirin is the commonest course of drug-induced bleeding. Aspirin exerts its haemorrhagic effects by inhibition of cyclo-oxygenase, an essential enzyme for platelet function.

Physical examination

In the physical examination the following must be particularly noted.

The type of skin bleeding

Petechial lesions alone suggest that the bleeding disorder is the result either of a vascular defect or a platelet abnormality. Petechial haemorrhages are very rare in disorders of coagulation. Should the skin bleeding be solely ecchymotic, a coagulation disorder is more likely. Frequently petechiae and ecchymoses coexist and this is more suggestive of a severe platelet deficiency.

The site of the bleeding

Although this does not by any means provide precise information of either type of bleeding or the disorder producing the bleeding, it may occasionally be helpful. For example, a haemarthrosis strongly suggests haemophilia A or B. Gastrointestinal haemorrhage in the neonatal period is suggestive of prothrombin deficiency, whereas in older children it is more suggestive of severe liver disease or extrahepatic portal hypertension.

Splenomegaly

The presence of an enlarged spleen in association with abnormal bleeding suggests that hypersplenism is probably causative, but the problem in this situation is the underlying cause of the splenomegaly rather than with the bleeding it produces. Hepatomegaly, splenomegaly and lymphadenopathy in association with bleeding strongly suggest leukaemia. The presence of an obvious anaemia usually implies more than a primary bleeding or coagulation disorder.

Miscellaneous

Bleeding in association with eczema is a feature of the Wiskott Aldrich syndrome; telangiectasia and mucosal bleeding are typical of hereditary haemorrhagic telangiectasia. Hyperelastic skin, hyperextensile joints and bruising are strongly suggestive of Ehlers-Danlos syndrome.

INVESTIGATION OF BLEEDING IN CHILDHOOD

It is again emphasized that a few simple laboratory tests will enable the diagnosis of most bleeding disorders to be made. The following tests are the most important:

Peripheral blood film and haemoglobin estimation

This is essential for the detection and estimation of the severity of any anaemia. At the same time the number and characteristics of both leukocytes and platelets will be determined. The white cell count may reveal a leukopenia or primitive forms may be present so that aplastic anaemia or leukaemia will be suspected. A platelet count will always be indicated. Thrombocytopenia may be associated with anaemia and immature white cells in leukaemia, with anaemia and leukopenia in aplastic anaemia or as a sole abnormality in thrombocytopenic purpura. In certain qualitative platelet disturbances the platelet count is usually depressed and giant platelets may be present (Bernard-Soulier syndrome).

Bleeding time (template)

Prolongation of the bleeding time is characteristic of thrombocytopenia (normal 2–7 minutes), Von Willebrand's disease and platelet function disorders. The bleeding time is characteristically normal in all other coagulation disorders.

Prothrombin time

This test measures both the prothrombin level and the adequacy of the entire extrinsic coagulation system. However, apart from the very rare congenital deficiencies of factors II, V, VII, and X, the prothrombin time is generally normal in inherited disorders of coagulation and this, if reduced, essentially measures acquired prothrombin (factor II) and/or factor VII deficiency.

Partial thromboplastin time

This test measures the adequacy of the intrinsic coagulation system. In the presence of a normal prothrombin time, prolongation of the partial thromboplastic time suggests a deficit in one of the following factors – XII, XI, IX, or VIII. By adding factor VIII or IX to the deficient plasma it is usually possible with this test to quickly identify the deficient factor as they are by far the commonest disorders. The PTT is the basis of the bioassay of the levels of the intrinsic coagulation factors.

Although a large number of clinical disorders are associated with bleeding most are rare and they will be suspected when the few common bleeding disorders are excluded on clinical grounds and by the tests described.

DISORDERS OF BLEEDING DUE TO VASCULAR DEFECTS

The commonest vascular defects seen in childhood are:

1. Anaphylactoid purpura
2. Infective states
3. Nutritional deficiency
4. A miscellaneous group.

Anaphylactoid purpura

Anaphylactoid purpura has been discussed elsewhere. The aetiology is still not clear but it is readily recognized

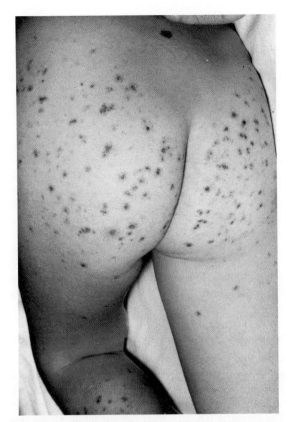

Fig. 43.1 Anaphylactoid purpura. The rash is typically distributed over the buttocks and backs of the legs.

clinically by the characteristic distribution of the rash over the buttocks and backs of the legs (Fig. 43.1). It is frequently accompanied by abdominal pain, melaena, joint swellings and occasionally by a glomerulonephritis. In anaphylactoid purpura the bleeding time, coagulation time and platelet counts are normal. (The Hess test is positive in only 25% of cases.) Thus, diagnosis must be made on the clinical picture alone. The outlook is excellent except for an occasional child who develops a progressive renal lesion. No specific therapy exists, although in children with severe abdominal pain corticosteroids may be helpful.

Infective states

The purpura associated with such disorders as meningococcaemia, other septicaemias and dengue haemorrhagic fever are the result of a severe angiitis. This lesion is probably the result of antigen-antibody complexes but further bleeding which accompanies these states is the result of activation of the coagulation mechanism producing the state of disseminated intravascular coagulation. The purpura in these states, although important in diagnosis, reflects but a small part of the underlying problem. Management involves that of the infection and of the associated vascular collapse.

Purpura fulminans

This is a rare form of non-thrombocytopenic purpura which may follow such infections as scarlet fever, varicella, measles and some other viral infections. It is usually manifest as rapidly spreading skin haemorrhages involving the buttocks and lower extremities and may be rapidly fatal. Recently, a number of vitamin K dependent proteins have been identified (Protein C, Protein S) which inhibit activated coagulation factors VIII and V. Protein C and S are activated by a platelet derived protein known as thrombomodulin. Congenital absence of either Protein C and S have been described in neonatal purpura fulminans.

Nutritional deficiency

Scurvy occurs in the artificially fed infant with inadequate vitamin C supplementation. The presentation is one with bleeding into the skin (bruises), under the periosteum and from the gums if the teeth have erupted. The infant is typically pale, lies immobile in the frog position and resents handling because of the subperiosteal bleeding. A radiograph of the wrist will demonstrate the characteristic dense lines as the metaphyses of the radius and ulna and the 'egg-shell'-like epiphyses. Treatment with vitamin C (100 mg–200 mg/day) reverses the clinical features within a week.

Miscellaneous

Bleeding from vascular wall defects is a feature of a group of rare disorders. These include hereditary haemorrhagic telangiectasia, polyarteritis nodosa, other vasculitides and uraemia. Anoxia, and thus damage to the capillary wall, is a not uncommon cause of purpura in the asphyxiated newborn. The bleeding that accompanies Cushing's syndrome, the Ehlers-Danlos syndrome and in cutis laxa is the result of defects in vascular supporting tissue.

BLEEDING DUE TO PLATELET DISORDERS

Platelets play an essential role in haemostasis in three ways.

1. They adhere to the subendothelial matrix and collagen to seal blood vessel leaks.

2. They aggregate in the area of vessel wall damage forming a plug.

3. Activation of coagulation is precipitated and takes place on the platelet plug surface.

Platelet deficiency is the most common of the platelet disorders, when the thrombocytopenia may be the primary and sole disturbance or it may be associated with disturbances in both the red cell and white cell series.

Idiopathic thrombocytopenic purpura (ITP)

Idiopathic thrombocytopenic purpura is the commonest of the primary platelet disorders in childhood. Both the chronic and acute forms have an immunological basis. The lifespan of platelets is markedly decreased and they are sequestrated and destroyed in splenic macrophages.

The diagnosis is established readily from the peripheral blood film and platelet count. Commonly the platelet count is below 50 000/mm3 and not rarely below 10 000/mm3. The red and white cell series are invariably normal. Other investigations of haemostasis are unnecessary. Bone marrow examination reveals normal numbers of megakaryocytes, but reduced platelet formation. The chief value of the bone marrow examination is to exclude the secondary causes of thrombocytopenia, for example leukaemia, other marrow infiltrations and aplastic anaemia.

The course of acute ITP in childhood is for spontaneous remission within 4–6 weeks in 75% of cases. In approximately 10–16% recovery may not occur for about 4–6 months. However, some children will recover in a year or so after periods of exacerbations and remissions. Some 10% of children presenting as ITP show no recovery of the platelet count. In these patients splenectomy produces an improvement in the platelet count in all patients and a normal platelet count in 90%.

Treatment

The treatment of ITP is controversial and relates to the use of observation alone, corticosteroids or high dose intravenous gammaglobulin. In children with acute onset of ITP the majority recover spontaneously and intervention is only required if there is persistent bleeding after bed rest or no increase of platelet count after 4 weeks of observation. In such circumstances the treatment of choice is high dose intravenous gammaglobulin which causes a rapid increase of platelet count without the undesirable side effects of steroids.

In patients with gradual onset of ITP in whom the platelet count does not rise above the base line after 3 weeks of observation high dose gammaglobulin can be administered repeatedly to maintain platelet counts above 20 000/mm3. If such therapy fails to control thrombocytopenia over a period of 6 months then the patient should be considered a candidate for splenectomy. Splenectomy is successful in curing persistent thrombocytopenia in 90% of children but has the disadvantage of hightened susceptibility to life threatening bacterial infection with the pneumococcus and *Haemophilus influenzae* organisms.

The use of corticosteroids can achieve the same result as high dose intravenous gammaglobulin. The well-known undesirable side effects of corticosteroids on immunity, growth and metabolism make them an unattractive alternative to high dose gammaglobulin.

Secondary thrombocytopenia

A large number of disorders exist in which thrombocytopenia is secondary. These disorders, which should always be considered in every case of thrombocytopenia, include:

1. Infiltration of the bone marrow where megakaryocytes are displaced by leukaemia or other neoplasms.
2. Aplastic anaemia. This may be congenital or acquired and has been discussed in Chapter 41.
3. Hypersplenism. An enlarged spleen from any cause may trap platelets or possibly produce a humoral substance which prevents maturation or release of platelets from the bone marrow. Common disorders associated with hypersplenism and bleeding include portal hypertension, thalassaemia and malaria. The thrombocytopenia here is associated with an active bone marrow and the features of the underlying disorder.
4. Autoimmune disorders: thrombocytopenia and abnormal bleeding are the result of platelet antibodies. This is particularly seen in systemic lupus erythematosus and rarely with some lymphomas.
5. Disseminated intravascular coagulation: the abnormal bleeding here results from the consumption of platelets and clotting factors. The causes include overwhelming infection, shock and tissue anoxia of various types. Management involves the treatment of the underlying disorder and replacement of coagulation factors and platelets and, in situations where the underlying disorder is difficult to control in a short time, heparin may be considered.

Bleeding due to qualitive platelet defects

In this group of rare disorders bleeding is the result of a functional platelet defect. They will be suspected in a child with abnormal bleeding in whom the bleeding time

is prolonged but platelet count is normal and large platelets will be noted on the blood film. The diagnosis of these disorders is dependent on platelet function studies which test release of platelet storage nucleotides and the ability of platelets to aggregate in response to the nucleotides.

The commoner disorders in this group are Glanzmann's disease, 'aspirin-like' syndrome and platelet storage pool disorders. Before undertaking platelet function studies one must ensure that there has been no ingestion of aspirin for at least 7 days, since aspirin interferes with platelet function.

BLEEDING DUE TO COAGULATION DISORDERS

These may frequently be suspected on clinical grounds because of large bruises or because of a history of prolonged bleeding following minor trauma, dental extractions or surgical procedures. Most of the coagulation disorders are heritable so a family history must be carefully taken. The diagnosis will be confirmed after the appropriate coagulation studies, mentioned above, have been performed.

Haemophilia A (factor VIII deficiency) occurs in 4–6 men per 100 000 of the population. Haemophilia B (Christmas disease, factor IX deficiency) occurs in 0.4–0.6 per 100 000 of the population. Factor XI deficiency (PTA deficiency) is even less common, and all the remainder are exceedingly rare.

The sequence of events in blood coagulation is an amplifying system in which each enzyme in turn activates an inert precursor factor to its active forms. The system is complex, and governed by a series of enhancing and inhibiting feedback loops. The most important inhibitor of the serine protease coagulation enzymes is antithrombin III. Congenital deficiency of antithrombin III is associated with deep vein thromboses in adolescence or early adult years. The most important inhibitors of the rate limiting factors in the coagulation cascade are Protein C and S. Their congenital deficiency causes purpura fulminans and venous thrombosis in infancy.

Figure 43.2 is a greatly simplified outline of the system, emphasizing the useful classification into intrinsic, extrinsic and common pathways, which correspond roughly to the steps used in the laboratory to elucidate a coagulation defect.

Haemophilia

The symptoms and signs of haemophilia A and B are similar and will be described together. As a rule

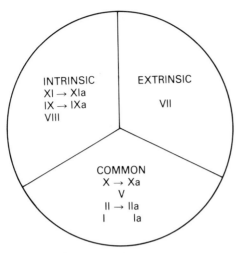

Fig. 43.2 Simplified outline of the coagulation system.

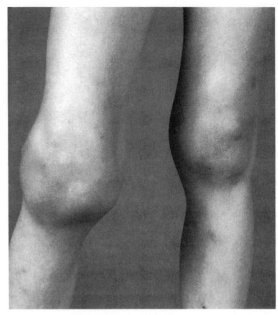

Fig. 43.3 Haemarthrosis of right knee in a boy with haemophilia.

haemophilia B is a milder disorder, but the degree of severity of haemophilia varies a great deal – mild cases being only recognized following surgical procedures. The degree of severity of haemophilia correlates inversely with the percentage of factor VIII in the patient's plasma. Both haemophilia A and B are transmitted as sex-linked recessives but classic haemophilia occurs sporadically in about 25–30% of patients, either because it arises as a mutant or because the disease has not been recognized previously in the family.

Usually patients present after the newborn period with either bleeding from minor mouth trauma or postcircumcision bleeding. It is remarkable that, despite the hazards of negotiating the birth canal head first, there is very seldom evidence of excessive bleeding or bruising in the newborn period. Bleeding from the umbilical cord is most uncommon. During the first year of life bleeding occurs mainly into muscles and subcutaneous tissues. In addition, when the child begins to walk there are episodes of joint bleeding. In early life the ankles are the most commonly involved but in older children the knees and elbows are common sites of bleeding. Certain sites of bleeding have the potential for particularly serious consequences. Bleeding into the forearm may occlude the neurovascular bundle and cause Volkmann's ischaemic contracture. Retroperitoneal bleeding may cause paralytic ileus and if the blood tracks down under the inguinal ligament there may be compression of the femoral nerve. Bleeding into the posterior pharyngeal wall may interfere with respiration and cause dysphagia. The most serious site of bleeding is intracranial. It is estimated that some form of intracranial vascular accident is the cause of death in 7%

of haemophiliacs. Haematuria is quite common in teenagers and adolescents and, although alarming, it is seldom serious.

The commonest and the most disabling symptom of haemophilia is joint bleeding (see Fig. 43.3) which eventually leads to synovial hypertrophy and the destruction of articular surfaces. Early painful arthropathies ensue which may need surgical treatment for control of pain and joint instability.

A major health and socioeconomic problem in some patients with haemophilia is infection with the human immune deficiency virus (HIV) which occurred in 50–90% of severe haemophiliacs receiving blood products in the years 1980–85. There has been deterioration of immune function in some of these patients and clinical AIDS has developed in 1.5–5% of infected haemophiliacs. The concurrent problems of external bleeding and HIV infection has lead to social and economic handicaps.

The management of the child with haemophilia

This can be best described by stressing major principles of therapy.

1. Correct the bleeding tendency. This is achieved by intravenous infusion of a factor VIII concentrate. In general, most bleeds can be arrested by increasing the plasma level of factor VIII to 30–60% of normal. Empirically it has been shown that 1 unit of factor VIII/kg bodyweight increases the factor VIII by 1–2%. Therefore, a dose of 15–30 units/kg bodyweight will arrest most haemorrhages. The half-life of factor VIII is 8–12 hours and in severe bleeds factor VIII may be administered 12-hourly for 3–6 doses. Unfortunately, the plasma used for production of factor VIII concentrates was contaminated with the human immune deficiency virus (HIV) during the years 1980–85. During this time a high percentage of severe haemophiliacs was infected with this virus. Factor VIII concentrates are now made from blood donations screened for the absence of HIV antibodies and as an additional safety factor the concentrates are heat treated to destroy the virus. Only appropriately screened and heat treated factor VIII concentrates are suitable for treatment purposes.

2. Treat pain. Replacement of factor VIII and immobilization of a painful limb are usually sufficient to control pain. In some instances this is insufficient for control of tense acutely painful joints. In such cases aspiration of the joint under factor VIII cover will alleviate the pain dramatically. Where aspiration is not practicable a narcotic analgesic may be required. These should only be given sparingly and on strong indication so as to prevent drug addiction.

3. Prevent deformity. This is achieved by splinting the limb in a position of function during the early painful phase of a bleed and by commencing active exercises as soon as pain has subsided. The exercise programme should be supervised by an experienced physiotherapist.

4. Assist normal intellectual and emotional development. This is best achieved by teaching the child self-reliance and relative independence of the hospital and subsequently the parent.

The introduction of home treatment programmes has been most successful in achieving this aim. Most if not all haemophilia centres now have active training facilities to teach parents and the older boys the techniques of factor VIII preparation and intravenous infusion. The indicators for early treatment are taught to the families and arrangements are made for one of the parents to be 'on call' so as to administer the factor VIII in school when necessary. Boys on home treatment gain confidence in being able to control the bleeding complications of their disorder and, through early treatment, they can continue school activities without frequent interruptions.

Some 10% of haemophiliacs develop antibodies to factor VIII. These patients require treatment in hospital. Generally, it is agreed that 60% of their haemorrhages can be controlled by the use of prothrombin complex

concentrates. In the remainder, haemostasis can usually be achieved by double doses of factor VIII.

Patients with Christmas disease are managed in a similar way to those with haemophilia. Replacement therapy is given with prothrombin complex concentrates at a dose of 20–40 units/kg bodyweight. The half-life of factor IX is usually 24 hours.

The specific preoperative management for coagulation disorders and the management of bleeding from specific sites will not be dealt with here. Schedules can be obtained from standard texts of haematology.

Von Willebrand's disease

This disorder is inherited as an autosomal dominant. The majority of patients are only mildly affected. With sensitive new methods of diagnosis it has been shown that von Willebrand's disease is the commonest congenital bleeding disorder. The disorder is due to an abnormality in the functional property of factor VIII which is required to allow platelets to adhere to the subendothelial matrix – the von Willebrand's factor. This property of factor VIII can be measured by the ability of platelets to aggregate in the presence of the von Willebrand's factor and an antibiotic known as ristocetin.

The diagnosis of von Willebrand's disease is suspected on the grounds of postoperative or posttraumatic bleeding with a history of mucosal haemorrhage, excessive bruising, and autosomal dominant inheritance. The clinical suspicion of von Willebrand's disease can only be confirmed by laboratory tests. The screening tests of haemostasis show a prolonged template bleeding time and in the patients with the severe form of the disease a prolonged PTT. The diagnosis can only be definitively established by assaying functional and immunological properties of factor VIII. The most specific test is a decrease in the level of von Willebrand's factor. There are various classifications of this disorder but they are provisional and are outside the scope of this book.

Haemorrhage in von Willebrand's disease should be treated by the use of the posterior pituitary hormone DDAVP or screened and heat treated factor VIII concentrate. DDAVP given intravenously can release stored von Willebrand's factor and provide a haemostatic effect for about 4 hours. It is only effective in the moderate and mild forms of this disease (Type I). Doses of DDAVP can be repeated at 12–24 hour intervals but not sooner since DDVAP works by releasing stored von Willebrand's factor and new synthesis and storage of that factor requires approximately 12 hours. The major advantage of DDAVP is its freedom from contamination with HIV.

Factor VIII concentrates are used when DDAVP has failed or in severe von Willebrand's disease. It is a safer product than cryoprecipitate because the latter cannot be heat treated. Usually, doses of factor VIII concentrate need not be repeated for 24–48 hours except in patients with very severe disease when they may need to be given 4–8 hourly.

Haemorrhagic disease of the newborn

This is a self-limiting disease usually presenting on the second or third day of life but rarely up to 4 weeks of age, and resulting from a deficiency of the coagulation factors dependent on their functional activity on vitamin K. The levels of factors II, VII, IX and X rapidly decline in the first 2–3 days of life and in some infants the decline is so extreme that spontaneous haemorrhage may occur. Melaena, haematemesis, umbilical cord bleeding and haematuria are the most common. Prophylactic treatment of the newborn infant with vitamin K virtually eliminates haemorrhagic disease of the newborn. In the management of overt haemorrhage 1 mg of vitamin K given intramuscularly or intravenously usually stops the bleeding within 2 hours. If this does not occur, if the bleeding is severe, or if intracranial haemorrhage has occurred, an infusion of 10–15 ml/kg of fresh plasma or fresh blood, will immediately correct the defect, if there is significant anaemia.

Vitamin K deficiency is uncommon after the neonatal period, but may be noted in association with bleeding in congenital biliary atresia or in other forms of severe liver disease.

FURTHER READING

Biggs R 1978 The treatment of haemophilia A and B and von Willebrand's disease. Blackwell Scientific Publications, Oxford

Ekert H 1982 Clinical paediatric haematology and oncology. Blackwell Scientific Publications, Oxford

Hardisty R M 1977 Disorders of platelet function. British Medical Bulletin 33: 207–212

Italia Working Group 1977 Spectrum of von Willebrand's disease: a study of 100 cases. British Journal of Haematology 35: 101–112

Rizza C R, Spooner R J D 1977 Home treatment of haemophilia and Christmas disease: five years experience. British Journal of Haematology 37: 53–66

Lusher J M, Shapiro S S, Palascak J E et al Haemophilia Study Group 1980 Efficacy of prothrombin-complex concentrates in haemophiliacs with antibodies to factor VIII: a multicenter therapeutic trial. New England Journal of Medicine 303: 421–425

44. The thalassaemias

Rae Matthews

Definition

The thalassaemia syndromes are genetic disorders characterized by a reduced rate of production of one or more of the globin chains of haemoglobin. The term 'haemoglobinopathy' is used for all inherited disorders of the structure and synthesis of globin and includes the thalassaemia syndromes as well as other conditions.

Human haemoglobin is a heterogeneous protein. Each type of haemoglobin appears as a tetramer consisting of two pairs of unlike polypeptide chains, each chain being associated with one haem molecule. During the transition from early fetal life to adult life, the predominant haemoglobin changes, the type of haemoglobin being determined by the predominant type of peptide chains (Fig. 44.1).

It is now known that the genes responsible for the production of these six different globin chains are located on chromosome 16 – zeta (ζ), and alpha (α) and on chromosome 11 – epsilon (ε) gamma (γ) beta (β) and delta (δ). It is now possible to identify the nature of the defect in many of these clinical conditions (Fig. 44.2).

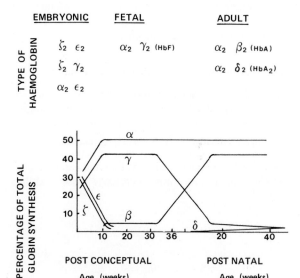

Fig. 44.1 Types and percentages of haemoglobin in embryonic, fetal and adult life.

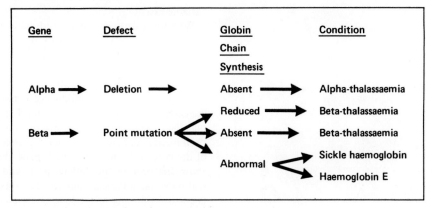

Fig. 44.2 Genetic disorders of haemoglobin – haemoglobinopathies.

357

Beta thalassaemia is commonly found in people who originate from the Mediterranean region, Middle East, the Indian subcontinent, southern Asia and Africa. It is the most common type of haemoglobinopathy seen in Australia.

A normal individual has two genes for the globin chain of haemoglobin. If one of these genes is not functioning at a normal rate, or is completely absent, that individual has the thalassaemia trait – also known as thalassaemia minor (carrier of thalassaemia).

If both genes are absent or non-functioning the patient has thalassaemia major – the homozygous form of thalassaemia, also known as Cooley's anaemia and Mediterranean anaemia. The inheritance is in a Mendelian autosomal recessive manner.

Beta thalassaemia trait (β thalassaemia minor)

This is the heterozygous condition, and is asymptomatic. The diagnosis is suspected by examination of the blood where microcytosis and hypochromia of the red cells is the main feature (Fig. 44.3). Confirmation of this diagnosis is achieved by estimation of the haemoglobin A_2 level, an elevation indicating thalassaemia minor. As iron deficiency also exhibits microcytosis and hypochromia of the red cells, it is important to distinguish between these two conditions. However, they may coexist, with the iron deficiency masking the β thalassaemia minor and preventing its diagnosis until the iron deficiency has been corrected. The importance of thalassaemia minor is in its genetic implications.

Beta thalassaemia major

Thalassaemia major results from the inheritance of two genes for β thalassaemia, i.e. the homozygous condition.

Pathophysiology

Because there is inadequate or no production of β chains, there is an excess of α chains. These chains cannot join with enough non-α chains but adhere to form intracellular inclusions. The inclusions result in ineffective erythropoiesis leading to anaemia, increased turnover of red cells resulting in an expanded marrow cavity and an expanded blood volume. Erythropoiesis in the liver and spleen leads to enlargement of these organs.

Clinical presentations

Usually, the presentation is in the first year of life but may be as late as the third or fourth year. Initially, these infants produce sufficient HbF to remain well and it is only when it becomes inadequate that they develop anaemia. The presenting symptoms include pallor, failure to gain weight, frequent infections, irritability and difficulties with feeding.

On examination, pallor is the outstanding feature accompanied by enlargement of liver and spleen of variable extent.

Without treatment, the child with β thalassaemia major becomes severely growth retarded, the mucous membranes pale and the skin pigmented. The abdomen becomes protruberant and poor musculoskeletal development leads to spindly arms and legs. Skeletal changes become severe, producing a characteristic facial appearance with bossing of the skull, hypertrophy of the maxillae, which tends to expose the upper teeth, prominent malar eminences and depression of the bridge of the nose. If treatment is inadequate skull radiographs show dilatation of the diploic space, and the subperiosteal bone has a typical 'hair on end' appearance. There is cortical thinning of the long bones and fractures may occur. Depending on the severity of the anaemia the child may survive for 5–10 years. With adequate treat-

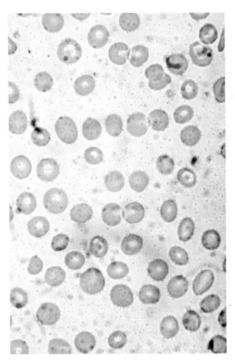

Fig. 44.3 Blood film. Thalassaemia minor: note microcytosis, hypochromia and the occasional target cell.

ment of thalassaemia major (see below) these clinical and radiological abnormalities will not be seen.

A few children (approximately 7%) are able to maintain a higher level of haemoglobin and fail to develop the ill-effects of ineffective erythropoiesis. These children are said to have thalassaemia intermedia and may develop the complications of any chronic haemolytic anaemia such as gall stones.

Diagnosis

The blood examination reveals a low haemoglobin accompanied by the following abnormalities in the red cells – hypochromia, basophilic stippling, microcytes, macrocytes, target cells and nucleated red cells (Fig. 44.4). An elevated HbF level confirms the diagnosis (usually 50–100%). Globin chain synthesis studies could differentiate between B° and B^{+} thalassaemia, β globin synthesis being completely absent in B° thalassaemia, but are not routinely performed.

Management

Any child who develops symptoms of anaemia during the first year of life is likely to be transfusion dependent.

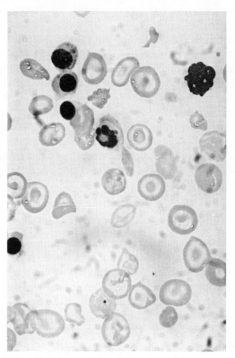

Fig. 44.4 Blood film. Thalassaemia major: note hypochromia, microcytes and large number of target cells, and also nucleated red cells.

Usually this occurs if the haemoglobin level drops below 7 g/dl.

If the presentation is later in life, factors such as hypersplenism and folic acid deficiency may be responsible for the anaemia and, once these are corrected, transfusions may not be necessary. When the haemoglobin is being observed over a period of time and does not rise above 7.5 g/dl, the child should be considered as transfusion dependent. If the haemoglobin is maintained between 7.5 and 9 g/dl, other parameters, such as degree of bone and marrow expansion, growth and development, become important in determining if regular blood transfusions are necessary to improve the quality of life.

Should the child show features of bone marrow expansion, the absorption of iron is likely to be at a greater rate than normal and will lead to haemosiderosis with eventual heart failure or liver disease, usually by the age of 20.

Once the decision to transfuse has been made the child should commence on a regular regime of transfusion at 4–5 weekly intervals with maintenance of haemoglobin levels above 10 g/dl.

As soon as practicable after commencement of transfusions, the child should commence chelation therapy, ideally before the serum ferritin level reaches 2000 ng/ml. Chelation therapy involves desferrioxamine infusions over 10-hourly periods by subcutaneous infusion using a syringe driver (pump), usually worn at night by young children though some young adults prefer to wear it during the day (Fig. 44.5).

Splenectomy may become necessary when transfusion requirements significantly exceed the expected requirements for the patient's size. Pneumococcal vaccine and prophylactic penicillin are required following splenectomy.

Patients with thalassaemia major should be reviewed regularly with particular regard to growth and general development. Other problems that need to be addressed include the social and psychological impact created by the chronic disease on both the child and family, attachment to hospitals and the dependency on medical care.

Prognosis

Better transfusion programmes have greatly improved the quality of life of these patients, so that they can lead normal lives, albeit with ongoing treatment. There is increasing evidence accruing to demonstrate that iron chelation therapy controls iron toxicity associated with iron overload in those patients who comply with this therapy. The availability of a safe and effective oral iron chelator would be a significant advantage.

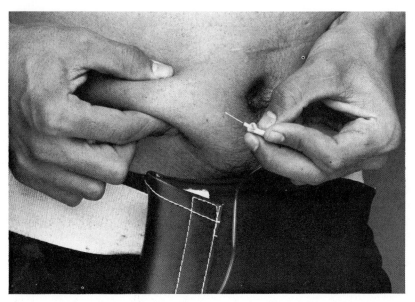

Fig. 44.5 Syringe drive (pump) in position for subcutaneous infusion of desferrioxamine.

HAEMOGLOBIN E/β THALASSAEMIA

This haemoglobinopathy occurs in people of South-East Asian origin, especially those from Thailand and Vietnam. This occurs when haemoglobin E is inherited from one parent and β thalassaemia from the other giving rise to a doubly heterozygous condition. Clinically, its presentation is similar to a moderately severe thalassaemia major. Diagnosis is confirmed by blood examination and haemoglobin electrophoresis. Many of these patients are transfusion dependent and require the same management as those with thalassaemia major.

THE ALPHA THALASSAEMIAS

These are less commonly seen. It is now known that four genes determine the formation of globin chains and thus there are four possible α thalassaemias corresponding to a loss or non-function of one to four of these genes.

The silent form

The loss of one α gene does not produce any abnormality in the morphology of the red cell, nor any abnormal clinical features.

Alpha thalassaemia trait

Loss of two α genes results in hypochromia and microcytosis but no anaemia.

Haemoglobin H disease

The loss of three α genes results in the formation of excess chains in childhood and adult life which form an unstable tetramer (β4). This accounts for 30–40% of the total haemoglobin. The clinical picture is similar to thalassaemia intermedia but the clinical severity is variable. Some patients may go through life with little or no disability. In others the disease may be as crippling as thalassaemia major. The blood film is similar to that of thalassaemia major with haemoglobin levels of 8–10% and a persistent reticulocytosis. Splenomegaly is usually present. Apart from maintenance of folic acid and the avoidance of oxidant drugs (e.g. phenacetin, primaquine, etc.), which aggravate the anaemia, no other treatment is necessary. The disorder is also aggravated by pregnancy and infections.

Haemoglobin Barts (hydrops fetalis syndrome)

There are no chains present and the haemoglobin pattern is Hb Barts (γ4) 70%, HbH (β4) 0–20% and haemoglobin Portland 10%. Survival in utero to 28–36 weeks is due to Hb Portland, which acts as an oxygen carrier in fetal life. These infants are almost always stillborn and grossly oedematous with hepatosplenomegaly. Those infants born alive usually die within an hour or two of heart failure.

HAEMOGLOBIN S

Haemoglobin S (HbS) is a β chain variant that results

from the substitution of glutamic acid at position 6 by valine. This results in a different structure to the haemoglobin, which, under hypoxic conditions causes the sickling phenomenon to occur, i.e. the red cells assume a sickle shape which may or may not be reversible.

Haemoglobin S (sickle-cell anaemia)

The incidence of the sickle-cell gene ranges between 5% and 20% in certain parts of Africa. It is also common in Cyprus, Greece, Italy, the Middle East and in populations who originate from these areas. It is a significant problem in the black population of the USA and the Caribbean.

In the heterozygous state (sickle-cell trait) the red cell size may be normal or a little reduced. Haemoglobin electrophoresis reveals a normal band of HbA and an abnormal band which may be either HbS or HbD. The definitive diagnosis is made by demonstrating sickling of the red cells (Fig. 44.6). In the sickle-cell trait the HbS level is 30–45%, HbF 1%, HbA_2 2–3% and HbA 55–65%. Individuals with sickle-cell trait are not anaemic, show no physical abnormalities and are usually asymptomatic.

Sickle-cell anaemia (HbSS)

Sickle-cell anaemia results from the inheritance of two sickle-cell genes, i.e. the homozygous condition.

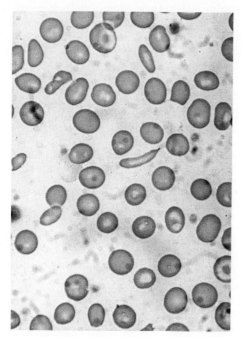

Fig. 44.6   Blood film. Sickle cell anaemia: note sickling.

Pathophysiology

Under certain conditions, such as deoxygenation and acidosis, the red cells change shape from biconcave discs to sickle or crescent shapes. In addition, the plasma of people with sickle-cell anaemia has increased viscosity. Viscosity increases rapidly in the presence of sickle cells leading to occlusion of vessels and tissue damage. As red cells containing sickle haemoglobin have a shorter than normal survival time in the circulation, a chronic haemolytic anaemia results. Increased erythropoiesis usually compensates for this, but at times this fails resulting in anaemia and increased haemolysis leads to jaundice.

Clinical presentation

Sickle-cell anaemia usually presents between the ages of 6 months and 4 years with signs and symptoms which may involve many systems. Thus, there may be considerable difficulty in diagnosis if the disease is not suspected. The most frequent presenting symptoms are pallor, jaundice, abdominal or limb pain and swellings of the hands and/or feet.

During the steady state, symptoms such as pallor and jaundice may be present for long periods of time. Intermittently, other symptoms called 'crises' may occur, e.g. pain, more extreme pallor or jaundice and evidence of infection such as fever, cough and headache. Crises may be haemolytic, infarctive, aplastic or associated with sequestration of the red cells in the spleen.

Diagnosis

The blood demonstrates a normochromic normocytic anaemia of moderate degree and a reticulocyte count of 10–20%. Sickling of the red cells is demonstrated by special tests and the diagnosis confirmed by finding sickle haemoglobin on haemoglobin electrophoresis. The level of HbS is usually 60–90%, HbA_2 approximately 2%, and HbF comprises the remainder. The higher the level of HbF the less severe the symptoms of the disease.

Management

The main emphasis is on the maintenance of the steady state by removal of those environmental factors known to precipitate a crisis. The following protective measures are recommended:

1. Good nutrition with regular folic acid supplements, especially during pregnancy.

2. Prevention of infections where possible, and prompt treatment of infections when these occur.

3. Maintenance of adequate hydration.

4. Prevention of vascular stasis. This may occur with tight clothing or the use of tourniquets applied during an operative procedure.

5. Avoidance of cold.

Treatment of crises

The treatment of crises requires hospitalization for control of pain, the maintenance of hydration and correction of anaemia. As most crises are precipitated by infection, this should be identified and vigorously treated.

Prognosis

The long-term outlook for patients with sickle-cell anaemia is steadily improving. Better general care and the availability of regular transfusions combined with iron chelation therapy, allows these patients to undertake most normal activities.

Sickle thalassaemia

This haemoglobinopathy occurs when the sickle gene is inherited from one parent and the β thalassaemia gene from the other, giving rise to a double heterozygous condition. Clinically the condition is similar to sickle-cell anaemia. Diagnosis is confirmed by blood examination and haemoglobin electrophoresis. The red cells are usually microcytic and hypochromic, target cells may be present, and sickling can be demonstrated. Examination of the parent's blood confirms sickle-cell trait in one and thalassaemia minor in the other.

The management of this condition is similar to that for sickle-cell anaemia.

GENETIC COUNSELLING

Before counselling an individual with a haemoglobinopathy an accurate diagnosis is essential. The subsequent discussion should outline the quality of life for that individual, and genetic implications for any offspring.

THE FUTURE

In the past decade, achievements in prenatal diagnosis and advances in management of the haemoglobinopathies have occurred at a great rate. Couples at risk of having children with these disorders now have a range of options from which to choose. Prenatal diagnosis has permitted selective abortions of affected offspring, although advances in the management of these disorders now creates a dilemma for some families.

Work continues to find a suitable oral iron-chelating agent. Bone marrow transplantations have been performed successfully in some patients. However, this approach is limited to patients with an HLA compatible sibling and the significant risks of rejection and graft versus host disease need to be overcome. The long-term risk of allogeneic bone marrow transplantation are as yet unknown.

Experimental work is addressing itself to the basic genetic defects in these disorders. Attempts have been made to use drugs for gene manipulation, e.g. 5-AZO cytodine, and gene transfer is being studied in experimental animals.

FURTHER READING

Cao A, Carcassi V, Rowley P T 1982 Thalassaemia: recent advances in detection and treatment. Birth defects: original article series, Vol 18, no 7. Alan R Liss, New York

Ekert H 1982 Clinical paediatric haematology and oncology. Blackwell Scientific Publications, Oxford

Modell B 1977 Total management of thalassaemia major.

Archives of Disease in Childhood 52(6): 489–500

Nathan D, Oski F (eds) 1987 Haematology of infancy and childhood, 3rd edn. W B Saunders, Philadelphia

Weatherall D J, Clegg J B 1981 The thalassaemia syndromes, 3rd edn. Blackwell Scientific Publications, Oxford

45. The problem of malignancy

Keith Waters

Malignant disease now ranks second to accidents as the major cause of death in children between 1 and 14 years of age. In children, malignancy most commonly affects the reticuloendothelial system with leukaemia and lymphoma accounting for 40–50% of all childhood malignancy. Primary CNS tumours form the next most common group (20%) with the embryonic tumours, neuroblastoma and nephroblastoma occurring with about equal incidence (6–8% each). Sarcoma of bone and soft tissue together account for 8–10%. All other types are relatively uncommon (Table 45.1).

Whilst malignant disease of childhood is uncommon, with a frequency of 10–12:100 000 children, a high index of suspicion is required of general practitioners so that early diagnosis and treatment may be initiated. The improvement in results obtained at present has been in large part the outcome of a multidisciplinary approach involving paediatric oncologist, surgeon, radiotherapist, radiologist and pathologist. Nonetheless, the general practitioner still has an important role in the overall management of the child and his family. Referral to a tertiary centre when the diagnosis is suspected is essential.

Table 45.1 Frequency of malignant disease in childhood

Malignant disease	Frequency (%)
Leukaemia	35
Primary CNS tumours	20
Lymphoma, both non-Hodgkin and Hodgkin	10
Wilms' tumour	6–8
Neuroblastoma	6–8
Sarcoma of bone – Ewing's and osteosarcoma	4
Rhabdomyosarcoma – soft tissue sarcoma	5
Teratoma	2
Histiocytosis	5
Retinoblastoma	1
Hepatic	1
Others	5

A not inconsiderable part of the management of malignant disease will be involved in providing the necessary emotional support to the child and family. Parents must initially be adequately informed of the nature of the disease, its course, treatment and prognosis and in a manner they can fully understand. The older child and teenager must also be informed honestly about the disease and its treatment, but always in a manner that is optimistic and stresses that the long-term gains far outweigh the short-term side effects. Physicians should not embark upon a treatment programme for malignant disease if they are not prepared to become involved in the many emotional problems that will inevitably occur. These problems will become even greater when recurrences occur and the goals of therapy change from those of cure to those palliation and quality of life questions become of prime importance.

Later, decisions concerning when and whether to terminate therapy will also require great patience and understanding on the part of the physician. Despite these remarks, the physician who is able successfully to handle the emotional problems involved in management, as well as the complexity of the actual therapy, will derive considerable personal satisfaction from caring for the patient and family despite the ultimate prognosis.

When death from malignancy is anticipated or becomes inevitable the child must be adequately supported. Not only the patient, but the parents and siblings are prepared for palliative care. Parents, relatives and close friends should be encouraged to visit so that the child is never left alone. Emotional and physical loneliness of the patient must be avoided. Provided that the whole family unit can cope, it may be preferable for the child to die at home in familiar surroundings and with the family. Here the help of a supportive family physician and palliative care nursing service is essential. Most children have an in-built denial of death and hence this continued support will enable the family to cope. Whether or not to inform the child of impending death is a very difficult question to answer and no fixed rules can be set. Many children in the terminal phase of their illness will acknowledge to their parents that they know they are dying, but may in their daily activities continue to 'deny' this to the last moment. With adolescents, it is probably best to admit the failure of treatment, but frankly and honestly reassure them that there is ready access to the unit, that effective analgesia is available and they will be allowed to retain their freedom and dignity. Emphasis must be placed upon emotional support at every level – parents, friends, nursing staff, paramedical staff and clergy, as well as the physician in charge.

A detailed description of staging and treatment of individual tumour types is beyond the scope of this chapter and the reader is referred to one of the many textbooks on paediatric haematology and oncology for this information.

ACUTE LEUKAEMIA IN CHILDHOOD

Leukaemia is a disease of unknown aetiology characterized by an abnormal proliferation of one of the leukocytic tissues, primarily of the bone marrow, but secondarily involving the peripheral blood and any other tissue of the body particularly the reticuloendothelial system. In children, tumours may arise primarily outside the bone marrow and subsequently enter the marrow and blood resulting in a disease clinically indistinguishable from acute leukaemia. Leukaemia is commonest in the 2–4-year-old age group and commoner in males than females. In children, 80% of leukaemia is acute lymphoblastic (ALL) and 20% is acute myeloid (AML) with chronic myeloid leukaemia accounting for only 1%.

Aetiology

Whilst in animals leukaemia can be induced by irradiation, chemical carcinogens and oncogenic viruses, the cause of leukaemia in man remains unknown but is probably multifactorial. Genetic factors may possibly play a role in only a minority of patients with leukaemia. Certain genetic diseases, all rare themselves, have been associated with an increased incidence of leukaemia. These include Down syndrome, D_1 trisomy syndrome, Klinefelter syndrome, congenital agammaglobulinaemia, ataxia telangiectasia, Wiskott-Aldrich syndrome and Fanconi's anaemia. Common to many of these disorders are congenital chromosome abnormalities. Preleukaemic conditions such as aplastic anaemia, myeloproliferative disorders, paroxysmal nocturnal haemoglobinuria and polycythaemia are very rare in children, as are exposure to chemical leukaemogenic agents such as benzene and chlorambucil.

Clinical manifestations

Often the child does not appear acutely ill at the time of presentation. Symptoms such as bleeding or easy bruising may have been present for only a few days, while vague skeletal symptoms may have been present for weeks or months. Pallor is the most common presenting feature and anorexia, malaise, irritability and low grade fever are often prominent symptoms. Infectious manifestations such as tonsillitis, pharyngitis, otitis media, skin sepsis and pneumonia are no different to those seen in the normal population. Petechiae and ecchymoses are common, as is epistaxis and bleeding from the mucous membranes. Bone and joint pain are the predominant and often only symptoms in as many as 20% of children and may lead to a mistaken diagnosis of rheumatoid arthritis or rheumatic fever. Lymphadenopathy, which is variable in extent, is seldom the initial presenting complaint and the nodes are discreet, firm, non-painful and non-tender. Liver and/or spleen enlargement, which is quite variable in extent, is present in most cases.

Rare manifestations include parotid or other salivary gland swelling, renal enlargement and skin infiltration. Gum hypertrophy and orbital chloromas may occur in the myeloid subgroups. Central nervous system infiltration as manifested by headache, papilloedema and cranial nerve palsies is very rare at presentation. Mediastinal gland enlargement on chest radiograph occurs in 10% of cases.

Laboratory findings

Anaemia and/or thrombocytopenia and/or blast cells in the peripheral blood are found in 80% of patients at presentation. The red cells are typically normocytic and normochromic. The initial total white cell count may be normal. In 25% the presenting count is less than $10^9/l$; in 50% 10–$50 \times 10^9/l$ and in 25% greater than $50 \times 10^9/l$. A relative and absolute granulocytopenia is common and is accompanied by a relative lymphocytosis.

Bone marrow examination is essential to establish the diagnosis of leukaemia with blast cells constituting 70–100% of cells present. The subtype of leukaemia is determined by a combination of morphology and cytochemical stains.

Immunological subclassification into common ALL, null cell ALL and T and B cell ALL should also be performed. Chromosome studies must also be performed as patients with translocations require more intensive treatment.

Management of acute leukaemia in childhood

At present 60–70% of children with ALL and 40–50% of children with AML can be confidently expected to be cured provided the child is managed at a specialized centre.

Acute lymphatic leukaemia

It is now well established that certain clinical and laboratory features at presentation may be used to predict the likely response to treatment (see Example 45.1). The most important features are the total white cell count at presentation, with a white cell count of less than $10 \times 10^9/l$ conferring a very good prognosis, 10–$100 \times 10^9/l$ an intermediate prognosis and greater than $100 \times 10^9/l$ a very poor prognosis; and age, with children aged 3–10 years having the best prognosis. Thus, children aged 3–10 years and having a white cell count of less than $10 \times 10^9/l$ can be expected to have a 70–80% chance of being able to cease therapy, whereas younger or older children with a white cell count of greater than $100 \times 10^9/l$ have only a 50–60% chance of being able to cease therapy.

Treatment involves general supportive measures as well as antileukaemic therapy. Before therapy the child must be thoroughly evaluated for the presence of infection and broad-spectrum intravenous antibiotics commenced if appropriate. Platelet transfusions should be given if there is active bleeding and packed cells to correct anaemia. Urea, uric acid and electrolyte levels should be determined. Before commencing

---

Example 45.1 Prognostic factors predicting disease-free survival in acute lymphatic leukaemia

Total white cell count at presentation
Age
Sex
Chromosome abnormality of leukaemic cell
Immunological subtype of leukaemia
Degree of splenomegaly
Degree of lymphadenopathy
Haemoglobin level at presentation
Platelet count at presentation
Mediastinal mass
CNS leukaemia at diagnosis
Rapidity of response to treatment

---

chemotherapy an adequate urine output should be ensured with intravenous fluids and alkalinization of the urine. Allopurinol is given if the white cell count is elevated or gross organomegaly, lymphadenopathy or hyperuricaemia is present.

Standard induction regimens would include the use of vincristine, prednisolone, and L-asparaginase, often with a fourth drug such as daunorubicin or cytosine arabinoside. Intrathecal methotrexate is also given during remission induction. The remission induction rate in ALL with multiple drugs ranges from 90–95% and is generally achieved within 4–6 weeks.

As the brain is a sanctuary site for leukaemia, CNS relapse terminated remission in as many as 60% of children before the use of CNS prophylaxis. Once remission is achieved CNS prophylaxis is instituted. The use of presymptomatic CNS therapy has reduced the CNS relapse rate to less than 10%.

Cranial irradiation and intrathecal methotrexate has been the standard form of CNS prophylaxis in most centres. Because of the long-term complications of poor school performance and short concentration span which occur in as many as 30% of cured patients, especially in children less than 5 years of age at diagnosis, many centres are now omitting cranial irradiation for all but high risk patients. Maintenance intrathecal methotrexate alone or together with high or moderate dose intravenous methotrexate have been used in place of cranial irradiation. Many protocols now include intensive systemic chemotherapy during CNS prophylaxis especially in higher risk patients.

There are a number of protocols for continuation therapy which will not be detailed. This is followed by more standard therapy with oral 6-mercaptopurine and methotrexate which may be given on an intermittent basis to lessen immunosuppression but without compromising its antileukaemic effectiveness. With these more intensive protocols antileukaemic therapy is ceased after 2 years of complete continuous remission.

After cessation of therapy the risk of relapse is 15–20% with the risk highest in the first 1–2 years after stopping. The remaining 80–85% of patients can be considered cured. Very late relapse may ocur, but relapse 4 years after ceasing therapy is exceedingly rare.

During remission the child is completely well and should be encouraged to lead a full and normal life. Episodes of myelosuppression may occur in association with bacterial or viral infections but opportunistic infection is rare.

The current trend in children with high white cell leukaemia (greater than $100 \times 10^9/l$) and/or mass disease is to treat them as stage IV non-Hodgkin lymphoma with more intensive therapy in an attempt to improve the poor prognosis obtained with standard ALL therapy.

Relapse. With modern therapy, relapse is usually detected on routine follow-up subsequent to an abnormality of the peripheral blood count. Routine regular bone marrow examinations are not necessary to detect early relapse but must be performed to document relapse. A fall in the platelet count is generally the most common finding. Rarely recurrence of initial symptoms may occur.

The prognosis of relapse during therapy is exceedingly poor despite the attainment of second remission. Less than 10% of children who relapse will be able to cease therapy, even though prolonged second or even third or fourth remissions may occur. This period is particularly stressful for the parents as cure is no longer possible. The physician will have to call on all of his resources, and of the support teams to cope with and meet the needs of both the child and family. Parents will need to be fully informed of the intended programme, the possible complications and the possible effects of therapy on the child. All questions must be truthfully answered and, in fact, should be actively encouraged. There will inevitably come a time when a decision to stop treatment must be made; parents must be completely involved and even encouraged to participate in this decision. Allogeneic bone marrow transplantation in second remission if an HLA identical sibling donor is available may lead to cure in 40–50% of patients.

Despite the marked improvement in prognosis, 20–30% of patients still die from ALL. Infection, bleeding and bone pain are common terminal complications. Disabling infection must be treated with adequate antibiotic therapy. Bleeding will usually respond to judicious use of platelet transfusion. Pain must be alleviated with analgesia of sufficient strength and frequency of administration. Morphine suspension and Proladone suppositories (oxycodone pectinate) are usually effective. Unnecessary investigations and procedures should be avoided. The family should be encouraged to nurse their children at home unless there are specific nursing or emotional problems or inadequate support services.

Acute myeloid leukaemia

The non-lymphoid subgroups of leukaemia have a much worse prognosis than the lymphoid group. Remission can be achieved in 70% of these children, but only with very intensive chemotherapy aimed at producing marked bone marrow hypoplasia. The mainstays of induction therapy are cytosine arabinoside and the anthracycline antibiotics, daunomycin and adriamycin. Patients who fail to remit usually die of infection or bleeding secondary to marrow hypoplasia.

With intensive chemotherapy 40–50% of children with AML can now be cured. Some centres report higher complete continuous remission rates with allogeneic bone marrow transplantation in first remission but only 25–30% of patients will have a histocompatible sibling.

LYMPHOMA

Non-Hodgkin lymphoma and Hodgkin lymphoma (or Hodgkin's disease) are not related diseases and manifest entirely different clinical patterns of behaviour in the child compared to the adult.

Non-Hodgkin lymphoma (lymphosarcoma)

Non-Hodgkin lymphoma (NHL) is more common in boys than girls. Certain features are unique to childhood, i.e. a high frequency of marrow and/or CNS involvement during the course of the disease; extreme rarity of nodular, well differentiated and mixed lymphocytic/histiocytic histological subtypes, and blurring of the distinction between lymphosarcoma with marrow involvement and true acute lymphocytic leukaemia of childhood.

A variety of pathological classifications have been devised most of which are unsuitable for paediatric use. One modification suitable for use in children is as follows:

1. Poorly differentiated diffuse lymphoblastic lymphoma
2. Undifferentiated non-Burkitt's
3. Burkitt's lymphoma
4. Large cell or histiocytic lymphoma.

Immunotyping reveals that approximately 50% of NHL is of T cell origin, whilst most of the remainder have a B cell neoplasm.

Clinical staging is essential and should be supplemented by appropriate organ imaging and bone marrow and CSF examinations.

Presentation is with painless enlargement of lymph nodes which may be regional or general. Mediastinal primaries account for 25% and may present with acute superior venal caval obstruction (a medical emergency) or a pleural effusion. They have a T cell immunophenotype and occur characteristically in preteen or early teenage males. Abdominal involvement of B cell origin accounts for 30–40% and characteristically presents as one of two extremes, either a localized readily removable tumour causing intussusception, or as massive intra-abdominal disease of indeterminate origin.

Surgery is limited to biopsy of involved nodes except for removal of localized abdominal lesions. Irradiation has no role in primary treatment as lymphosarcoma is never a localized disease. Its role is in CNS prophylaxis as for ALL. Chemotherapy is the mainstay of treatment with many drugs being active. There is no role for single agent therapy and most regimens combine agents such as vincristine, prednisolone, cyclophosphamide, anthracyclines, moderate or high dose methotrexate, cytosine arabinoside and L-asparaginase used in an intermittent fashion.

Cure rates of 80–90% are achieved in patients with stage I and II disease and 50–60% in stage III and IV disease. The patients with the worst prognosis are those with widely disseminated abdominal disease.

Hodgkin's disease

Hodgkin's disease is uncommon in children, being particularly rare in children less than 5 years of age; boys are affected more than girls. Its aetiology is unknown.

Clinically it presents as painless enlargement of a lymph node or group of nodes with the cervical nodes being most commonly affected. Splenomegaly and/or hepatomegaly may be present but do not necessarily indicate infiltration by Hodgkin's disease.

Diagnosis is established by biopsy of an involved node with four histological types described, i.e. lymphocyte predominant, nodular sclerosing, mixed cellularity and lymphocyte depleted. Staging is by clinical examination, organ imaging and bone marrow aspirate and trephin only.

Whilst irradiation therapy has been responsible for the dramatic improvement in results in adults with Hodgkin's disease, it must be remembered that this has significant side effects on growth of bone, soft tissue and muscle in children. The current trend in childhood Hodgkin's disease is, therefore, to rely on chemotherapy as the mainstay of treatment, either used alone, or with radiotherapy on a limited supplementary basis only.

Combination chemotherapy with nitrogen mustard, vincristine, prednisolone and procarbazine (MOPP) is the cornerstone of treatment of Hodgkin's disease in both children and adults. Apart from myelosuppression and immunosuppression, MOPP is a potent cause of sterility in adults. To what degree MOPP will affect ultimate fertility of prepubertal children remains to be documented.

The prognosis of childhood Hodgkin's disease is excellent with an 80% 5-year disease-free survival of all stages being reported.

HISTIOCYTOSIS X

The term histiocytosis X has been coined to encompass Letterer-Siwe disease, Hand-Schuller-Christian disease, and eosinophilic granuloma, on the basis that they are variants of a single disease entity of unknown aetiology. The disease is peculiar to childhood being characterized by proliferation of fixed tissue histiocytes, associated with varying degrees of lymphocytic and eosinophilic infiltration and destruction of surrounding tissues. Whether it is a malignant disorder, a disorder of immune regulation, an abnormal response to an unknown infectious agent remains to be determined. The diagnosis is usually confirmed by biopsy of a bony lesion or the skin. Rarely lymph node biopsy is required.

Letterer-Siwe disease

This disease presents in infancy with a characteristic seborrhoeic scalp rash and a fine petechial-like trunk rash in association with hepatosplenomegaly and lymphadenopathy. Fever, weight loss, diarrhoea and pulmonary involvement may follow. Previously the prognosis was very poor. Therapy with multiple agents such as vinblastine, prednisolone, cyclophosphamide and methotraxate has led to a vastly improved prognosis with 70–80% of children surviving. Letter-Siwe disease needs to be distinguished from the clinically similar but exceedingly rare disorder of haemophagocytic reticulosis, which often has a familial basis.

Hand-Schuller-Christian disease

This usually presents between 2 and 8 years but the classic triad of diabetes insipidus, exophthalmos and skull lesions is rarely seen. Diabetes insipidus is due to involvement of the posterior pituitary stalk or hypothalamus and the exophthalmos which may be unilateral or bilateral is due to retro-orbital infiltration. The common sites of bone lesions are the calvarium, mastoids, mandible and sinuses. Chronic otitis media is a frequent development. Abnormal dentition, premature eruption of teeth or four quadrant mouth ulcers which are quite typical of histiocytosis X may also be seen.

Therapy is best given with chemotherapy, usually vinblastine and prednisolone, with good response. Surgical dental treatment may be necessary to control the oral lesions. Despite resolution of the skull lesions, the diabetes insipidus may be permanent requiring replacement therapy with DDAVP. Because of the long-term effects of irradiation therapy on bone growth, irradiation therapy is seldom indicated.

Eosinophilic granuloma

This usually presents in children aged above 8 years either with single or multiple bony lesions without soft tissue involvement. Biopsy of the lesions confirms the diagnosis and curettage is curative. If multiple bony lesions are present chemotherapy may be necessary.

Atypical presentations may occur in all age groups. Five-year disease-free survival rates of 70–80% are now seen in all types following appropriate therapy. Relapse may occur but usually responds to retreatment.

SOLID TUMOURS IN CHILDHOOD

The improved results seen in childhood cancer are due to introduction of a multidisciplinary clinic, where clinical staging is determined and advice is given as to which diagnostic procedures are most appropriate. Surgery may range from needle biopsy to excisional biopsy to complete removal of the affected organ. Definitive surgery may be delayed until after initial chemotherapy has made the tumour more readily resectable. Pathological findings and histological subtype will determine final stage and treatment required. Chemotherapy forms the back bone of most treatment programmes, with irradiation therapy having a more supplemental or no role in modern therapy. For most solid tumours stage I refers to local totally resectable tumour; stage II to local tumour with microscopic extension to the edge of excision; stage III to surgically irremovable tumours or those with disseminated disease.

At presentation treatment should be undertaken with curative intent even for those patients with metastatic disease.

Wilms' tumour (nephroblastoma)

This highly malignant tumour arises in the kidney. It usually presents in the first 5 years of life. Certain congenital anomalies such as hemihypertrophy, aniridia, Beckwith syndrome and genitourinary abnormalities are associated with an increased frequency of Wilms' tumour.

Most patients present with an abdominal mass, occasionally in association with abdominal pain. Haematuria is uncommon. Hypertension may occur but is rarely a presenting feature. The differential diagnosis includes polycystic kidneys, hydronephrosis, neuroblastoma, hepatoblastoma and, rarely, in left-sided cases splenomegaly.

The diagnosis is established by abdominal ultrasound, IVP being less important. Chest radiograph is necessary for staging. Surgical removal of the involved kidney with biopsy of para-aortic nodes and inspection of the other kidney and liver is the first step in treatment. The frequency and intensity of chemotherapy will vary depending upon both the stage and histological subtype. Vincristine, actinomycin-D, adriamycin and, rarely, cyclophosphamide are the drugs used. Irradiation therapy is only necessary for certain stage III and IV patients. At present 2-year disease-free survival rates are 80%. A subgroup of patients with 'unfavourable histology', comprising approximately 10% of all cases of Wilms' tumour, has been identified which has a universally poor outcome irrespective of stage of presentation or treatment given.

Neuroblastoma

This tumour may arise anywhere in the sympathetic nervous system or adrenal medulla, both of which have similar origins embryonically. Abdominal tumours account for 50%, most being adrenal in origin. Thoracic lesions are paravertebral in origin and may be massive in size before producing symptoms. The disease is metastatic at presentation in 70% of patients and in about 10% the primary site of origin is not found. Most occur in children less than 5 years and the following are the most common modes of presentation:

1. With fever, anaemia, vomiting and 'malignant malaise'.
2. With an abdominal mass often associated with the above symptoms.
3. With symptoms due to compression of neighbouring structures, for example paraplegia with dumbell paravertebral lesions, or retention of urine with pelvic primaries.
4. With bone pain, limp, refusal to walk, a nodule in the skull or proptosis, i.e. secondary to metastatic disease.
5. With lymphadenopathy.
6. Occasionally with chronic diarrhoea due to secretion of vasoactive intestinal peptides.
7. Very rarely with opsomyoclonus and ataxia.

Histologically neuroblastoma is a malignant small round cell tumour. Neurofibrils and rosettes may occur in the more differentiated ganglioneuroblastoma. Ganglioneuroma is the benign counterpart of neuroblastoma where benign conversion may have occurred by an as yet unknown process.

The diagnosis is confirmed by a positive bone marrow examination plus an elevated 24-hour urinary catecholamine and vanillyl mandelic acid (VMA) level. If both these two findings are not present, surgical biopsy will be required. Isotope bone scan will complete staging procedures.

In neuroblastoma age and stage are closely related, with the more favourable stage I and II lesions tending to occur in children less than 1 year. Surgical resection is usually the only therapy necessary for these early stages where an 80–90% disease-free survival can be expected. Chemotherapy is the preferred treatment of stage III and IV disease with vincristine, cyclophosphamide and adriamycin. Cis-platinum, VM-26 (Teniposide) and DTIC (Dacarbazine) are also active agents. Despite improvements in therapy, cure is still not possible, with stage III patients having a 10–20% survival and stage IV less than 10% survival. Recurrence nearly always occurs within 12 months of diagnosis. Irradiation therapy may be necessary to relieve severe bone pain or alleviate obstructive symptoms.

Mention should be made of the IV-S stage of neuroblastoma with metastatic spread limited to skin and/or liver and/or bone marrow but not bone in a child less than 6 months (the 'blueberry muffin' baby), where spontaneous resolution may occur in as many as 60% of patients. Apart from age and stage other prognostic factors are histology, levels of serum ferritin and non-specific enolase. Current data suggests amplification of the N-myc oncogene may be the most significant prognostic factor with highest levels conferring the worst prognosis.

Soft tissue sarcoma

Apart from rhabdomyosarcoma soft tisue sarcomas are rare in children. Rhabdomyosarcoma represents 4–8% of malignancies in children less than 15 years. Orbital and head and neck primaries account for 30%, extremities for 23%, genitourinary for 18% and trunk for 8%. The presenting signs and symptoms will vary according to the site of origin. Excisional biopsy is preferred, provided this is non-mutilating and does not compromise organ function. Adequate staging is essential to determine therapy which will primarily involve chemotherapy. Survival depends upon stage ranging from 80–90% in stages I and II, 30–50% in stage III and 10–20% in stage IV. Other soft tissue sarcomas are treated primarily by surgery with adjuvant chemotherapy having a less certain role. Late metastasis is a problem in certain subtypes, for example synovial sarcoma.

Bone sarcoma

Pain and swelling, often present for many weeks, are the usual presenting features. A biopsy is necessary to confirm the diagnosis and chest radiograph, CT lung scan and isotope bone scan are necessary to accurately stage. Over 50% of osteosarcomas arise in the lower femur or upper tibia. Ewing's sarcoma may occur in any site but pelvic lesions are usually extremely large at the time of diagnosis. In both types the prognosis has been markedly improved with modern therapy, the 5-year disease-free survival rate being increased from 10–15% to 60–70%. In patients with metastatic disease on presentation, the prognosis remains poor.

Chemotherapy forms the mainstay of treatment. In Ewing's sarcoma intensive chemotherapy will usually lead to resolution of the primary tumour, which should then be resected if it is an expendable bone, reserving irradiation therapy for those tumours which are not resectable. In osteosarcoma some centres are exploring the role of limb preservation, following initial chemotherapy, rather than amputations. Resection of pulmonary metastases may lead to long-term survival in 30% of patients with osteosarcoma, whether they develop during or after initial chemotherapy.

Hepatoblastoma

This tumour usually presents as a painless large abdominal mass. An elevated serum alphafetoprotein strongly suggests the diagnosis. Partial hepatectomy, if possible, is curative in the majority of patients with limited disease. Intensive chemotherapy may convert an inoperable lesion to an operable one. The prognosis for patients with irresectable or metastatic disease remains poor.

Teratoma

The most common site of origin is the sacrococcygeal area, but ovarian, testicular and mediastinal sites are also seen. Most are benign and surgical removal is indicated. Malignant teratoma often has a grossly elevated serum alphafetoprotein and should be excised completely, if possible, or following initial chemotherapy and then given adjuvant chemotherapy. With the newer agents cis-platinum and bleomycin, malignant teratoma is no longer a fatal disease and cures may be achieved even in patients with metastatic disease.

CEREBRAL TUMOURS

Excluding the leukaemias, intracranial neoplasms are the commonest malignancies in childhood. The clinical presentation depends to a large extent on the site of the tumour. Approximately three-quarters of childhood in-

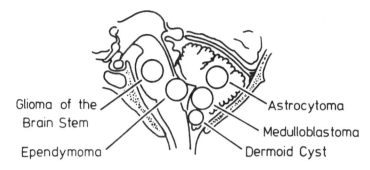

Fig. 45.1 Distribution of the main types of tumour of the posterior cranial fossa. (Reproduced with permission, Jones & Campbell 1976.)

tracranial tumours are situated either in the posterior fossa or, somewhat less frequently, close to midline structures in the third ventricle region. The distribution of the main types of posterior fossa tumour is shown in Figure 45.1. Craniopharyngioma, optic nerve or chiasm glioma, and dysgerminoma are the more common of the anteriorly placed deep midline tumours. Astrocytomas and ependymomas of the cerebral hemisphere make up the majority of the remaining supratentorial tumours. Meningiomas and secondary cerebral tumours which are common in the adult are rarely seen in childhood.

The early signs and symptoms of cerebral tumours in childhood may be few and difficult to elicit, for example, visual impairment and diplopia, both of which may not be appreciated by the young child. The following are the commoner modes of presentation of cerebral tumour. It is not surprising that evidence of raised intracranial pressure is the predominant presenting manifestation, because the posterior fossa and deep midline tumours commonly obstruct the CSF pathways.

1. Signs and symptoms of raised intracranial pressure

Headache, which typically occurs on or soon after waking and which may be frontal or occipital in site, is by far the most important symptom. The headaches characteristically increase in frequency and severity with the passage of time but are not day-in day-out headaches.

Morning vomiting, and sometimes nausea, commonly accompanies the headaches. Drowsiness is a late feature. Papilloedema is common except in the young infant as it very rarely occurs before closure of sutures. A 'cracked-pot' percussion note may be elicited in young children with sutural separation by placing the ear close to the child's skull near the point of percussion along the coronal suture.

2. Signs and symptoms of involvement of posterior fossa structures

Ataxia may be due to either involvement of the cerebellum or cerebellar tracts and is typically truncal ataxia in medulloblastomas, which are situated in the midline vermis. Lateralized cerebellar signs, for example, incoordination and intention tremor, suggest a lateralized astrocytoma, a tumour with a very favourable prognosis. Multiple cranial nerve palsies suggest a brainstem glioma. They are usually accompanied by incoordination and gait disturbance due to involvement of cerebellar and corticospinal tracts. Defective upward gaze is seen with tumours in the pineal region and is due to pressure on the superior colliculus region of the brain stem.

3. Signs and symptoms of deep midline tumours around the third ventricle

Both craniopharyngioma and optic nerve glioma may cause severe impairment of visual acuity, in one or both eyes, or visual field defects. However, classical bitemporal hemianopia is relatively rare. A variety of endocrinological features may be present because of involvement of the pituitary-hypothalamic axis. Diabetes insipidus and growth failure are the more common of these. Occasionally severe wasting and anorexia result from an hypothalamic tumour, producing the 'diencephalic syndrome'.

4. Epilepsy

Epilepsy is an uncommon mode of presentation of cerebral tumours in childhood. However, the possibility of a tumour should be considered in focal epilepsy, other than typical benign focal epilepsy of childhood, and in any child whose epilepsy is progressively more difficult to control. Some of the hemisphere gliomas which may present as epilepsy run a relatively benign course over very many years.

Investigation of suspected intracranial tumour

Computerized axial tomography should be carried out in any child suspected of having an intracranial tumour, or other cause of raised intracranial pressure. Cranial ultrasound is a useful screening procedure in infants with an open fontanelle.

Treatment of intracranial tumours

For patients with low grade astrocytoma surgical excision may be all that is required. High grade lesions require irradiation therapy in addition to surgery. Brain stem gliomas are treated with irradiation alone. Posterior fossa medulloblastoma and ependymoma require craniospinal irradiation after surgical excision. Long-term complications of growth failure due to arrest of spinal growth and growth hormone deficiency are major problems especially in younger children. The role of adjuvant chemotherapy is beginning to be explored in medulloblastoma and ependymoma.

Retinoblastoma

Retinoblastoma usually presents with leukokoria (cat's eye reflex) or squint. In Western countries exophthalmos and metastatic disease are very rare presenting features. In those with a positive family history, lesions may be detected at a very early stage by regular follow-up. Enucleation of unilaterally affected eyes and the more affected eye in bilateral cases is the preferred treatment. Cryotherapy and photocoagulation may be used to treat small lesions. Irradiation therapy, with its long-term side effects, is required for larger tumours.

FURTHER READING

Behrendt H, Van Bunningen N F M, Van Leeuwen E F 1987 Treatment of Hodgkin's disease with or without radiotherapy. Cancer 59: 1870–1873

Breslow N, Churchill G, Beckwith J B et al 1985 Prognosis for Wilms' tumour patients with non-metastatic disease at diagnosis – results of the second national Wilms' tumour study. Journal of Clinical Oncology 3: 521–531

Camitta B M, Lauer S J, Casper J T et al 1985 Effectiveness of a six drug regimen (APO) without local irradiation for treatment of mediastinal lymphoblastic lymphoma in children. Cancer 56: 738–741

Clavell L A, Gelber R D, Cohen H J et al 1986 Four agent induction and intensive asparaginase therapy for treatment of childhood acute lymphocytic leukaemia. New England Journal of Medicine 315: 657–663

Ekert H 1982 Clinical paediatric haematology and oncology. Blackwell Scientific Publications, Oxford

Ekert H, Waters K D 1983 Results of treatment of 18 children with Hodgkin's disease with MOPP chemotherapy as the only treatment modality. Medical and Paediatric Oncology 11: 322–326

Evans A E, D'Angio G J, Propert K et al 1987 Prognostic factors in neuroblastoma. Cancer 59: 1853–1859

Goorin A M, Abelson H T, Frei E III 1986 Osteosarcoma: 15 years on. New England Journal of Medicine 313: 1637–1643

Grier H E, Weinstein H J 1985 Acute non-lymphocytic leukaemia. In: Altman A J (ed) Paediatric oncology. Paediatric Clinics of North America, Saunders. Philadelphia, p 653–668

Jones P G, Campbell P E (eds) 1976 Tumours of infancy and childhood. Blackwell Scientific Publications, Oxford

King D R, Clatworthy H W 1981 The paediatric patient with sarcoma. Seminars in Oncology 8: 215–221

Matus-Ridley M, Raney Jr R B, Thaweroni H, Meadows A T 1983 Histiocytosis X in children. Patterns of disease and results of treatment. Medical and Paediatric Oncology 11: 90–105

Philip T, Pinkerton R, Biron P et al 1987 Effective multiagent chemotherapy in children with advanced B cell lymphoma who remain high risk patients. British Journal of Haematology 65: 159–164

Sutow W W, Fernbach D J, Vietti T J 1984 Clinical paediatric oncology. Mosby, St Louis Woods W G, Tuckman M 1987 Neuroblastoma: the case for screening infants in North America. Pediatrics 79: 869–873

Disorders of the nervous system

46. Convulsions and epilepsies

I. J. Hopkins

Few events are more alarming to parents than their child having a first convulsion. Many parents have thought their infant or child had died in what has, in retrospect, been nothing more than a breath-holding attack or febrile convulsion. Convulsions are very common in childhood, with several studies indicating that about 7% of children have a suspected or verified seizure of some type in the early years of life. Fortunately, most seem to 'outgrow' their disorder, and do not have epilepsy, which is simply defined as chronically recurring afebrile seizures. The prevalence of epilepsy in later childhood and adult life is only about one-fifth that of convulsions in early childhood.

There are many different ways of classifying convulsive disorders. The International League Against Epilepsy classification of seizure types, based on clinical and EEG observations (1981) recognizes two main categories – partial seizures and generalized seizures (see Example 46.1). Partial seizures originate in part of the brain – one hemisphere – whereas generalized seizures commence synchronously in both hemispheres. A third group is recognized, consisting of those that at present cannot be fitted into either of the above. Many seizures in infancy fall into this category.

Complementary to a classification of seizure types is a classification of epilepsy or seizure disorder syndromes. An epilepsy syndrome has broader implications, both with regard to possible aetiology, associated clinical features such as intellectual disability, prognosis and therapy. In some epilepsy syndromes more than one seizure type may occur. For instance, in febrile convulsions generalized tonic-clonic convulsions occur most commonly, but some infants will have partial seizure or atonic limp attacks as their febrile convulsions. There are different ways of classifying epilepsy syndromes, one of which is shown in Example 46.2, which lists some of the more common epilepsy syndromes of childhood according to the usual age of onset of seizures.

Example 46.1 Classification of seizure type, based on a combined study of clinical and EEG features

Partial (focal)
1. Simple
   focal motor, and/or sensory, psychomotor, but conscious state preserved.
2. Complex
   similar but impaired conscious state
3. As above but becoming generalized

Generalized
Tonic-clonic
Absence
Myoclonic
Clonic
Tonic
Atonic.

Example 46.2 Classification of some of the more common epilepsy syndromes of childhood

Neonatal seizures
Due to hypoxic ischaemic encephalopathy, metabolic disturbance, infections and brain malformations

Infancy
Febrile convulsions, 'breath-holding', infantile spasms

Early childhood
Myoclonic epilepsies, including Lennox-Gastaut syndrome

Mid-late childhood
'Idiopathic' or primary generalized epilepsy, benign focal epilepsy, temporal lobe epilepsy

---

NEONATAL CONVULSIONS

Convulsions in the neonatal period differ from convulsions in the other age groups because of special aetiological factors, different clinical manifestations and special considerations with regard to anticonvulsant therapy.

Aetiology

1. Hypoxic – ischaemic encephalopathy. Various abnormalities of the pregnancy, labour and delivery, including placental malfunction, may be present singly or in combination. Fetal distress and neonatal asphyxia are the usual clinical pointers to this aetiology.

2. Metabolic disturbance. Hypoglycaemia, hypocalcaemia and, less frequently, hypomagnesaemia are the most common metabolic causes of neonatal convulsions. Inborn errors of metabolism, including pyridoxine-dependency, are much rarer causes.

3. Infections. These may be transplacentally acquired in utero, e.g. cytomegalovirus (CMV), toxoplasmosis, herpes, or acquired postnatally, e.g. bacterial infections such as meningitis, septicaemia.

4. Developmental structural anomalies of the brain.

Clinical features

Classical grand mal seizures with tonic and clonic phases are rarely seen in the newborn. Repetitive clonic jerking, which may be generalized, focal, or multifocal, and tonic spasms, in which the baby stiffens usually with an extensor posture, and becomes cyanosed, are the common types. Other findings vary widely depending on the cause of the convulsion. Concurrent video and EEG recording has shown that neonatal seizures may be very ·subtle in their clinical manifestations and not always accompanied by EEG changes typical of seizures in older infants and children.

Treatment

This will depend very much on the diagnosis, arrived at after blood sugar, serum calcium and magnesium estimations, CSF examination, and viral studies. Pending the results of investigations, it is also advisable to give pyridoxine 50 mg intravenously or intramuscularly if seizures are recurring even in those infants in whom evidence of intrauterine hypoxia or birth asphyxia has been present. If the results of investigations are not available and seizures are continuing, a therapeutic trial of intravenous glucose, intravenous calcium, and intramuscular magnesium sulphate should also be considered. Phenobarbitone in an initial dose of 15 mg/kg is suggested as the best initial anticonvulsant, but phenytoin is also an effective anticonvulsant in many newborn infants with seizures. Blood level monitoring of anticonvulsants is essential in the maintenance therapy of newborn infants.

CONVULSIVE DISORDERS IN INFANCY

Febrile convulsions

Fever and convulsions may be present concurrently with infections involving the central nervous system, such as meningitis or encephalitis, and with an intercurrent infection in epilepsy of many different types. In prolonged convulsions or frank status epilepticus due to any cause, a rise in temperature is also likely to occur. However, most commonly, fever and convulsions occur together in the condition called febrile convulsions (FC), in which there seems to be simply a lowered threshold to convulse in the presence of fever. Varying definitions of FC are used, but in recent literature a rather broader definition is used in which a child is considered to have a FC if:

1. There is neither clinical nor laboratory evidence of an infective process directly involving the central nervous system, e.g. meningitis, encephalitis, causing the febrile illness.

2. Seizures have occurred only when the temperature is 38°C or higher, in a child who at no time has had convulsions in the absence of fever.

Recent studies have shown that FC occur in approximately 3% of the population, and that in approximately one-third of cases the FC are recurrent. Approximately 3% of children with FC have later afebrile convulsions, i.e. epilepsy.

Aetiology

Why some apparently normal infants convulse with fever, and others do not, is unknown, except that genetic factors are important, as a family history of FC is present in more than 30% of children studied in most series.

Clinical features

The convulsions are of the typical grand mal type in most cases, although some more abortive types of grand mal seizure without both tonic and clonic phases are seen. Atonic fits and focal features may be present in some cases. Although the great majority are brief seizures lasting only several minutes, occasional patients have prolonged seizures of over 15 minutes' duration, and frank status epilepticus occasionally occurs. The great majority of FC occurs between 6 months and 2 years of age.

Prognostic indicators for further febrile convulsions and later afebrile seizures

Recurrence of FC is particularly likely to occur if the first fit occurs in early infancy. If the first FC occurs below the age of 12 months, a further FC is almost twice as likely to occur than if the first FC occurs at the age of 3 years or older, especially if the infant is female.

Although only a small proportion of children who have FC will have epilepsy later in life, the prevalence of epilepsy is increased approximately four-fold in patients who have had febrile convulsions compared with those who have not. The following have been shown to be risk factors for later occurrence of epilepsy:

1. Abnormal developmental or neurological status
2. Focal features present during the febrile convulsion or in the postictal period
3. Prolonged febrile convulsions (more than 15 minutes' duration)
4. Recurrent febrile convulsions within the one febrile illness
5. A positive family history of afebrile convulsions in first degree relatives.

Treatment

1. Acute management of the febrile convulsion. The cause of the febrile illness is treated on its own merits and measures to lower body temperature with the administration of an antipyretic and gentle cooling are employed. The convulsion will have ceased in the great majority of cases before medical help is obtained. If not, prompt and vigorous treatment of a persisting convulsion is of the utmost importance. Intravenous or rectal diazepam is the usual initial measure, although if the convulsion is resistant to this line of treatment the child should be admitted to an intensive care unit and treated with intravenous thiopentone and assisted ventilation, with EEG monitoring if possible.

The possibility of meningitis should always be considered and spinal puncture carried out in a first FC unless a clear cause is found for the fever and signs of meningism are unequivocally absent. A spinal puncture should always be considered in any child having had a recent FC who seems more seriously ill than would be expected.

2. The role of prophylactic anticonvulsants. There is no universal agreement on the role of anticonvulsants in the prevention of further FC and epilepsy. Phenobarbitone and sodium valproate have both been shown to reduce the recurrence rate from 30–50% to ap-

proximately 10%. Unacceptable side effects, especially irritability, are present in approximately 20% of infants who have maintenance phenobarbitone. The risk of hepatotoxicity with sodium valproate is highest in infancy and thus, while effective, it is not recommended for prophylactic use in what is generally a benign condition. It has been shown that phenytoin, administered as a maintenance anticonvulsant, is ineffective in preventing febrile convulsions. Insufficient studies are available with carbamazepine to assess its role. Intermittent oral use of phenobarbitone in conventional dosage when fever is recognized has also been found ineffective. Prompt attempts at reducing body temperature, with cooling and paracetamol, are most important in seizure prophylaxis and the use of rectal diazepam when fever is recognized in a child who has had a previous FC has also recently been advocated. However, both these measures will only be partially successful, as approximately one-third of all patients with FC are not recognized as being febrile or unwell before the onset of a seizure.

It is the author's usual practice not to use a maintenance anticonvulsant for prophylaxis after a first or second FC, but to consider it if further attacks occur, especially if one or more of the risk factors listed above for recurrence of FC or the occurrence of later epilepsy is present. However, at the present time there is no definite evidence that the prevention of recurrent FC alters the likelihood of epilepsy occurring later. Less well-defined factors, such as the parents' anxiety regarding the use of anticonvulsants versus their anxiety about FC recurrence, and the ready availability or otherwise of medical help if a further FC occurs, should be taken into consideration in the management of individual patients.

Infantile spasms (West's syndrome)

This form of epilepsy occurs in the first year of life and is of sinister significance because the attacks are often difficult to control and are frequently accompanied by severe mental retardation. The EEG usually has a very disorganized pattern of generalized high-voltage slow wave, sharp wave and spike components called hypsarrhythmia (Fig. 46.1). This term is best restricted to EEG usage, although it is sometimes used loosely as a clinical diagnostic term to embrace the clinical entity of infantile spasms. The terms salaam spasms, jackknife seizures, and massive myoclonic seizures of infancy are also sometimes used synonymously with the term 'infantile spasms'.

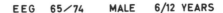

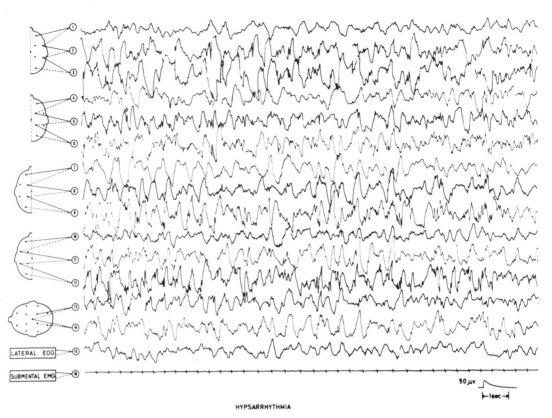

Fig. 46.1 The EEG pattern of hypsarrhythmia, showing continuous high amplitude, irregular sharp waves, spikes and slow waves of generalized distribution.

Aetiology

This form of infantile epilepsy has many different causes and, rather than indicating involvement of specific structures by particular pathological processes, the common factor is probably the timing and diffuse nature of a severe insult to the immature nervous system. In about half the cases no aetiological factor is obvious and development has been normal until the onset of spasms. In some of these cases pertussis immunization has been incriminated, but it is now thought that adverse response to pertussis immunization accounts for only very rare cases of infantile spasms. In about one-third of cases there is a history of some abnormal event in the prenatal or perinatal periods. Tuberous sclerosis is present in 5–10% of patients. In a small proportion there is evidence of a CNS developmental abnormality, e.g. agenesis of the corpus callosum, arrhinencephaly, and cases have been described with phenylketonuria, Sturge-Weber syndrome, Tay Sachs' disease, hypoglycaemia and pyridoxine dependency.

Clinical features

Males are affected twice as commonly as females. The onset is usually between 3 and 8 months of age, and in the idiopathic group development has been quite normal to that time. The common type of flexor or salaam spasm, which can be a myoclonic or brief tonic seizure, consists of sudden drawing up of the legs on the abdomen and hunching forward of the neck and shoulders. The arms are often flung out in extension. Opisthotonic spasms are less common. Each spasm may be accompanied by a cry, and, not infrequently, the condition is misdiagnosed as colic. The suddenness of the spasm in some cases has led to the term 'lightning fits'. Spasms characteristically occur in clusters of several within a minute or two, and such episodes may be repeated many times a day. In the symptomatic group development may already be delayed when spasms commence, whereas in the idiopathic group there is nearly always a sudden regression of intellectual, social and motor achievements when spasms are first noted.

Treatment

In most cases the spasms can be controlled by the administration of corticosteroids or ACTH (e.g. prednisolone 2 mg/kg a day for 1–2 months and then slowly reduced). If orally administered steroid is unsuccessful, ACTH 40 units daily should be tried even though this will necessitate daily injections. In a small percentage of cases treatment with steroids or ACTH also appears to reverse the regression in development. Clonazepam and other bendodiazepines are also frequently successful in controlling the spasms, and sodium valproate is also worthy of trial in infants not responding to other medication. However, such anticonvulsant drugs do not reverse the mental retardation.

Prognosis

Even in the absence of treatment, the spasms tend to cease spontaneously by 2–4 years of age, but other types such as grand mal seizures, may replace the spasms. Gross motor function is usually delayed but eventually most patients learn to sit and walk, although co-ordination is generally poor. Intellectual disability is present in 70–80% even with early and adequate therapy. The behaviour of the severely retarded patient is frequently autistic and difficult.

Reflex hypoxic seizures (breath-holding attacks)

Although the majority of 'breath-holding attacks' are mild, more severe attacks may terminate with loss of consciousness or a grand mal convulsion. They are not a form of epilepsy but are not infrequently misdiagnosed as such.

Aetiology

Although the precise pathophysiology is not well understood there appears to be a basic difference between 'blue' breath-holding attacks and 'white' breath-holding attacks. With 'white' breath-holding attacks, it has been shown that marked bradycardia or frank cardiac arrest of brief duration occurs. It has been demonstrated that such patients have an abnormally sensitive response to carotid sinus and eyeball pressure, with the production of marked bradycardia or temporary cardiac arrest.

In contrast, patients with the cyanotic variety show a later and much less conspicuous lowering of heart rate during their attacks.

Clinical features

Although attacks usually occur late in the first, second,

or third year of life they may occur from the earliest months of age. Crucial to diagnosis is the recognition that attacks are precipitated by either physical trauma such as a knock or a fall, or emotional trauma such as a fright, anger or frustration. The attack usually commences with crying, but this may be very shortlived or absent. Apnoea then occurs, with either cyanosis or extreme pallor. The attack may terminate without apparent loss of consciousness, or the child may fall limp and unconscious or more rarely have a brief tonic seizure or a tonic-clonic convulsion. Incontinence may occur with such a convulsion.

Many a parent has thought that their child has died during a breath-holding attack. This is not surprising when a child stops breathing, becomes limp, unconscious and deathly white. However, recovery is usually rapid, although some children are drowsy and lethargic for some time after the episodes.

Prognosis

This is excellent. Attacks usually cease by the third or fourth year of life, or earlier, but occasionally not until 6 or 7 years. They are not a cause of convulsions, mental retardation, or cerebral damage in later life.

CONVULSIONS IN THE PRESCHOOL AGE GROUP

Lennox-Gastaut syndrome and other varieties of myoclonic epilepsy.

These comprise a heterogeneous group, both with regard to aetiology and clinical features of the attack. There is commonly a mixed seizure pattern, with 'small attacks' predominating e.g. myoclonic, tonic and atypical absence seizures. These brief attacks are clinically distinct from typical absences of true petit mal epilepsy (see below), and also in their EEG patterns and their less satisfactory response to anticonvulsants.

Aetiology

Although cases of myoclonic epilepsy of early childhood frequently fall into the idiopathic group, they may also be due to well-defined conditions such as perinatal hypoxic-ischaemic brain injury, metabolic disturbance, e.g. phenylketonuria, hypoglycaemia, degenerative diseases of the brain, such as cerebral lipidoses.

Clinical features

Brief spasms or myoclonic jerks may occur with or

without loss of consciousness. Head nods and drop attacks, in which there is a sudden loss of postural control so that the child falls, often with only momentary loss of consciousness, are the most common type. Brief tonic spasms may occur, with nocturnal tonic spasms being a feature of the Lennox-Gastaut syndrome. Many patients also have tonic-clonic grand mal seizures. Mental retardation is almost invariably present in the Lennox-Gastaut syndrome, but not in some more benign varieties of myoclonic epilepsy.

Myoclonic, minor or 'non-convulsive' epileptic status also occurs. There is partial depression of consciousness so that the child appears vague and inattentive, or even deaf. Irregular and small amplitude myoclonic jerks of the extremities and nods of the head are usually present. These myoclonic intrusions may be responsible for the incoordinate and 'ataxic' gait that is present. Status epilepticus of this type may last from hours to days or weeks.

Prognosis

In most cases this is poor because of difficulty in controlling seizures, and the frequent association of retarded intellectual development. If an aetiological diagnosis can be made this enables a more precise prognosis to be given.

Treatment

Sodium valproate is the drug of choice, but is not successful in all cases. Benzodiazepines are the next best choice. It is often necessary to try many different anticonvulsants, and frequently it is not possible to obtain complete seizure control. If anticonvulsants are unsuccessful, the ketogenic diet should be considered. ACTH and corticosteroids may also be used in the resistant case, as described above for infantile spasms. Intravenous diazepam is usually successful in terminating minor epileptic status.

CONVULSIONS IN THE SCHOOL-AGE CHILD

Primary generalized (idiopathic) epilepsy

This term is used to delineate a group of patients in whom there is no demonstrable structural or metabolic disease. Genetic factors are thought to be important in aetiology. The empirical risk, whether of the grand mal or petit mal type is approximately 8% amongst siblings and offspring of affected individuals.

Clinical features

The seizure types associated with this variety of epilepsy are particularly grand mal tonic-clonic seizures and petit mal absences. There is some evidence to suggest that benign focal epilepsy of childhood (see below) and some cases of myoclonic epilepsy, may also fall within this general category.

Generalized tonic clonic (grand mal)

Although these may arise from a very wide range of structural and metabolic processes affecting the brain, they also commonly occur in the absence of any demonstrable cause. In tonic-clonic seizures there is initially a generalized stiffening of the whole musculature with temporary cessation of respiration (the tonic stage). The patient will fall if in the erect position as the onset is usually dramatically sudden: head injuries occasionally occur. With the onset of respiration, generalized coarse jerking (the clonic stage) commences. This lasts a variable period, usually a few minutes only, but rarely may last up to an hour or longer. This clonic stage is followed by a period of confusion after which the child commonly falls in to a deep sleep for an hour or so. On awakening there may be a headache, but there is no memory for the event.

Auras do not occur in generalized tonic-clonic convulsions of primary generalized epilepsy. If present they are an indication that the seizure is of partial origin, even though a secondarily generalized seizure may occur.

Treatment

Phenytoin or carbamazepine are the drugs of first choice. Because accentuation of acne and gum hypertrophy may occur, phenytoin is not popular for children around the age of puberty. In unresponsive cases sodium valproate is indicated.

Prognosis

In the idiopathic form control is usually possible and satisfactory but several years should elapse before the drug is withdrawn and phased out over many months.

Absence (petit mal) seizures

In the great majority of cases typical absences are a manifestation of primary generalized epilepsy, although very rarely patients have had typical petit mal absences in association with a cerebral tumour or lipoid storage disease.

Clinical features

Petit mal attacks usually commence between 5 and 10 years of age, and are very rare under the age of 3 years. They continue into adult life in a minority of cases. Females are more commonly affected than males. An absence consists of sudden cessation of activity, with staring into space for a short period, usually 5–10 seconds. Blinking, upward deviation of the eyes, slight mouthing movements, and some hand movements may occur. The child does not fall with petit mal attacks and is rarely incontinent. Attacks can usually be brought on by hyperventilation; this is of value in clinical diagnosis and during electroencephalography, as the attacks and accompanied by a very characteristic EEG pattern of 3 per second spike and wave generalized discharges (Fig. 46.2). Many attacks may occur in a day, and occasional-

ly they may be almost continuous so that true petit mal status, when a child is out of touch with his surroundings, appearing inattentive and confused for hours or days at a time, may occur.

Treatment

Ethosuximide (Zarontin) and sodium valproate (Epilim) are the specific drugs for petit mal. Because more than 50% of children with petit mal attacks also have a grand mal attack at some time, there is an increasing tendency to use sodium valproate so that both minor and major seizures can be controlled with a single drug.

Prognosis

Petit mal is sometimes said to be a self-limiting disease, invariably ceasing soon after adolescence. However, in some series at least 25% of cases have some attacks in early adult life, although it is rare after the age of 30 years. Intellectual development is usually normal.

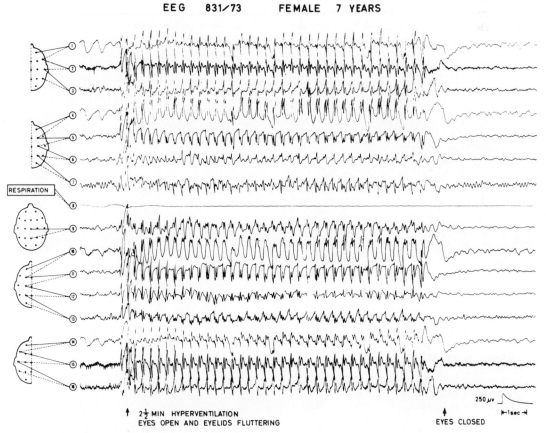

EEG   831/73   FEMALE   7 YEARS

RESPIRATION

250 μv

↑ 2½ MIN HYPERVENTILATION
EYES OPEN AND EYELIDS FLUTTERING

↑ EYES CLOSED

|←1sec→|

Fig. 46.2 The EEG of classical petit mal. This paroxysm of generalized regular 3 Hz spike and slow wave activity was accompanied by a clinical absence.

Benign focal epilepsy of childhood with centrotemporal spikes

This is one of the most common forms of epilepsy in mid-childhood and is more common than petit mal. It is sometimes called Sylvian or Rolandic spike epilepsy.

Aetiology

In spite of the well-defined focal EEG changes noted below, focal structural pathology is not demonstrable. Some authorities consider that it is genetically determined, and possibly related to primary generalized epilepsy.

Clinical features

Onset is usually between 5 and 10 years of age, and the focal seizures most commonly involve the face. At times the focal disturbance is limited to paraesthesiae of the side of the face, mouth and tongue. Motor seizures are most commonly twitching of one side of the face, or jerking movements of the jaw. Mouthing movements, inability to speak or gurgling noises, and salivation, may be conspicuous. Consciousness may be unimpaired but,

in some cases, there is usually inability to speak during the attacks. Attacks are most commonly nocturnal and, for this reason, it is at times not possible to get a good description of the characteristic features. An important aid to diagnosis is the characteristic EEG finding of well-defined focal spike discharges in the temporal-frontal-parietal region (Fig. 46.3).

Treatment

This form of epilepsy usually responds well to phenytoin or carbamazepine.

Prognosis

Prognosis is excellent, not only because of the good response to anticonvulsants, but because seizures normally cease by the age of 15–16 years.

Temporal lobe epilepsy

Aetiology

In childhood temporal lobe epilepsy is most commonly due to gliosis (sclerosis) of the hippocampal region,

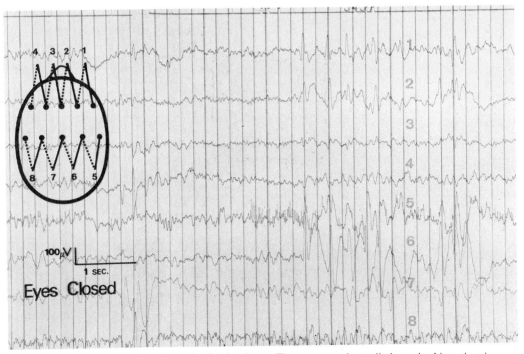

Fig. 46.3 The EEG in a child with benign focal epilepsy. The most prominent discharge in this patient is from the right centrotemporal region, although an independent discharge is also present in the left frontocentral region.

sometimes called mesial temporal sclerosis. The cause of mesial sclerosis is uncertain, although in some cases it is associated with prolonged febrile convulsions in early childhood. Developmental malformations of the temporal lobe, angiomas, and tumours together account for about one-third of the cases that are examined pathologically and, in a small percentage, no structural abnormality can be demonstrated.

Clinical features

Classical clinical descriptions of temporal lobe epilepsy are occasionally encountered in the first 5 years and thereafter with increasing frequency through the next two decades. The seizures are usually of complex partial type, but vary greatly in detail. There may be complex psychic perceptual disturbances such as unreal dream states, feeling of familiarity (déjà vu), fear, distortion of visual images, e.g. micropsia and macropsia, and olfactory hallucinations. Motor phenomena are semiorganized but purposeless, e.g. repeated buttoning and unbuttoning of a coat, lip smacking and swallowing, fidgeting hand movements. Autonomic disturbance may be evident, e.g. facial flushing or pallor, belching, abdominal pain or discomfort. Occasionally temporal lobe attacks may be nothing more than an 'absence', but with a careful history, these can usually be distinguished from petit mal because of their longer duration and less abrupt return to a normal level of consciousness. Behavioural problems are very common in temporal lobe epilepsy, although there are no unique features to the type of behavioural disturbance that occurs. However, behavioural disturbance and rage reactions are very rarely part of actual seizures; they are interictal accompaniments of temporal lobe epilepsy rather than ictal events.

Treatment

Carbamazepine is the drug of first choice in temporal lobe epilepsy, followed by phenytoin. Temporal lobectomy has a definite role in the treatment of intractable temporal lobe epilepsy, in childhood, but only after very detailed evaluation of such patients in centres experienced in the evaluation of children for epilepsy surgery.

Prognosis

Unfortunately, this is not very good because of the difficulty in obtaining complete seizure control in many patients, and because of associated behavioural and learning difficulties that may be present. Spontaneous 'cure' as occurs in benign focal epilepsy of childhood is seldom seen in temporal lobe epilepsy.

MANAGEMENT OF CONVULSIONS

General principles

1. The underlying cause must be sought by appropriate investigations and treated on its own merits. Metabolic disturbance, especially hypoglycaemia and hypocalcaemia should always be considered, especially with convulsions having onset in infancy. Plain skull radiographs have little place in the investigations of convulsions since the advent of CT scan. CT scan is indicated in focal epilepsy, except for classical cases of benign focal epilepsy of childhood. Electroencephalography is seldom of value in the assessment of febrile convulsions, but in other recurring convulsive disorders it may be helpful in distinguishing partial from generalized seizures and in distinguishing various types of seizure disorders, e.g. petit mal absences from absences of temporal lobe epilepsy, or the Lennox-Gastaut syndrome. In this way the EEG may assist in making the correct decision as to an appropriate anticonvulsant. In difficult problems, concurrent long-term video and EEG monitoring to obtain recordings during attacks may provide additional information that is of great assistance in diagnosis and treatment.

2. The appropriate anticonvulsant can usually be predicted from the clinical type of seizure disorder (Table 46.1). However, in patients whose epilepsy is difficult it is often necessary to change drugs and adjust dosage before control is obtained. This possibility should be explained to patients and parents at the outset so that they are not disheartened and dissatisfied if the first anticonvulsant used is not successful.

3. The majority of patients can be controlled with one

Table 46.1 Anticonvulsants that are most likely to be successful with different types of seizures

Seizure type	Anticonvulsant
Partial (focal)	
Focal motor	Carbamazepine, phenytoin, primidone
Complex partial	Carbamazepine, phenytoin
Generalized	
Tonic-clonic	Carbamazepine, phenytoin, sodium valproate, primidone
Absence (true petit mal)	Ethosuximide, sodium valproate
Myoclonic	Sodium valproate, nitrazepam, clonazepam
Atypical absence	
Tonic	
Infantile spasms	Prednisolone/ACTH, nitrazepam

anticonvulsant drug. Very few patients are better controlled on more than one anticonvulsant than on single drug therapy.

4. Individuals vary greatly in their dosage requirements and tolerance to anticonvulsants. Almost all anticonvulsants produce 'side effects' of the type more commonly associated with alcohol and sedatives if given in excess (Example 46.3). Less common are side effects of an idiosyncratic type. Except in status epilepsy and severe convulsions, appropriate drugs are commenced singly and in low dosage and then increased to a level where control is obtained or side effects appear.

5. Use of serum levels for monitoring anticonvulsants is particularly indicated if seizure control is inadequate or if side effects attributable to anticonvulsants are

---

Example 46.3 Side effects of anticonvulsants

Overdose
Drowsiness, impaired co-ordination, ataxia and nystagmus, dysarthria and confusion occurs with many anticonvulsants.

Idiosyncratic
Any rash, hepatic, renal, gastrointestinal and haematological dysfunction or behavioural change should be considered as possibly due to the anticonvulsant.
Particular problems are:

Phenytoin:	Skin rash (Morbiliform) and serum sickness-type illness
Carbamazepine:	Skin rash, irritability, depression
Valproate:	Acute hepatic failure, pancreatitis
Clonazepam:	Severe behavioural changes, increased bronchial secretions

---

suspected. However, they are not of equal value for all drugs. Barbiturate and phenytoin levels correlate well with both seizure control and side effects; a lesser correlation is present with carbamazepine and valproate. There is little role for blood level monitoring with ethosuximide and the benzodiazepines. Blood level monitoring is of particular value in mentally retarded children and young infants who are not able to describe side effects. Blood levels are also useful in checking compliance.

6. Several years of freedom from seizures are desirable before anticonvulsants are ceased, and this is best done slowly over a period of months.

7. It is necessary to consider a patient and his total environment, and not only the seizures and a prescription for anticonvulsant medication. Problems pertaining to appropriate and adequate education and vocational training, and the management of emotional disorders associated with epilepsy may be more difficult to manage than the actual convulsions.

FURTHER READING

Aicardi J 1986 Epilepsy in children. Raven Press, New York
International League Against Epilepsy 1981 Commission on classification and terminology. Epilepsia 2: 493
O'Donohue N V 1979 Epilepsies of childhood. Butterworths, London
Nelson K B, Ellenberg J H 1981 Febrile seizures. Raven press, New York
Vajda F J, Donnan G A 1984 Refractory epilepsy. Proceedings Austin Hospital Epilepsy Workshop October 1983. York Press, Melbourne

47. Cerebral palsy and cerebral degeneration

Robert Ouvrier, Kevin J. Collins

Cerebral palsy may be defined as a permanent disorder of movement, posture, or both, beginning before birth or in early infancy and characterized by hypotonia, spasticity, ataxia or involuntary movements, either singly or in various combinations. The dysfunction is caused by impairment of the brain and is not episodic or progressive.

Incidence

An incidence of approximately 2:1000 was found by Hansen in Denmark. Birth prevalence rates in Western Australia are between 2.0 and 2.5 per thousand live births. Although there are minor fluctuations in prevalence from year to year there is no convincing evidence of a change in frequency. In the United States Collaborative Perinatal Project, 128 of 40 057 children had either died from or were afflicted by moderate to severe cerebral palsy by the age of seven years.

In an area of 100 000 population, seven infants destined to have cerebral palsy are born each year. Of these, one will die, one will be overwhelmingly incapacitated by neuromotor difficulties, two will be incapacitated by severe mental retardation, two will be moderately disabled and one will have so mild a deficit as not to require special treatment.

Aetiology

Cerebral palsy can result from a cerebral malformation, an hypoxic insult or other injury of prenatal origin, from a destructive or hypoxic process of perinatal or early postnatal onset or from a combination of a malformation and perinatal damage acting together.

Malformations

Severe disturbances of brain development such as anencephaly may result in intrauterine or early postnatal death.

Failure of the cortex to develop the normal sulci and gyri (lissencephaly or agyria) is accompanied by disordered development of the neuronal layers of the cortex. The clinical picture is usually one of severe psychomotor retardation, failure to thrive and seizures. Spastic quadriplegia or atonic diplegia may be present. Such infants frequently die in their first year.

Holoprosencephaly is a major brain malformation in which the primary cerebral vesicle or telencephalon fails to cleave and extend bilaterally into separate cerebral hemispheres. Severe retardation, seizures and varying degrees of spasticity or rigidity are the usual clinical accompaniments.

In schizencephaly, bilateral cleft-like defects extend from the cerebral cortex of the hemispheres to the underlying ventricular cavity. Spastic quadriparesis is frequently associated.

Certain brains show macro- (or pachy-) gyria where the gyri are excessively enlarged. At other times, multiple small gyri occur – micropolygyria. Such defects are due to an insult occurring before the fifth month of fetal life. The clinical picture varies depending on the extent of the lesion but may be associated with spastic or hypotonic forms of cerebral palsy.

Many infants with cerebral palsy have microcephaly, although this is not always a cause of motor signs.

Porencephaly is a frequent cause of localized forms of cerebral palsy such as hemiplegia. Porencephaly may be the result of dissolution of brain tissue in utero, following an intrauterine vascular accident or from intrauterine encephalitis, e.g. toxoplasmosis or cytomegalovirus infection, especially when associated with raised intracranial pressure.

The most extreme form of porencephaly is hydranencephaly where the entire cerebral hemispheres are replaced by a fluid-filled cystic cavity which transilluminates brilliantly when a torch is applied to the head. These infants appear superficially normal at birth but are soon found to have severe spastic quadriparesis, blindness and fits and usually die before the third year of life.

Perinatal causes of cerebral palsy

Considering the nature of the birth process, it is not surprising that trauma to the brain occurs. However, with modern obstetrics this appears to be a less important cause of cerebral palsy. The use of vitamin K derivatives by injection on delivery has markedly reduced the incidence of intracranial bleeding due to haemorrhagic disease of the newborn. Thus, neonatal subdural haematomas are now extremely rare.

Physical damage to the brain during birth contributes significantly to perinatal mortality, but is much less commonly a cause of permanent neurological deficits than is hypoxia with its related metabolic accompaniments. Little, a nineteenth century physician, clearly recognized this fact in his important contribution to the understanding of the aetiology of cerebral palsy. In addition, it is likely that prolonged hypoxia in utero is more dangerous than acute, relatively severe (but brief) episodes of hypoxia occurring during the actual delivery.

Apart from hypoxic injuries, infants occasionally suffer from damage to the great vessels in the neck due to excessive twisting of the cervical spine during labour.

Postnatal causes of cerebral palsy

Any conditions causing structural damage to the brain after birth, e.g. trauma, infection and hypoxia, are capable of causing cerebral palsy.

Bilirubin encephalopathy, which results in kernicterus, has diminished markedly in frequency. Here the maximum damage is in the basal ganglia, the cerebellum, the hippocampus and medulla. It is likely that some degree of anoxia or other metabolic neuronal disturbance is necessary to produce the syndrome, in addition to the high level of unconjugated bilirubin.

In those patients who recover from the acute illness, the clinical picture is of athetosis, sometimes with high-tone hearing loss and abnormalities of ocular movements.

Clinical features

The diagnosis of cerebral palsy is sometimes possible in the neonate, but is frequently delayed, especially in the mildly affected case when it is most often made in the second year of life because of gait abnormalities. In Australian studies, approximately 50% of cases are diagnosed in the first year of life and 70% by the end of the second year.

From the neurological point of view, the diagnosis is made on several grounds:

1. Persistence of abnormal reflex patterns.

2. Presence of spasticity or hypotonia with other neurological abnormalities attributable to disease of the brain or spinal cord.

3. A clinical evolution consistent with essentially static central nervous system pathology.

About half the patients considered to have cerebral palsy at one year are free of motor handicap by the age of seven, but about 20% of these have an IQ below 70.

Cerebral palsy is classified mainly according to the pattern and distribution of the neurological involvement (Table 47.1).

Table 47.1 Classification of cerebral palsy

Type	%
Spastic cerebral palsy	64.6
Quadriplegia	19
Diplegia	2.8
Hemiplegia	40.5
Monoplegia	0.4
Triplegia	1.9
Extrapyramidal	22.3
Mixed and other forms	13.1
(Atonic, ataxic CP etc.)	

The above figures are taken from the series of Crothers & Paine (1959) and will differ in various localities, depending on the incidence of prematurity and kernicterus.

SPASTIC CEREBRAL PALSY

Aetiology

In the spastic forms of cerebral palsy, the following aetiological factors are important:

1. Prematurity. In one study 8.6% of cerebral palsy children weighed 1500 g or less at birth compared to 0.4% of a control series. Of cases of spastic paraplegia, more than one-half weighed less than 1500 g at birth and about three-quarters weighed 2500 g or less. Prematurity is a predisposing factor to periventricular leukomalacia in which necrosis is found in the white matter close to the lateral ventricles. This lesion is thought to be responsible for much of the spastic cerebral palsy observed in preterm infants.
2. Multiple births.
3. Prolonged labour or traumatic delivery.
4. Asphyxia neonatorum – spastic quadriparesis.
5. Intra-uterine growth retardation.

Clinical features

In the neonatal period, the infant destined to show severe spasticity may rarely already exhibit hypertonia and hyperactive deep tendon reflexes; respirations may be abnormal and feeding problems are frequent. Seizures, degrees of coma, disturbed oculomotor function or severe hypotonia herald a bad prognosis. More frequently, hypotonia is seen in the neonatal period with absent or poor suck, weak or absent Moro and other primitive reflexes and a general poverty of movement. Head lag is excessive and the traction response to pulling up by the arms is poor. Reflexes may be depressed, normal or excessive with sustained clonus. The child is often irritable or oversomnolent.

As the condition evolves over the next few weeks, there is a gradual transition from generalized hypotonia to spasticity. If more marked in the legs, as is the case in paraparesis, the knee and ankle jerks are excessively brisk with sustained clonus. A few normal infants have up to 10 beats of clonus until the age of 6 months. Scissoring and tonic extension frequently appear in vertical suspension.

SPASTIC QUADRIPARESIS

In the more severe forms (Fig. 47.1) involvement of the arms is shown by persistent fisting of the thumb with hypertonia and hyper-reflexia. When rigidity predominates (as opposed to spasticity), the reflexes may be difficult to elicit. The infant does not reach and will not remove a cloth from the face (normally performed by 6 months of age).

In some infants there is a phase lasting several months in which intermittent extensor spasms occur. These may be severe, leading to opisthotonos. They are distressing for the child and the parents. They can be much alleviated by physiotherapy and suspension in a hammock or positioning in a 'bean bag'.

SPASTIC DIPLEGIA

Spastic diplegia is the form of cerebral palsy in which the lower limbs are more affected than the upper. The term spastic paraplegia is sometimes used when there is minimal or no involvement of the upper limbs. This picture is common in the premature infant. In this situation it is important to look for sensory signs and sphincter involvement; if present, they suggest conditions other than cerebral palsy, e.g. spinal cord tumours.

Mild cases of diplegia may go unrecognized causing general clumsiness, frequent falls and lack of agility. The toes tend to be worn out on the shoes. Such children have great difficulty hopping and running. The normal child can hop by 4 years of age and should be able to perform 20 consecutive hops on one foot by 6 years. Tendon reflexes are brisk and the plantar responses extensor. Occasionally this group may present with shortening of the tendo-Achilles and minimal signs of spasticity. The differential diagnosis is idiopathic shortening of the tendo-Achilles. In more severe cases, there is delay in walking, and then a characteristic shuffling gait with flexion and adduction of the hips and flexion of the knees.

The older diplegic child may demonstrate poor growth and vasomotor changes in the lower extremities.

HEMIPLEGIA

In the majority of these affected, hemiparesis is present from birth but only slowly becomes evident in the first year or two of life. In the remainder, the hemiparesis develops as an acute postnatal event – 'acute infantile hemiplegia' – a neurological syndrome due to a wide variety of causes.

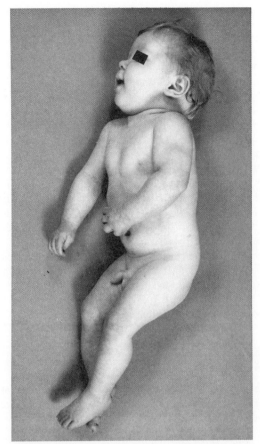

Fig. 47.1 Infant with spastic quadriplegia. Note the abnormal attitude of all four limbs and in particular scissoring of the lower limbs.

Congenital hemiplegia is only rarely recognized at birth. Most commonly parents note a too early establishment of hand preference. Any infant showing persistent preference for one hand under the age of 9 months is almost certainly abnormal. In fact, many infants do not establish hand dominance before the age of 2 years. Simply placing a cloth over the face and restraining each hand successively will establish a paresis of one hand beyond the age of 5 or 6 months. The corresponding leg may be kept straight and is often kicked less than its fellow. Growth arrest in the affected side may be apparent after 6 months of paresis and there will be the expected tone and reflex changes. In addition, the parachute response is asymmetrical. There is slight predominance of right-side involvement in most series.

Sensory abnormalities are detectable in the affected limbs in about two-thirds of patients – mainly, as expected, affecting cortical modalities such as stereognosis, two-point discrimination and joint position sense, which require intact pathways to the cortex.

Monoplegias and triplegias show combinations of the above features in the affected area(s) of the body.

EXTRAPYRAMIDAL FORMS OF CEREBRAL PALSY

These conditions are characterized by the presence of a variety of involuntary movements, especially athetosis and choreoathetosis.

Aetiology

Aetiological factors include:

1. Prematurity (in about 15%)
2. Cerebral malformations
3. Asphyxia neonatorum
4. Hyperbilirubinaemia (kernicterus).

Clinical features

The clinical picture evolves gradually, from hypotonia with active reflexes in infancy to choreoathetosis during childhood. It is very uncommon to detect significant athetosis before the age of 9 months. (However, it should be noted that many normal infants have slight involuntary movements resembling chorea in the first 6 months of life.)

The asymmetric tonic neck reflexes are frequently abnormally persistent in this group of infants. Eventually, the characteristic athetoid (writhing) movements of the limbs develop along with suggestive postural abnor-

malities. An example is tonic extension of the great toe and a tendency, when reaching for an object, to hyperextend the fingers while pronating and flexing the wrist. At times the movements may be so severe as to render the child virtually helpless. Because of the involvement of muscles subserving speech, defects of the latter are common and often severe. Poor swallowing leading to drooling of saliva is common in this disorder as in spastic quadriparesis. In this group intellectual development is often normal.

MIXED FORMS OF CEREBRAL PALSY

Many children with cerebral palsy exhibit a mixture of spasticity and ataxia or extrapyramidal movements. Some patients develop dystonia – excessive muscular contraction of antagonistic groups of muscles during attempts at voluntary activity. The onset of dystonia or involuntary movements may sometimes occur many years after cerebral palsy is diagnosed.

Atonic diplegia

In a small percentage of patients, hypotonia persists instead of evolving into spasticity or athetoid cerebral palsy. In contrast to hypotonia due to disease of muscle or peripheral nerve, the deep tendon reflexes are normal or hyperactive and the plantar responses extensor. Mental deficiency may be severe and seizures are fairly frequent in this group.

Ataxic cerebral palsy

In this relatively uncommon form, ataxia due to cerebellar malformation or damage is the conspicuous feature. Hypotonia is frequent and nystagmus or disturbances of conjugate extraocular movements are also seen. Because of the frequent confusion with other conditions, e.g. peripheral neuropathy and certain degenerative disorders of the brain, this tends to be a diagnosis of exclusion. Thus the child requires careful neurological evaluation.

Ataxic diplegia

A combination of ataxia with signs of spastic diplegia is called ataxic diplegia. It is most commonly seen in association with inadequately treated hydrocephalus, under which circumstances it should not really be regarded as a form of cerebral palsy.

COMPLICATIONS AND ASSOCIATED CONDITIONS

Intellect

The incidence of intellectual deficit varies with the severity of the cerebral palsy. It is very high in spastic quadriparesis and in mixed forms of cerebral palsy. Approximately two-thirds of hemiplegic patients have normal or borderline intelligence. Of the remaining one-third, the majority are only mildly retarded. Those with a relatively pure paraplegia or athetosis are most commonly of normal intellect. There is a tendency to underestimate the intelligence of athetoid patients in early life. Intelligence in the ataxic and hypotonic forms is variable. Severe motor deficits may at times interfere with the demonstration of normal intellect, thus great care with prognosis is indicated. The head circumference and the speech development is more important prognostically in the individual case than the type of cerebral palsy. Visuospatial and auditory perceptual handicaps often contribute to learning difficulties.

Convulsions

Approximately 25–35% of cerebral palsy patients have seizures. In the series of Crothers & Paine (1959), 55% of postnatally acquired hemiplegics developed convulsions as compared to 29% of congenital hemiplegics. In the same series, 13% of spastic quadri- and triplegics had convulsions. This paradoxical lower rate of seizures in tetraplegics has been mentioned by other authors. Varied seizure patterns are seen. These include infantile spasms, grand mal, focal and psychomotor seizures. Status epilepticus sometimes occurs and may cause deterioration in the overall clinical picture.

Visual and auditory abnormalities

About 40–60% of patients with cerebral palsy have visual defects. The commonest abnormality is strabismus, mainly esotropia, which is found in about 50% of the patients with eye problems. Its cause is poorly understood. Homonymous hemianopia, defects of conjugate ocular gaze and nystagmus are often seen. Retinopathy of prematurity may result in blindness in addition to the motor handicap. Optic atrophy is seen in a minority of patients.

Hearing is impaired in about 10% of patients.

Orthopaedic complications

Because of the spasticity, muscle contractures are frequent. The Achilles tendons and hip flexors and adductors are most obviously involved in the lower limbs while the elbow, wrist and finger flexors are most often involved in the arms. Untreated adduction deformity of the hip may lead to dislocation of the joint with subsequent deformity and pain.

Growth discrepancies may lead to pelvic tilt; scoliosis may also develop.

Speech and feeding difficulties

Severely affected patients with quadriparesis, in particular, often have a pseudobulbar paresis with consequent swallowing difficulties, dysarthria and drooling. In many cases, this leads to aspiration of saliva and food with consequent pulmonary infection. Reflux oesophagitis is common and may lead to blood loss and stricture formation. A complication of choreoathetoid cerebral palsy is hiatus hernia, which causes an exacerbation of choreoathetoid movements ('dystonic dyspepsia'). Sometimes cure of the hernia markedly alleviates the involuntary movements.

Speech defects occur in about 50% of patients.

Psychological complications

There has been a strong emphasis on physical forms of therapy in the management of cerebral palsy. However, psychological disorders, resulting from lack of confidence, parental overprotection and community attitudes, often prevent the cerebral palsied children from attaining their physical potential. These problems, which are an inevitable result of cerebral palsy, will require sympathetic management from personnel specifically trained to meet the needs of these children. Their families will also need much support to enable them to cope with many problems which inevitably occur within the home. Only about one-third of hemiplegic patients are economically productive. One-quarter of patients with extrapyramidal disorders are ultimately able to work competitively. In the series of Crothers & Paine (1959), none of the adults with spastic quadriplegia was usefully employed. Sheltered workshops are improving this situation.

TREATMENT

The management of cerebral palsy is complex and involves multiple disciplines. However, it must be appreciated that a cure is not possible. The child must be educated and rehabilitated to make the utmost use of the resources that remain after the initial brain injury.

As in any complex medical disorder, there should be one physician who should supervise all aspects of care and act as the parents' and child's advocate.

Motor aspects

Spastic children tend to develop contractures. This tendency can be counteracted by surgical and non-surgical means. Tendons that are tight can be stretched by passive and active exercises. Stretching exercises will rarely, however, reverse significantly established contractures. There has been a move away from bracing and indications for this are now very limited. Occasionally the application of serial plasters to the ankles will dramatically improve shortening of the Achilles tendon. A variety of surgical procedures has been devised for the correction of tendon contractures that do not respond to medical measures. Lengthening of the Achilles tendon and tenotomy of the hip adductors are the most commonly performed and successful procedures. Physiotherapy is of limited value in the management of the hemiplegic hand. The results of surgical therapy are also often disappointing; function is rarely improved and cosmetic appearance often only transiently benefited. When hemisensory deficits or neglect are present, the hand will never be more than an assistant to its unaffected fellow. Arrest of growth in an affected limb is not improved by any mode of treatment.

At the appropriate stage of development and function, generally early in life, a co-ordinated programme of physical and occupational therapy is undertaken. This will help contribute to the learning of fundamental motions and functions to perform useful and enjoyable tasks. Occupational therapy shows the child how and where performances can be improved in order to be more efficient and less awkward. However, objective proof of the value of many of these programmes is rather limited. Athetosis and other forms of dyskinesia are affected only slightly, if at all, by exercises.

Drug therapy

Medications have been largely unsuccessful in reducing spasticity or influencing the abnormal movements of cerebral palsy, unless given in doses which cause a high incidence of side effects. The management of seizures requires the daily use of anticonvulsants (see Ch. 46).

Neurosurgery

In general, this has a limited role in cerebral palsy. Cerebellar and thalamic lesions are sometimes made stereotactically for athetosis or dystonic complications with only occasional impressive improvement.

On rare occasions, surgical ablation of seizure foci or even hemispherectomy will cause considerable improvement in seizure control.

The use of chronic electrical stimulation of the cerebellum has not fulfilled the expectations that it originally aroused.

Excessive salivation

Drooling is often unsightly and embarrassing for patient and family. This can be very satisfactorily relieved by an operation in which the submandibular salivary glands are removed on one side and the chorda tympani is sectioned on the opposite side.

This operation should be reserved for severe cases older than 6 years of age.

Education

Often it will be necessary for these children to attend special schools as many will be unable to handle the regular school programme because of the severity of the handicap. On the other hand, children with mild hemiplegias and otherwise mild cerebral palsy should be encouraged to attend regular schools. It should be stressed that current attitudes are to integrate as many cerebral palsied children as possible into regular schools.

Employment

As these children mature employment will be a big consideration. About 25% of cerebral palsied children who reach adult life can be employed within the community. A percentage of others who are of normal or near normal intelligence cannot compete in open employment because of the physical disabilities. These will require a sheltered employment. Thus, community facilities will be required to supply job opportunities for this group.

CEREBRAL DEGENERATIONS

This section will address the problem of the child who presents because of concern about regression in previously normal development, or with apparent worsening of a pre-existing neurologic disorder. In infants and young children, attention may focus on loss of previously acquired skills in the areas of gross and fine motor, personal-social and language skills introduced in Chapter 11, while a decline in school performance may lead to referral of the older child.

An approach to this problem will be outlined, with brief reference to examples of the many disorders which may present in this way. Some of these disorders are mentioned in Chapter 28. Broader management issues are covered in Chapters 17 and 18, and will not be discussed here. The suggested reference texts provide a more detailed account of the wide range of neurodegenerative conditions. The diagnostic process is presented here as a series of five questions.

Is there evidence of regression or lack of progress in any area of development?

This is sought in a sequential history of progress in each area of development, supplemented by questions such as 'How is your child's speech now, compared with this time last year? Is there any area where the child has gone backward or shown no progress at all?'

A clear ongoing loss of former skills as shown in the latter part of Curve C in Figure 47.2 raises obvious concern about a progressive disorder, but this may be less certain during the earlier 'plateau' phase before actual regression appears.

This is to be distinguished from the pattern of abnormally slow but consistent progress shown in Curve A,

and commonly found in the child with intellectual disability or 'cerebral palsy'. This child may be seen as falling behind other children in abilities, although in fact continuing to acquire new skills, but at a slower pace, due to a static brain disorder arising in the prenatal or perinatal period.

A variation on this pattern, seen in Curve B, occurs in the child whose initially normal progress is interrupted by an acute injury or illness (e.g. meningitis) causing brain damage with subsequent slower development. Could the apparently progressive symptoms be due to a static disorder complicated by other factors? Such factors are often amenable to treatment, and include:

1. Frequent seizures, especially subtle myoclonic and atonic episodes which may severely impair alertness and co-ordination.

2. Drug toxicity, particularly from anticonvulsants.

3. Psychological or emotional factors, including depression, withdrawal and psychosis. A particular problem is the tendency for autistic children to show arrest or regression in social and language skills during the second year of life.

4. Joint deformities due to soft tissue contractures in spastic 'cerebral palsy', leading to worsening of postural stability and gait.

If this is a progressive disorder, what is its distribution in terms of brain anatomy?

Important anatomic patterns to consider are:

1. One lesion. Progressive hemiparesis, perhaps associated with focal seizures, suggests a cerebral hemisphere tumour, while spinal cord tumours may produce progressive weakness and spasticity affecting the lower limbs either alone or with variable upper limb involvement, thus imitating diplegic 'cerebral palsy'. This clinical pattern, sometimes with associated ataxia, is also seen in slowly progressive hydrocephalus even in the absence of a cerebral neoplasm. The triad of cranial nerve palsies, corticospinal tract signs and ataxia suggests a brain-stem glioma. Most other childhood tumours of the nervous system raise clear concern because of symptoms of raised intracranial pressure, but the insidious visual loss associated with optic nerve glioma and craniopharyngioma is often not recognized as a progressive problem until late in its course.

2. One functional system or group of systems. The prototype of 'system degenerations' is Friedreich's ataxia. In this disorder, abnormalities of spinocerebellar, corticospinal and sensory tracts arise in the second decade of life. In other cerebellar ataxia syndromes, there is involvement not only of neural pathways but of other body organs as with ataxia telangiectasia in which

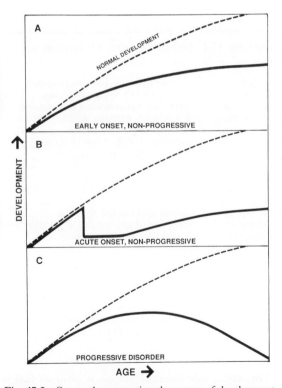

Fig. 47.2 Curves demonstrating the course of development over time in a child with static (**A** and **B**) and progressive neurological disease (**C**) compared with expected normal development. The actual age scale will vary, and a different curve may apply to each aspect of development in each child or disease process.

chromosomal breaks, immunologic defects and skin lesions occur. A system disorder involving basal ganglia or extrapyramidal motor function may be inferred from the signs of dystonia, rigidity and choreoathetosis. The important example in this category is Wilson's disease, which is treatable with penicillamine. Peripheral neuromuscular diseases, which may also be regarded as system disorders, are discussed separately in Chapter 48.

3. A multifocal process, with several discrete lesions in the brain. This is exemplified by recurrent cerebral infarctions associated with cyanotic congenital heart disease. In the absence of cardiac disease, repeated cerebral vascular occlusions are suggestive of moyamoya disease, a well recognized but poorly understood syndrome. Angiography here shows progressive occlusion of the major cerebral arteries, with a curious network of fine collateral vessels in the basal ganglia.

There has been increasing recent interest in a group of disorders, known collectively as mitochondrial encephalomyopathy. One form of this may present with repreated stroke-like episodes and multifocal brain lesions associated with lactic acidosis and abnormal mitochondria in muscle. Recurrent 'strokes' may also occur due to inborn errors of metabolism involving amino acids (homocystinuria), and lipids (Fabry's disease). It should be noted that while multiple sclerosis is a major cause of multifocal lesions in young adults, it is seldom seen in childhood.

4. A diffuse degenerative disorder of the nervous system. Diseases causing widespread loss of neurologic function are generally separated into those which begin by affecting predominantly cortical grey matter, or nerve cell bodies and those in which white matter, or nerve sheath myelin, is primarily involved. While this distinction is of value as a clinical starting point, many disorders are not easily classified in this way.

Diffuse disorders of grey matter. These tend to cause seizures (often myoclonic) and early loss of intellectual function, with progressive impairment of language, comprehension and memory. In addition, involvement of nerve cells in the retina leads to a variable pattern of visual loss. This clinical syndrome is seen in several of the lipid storage disorders, of which Tay-Sachs' disease is the best known. Subacute sclerosing panencephalitis, noted in Chapter 29 as an infrequent complication of measles, evolves as a sequence of behavioural change, intellectual decline, myoclonic jerks and later rigidity.

Diffuse disorders of white matter. By involving the corticospinal tracts, these tend to present with early motor impairment and spasticity, and may initially masquerade as 'cerebral palsy'. Impaired vision reflects disease in optic pathways, and is variable. The clinical findings become more complex if peripheral nerve myelin is also involved, as occurs in two lipid storage disorders, Krabbe's disease and metachromatic leukodystrophy.

The preceding two questions will often be resolved after a careful clinical history and examination, but the remaining steps in diagnosis require knowledge of a growing number of recognized but rare diseases. In practice, this will involve specialist consultation.

Which disorders are known to occur in children of this age, and to produce the other clinical features present in this child?

Individual neurodegenerative diseases tend to have a characteristic age of onset. It is useful to consider broad age ranges, such as early infancy, late infancy and later childhood, in narrowing the diagnostic field. Next, by cross-matching possible diagnoses against associated clinical findings (enlargement of liver and spleen, ocular abnormalities or unusual facial features), the physician may further refine the search and select the most relevant diagnostic tests (see Example 47.1).

Example 47.1 Several disorders of different age groups

1. Early infantile *Gaucher's disease*. This lipid storage disorder would be suspected in a 6-month-old baby whose neurologic regression was associated with marked neck retraction and a palpably enlarged spleen.
2. A 10-year-old boy with personality change, scholastic deterioration and vomiting. The detection of cortical visual loss and skin pigmentation would suggest *adrenoleukodystrophy*, a disorder of fatty acid oxidation.
3. A 2-year-old girl with a history of normal development in the first year, followed by regression in language development, loss of purposeful hand skills and the emergence of curious rubbing and wringing movement of the hands, and hyperventilation is highly suggestive of *Rett's syndrome*. This is a recently recognized clinical condition of uncertain aetiology.
4. A 2-year-old infant with previous delay in motor development, presenting with intermittent sighing respirations, prolonged apnoeic pauses in sleep and pale optic discs would be strongly suspected of having *Leigh's disease*. This disorder is characterized by multiple symmetric brain-stem lesions and is associated with metabolic errors affecting lactate and pyruvate production.

This admittedly idealized process is often all that is needed to establish a diagnosis, but when it is not, it is useful next to turn from clinical features to pathophysiology.

Are any other, less evident, diagnoses suggested by a systematic review of known mechanisms of disease?

We now complement the previous selective clinical correlation by considering in turn the major categories of:

1. Disease process, including metabolic errors, neurocutaneous disorders, slow virus infection, and chronic intoxications.
2. Biochemical substrates, such as lipids, vitamins and minerals, and
3. Cellular organelles – lysosomes, peroxisomes and mitochondria, with their respective disorders.

This search may yield a further 'short list' of possible diagnoses which the clinician was aware of, but had not considered until now, usually because of limited recent experience with them.

Are there any treatable disorders among the diagnoses being considered in this child?

This important question may alter the priority of further investigations, since a potentially treatable disorder, even if unlikely, must be rigorously excluded at an early stage. The major groups to recognize are:

1. Neoplasms and other space-occupying lesions, involving the brain, spinal cord or optic nerves. Of this group, slowly progressive spinal cord lesions deserve special emphasis, because they are often not suspected until late in their course.
2. Subacute and chronic infections of the nervous system, including tuberculous and cryptococcal meningitis.
3. Intoxication, due to lead poisoning, glue-sniffing, prescribed medications and the occasional instance of chronic drug administration by a disturbed parent.
4. Inborn errors of metabolism. The use of a modified diet in phenylketonuria is well known, but is also of potential value in less common disorders. Removal of toxic substances is exemplified by copper chelation in Wilson's disease, mentioned earlier. In seizures due to pyridoxine dependency and in other vitamin dependency syndromes, large doses of vitamins may effectively compensate for the metabolic defect.
5. Deficiency states, especially of vitamins required for normal growth and function of the nervous system.

Although effective treatment is not currently available for most of the degenerative neurologic disorders of childhood, accurate diagnosis remains essential as the basis for genetic counselling, and for offering a realistic prognosis. Finally, a specific diagnosis or 'answer' is of great value to parents in coping with the distress of having a disabled child.

REFERENCES

Crothers B, Paine R S 1959 The natural history of cerebral palsy. Harvard University Press, Cambridge, Massachusetts
De Vivo D C, Di Mauro S, Johnston W G, Rapin I 1987 The nervous system. In: Rudolph A M (ed) Pediatrics. Appleton and Lange, Norwalk Connecticut, 1719–1754

FURTHER READING

Brett E M (ed) 1983 Paediatric neurology. Churchill Livingstone, Edinburgh
Hansen E 1960 Cerebral palsy in Denmark. Munksgaard, Copenhagen
Nelson K B, Ellenberg J H 1979 Neonatal signs as predictors of cerebral palsy. Pediatrics 64: 225–232
Nelson K B, Ellenberg J H 1982 Children who outgrew cerebral palsy. Pediatrics 69: 529–536
Stanley F J, Watson L, Mauger S 1987 Second report of the Western Australian Cerebral Palsy Registrar. January
Taft L T 1979 New insights into cerebral palsy. Pediatric Annals 8: 573–619
Wright T, Nicholson J 1973, Physiotherapy for the spastic child; and evaluation. Developmental Medicine and Child Neurology 15: 146–160

48. Neuromuscular disease

L. K. Shield

The peripheral neuromuscular diseases of childhood, while individually uncommon, collectively constitute a major cause of morbidity and mortality. Disorders such as Duchenne muscular dystrophy and severe chronic spinal muscular atrophy are amongst the most distressing disorders in terms of their physical, social and emotional impact on the child and family. While most of these disorders remain incurable (but not untreatable) there are cogent reasons for establishing a diagnosis as early as possible, as an early accurate diagnosis allows a rational approach to management, enables one to offer appropriate prognostic information and, most impor-

tantly, allows accurate genetic counselling. The relative frequencies of the major neuromuscular diseases at the Royal Children's Hospital, Melbourne are shown in Figure 48.1.

The diagnosis of peripheral neuromuscular disease in childhood requires the following two separate steps:

1. Recognition that a child's presenting symptoms or signs may be due to peripheral neuromuscular disease

While weakness and hypotonia are typical signs, parents do not usually consult a doctor with a complaint that their child is weak. The parents of 20 older

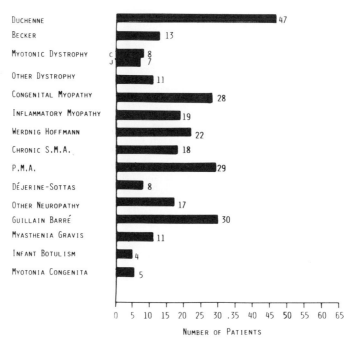

Fig. 48.1 Neuromuscular diseases seen at the Royal Children's Hospital, Melbourne, over a 6.5-year period. Abbreviation:
C = congenital; J = juvenile; SMA = spinal muscular atrophy;
PMA = peroneal muscular atrophy.

children, subsequently shown to have proximal muscle weakness due to a number of different myopathic conditions, shared the following concerns:

- Trouble walking and running
- Poor at sports
- Cannot keep up with peers
- Poor co-ordination
- Tires easily
- Falls frequently.

Other modes of presentation include a known family history of neuromuscular disease; weakness, hypotonia, respiratory difficulty or feeding difficulties in the neonatal period; delayed motor milestones; abnormal gait (particularly toe walking); orthopaedic abnormality such as foot deformity and scoliosis. Some patients present with non-neuromuscular problems such as mental retardation or delayed language development (e.g. Duchenne muscular dystrophy).

2. Anatomical, electrophysiological, biochemical and histopathological identification of the neuromuscular lesion

A logical approach to differential diagnosis can be taken by thinking of disorders that may affect the anatomical constituents of the neuromuscular apparatus, namely:

- Anterior horn cell
- Anterior and posterior nerve roots
- Peripheral nerve (motor, sensory, autonomic)
- Neuromuscular junction
- Muscle.

It should not be forgotten that central nervous system disorders and metabolic diseases may also have a significant influence on the effective functioning of the peripheral neuromuscular system.

Table 48.1 summarizes the clinical clues that help localize the site of the lesion, but in the final analysis the definitive diagnosis of a peripheral neuromuscular disease rests on a combination of:

- Family history
- Clinical history
- Clinical examination
- Serum enzymes – particularly creatine kinase (CK)
- Electrophysiology (e.g. nerve conduction study, electromyography, repetitive nerve stimulation)
- Histology of muscle and/or nerve
- Metabolic studies (e.g. muscle glycogen, carnitine assay).

With only few exceptions, pathological examination of muscle and/or nerve should be undertaken as the implications of a neuromuscular disease diagnosis are so

Table 48.1 Clinical clues helpful in establishing the site of the lesion in neuromuscular disease

Weakness	AHC Proximal	PN Distal	NMJ Proximal, cranial nerve	M Proximal
Hypotonia	++	+	±	++
Hyporeflexia	±	early	±	late
Fasciculations	+++	+	–	–
Sensory disturbance	–	±	–	–
Myotonia	–	–	–	±
Autonomic dysfunction	–	±	–	–
Muscle enlargement	–	–	–	±

Abbreviations: AHC = anterior horn cell; PN = peripheral nerve; NMJ = neuromuscular junction; M = muscle.

great for the child and immediate family (and sometimes the extended family) that there is no room for error. In the event of death of a child, an autopsy examination should be undertaken to confirm the antemortem diagnosis.

CLASSIFICATION

The classification of neuromuscular diseases has always been difficult but a practical approach is given below.

Anterior horn cell

- Acute (e.g. poliomyelitis)
- Chronic (e.g. spinal muscular atrophy)

Peripheral nerve

- Acute neuropathies (e.g. Guillain–Barré syndrome)
- Chronic neuropathies (e.g. peroneal muscular atrophy)

Neuromuscular junction

- Acute (e.g. infant or wound botulism)
- Chronic (e.g. myasthenia gravis)

Muscle

- Acute myopathies (e.g. toxic rhabdomyolysis)
- Chronic myopathies:
    congenital myopathies
    progressive muscular dystrophies
    myotonic disorders
    inflammatory myopathies

metabolic-storage myopathies
endocrine myopathies
other.

ANTERIOR HORN CELL

Acute disorders

Poliomyelitis

This disorder is now rare in developed countries. It should still be considered where there is acute onset of flaccid paralysis of lower motor neurone type of a single limb, or with patchy asymmetrical distribution, particularly if associated with fever, vomiting, neck or spine stiffness and muscle pain or spasm.

Other

Other acute disorders are also rare, but a clinical syndrome of asthma with flaccid paralysis of a limb resembling polio and probably secondary to anterior horn cell dysfunction has been recognized (Hopkins syndrome). Coxsackie- and echovirus infections have occasionally produced weakness thought to be of anterior horn cell origin.

Chronic disorders

In childhood, the chronic, usually inherited disorders, pathologically characterized by degeneration of the anterior horn cells and clinically associated with muscle weakness that is progressive at least for a time, are called the spinal muscular atrophies. Several different clinical syndromes are recognizable, the important ones being:

1. Infantile spinal muscular atrophy
   (Werdnig-Hoffman disease).
2. Chronic childhood spinal muscular atrophy.

Infantile spinal muscular atrophy (Werdnig-Hoffman disease)

This occurs in approximately 1 in 25 000 live births and is usually inherited as an autosomal recessive disorder. The earliest symptom may be decreased fetal movements in late pregnancy. Presentation is either at birth with hypotonia, weakness, joint deformity, respiratory difficulty or later with apparent failure to thrive, poor feeding, cough and cry and with marked hypotonia and limb weakness. Patients with this form of spinal muscular atrophy invariably come to medical attention before 6 months of age. The onset of symptoms is sometimes relatively rapid and when first seen the child is often surprisingly severely weak. Weakness, although

generalized, is maximal in the shoulder and hip girdle muscles. Intercostal muscle weakness leads to chest deformity, poor cough and weak cry and the respiratory pattern becomes diaphragmatic (Fig. 48.2). Deep tendon reflexes are absent. Fasciculations of the tongue are an important clinical clue to the diagnosis, but this is sometimes an exceedingly difficult sign to be certain about and one can only be confident of the presence of fasciculations if the baby is relaxed and there are no major movements of the tongue. Facial weakness is only mild and extraocular movements remain full, giving the babe an alert appearance. The disease is progressive and death, usually from respiratory failure and pneumonia, occurs by 18 months of age in 95% of patients.

Chronic childhood spinal muscular atrophy

Although the pathological changes are similar to those seen in Werdnig-Hoffman disease, chronic childhood

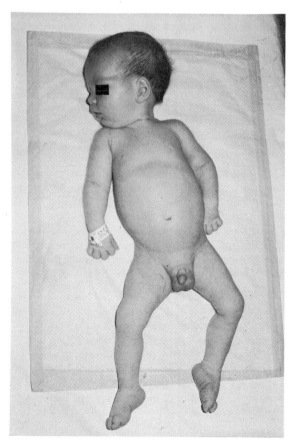

Fig. 48.2 Werdnig-Hoffman disease; note 'frog posture', appearance of distended abdomen from diaphragmatic respirations, and claw hand deformity.

spinal muscular atrophy is thought to be genetically and clinically distinct from the infantile (acute) form. Autosomal recessive inheritance is present in most families. Chronic childhood spinal muscular atrophy is at least as common as the Werdnig-Hoffman form.

In 75% of patients the clinical onset is before 15 months of age and in 95% before 3 years of age. Nearly 50% of .these patients never walk. Only 20% are still walking unaided by 10 years and only 5% by 20 years of age. Survival varies from 18 months through to adult life. Patients with a relatively late onset and a moderately benign clinical course have often been classified as the Kugelberg-Welander syndrome.

The clinical picture is one of severe generalized weakness and wasting, sometimes with a proximal predominance. Deep tendon reflexes are decreased or absent and often there are fasciculations of the tongue. The facial muscles may be weak but eye movements remain normal and the patient is usually normal intellectually. The main management problems include the prevention of orthopaedic deformity, especially spinal deformity, and the management of the respiratory complications of muscle weakness.

PERIPHERAL NERVE

Many different acute, subacute and chronic peripheral neuropathies have been described in childhood. They may be inherited or acquired, they may involve motor, sensory, autonomic fibres or commonly mixtures of all three. Pathologically they may be associated with combinations of demyelination and axonal degeneration. Some central nervous system degenerative disorders, such as Krabbe's disease and metachromatic leukodystrophy, may also have a peripheral neuropathy component. The commonest significant clinical problems are the Guillain-Barré syndrome and the peroneal muscular atrophy (Charcot-Marie-Tooth) syndrome.

Guillain-Barré syndrome (postinfectious polyneuropathy)

This may occur at any age, although it is rare in infancy. An infection, commonly an upper respiratory tract infection, precedes the neurological syndrome in about 50% of cases. Clinical features are similar to those seen in adults with progressive, relatively symmetrical lower motor neurone paralysis commencing in the lower extremities and ascending to involve upper extremities, muscles of respiration and cranial nerve innervated musculature. Areflexia, muscle pain or tenderness and back pain or stiffness are accompanying features. Sensory symptoms are usually not prominent. Autonomic dys-

function may take the form of urinary retention or incontinence or fluctuations in blood pressure. Weakness may progress rapidly over one or two days or more slowly over one or two weeks. Involvement of respiratory muscles and those involved in swallowing poses a serious threat to life and careful observation and monitoring is required until recovery begins, usually within one or two weeks of cessation of the phase of deterioration. Artificial ventilation for periods up to eight weeks may occasionally be required. Recovery continues over weeks to many months, with most children returning to normal function. Some more severely affected children may have residual distal weakness and require ankle flexion orthoses.

Diagnosis is based on the clinical features with elevation of the cerebrospinal fluid protein with only a few, if any, leukocytes. A nerve conduction study may be useful in difficult diagnostic situations. Plasmapheresis, if used early, may hasten recovery but otherwise treatment is supportive. Relapses may occur but are uncommon.

Peroneal muscular atrophy (Charcot-Marie-Tooth) syndrome

This group of disorders (recently termed hereditary motor and sensory neuropathy) constitutes the commonest chronic inherited neuropathy syndrome in childhood. Subclassification of the syndrome is based mainly on electrophysiological and pathological criteria, although some clinical differences between the subgroups have been noted. Most families show autosomal dominant inheritance but autosomal recessive forms occur. 60% of all patients with peroneal muscular atrophy have onset of symptoms in the first decade of life, many in the first five years.

Foot deformity (commonly pes cavus), distal weakness in the lower extremities with prominent loss of foot dorsiflexion and eversion, hyporeflexia and sensory loss are typical clinical features. However, presenting features in childhood can be quite different. Some relatively asymptomatic children present because of their family history. In others, gait disturbance, particularly toe walking, frequent falling and poor co-ordination are presenting problems. Foot deformity is the main reason for seeking medical attention in no more than 50% of patients. Weakness and wasting in the legs may progress slowly and distal weakness in the upper extremities is sometimes seen. Thickened peripheral nerves can occasionally be palpated.

The diagnosis of peroneal muscular atrophy is confirmed by a nerve conduction study. A full family history is necessary and it is important to examine and perform a nerve conduction study on both parents before offering genetic counselling as affected family members may be relatively asymptomatic.

No medical treatment is available but orthopaedic procedures to correct foot deformity are often required. Progression is only relatively slow with patients leading a fairly full life, albeit sometimes with gait difficulties and ataxia.

NEUROMUSCULAR JUNCTION

Infant botulism

Infant botulism is the result of production in the gastrointestinal tract of a powerful exotoxin from *Clostridium botulinum*. It differs from the botulism syndrome associated with food poisoning in which the disease is due to ingestion of preformed toxin from contaminated food. In infant botulism the botulinum spores are ingested but the only food with which any correlation has been found is honey. The disease occurs usually in infants under 9 months of age.

Constipation for days or weeks precedes the onset over hours or 1 or 2 days of hypotonia, weakness, hyporeflexia and ptosis. In addition, feeding and swallowing difficulty, poor cough, weak cry and respiratory insufficiency will be noted. Extraocular movements may be impaired and dilated sluggishly reacting pupils (internal ophthalmoplegia) are often seen. Deterioration may be so rapid that some cases may resemble the 'sudden infant death syndrome'. Many patients require artificial ventilation, some for up to 1–2 months.

Diagnosis is based on recognition of the clinical syndrome supported by isolation of the organism and its toxin from the faeces. Treatment is supportive and botulinum antitoxin has not yet been shown to be helpful. The prognosis is excellent with full recovery unless complications, such as cerebral hypoxia from respiratory arrest, intervene. For this reason, prompt recognition and transfer to a facility capable of long-term ventilatory support is mandatory.

Myasthenia gravis

About 10% of patients with myasthenia gravis have onset of their disorder in childhood. A number of clinical syndromes are recognized.

Myasthenia in most children appears to have an autoimmune basis with antibody directed against acetylcholine receptors on the postsynaptic membrane of the neuromuscular junction. Onset may be at any time from the second year of life onwards. Symptoms are present for less than one month in the majority of patients and

it is important to note that many have an episode of respiratory failure if untreated. Symptoms and signs are similar to those in adults with myasthenia although relatively more prepubertal patients have only ocular problems. Ptosis, eye movement disorder, diplopia, difficulty chewing and swallowing, slurred speech with or without predominantly proximal limb muscle weakness of recent onset should raise the suspicion of myasthenia gravis. Fatigability, the hallmark of myasthenia, is usually, but not invariably, prominent.

A child suspected of having myasthenia gravis should undergo a diagnostic assessment as a matter of urgency. The diagnosis is based on clinical observation of fatigability often best seen in the upper eyelid, response to intravenous or intramuscular injection of an anticholinesterase agent such as edrophonium (Tensilon) or neostigmine, repetitive nerve stimulation and assay of acetylcholine receptor antibodies. Symptomatic relief may be obtained by oral administration of an anticholinesterase, commonly physostigmine (Mestinon). Corticosteroids, thymectomy and plasmapheresis have a role in selected circumstances.

Although myasthenia gravis in childhood is a serious and potentially fatal disorder, the disease remits in some children with only a minority having serious long-term problems.

Transient neonatal myasthenia gravis occurs in about 10% of babies of mothers who have the disease. A number of syndromes of congenital myasthenia gravis in the offspring of non-myasthenic mothers have also been described.

MUSCLE

Disorders primarily involving muscle are termed myopathies. The term muscular dystrophy should be reserved for some relatively specific clinico-pathological entities as described below.

Acute myopathies

Myopathic disorders leading to acute onset of muscle weakness are uncommon in childhood. Acute onset of severe weakness may be due to exogenous factors, such as snake bite or drug-induced rhabdomyolysis. Endogenous causes include metabolic disorders such as the periodic paralyses, glycogenoses, carnitine palmityl transferase deficiency and severe diabetic ketoacidosis. Severe destruction of muscle is sometimes seen with collagen vascular diseases. The dominantly inherited, often fatal syndrome of malignant hyperthermia during anaesthesia is associated with muscle necrosis and myoglobinuria. Rhabdomyolysis with myoglobinuria appears occasionally after an upper respiratory tract infection or exercise.

Chronic myopathies

Congenital myopathies

This term is applied to a group of disorders, often inherited, characterized by onset of weakness and hypotonia at or shortly after birth. At times the onset may not be until the later decades of life. Weakness may be either mild or severe and tends to be only slowly progressive although exceptions occur. Pathologically the disorders are recognizable by structural changes in individual muscle fibres or variations in the number or size of the muscle fibre types.

A large number of congenital myopathies are recognized and more are being documented each year. Some of the well-recognized disorders include central core myopathy, nemaline myopathy and congenital fibre type disproportion.

Progressive muscular dystrophies

The muscular dystrophies are genetically determined disorders primarily affecting skeletal muscle although other tissues may also be involved. Histologically the muscle shows variation in fibre size, degeneration and regeneration, a high internal nuclear count, splitting of fibres and proliferation of connective tissue and fat. The primary biochemical cause of Duchenne muscular dystrophy was not known until the recent discovery of absence of a muscle protein named dystrophin.

The clinical features of some muscular dystrophies are described below.

1. Duchenne muscular dystrophy (*pseudo-hypertrophic muscular dystrophy of childhood*). This is the commonest serious muscle disorder commencing in childhood and ranks high in the list of devastating childhood diseases as reflected by its effect on the child, the family, and the requirements for community resources. Duchenne dystrophy occurs only in males (with rare exceptions) and is inherited as an X-linked recessive trait with an incidence of 1 in 5000 live male births. Two-thirds of patients have a family history of muscular dystrophy or are isolated cases with an unsuspecting female carrier in the family, while one-third appears to arise as spontaneous mutations.

While delayed developmental progress occasionally is noted in the first year of life, the first symptoms are usually not seen until 18 months to 4 years of age. The average age at diagnosis in south-east Australia is 5.75 years. Early symptoms include delayed motor development with 50% not walking before 18 months of age. Abnormal gait including toe walking, the inability to run normally, difficulty in climbing and in rising from a sitting or lying position, and frequent falling are other prominent early features. Also, 20% of patients have delayed mental or language development as significant early features.

Proximal muscle weakness accounts for the motor difficulties noted above and is demonstrated by Gower's sign (Fig. 48.3). This sign is not specific for Duchenne dystrophy and is seen in any condition producing proximal muscle weakness. The calf, quadriceps and triceps muscles are commonly enlarged (pseudo-hypertrophy) and firm.

Between 4 and 6 years of age, parents often note apparent improvement in mobility, presumably as normal muscle development outstrips the disease process. Ultimately, however, relentless decline in function occurs with increasing proximal and distal weakness in extremity and truncal musculature, leading to a progressively waddling gait, increasing lumbar lordosis and increasing equinus foot deformity. The knee jerk becomes depressed while the ankle jerk is retained until late. Independent mobility is lost usually between 9 and 13 years of age. Weakness and wasting progress, with spinal deformity and progressive decline in pulmonary function dominating the clinical picture until death between 15 and 25 years. Death is usually due to respiratory complications although cardiac failure or arrhythmias may sometimes contribute.

Non-progressive intellectual impairment is associated with Duchenne dystrophy with the mean IQ being approximately 85.

The diagnosis of Duchenne muscular dystrophy should be based on the family history (if any), clinical features, serum creatine kinase, electromyography and muscle biopsy. Pathological confirmation of the diagnosis is essential except where the diagnosis has been confirmed in another family member. The creatine kinase is a reliable screening test and is invariably grossly elevated in a child with Duchenne dystrophy, even from the neonatal period. Conversely, a normal creatine kinase test excludes the later development of Duchenne dystrophy. Effective genetic counselling can only be offered if the first case in the family is diagnosed before other affected males are born. The early diagnosis of Duchenne dystrophy can be facilitated by using the following criteria for ordering serum creatine kinase estimations in males:

1. Known or suspected family history of muscular dystrophy.

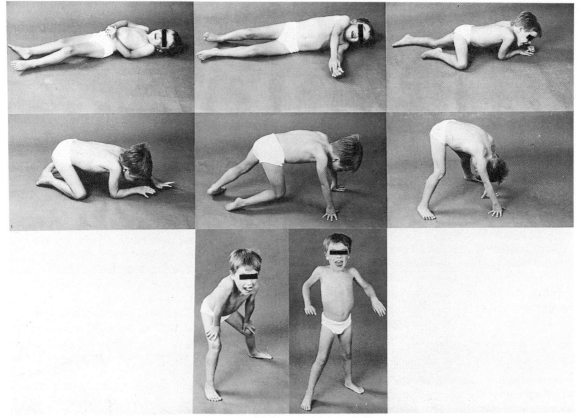

Fig. 48.3 Gower's sign in a patient with Duchenne dystrophy, illustrating the sequence of manoeuvres required to rise from the supine position. (Reproduced with permission Williams 1982.)

2. Unexplained delayed motor development including not walking before 18 months of age.

3. Unexplained gait disturbances including toe walking.

4. Unexplained delay in mental or language development.

The male offspring of a known carrier have a 50% risk of having a Duchenne dystrophy while 50% of female offspring will be carriers themselves. Detection and counselling of female carriers is a most important aspect of family management. The serum creatine kinase is mildly elevated in about 60% of carriers. DNA technology can now be applied to offer carrier detection and antenatal diagnosis, either through the detection of deletions from the X chromosome or by linkage analysis.

There is no cure for muscular dystrophy at the present time. Management involves a very positive approach to satisfying the emotional, social and educational needs of the child and his family along with judicious use of physiotherapy, orthotic devices and surgery for orthopaedic deformity.

2. Becker muscular dystrophy. This type closely resembles Duchenne dystrophy but tends to be later in onset and slower in progression. The early symptoms and signs are very similar to those of Duchenne.

3. Facioscapulohumeral syndrome (FSH). This refers to a group of disorders with various underlying pathological processes having in common maximal muscle weakness in facial, periscapular and humeral musculature. Many patients have an underlying myopathic process and hence the common terminology of facioscapulohumeral (FSH) dystrophy. However, many patients with similar clinical features have been shown to have pathological changes consistent with spinal muscular atrophy or congenital myopathy.

The FSH syndrome is usually relatively mild with very slow, if any, progression and is compatible with long-term survival. Onset is commonly in adolescence or early adult life although occasionally the onset can occur in very early childhood.

Facial muscle weakness leads to difficulty closing the eyes, blowing out the cheeks, whistling or sucking through a straw. Shoulder girdle weakness produces difficulty lifting the arms above the head and there is winging of the scapulae. Upwards and forwards riding of the scapula gives a characteristic appearance to the shoulder region. Foot drop is not uncommon. Inheritance is usually autosomal dominant.

Myotonic disorders

These are a clinically heterogeneous group with myotonia being the unifying clinical feature. Myotonia is the inability of muscles to relax after voluntary contraction or stimulation. Myotonia can be detected during attempted relaxation of a voluntary contraction (such as after shaking hands or eyelid closure), or by percussion of the thenar eminence, or by electromyography. Older children may describe myotonia as stiffness or cramping.

Myotonia congenita and myotonic dystrophy are the main disorders but other myotonic syndromes such as paramyotonia congenita and chondrodystrophic myotonia (Schwartz-Jampel syndrome) occur.

Myotonia congenita (Thomsen's disease). Autosomal dominant or autosomal recessive inheritance may occur. Onset is in infancy or early childhood with symptoms due to myotonia such as stiffness, difficulty initiating rapid movements and sometimes feeding difficulties. Muscle hypertrophy is a common feature, giving the child a Herculean look. The myotonia decreases with continued activity and may be aggravated by cold. Improvement occurs with increasing age. Symptomatic relief of myotonia with phenytoin, quinine or procaine amide is occasionally required.

Myotonic dystrophy (Steinert's disease). Myotonic dystrophy is inherited in an autosomal dominant fashion but an affected parent may be relatively asymptomatic and not diagnosed until detailed examination and investigation is undertaken. The abnormal gene is on chromosome 19 and linkage analysis is useful in some families for presymptomatic and antenatal diagnosis.

1. *Juvenile type:* the clinical features are similar to those seen in adults with distal muscle weakness, wasting and myotonia, an expressionless face due to facial muscle weakness and ptosis. Cataracts, frontal alopecia, testicular atrophy, cardiopulmonary insufficiency and dementia may occur with increasing age.

2. *Congenital type:* a syndrome of hypotonia, weakness, arthrogryposis, feeding difficulty, respiratory difficulty and marked facial weakness all present at birth along with other dysmorphic features has been recognized in families with myotonic dystrophy. Invariably the mother is the affected parent. There is a high incidence of mental retardation.

Inflammatory myopathy

Acute viral myositis. Patients with acute viral myositis have been described. The outlook is good and it is important to distinguish these patients from those with chronic polymyositis or dermatomyositis. One clinically recognizable syndrome is that of acute onset of pain and tenderness of the gastrocnemius and soleus complex several days after an upper respiratory tract infection, often with influenza B virus. Recovery occurs in a few days.

Chronic inflammatory myopathy. This may occur as an idiopathic disorder and is termed polymyositis or dermatomyositis, or may occur as part of a recognized collagen vascular disease. The clinical features are discussed in Chapter 73.

Metabolic-storage myopathies

A large number of individually uncommon metabolic disorders may produce problems such as episodic, acute or chronic muscle weakness, hypotonia, stiffness or cramping, exercise intolerance or myoglobinuria. Symptoms are sometimes accentuated or precipitated by exercise, rest after exercise, fasting or excessive carbohydrate intake.

The underlying metabolic defects are usually in glycogen metabolism (e.g. the glycogenoses, such as Pompe's disease), lipid metabolism (e.g. carnitine deficiency, carnitine-palmityl transferase deficiency), potassium metabolism (the periodic paralyses associated with hyper-, hypo- or normo-kalaemia), or a variety of mitochondrial functions (e.g. myopathies associated with cytochrome oxidase deficiency and Kearn-Sayre syndrome of progressive external ophthalmoplegia).

Knowledge of the underlying metabolic causes of many of the myopathies and muscular dystrophies is progressively increasing.

Endocrine myopathies

Peripheral neuromuscular disease symptoms may occur in patients with hypothyroidism, hyperthyroidism and adrenal dysfunction. Excessive doses of corticosteroids may produce proximal muscle weakness.

Other

'The floppy infant syndrome'. Muscle hypotonia (or floppiness) is a common problem in infancy and may be secondary to a large number of unrelated conditions. Muscle tone is assessed by observation of posture, assessment of the resistance of joints to passive movements and of the range of movement of joints. The maintenance of normal muscle tone depends not only on the integrity of the peripheral neuromuscular system but also on the spinal cord and higher centres. Indeed, disorders affecting the central nervous system are more frequently the cause of the floppy infant syndrome than peripheral neuromuscular causes (see Chapter 47).

When an infant or young child is found to be significantly hypotonic, further assessment is indicated. The first question to be asked is whether the hypotonia is 'central' or 'peripheral' in origin. Theoretically it should be easy to answer this question as hypotonia of peripheral nervous system origin is usually associated with significant weakness (e.g. as in Werdnig-Hoffmann disease) while 'central' hypotonia is usually not associated with significant weakness (e.g. as in Down syndrome). Practically, however, the differentiation in early childhood can sometimes be quite difficult. At times, there can be a combination of peripheral and central causes of hypotonia in one child.

Apart from the absence of significant weakness, clues to a central cause of hypotonia may be a history of adverse perinatal events, abnormal behaviour in the neonatal period, delayed mental development, seizures, abnormality of head size or shape and the presence of normal or brisk deep tendon reflexes. Hypotonia of peripheral nervous system origin is often, but not invariably, accompanied by hyporeflexia in an alert baby with normal mental development.

FURTHER READING

Dubowitz V 1978 Muscle disorders in childhood. In: Dubowitz V (ed) Major problems in Paediatrics, Vol 16. Saunders, London
Dubowitz V 1980 The floppy infant, 2nd edn. Clinics in Developmental Medicine No. 76. Heinemann, London
Williams P F 1982 Orthopaedic management in childhood. Blackwell Scientific Publications, Oxford

49. The child with a large head

Geoffrey Klug

Hydrocephalus refers to a group of conditions characterized by an increase in CSF volume associated with ventricular dilatation and elevation of intraventricular pressure. This is in contrast to cerebral atrophy where increased ventricular volume is unrelated to pressure changes. An understanding of the formation, circulation and absorption of the CSF is important in order to appreciate the various mechanisms that can lead to hydrocephalus (Fig 49.1). CSF is formed within the ventricles by both active and passive processes. Radioisotope studies indicate that proteins and electrolytes are actively secreted by the choroid plexus, while water and other substances diffuse from the plasma into the CSF across the ependyma and other membranes. The rate of CSF formation has been estimated to be approximately 0.35 ml/min (500 ml/day).

It is slightly lower in hydrocephalic children (0.30 ml/min). Normally, only a small proportion of the fluid is reabsorbed through the ependyma, the bulk flow is through the ventricular orifices into the subarachnoid space. The circulation is not completely unidirectional but has an ebb and flow movement, the propelling force arising from the expansile-retractile pulsations of the choroid plexus. The CSF leaves the ventricular system through the foramina of Magendie and Luschka of the 4th ventricle into the basal cisterns. Some of the fluid passes down the spinal canal and the remainder circulates upwards over the lateral surface of the brain where some absorption takes place at the perineural sheaths or through subpial vessels. The subarachnoid villi, which communicate with the venous channels of the dura, are considered to be the sites of maximal absorption.

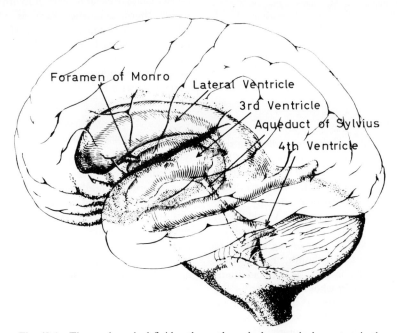

Fig. 49.1 The cerebrospinal fluid pathway through the ventricular system in the normal brain.

AETIOLOGY OF HYDROCEPHALUS

Hydrocephalus occurs when there is an imbalance between formation and absorption of CSF. Impaired absorption is almost always due to some degree of obstruction along the CSF pathways. If the passage of CSF is obstructed within the ventricular system the resultant hydrocephalus is labelled non-communicating, while if obstruction exists in the surface pathways the hydrocephalus is described as being communicating. In all cases the imbalance is only of a minimal degree and most CSF will continue to be absorbed. The condition occurs when the imbalance persists and leads, over a period of time, to a progressive increase in CSF volume. The rate of this volume change will vary from patient to patient, and depends in large part on the degree of obstruction. The lesions that commonly produce hydrocephalus are listed in Table 49.1.

Table 49.1 Classification of hydrocephalus

A. Non-communicating	B. Communicating
1. Aqueduct stenosis or atresia a. sporadic b. familial	1. Arnold Chiari malformation a. with myelomeningocele b. without myelomeningocele
2. Obstruction at the 4th ventricle a. Dandy-Walker syndrome b. arachnoiditis	2. Encephalocele
3. Obstruction due to mass lesions a. neoplasm, cysts b. haematoma c. Galenic vein aneurysm	3. Meningeal adhesions a. postinflammatory b. posthaemorrhagic
4. Ventricular inflammations – rare	4. Choroid plexus papilloma

Aqueduct obstruction

This is the commonest site of intraventricular obstruction in infants with congenital hydrocephalus. When obstruction is complete, the aqueduct is replaced by multiple blind channels or a membrane lined by ependyma. It may occur as an isolated anomaly or be associated with myelomeningocele and the Arnold Chiari malformation. Aqueduct obstruction is sometimes inherited as a sex-linked trait. Accompanying features in this group include a short flexed thumb, mental retardation and other cerebral abnormalities. In addition, there is a group of patients in whom narrowing of the aqueduct may be slowly progressive, the child remaining well for several years before obstructive symptoms appear, sometimes with dramatic suddenness. Histologi-

cally, subependymal gliosis around the aqueduct is demonstrable. Although neurofibromatosis has been recorded in a few cases, there is little known of the pathogenesis of this lesion. In the experimental animal aqueduct gliosis can be produced by innoculating mumps, papova and other viruses into the brain.

Dandy-Walker syndrome

The cystic dilatation of the 4th ventricle, classical of this malformation, is associated with atresia of the exit foramina of the 4th ventricle. The cerebellum is hypoplastic, particularly in the region of the vermis and other structural brain anomalies may coexist. Hydrocephalus may be present at birth or develop subsequently. The diagnosis is suggested in typical cases by the shape of the skull and the presence of cerebellar signs.

Arnold Chiari malformation

This consists of downward displacement and elongation of the hind brain with herniation of the medulla, cerebellar vermis and inferior part of the 4th ventricle into the upper cervical canal. The neural structures are so tightly packed and adherent in the region of the foramen magnum that CSF flow is impaired usually within the subarachnoid space. This malformation is frequently associated with cranium bifidum, myelomeningocele and cervical hydromyelia. Less commonly, bony anomalies such as platybasia and the Klippel-Feil deformity are found. Hydrocephalus usually develops in early infancy. In some the abnormality may remain relatively silent for years, to manifest later as tetraplegia, lower cranial nerve palsies, ataxia and nystagmus with or without evidence of intracranial hypertension.

Intracranial mass lesions

This should always be considered in any child in which head enlargement develops in late infancy or childhood. The majority of childhood tumours arise in the posterior cranial fossa and include medulloblastoma, astrocytoma and ependymoma. Because of their close proximity to the 4th ventricle increased intracranial pressure develops early in the course of the illness, and papilloedema is invariably noted. Ataxia, incoordination, and nystagmus are helpful pointers to the diagnosis. Other space-occupying lesions encountered in childhood include craniopharyngioma, gliomas, pinealomas, and arachnoid cysts. In supratentorial lesions, CSF obstruction is a late event so that neurological or endocrinological abnormalities often precede symptoms of raised intracranial pressure. Less commonly cerebral tuberculoma, torular meningitis, an aneurysm of the vein of Galen simulate intracranial neoplasms. The latter should be suspected if, in addition to hydrocephalus, a loud intracranial bruit, high output failure and vascular naevi are also present in the same patient.

Meningeal adhesions

Hydrocephalus, resulting from postinflammatory adhesions and fibrosis, is common, particularly as there is improved survival in patients suffering from neonatal meningitis. The hydrocephalus, which is usually communicating, may develop during the acute infection or gradually appear during the convalescence. In these infants, neurological deficit, mental retardation and seizures are usually the result of the infective process, but the hydrocephalus, if not relieved, will aggravate the brain damage. Progressive hydrocephalus sometimes develops in low birthweight babies, who survive intraventricular or subarachnoid haemorrhage. In older children the presence of blood in the CSF from any cause, may incite such changes with subsequent development of hydrocephalus.

Choroid plexus papilloma

This is a rare but important cause of hydrocephalus. This benign neoplasm is confined almost entirely to childhood. At the time of presentation, papilloedema is found in about half of these hydrocephalic children, indicating the rapidity of increase in intracranial pressure. Although ventricular enlargement can be explained on the basis of obstruction to the CSF circulation in a few cases, in the majority the hydrocephalus is produced by excessive fluid secreted by the tumour. It is also believed that recurrent haemorrhage from the tumour may play a role. Generally total excision of the tumour leads to a resolution of the hydrocephalic process.

APPROACH TO CLINICAL DIAGNOSIS

The clinical appraisal of the hydrocephalic child involves the establishment of the diagnosis, elucidation of the aetiology, assessment of neurological and mental functions and the search for other associated malformations.

In the history, it is essential to determine the age and rapidity of onset of hydrocephalus and its rate of progression. In most clinical situations the child presents with a chronically large head, which may already be apparent at birth or at a few months of age.

Despite the obviously large head, many babies thrive well and make normal developmental gains, except for poor head control. Other infants with hydrocephalus, however, feed poorly, are irritable, vomit excessively and fail to gain weight. In infants with congenital hydrocephalus, the birthweight, nature of delivery and the neonatal course should be noted. In addition, inquiring into the history of similar illness in an elder sibling and to the possibility of intrauterine infection is relevant.

Hydrocephalus which develops in an older and previously normal child, should alert to the possibility of a posterior fossa neoplasm. Because ventricular dilatation is generally subacute in children with cerebellar tumours, symptoms of raised intracranial pressure are often associated with changes in behaviour, a clumsy gait, abnormal articulation, tremors and incoordination. If elevation of ventricular pressure occurs abruptly, attacks of nausea, vomiting, head retraction and extensor spasms are prominent. In these very ill children, symptoms of intracranial hypertension may be obscured by those of the primary illness, such as cranial infection and haemorrhage. It is important in all cases to ascertain any neurological symptoms and to date the onset of head enlargement and to chart the developmental progress of the child.

Physical examination

Classically, hydrocephalus is recognized by a progressive increase in occipitofrontal head circumference, out of proportion to other bodily dimensions (see Fig. 49.2). A single head circumference which greatly exceeds the 97th percentile strongly suggests the existence of the disease. Where head enlargement is equivocal, and neurological abnormality absent, serial head measurements will often indicate the need for further diagnostic studies. It must be emphasized that, once enlargement of the skull is clinically obvious, the ventricles are already grossly dilated and the cerebral cortex thinned out. Clinical signs which frequently precede actual enlargement of the head include a large and bulging fontanelle, thinning of the bones of the calvarium and widening of the coronal, sagittal and lambdoidal sutures. With advancing hydrocephalus the scalp thins out and becomes shiny and pale, hair appears sparse, and superficial scalp veins become distended. Finally, the brow overhangs the small triangular face, there is upwards retraction of the eyelids and the eyes are fixed in a downward gaze demonstrating the 'setting sun' phenomenon. Despite the enormous head size, papilloedema is uncommon in congenital hydrocephalus. The

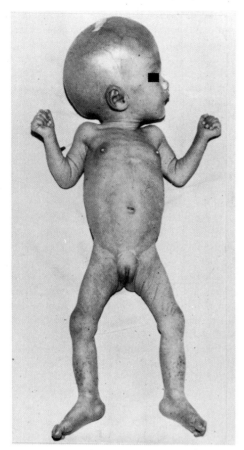

Fig. 49.2   Gross hydrocephalus in an infant.

shape of the skull should be noted. A large protruding occiput is typical of a Dandy-Walker cyst, while an asymmetrical head may be due to unilateral obstruction at the foramen of Monro. In addition, auscultation for a cranial bruit should be performed over the eye balls and over the calvarium. Transillumination of the skull in a darkened room is a useful procedure. To be reliable, the observer should familiarize himself with the normal pattern obtained with a particular transillumination lamp. The whole calvarium transilluminates brilliantly if the cerebral mantle is either absent or excessively thinned out. Porencephalic and other cysts and subdural effusions also produce focal or generalized areas of abnormal transillumination.

Many mildly affected hydrocephalic children have a remarkably normal development and minimal neurological deficit. Gross abnormalities in a child with mild hydrocephalus are usually related to the underlying disorder which caused the hydrocephalus. However,

prolonged stretching and compression of neural structures will ultimately lead to profound neurological damage. Where increase in intracranial pressure is rapid, and there has not been a compensatory increase in head size, the highly irritable child frequently gives a short, high-pitched 'cerebral cry'. During these screaming episodes, decerebrate posture may be evident. In the older child with 'arrested' hydrocephalus, it is important to evaluate the mental and psychological status. These children are typically talkative, jovial and euphoric (cocktail party syndrome) but their capacity for concentration, comprehension, enterprise and abstract thinking is often deficient. Manifestations of long-standing hydrocephalus include a variety of endocrinological and metabolic disorders such as precocious puberty, diabetes insipidus and abnormal thermoregulation. Various anomalies, particularly neural tube defects, skeletal defects and cutaneous naevi, are known to coexist with obstructive hydrocephalus, and a careful search must be made to exclude them, for they not only frequently indicate the underlying cause of the hydrocephalus, but their presence will greatly influence decisions regarding treatment.

Investigations

The child's assessment based on the history and examination will often enable a diagnosis of hydrocephalus to be made with some degree of certainty. However, in all cases investigations are required to confirm the diagnosis, determine the extent of the disorder and if possible define the aetiology. Investigations are also of assistance in deciding the need or otherwise for active treatment and also as a means of assessing the success or otherwise of treatment.

Plain skull radiograph

Such an investigation may show evidence of raised intracranial pressure. Sutural separation, thinning of the vault and demineralization may be present and in the older child excessive gyral markings may occur. The skull shape may be characteristic of particular types of hydrocephalus. If hydrocephalus is due to stricture of the aqueduct the posterior fossa tends to be small and flat, while with the Dandy-Walker syndrome this fossa is large with a high torcula. Intracranial calcification may indicate the presence of a tumour or a prior infective episode.

Ultrasound

The widespread use of ultrasound scanning (Fig. 49.3)

has in recent times greatly facilitated the assessment of infants with suspected hydrocephalus. Real-time ultrasound imaging through the open fontanelle provides a clear demonstration of the ventricles and may well-define other structural anomalies. This non-invasive risk-free investigation can be undertaken with little or no sedation, and can be repeated as often as required. With closure of the fontanelle satisfactory imaging can no longer be obtained.

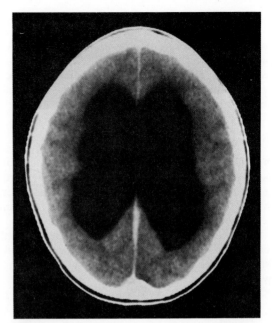

Fig. 49.4 CT scan demonstrating gross ventricular dilatation in hydrocephalus.

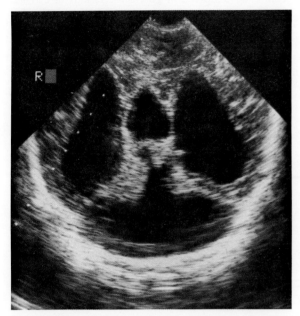

Fig. 49.3 Frontal view at real-time ultrasound study showing markedly dilated lateral ventricles on either side of a large posterior fossa cyst in a patient with Dandy-Walker malformation.

Computerized tomography

In the older child, and occasionally infants where more detail is required, CT scanning (Fig. 49.4) is the method of choice. Radiographs used in this manner provide extreme detail of the intracranial anatomy and the images may be enhanced by the injection of contrast material. Many children can be assessed by this method without sedation while others will require such preparation or occasionally a general anaesthetic. The radiation involved in a single scan is of an acceptable degree but a limitation should be placed on repeated studies.

Magnetic resonance imaging

This investigation is rarely undertaken as a primary investigation but may be of value in defining the cause of

the condition. Small tumours in the region of the aqueduct causing obstruction to CSF flow may not be visualized by a CT scan but are clearly defined by an MRI study.

Ventricular and lumbar puncture: CSF

Before the advent of the above imaging methods, investigation involved the use of invasive techniques which were associated with some morbidity. A ventricular puncture via the fontanelle or a burr hole was used to remove CSF and replace the fluid with air (air ventriculography). Less commonly, air would be introduced via a lumbar puncture (lumbar air encephalography). With either technique the introduced air would clearly define the relevant anatomy. These techniques are now rarely used for radiological purposes but remain of value when it is essential to obtain samples of CSF before treatment. Ventricular puncture is often preceded by subdural taps to detect the presence of fluid in that site.

Other investigations

The injection of radioisotopes into the CSF has provided useful information about CSF flow patterns. On very rare occasions such a study may be used to try and decide if treatment is required in a particular patient.

Angiography is rarely used but may be of assistance in defining the nature of an intracranial mass lesion. Continuous monitoring of intracranial pressure is infrequently employed, but again may be of assistance in deciding the need or otherwise of definitive surgical treatment. Psychometric evaluation is also occasionally employed for the same purpose.

Differential diagnosis

In a child presenting with features suggestive of an acute increase in intracranial pressure, the possibility of drug intoxication (tetracycline, vitamin A, nalidixic acid, etc.), lead encephalopathy, subdural haematoma, and Reye's syndrome should be considered.

When there is history of head injury together with convulsions, anaemia and a bulging fontanelle, a subdural haematoma is likely; the diagnosis is established by subdural taps or scanning.

When enlargement of the head is present at birth, or is insidious in onset, the following diagnoses should be entertained.

Skeletal defects

The head enlargement may be more apparent than real in a child who is dwarfed from intrauterine growth retardation. In the Russell-Silver dwarf, the 'pseudo-hydrocephalus' is associated with skeletal hemiatrophy, skin pigmentation and clinodactylism. The situation is more complex in the child with achondroplasia. In some, the disproportionately large head in relation to the trunk has been attributed to megalencephaly, while in a few, progressive ventricular dilatation is due to obstruction at the foramen magnum. Other disorders associated with abnormal head size include the mucopolysaccharidoses, craniocleidodysostosis, osteopetrosis and osteogenesis imperfecta. These conditions are easily recognizable from their physical features and characteristic changes on radiological examination.

The large dolichocephalic head in 'cerebral gigantism' may be mistaken for hydrocephalus and imaging may, in fact, reveal large ventricles, but ventricular pressure is normal. Other clues to the diagnosis are a dull mentality, incoordination, coarse facial features with hypertelorism and a downward slant to the eyes.

Megalencephaly

This refers to a brain which is oversized and overweight. The diagnosis from true hydrocephalus is possible only during scanning, when normal sized ventricles are demonstrated. A large head of this type may be related to familial factors and assessment of head size in close relatives is always appropriate. Head enlargement in metabolic megalencephaly is a late manifestation of many cerebral degenerations.

Hydranencephaly

Hydranencephaly is a condition of uncertain aetiology in which the cerebral cortex is represented by a thin membrane composed of glial cells. Islands of cerebral cortex are sometimes scattered in this tissue. The 3rd ventricle, basal ganglia, brain stem and cerebellum are present but reveal morphological abnormalities. The head size is usually normal at birth but increases rapidly within a few weeks of life. Neurological function may initially be deceptively normal. Within a short time, gross neurological abnormality is evident from the rigid muscle tone, tremors and persistence and exaggeration of primitive reflexes. In addition, the child sleeps excessively, is irritable, feeds poorly and has unstable thermoregulation. Optic atrophy is common and the head transilluminates readily. In most, electroencephalography reveals a flat tracing or a few low voltages over islands of cerebral cortex.

TREATMENT

The indications for treatment are based on a clear understanding of the natural history of the disorder. Three patterns may be described.

1. In a majority of patients the ventricles will continue to enlarge and the overlying brain will become stretched, compressed and thinned. If the process starts in infancy before the skull bones have developed significant attachment to each other, massive head enlargement will result and under these circumstances significant brain damage will result. This type of progression will be detected by the presence and persistence of signs of raised pressure, an excessive rate of head growth and, less commonly, by the finding of neurological abnormality and developmental delay. Serial imaging will confirm progression of ventricular dilatation. In this group treatment is essential if brain damage is to be avoided or minimized.

2. In a lesser number of patients limited enlargement of the ventricles will occur and then cease. The ventricles remain somewhat larger than normal but there are no clear signs of raised intracranial pressure and brain function appears normal. The term 'compensated hydrocephalus' has been applied to this group. The head may be large but the rate of growth will either be normal or only slightly excessive and serial images will

show no significant alteration in ventricle size. With this pattern, decisions regarding treatment are less well defined. If the degree of dilatation is mild to moderate there is no good evidence that treatment will favourably influence the outcome. Under these circumstances frequent assessment is required to ensure that stability is maintained. With large but stable ventricles, intervention is not indicated.

3. With the widespread use of head imaging techniques, it has become apparent that hydrocephalus may be a temporary state in certain circumstances. Post-haemorrhagic hydrocephalus in the low birthweight infant is often of this type as is the disorder complicating certain forms of meningitis. In these patients it appears likely that the CSF pathways have regained their patency. These patients are usually defined by repeating imaging. Such studies would show reduction in size of ventricles to the norm and this satisfactory state would be associated with the disappearance of all physical signs of progressive hydrocephalus. Obviously no long-term treatment is required in this group, but intermittent removal of CSF by either a lumbar puncture or ventricular puncture may help resolve the process and prevent any excess ventricular dilatation during the period before effective CSF flow via normal pathways is established. On occasions a reservoir may be inserted into a lateral ventricle to facilitate such intermittent removal. In addition, drugs which reduce CSF produc-

tion have been used with the same intent. Acetazolamide is a carbonic anhydrase inhibitor which decreases the active production of CSF by the choroid plexus while isosorbide is an osmotic diuretic which also interferes with CSF formation.

Operative treatment

The definitive treatment of the condition is a surgical procedure. Many different techniques have been employed with the aim of either re-establishing normal or near normal CSF pathways or by diverting the CSF to some other site in the body. Either method will allow the intracranial anatomy to revert to normal. Of these two basic techniques the second is far more commonly used.

1. Ventriculoperitoneal shunt

This is the most frequently performed operation in paediatric patients with hydrocephalus. A Silastic catheter is placed in a lateral ventricle via a burr hole and the other end of the tube is passed subcutaneously to the abdomen and then placed in the peritoneal cavity. A valve is frequently interposed and an adequate length of tube is placed in the peritoneal cavity to allow for growth. The peritoneum effectively absorbs CSF (Fig. 49.5).

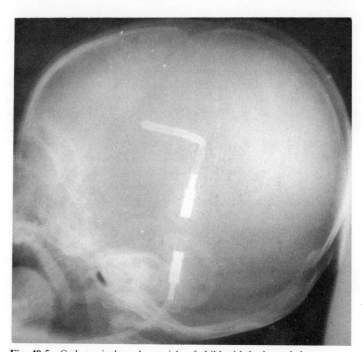

Fig. 49.5 Catheter in lateral ventricle of child with hydrocephalus.

2. Ventriculoatrial shunt

In this procedure the lower end of the shunt is passed via a neck vein to the right atrium. The catheter is so designed that CSF can pass often from the catheter tip but blood not flow back in to the lumen. The turbulent blood flow in the atrium prevents thrombus formation around the catheter. This operation is not frequently undertaken in patients as maintenance involves the lengthening of the atrial catheter on several occasions.

3. Other shunts

CSF is very occasionally diverted from a ventricle to the pleural cavity. In communicating hydrocephalus CSF may be drained from the lumbar subarachnoid space to the peritoneal cavity. This procedure, known as a spino-peritoneal or lumbo-peritoneal shunt, may work well in certain patients. Of historic interest are other procedures in which CSF was drained to such structures as a ureter, gall bladder and Fallopian tube. The failure rate of these procedures was found to be unacceptably high.

Removal of a mass lesion causing CSF obstruction such as a neoplasm or haematoma is obviously the most direct and logical way of treating hydrocephalus. In many patients such can be achieved while in others removal may not be feasible and a shunt is still necessary. On occasions a shunt may be inserted to relieve high intracranial pressure and allow a patient's condition to improve before such a major procedure is undertaken. In non-communicating hydrocephalus the creation of a communication between the ventricles and subarachnoid space is infrequently undertaken. Such operations as third ventriculostomy and ventriculocisternostomy are of this type. General acceptance has not been achieved as the success rate is not high and the procedures involve some increased risk.

Excision of the rare choroid plexus papilloma generally leads to resolution of hydrocephalus, but again, on occasions, a shunt may be required as well.

Postoperative care

It is important to emphasize that the undertaking of the operation is but one step in the care of a child with hydrocephalus. Of equal importance is the need to maintain an optimal state of function of the shunt. With this in mind it is essential that the child's parents have a reasonable understanding of the disorder and the essential nature of the treatment. It is only with such explanation that they can appreciate the need for prolonged follow-up.

In the first 2 years of life the child with a shunt should be reviewed at least 3–4-monthly intervals while in later years 6–12-monthly intervals are appropriate. During such reviews the aim must be to ensure that the shunt is functioning in a satisfactory manner and that the hydrocephalic condition is under control.

Complications of treatment

The operation is generally well tolerated with infrequent early difficulties. The main long-term problems are related to shunt obstruction and infection. Obstruction is the most common complication and the relevant frequency of its occurrence is responsible for much morbidity and very rarely mortality.

Obstruction is usually due to blockage of the tubing, which can occur at any site, and it also may result from disconnection or breakage of the catheters. With failure of the shunt the symptoms and signs of hydrocephalus will recur and the pattern tends to follow one of three courses.

The most common presentation of a child with a blocked shunt is that of a vague illness. Irritability and vomiting are frequent and headache may be present. The symptoms are very similar to those of many childhood illnesses and difficulties are often experienced in trying to decide if the symptoms are a consequence of shunt malfunction or an unrelated illness. Definite signs of raised intracranial pressure, if present, are of great assistance but are often not readily ascertained. Palpation of the shunt mechanism may also frequently be inconclusive.

In a small number of patients blockage can be followed by a rapid rise in intracranial pressure which is reflected in a dramatic deterioration in the patient's condition. A decline in conscious state, pupillary signs, abnormal motor responses and variable changes in vital signs are all signs of such a change and indicate the urgent need for surgical correction of the shunt obstruction. Delay in such a situation may lead to a fatality.

In a second small group symptoms may be minimal or even non-existent and the obstruction with raised pressure will only be detected by careful examination and possibly by the use of radiological techniques. Detection of such a problem is of great importance as, if left untreated, the chronic raised intracranial pressure may in time produce optic atrophy with resultant premature impairment of visual acuity. Such a chronic situation may also be associated with subtle changes of psychological function.

The treatment of shunt obstruction is usually a simple procedure and involves the replacement of the defective component. A small number of patients unfortunately suffer from repeated episodes of obstruction and management can be difficult and involve many variations of shunt equipment and of surgical technique.

Colonization of the shunt occurs in small numbers of patients with a reported incidence, varying widely, but usually at the 5–10% figure. The causal organism is usually a coagulase negative Staphylococcus but on occasions *Staphylococcus aureus*, streptococci, *Escherichia coli* and other Gram-negative organisms may be responsible. Generally, infection occurs within a short time of a shunt operation, but it may not appear until many months or even years have elapsed since the last procedure. Operative contamination is responsible for early infection while in later infection it is believed that such colonization may follow a transient bacteraemia. The latter may follow minimal surgical procedures and many authorities consider that such procedures undertaken on a child with a shunt should be 'covered' by an appropriate antibiotic.

Most commonly such infections are indolent with no evidence of any local infection in the vicinity of the shunt apparatus. Symptoms are often vague and the signs of low grade infection are mistakenly attributed to other causes. In a child with a shunt the presence of a low grade fever, mild constitutional upset and changes in the blood picture suggestive of infection could well indicate such a complication. Blood cultures may be informative but the only positive way of confirming such a diagnosis is by the aspiration of CSF from the valve system and obtaining a positive culture. Long-standing unrecognized shunt infections may be associated with other findings such as hepatosplenomegaly and so-called shunt nephritis. The latter may be recognized by the finding of proteinuria.

Treatment of shunt infections with antibiotics alone has a low success rate and eradication involves the removal of the entire system with concomitant use of an appropriate drug. After a short time a new shunt can be reinserted with only a small risk of reinfection. In the interim between shunts hydrocephalus can usually be controlled by either intermittent removal or continuous external drainage of CSF.

Results of treatment

With the present forms of surgical treatment the outlook for many children with hydrocephalus is excellent. Such an outcome would be expected in a patient who is found to have hydrocephalus with no significant associated cerebral anomalies and in whom the condition is detected at a relatively early stage and where treatment is appropriate and well maintained. Such children are fully capable of, and are encouraged, to lead a completely normal life. In many children hydrocephalus is associated with structural anomalies of the brain of either a congenital or acquired nature and such anomalies may be responsible for a poor outcome. Despite adequate control of hydrocephalus, such children may have permanent physical and intellectual problems.

FURTHER READING

Lorber J, Priestley B L 1981 Children with large heads: a practical approach to diagnosis in 557 children, with special reference to 109 children with megalencephaly. Developmental Medicine and Child Neurology 23: 495–504

McComb J G 1983 Recent research into the nature of cerebrospinal fluid formation and absorption. Journal of Neurosurgery 59(3) 369–383

Milhorat T H 1978 Pediatric neurosurgery, Williams & Wilkins, Baltimore 91–135

50. Neural tube defects

A. D. Bryan

Neural tube defects (NTD) is the term given to a group of malformations involving the brain and/or the spinal cord in association with varying degrees of absence or malformation of the overlying tissues – meninges, bone, muscle and skin.

INCIDENCE

Neural tube defects are the commonest, major congenital abnormalities affecting the nervous system. The incidence varies in different countries with the highest rates occurring in Northern Ireland, the west of Scotland, and South Wales, where the incidence has been recorded variously between 4 and 16 per 1000 live births. Recently, the incidence of spina bifida in the State of Victoria, Australia, was noted to be 1.59 per 1000 live births.

Recurrence risks in families have been documented extensively. Risk of recurrence, following the birth of the first child with a neural tube defect, is of the order of 1 in 25. A recurrence after two affected children is of the order of 1 in 8.

Neural tube defects are commoner in females, in lower socioeconomic groups and the incidence appears lower in Jewish and black people. Neural tube defects are a common association of spontaneous first trimester miscarriages.

EMBRYOLOGY AND PATHOGENESIS

Among the most important processes in the development of the central nervous system is the change from a flat neural plate (on the dorsal surface of the embryo) to an internal neural tube (Fig. 50.1). The internalization of the central nervous system is complete by the 28th day of gestation. It is thought that neural tube defects result from failure to midline fusion anywhere along the dorsal surface of the embryo. The mechanism of this failure of fusion is not clear. For reasons that are not altogether clear, incidence of neural tube defects is increasing in many societies. Genetic factors clearly play

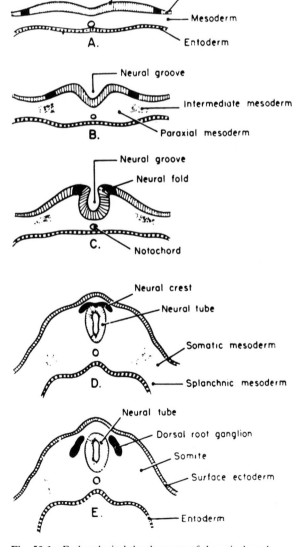

Fig. 50.1 Embryological development of the spinal cord.

412

a major role in some societies, for example, the high incidence in the Celts of South Wales, the west of Scotland and in Northern Ireland.

It has been suggested, recently, that vitamin supplement (in particular of folic acid) may reduce the incidence of recurrence or occurrence in high-risk populations. Dietary factors may or may not play a major part in low risk populations.

Many other aetiological clues have been examined in the last 20 years.

CLINICAL FEATURES

Neural tube defects may be classified as in Example 50.1.

Example 50.1 Classification of neural tube defects

1. Anencephaly
2. Cranium bifidum
   a. Cranial meningocele
   b. Encephalocele
3. Spina bifida occulta
4. Spina bifida cystica
   a. Myelomeningocele
   b. Meningocele
5. Sacral agenesis

Anencephaly

Anencephaly is obvious at birth presenting as an opened malformed skull and brain. Many individuals with this condition are stillborn. Clearly no treatment is indicated. The families require a great deal of emotional support at this time.

Cranium bifidum

Cranial meningocele

In this situation the underlying brain is normal, but a meningeal sac protrudes through a skull defect.

Encephalocele

In this situation a midline sac protrudes which may contain brain. Hydrocephalus is a common association.

Spina bifida occulta

Here one to three vertebral arches are incomplete posteriorly but the overlying skin is intact. Most often it is diagnosed accidentally, e.g. as the result of a radiograph of the spinal column for other reasons such as an intravenous pyelogram. Up to 10% of people who have had radiographs in this random fashion have been demonstrated to have spina bifida occulta. While the vast majority of individuals with spina bifida occulta have a normal spinal cord, a number of abnormalities of the spinal cord have been described.

Occasionally ectodermal abnormalities are associated with spina bifida occulta. These include a dermal pit, a depression with a tuft of hair or a fatty swelling (Fig. 50.2). Occasionally, this ectodermal component communicates with the dura so that there is some risk of intraspinal infection. The fatty swelling described above may be a lipomeningocele and, although this condition is uncommon, full neurological examination is warranted in the presence of any associated ectodermal abnormality. It is also important to ensure that any pit associated with spina bifida occulta is not a dural sinus.

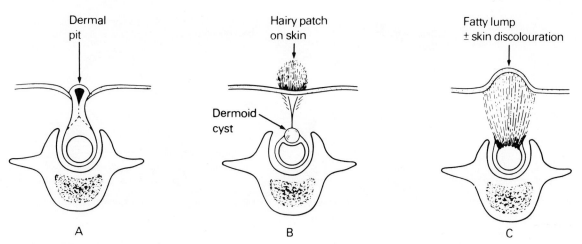

Fig. 50.2 Schematic representation of spina bifida occulta. (**a**) – Dermal sinus; (**b**) – Intraspinal cyst pressing on the cord. (**c**) – Lipomatous mass infiltrating the cord elements.

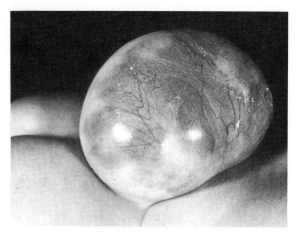

Fig. 50.3   A lumbosacral myelomeningocele

Spina bifida cystica

This is almost always obvious at birth when, most frequently, a midline sac protrudes through a spinal defect (Fig. 50.3). Such a defect may occur anywhere along the length of the spinal column, with the lumbar and lumbosacral regions being the most frequent. Abnormal spinal cord tissue and nerve roots may be readily apparent.

Pathologically and clinically, spina bifida cystica can be divided into two main groups:

a. myelomeningocele (Fig. 50.4) in which vertebral column skin, meninges and spinal cord are involved, and

b. meningocele, in which the spinal cord is not involved (Fig. 50.5).

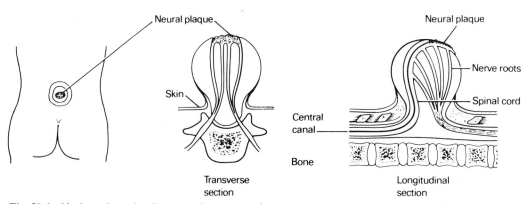

Fig. 50.4   Myelomeningocele: diagrammatic representation.

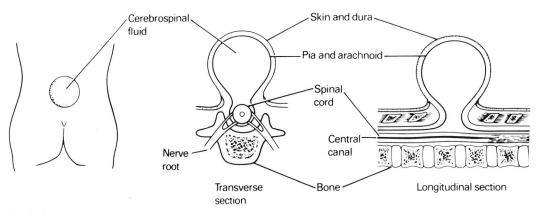

Fig. 50.5   Meningocele: diagrammatic representation.

Myelomeningocele – myelocele

That neural tissue is involved in this malformation is confirmed by the presence of:

Voluntary muscle paralysis, which is mainly but not entirely of lower motor neurone type, and manifest clinically by flaccid paralysis and limb deformity below the level of the lesion.

The degree of functional impairment here is dependent on the level of the lesion with a progressive worsening of the function the higher the level. The exception to this rule is that cervical lesions usually only have minor paralysis involving the upper rather than the lower limbs.

Sensory loss in the dermatomes below the lesion. Almost all children have a substantial problem with skin sensory loss. The loss involves almost always the sacral segments because most spina bifida lesions are lumbar and lumbosacral. The sacral segments include the weight-bearing surfaces of the feet and buttocks, resulting in a very great risk of pressure sores in these areas; in fact, almost 100% of individuals have had pressure sores by 18 years of age although they are uncommon in infancy.

Bladder paralysis due partly to disturbance of autonomic function but also to disturbance of pelvic floor voluntary muscle intervention. Involvement of the bladder manifests clinically in a variety of ways (Fig.50.6), for example:

a. as a flaccid bladder with no reservoir function, poor urinary stream and/or constant dribbling;

b. as a large palpable bladder with a high residual volume with, at times, a good urinary stream. Dribbling or urine may or may not occur here.

Rectal paralysis. Again this relates to involvement of the autonomic nervous supply to the rectum and paralysis of the voluntary muscles of the pelvic floor. Clinical manifestations vary, for example;

a. on the one hand, rectal capacity may be small and small pellets of dried faeces are passed on a regular basis throughout the day and constipation is not a feature;

b. on the other hand, some children have a larger rectum with substantial capacity in which chronic constipation may pose major problems.

As bowel and bladder innervation are also sacral in origin, it is the rare individual who escapes significant problems in either of these two areas.

Cerebral manifestations. In addition to the spinal component there is a major intra-cranial involvement in most children with spina bifida. The Arnold Chiari malformation (see Ch. 49) is the most significant lesion clinically, largely but not solely because of its relationship to the development of hydrocephalus. In addition,

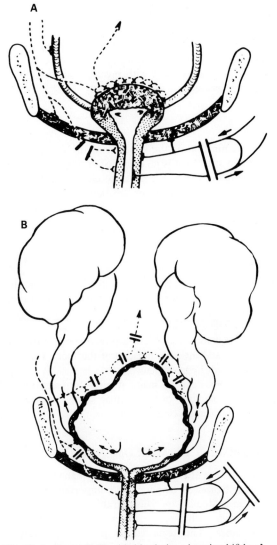

Fig. 50.6 **A** and **B** The bladder lesions in spina bifida. **A** – Low pressure bladder with decreased sphincter tone – note normal calibre ureters and interrupted autonomic nerve pathways. **B** – High pressure bladder – increased sphincter tone and detrusor activity – note bilateral megaureters and hydronephrosis and interruption of autonomic nerve pathway.

there are a number of complex neuropathological lesions in the brains of most persons with spina bifida; the clinical significance of these are not apparent at this time.

Hydrocephalus. This occurs in approximately 90% of children with spina bifida cystica. The Arnold Chiari malformation accounts for most cases with aqueduct stenosis (see Ch. 49) accounting for most of the remainder. Of the 90% of children who develop hydrocephalus, approximately 70% have a progressive form. It is this progressive hydrocephalus which requires surgery with the insertion of a shunt. Hydrocephalus may be obvious clinically at birth or may be demonstrated by brain ultrasound and/or CT scan. About 15% of individuals with myelomeningocele have grand mal epilepsy.

Meningocele

If, on examination of the infant (and the pathology of the excised sac) there is no evidence of neural tissue involvement, the lesion is a meningocele (see Fig. 50.5). There will be no limitation of function. There is still an increased risk of recurrence of an NTD in subsequent children.

Sacral agenesis

Sacral agenesis is a rare condition in which the sacrum is absent and is replaced by a bar of bone. Sacral level lower motor neurone paralysis is present to varying degrees, affecting bladder and bowel function and the extensors and abductors of the hip (and very occasionally, the calf, and intrinsic muscles of the foot). It is not associated with hydrocephalus.

The diagnosis can be made at birth by palpation of the defect, radiology of the lumbar spine and sacrum and full neurological examination.

MANAGEMENT OF MYELOMENINGOCELE

A team is essential for the proper management of myelomeningocele. The parents are important members of the team. Medical specialists in this team include the neurosurgeon, orthopaedic surgeon and urologist in the first instance. The team leader is most properly a paediatrician with special skills in the field of child development and rehabilitation. The team leader will co-ordinate the various activities to support the parents and child through the many problems – physical and psychological – that invariably arise. The physiotherapist, occupational therapist, orthotist, psychologist, and medical social worker, together with trained nursing staff, both hospital and community based, and teachers are important members of this team.

The team has three major goals:

1. To promote good health in the short and long term.
2. To promote maximum function in the child so that, as nearly as possible, normal developmental se-

quences and timing can be followed to enable maximal independence for the child and family.
3. To promote good family functioning.

Specific problems in the management of the newborn with spina bifida

It is possible to predict with considerable accuracy the potential for future impairment in a number of areas. These include ambulation and subsequent mobility, likely bowel and bladder function and hydrocephalus with its likely sequelae. A more difficult area is to predict the effects these impairments will have on the lifestyle of the individual and family. Also, it is possible to recognize early those lesions which are inoperable because of massive bony deformity and extensive skin loss which would prevent closure of the defect.

The specific problems are:

1. Children with high lesions (thoracic and thoracolumbar), significant hydrocephalus at birth, major kyphosis or other significant problems (either congenital or acquired) have a significantly increased mortality in early life and substantial morbidity if they survive. In these circumstances, in discussion with the family, conservative supportive care may be recommended. If the infant survives the perinatal period, elective surgical care may be indicated.

In the absence of such adverse factors, in discussion with the family, early surgical repair/removal of the lesion is usually recommended.

2. Careful serial evaluation of head circumference and ventricular size by ultrasound or CT scan will indicate if hydrocephalus is developing. Once it is established that progressive hydrocephalus is present, a shunt operation is recommended.

3. Baseline orthopaedic, urology and neurosurgery assessments provide the basis for ongoing discussions with the family and management of the condition. Occasionally, active orthopaedic or urological intervention is required for, e.g. dislocated hip joints or urinary obstruction.

4. It is critical to begin to establish an empathic, therapeutic relationship with the parents in the newborn period, which forms the foundation for ongoing support throughout childhood.

Ongoing management issues

The neurogenic bladder

The aims of management of the paralysed bladder are to minimize urinary infections and ill health, prevent chronic renal disease and enable the child to be dry by kindergarten or school entry.

Urinary infections are common. Because of loss of sensation there may be no localizing symptoms. Pathological examination of urine specimens is the only reliable diagnostic tool.

In the past, ileal conduits were constructed in an attempt to achieve these aims. Early results were encouraging but long-term follow-up has revealed increasing medical and social problems in many adolescents and adults. However, most young adults continue to rely on an ileal conduit for continence. A few have had urinary diversion and use catheters for continence.

In the past decade clean intermittent catheterization (CIC) has been the first line of management. Most children have substantial improvement in continence with this technique. Even though a few iatrogenic infections may occur using this technique, the overall rate of bladder infection is less.

In some cases, particularly if vesico-ureteric reflux is present, low-dose prophylactic antibiotics are given in the long term.

A proportion of children remain wet on CIC. More recently, bladder augmentation and artificial sphincter operations have helped these children.

The neurogenic bowel

The principal goal in the management of the neurogenic bowel is for the individual to be able to defaecate at a time and place of his choosing and to be clean in between. Gross constipation with megacolon, faecal impaction and overflow incontinence is the major risk in spina bifida. This will be prevented by emptying the bowel regularly. Even in the absence of sensation, sitting on the toilet and pushing is often all that is required. Laxatives and dietary manipulation may be necessary and a bowel wash-out may be required either regularly or occasionally. This latter procedure should also be done in the home, by the parents in the first instance and later by the child.

Mobility

The outlook for walking clearly depends upon the level of the spinal cord lesion. For example, an infant with a lesion at T12 or above will have no active movements in the legs, although ambulation is possible in early childhood using long braces and crutches. Most of these individuals, however, will elect for a wheelchair, certainly by adult life. A child with a lesion at L4 will have good quadriceps function and may walk with below knee braces. Children with lower lesions will have an even better prognosis for walking in childhood and adult life. Surgery, including tendon transfers and correction of deformity may improve the prognosis for mobility.

Training for walking and the fitting of appropriate splints will commence between the ages of 2 and 3 years. Again it is emphasized that trophic ulcers are an ever-present risk in spina bifida so that care of the skin and, in particular, correct fitting of splints is essential.

Deformity

A major aim in management is to prevent or correct deformity, particularly if it affects function or predisposes to pressure sores. Surgical procedures will be necessary in many cases. This will particularly apply to the management of talipes and fixed flexion deformities in the legs, to the correction or prevention of hip dislocation and correction of various spinal deformities, e.g. kyphoscoliosis.

Skin care

Skin problems, particularly pressure sores and burns, are a major cause of morbidity and hospitalization, particularly in adolescence and adult life. Prevention through education and careful monitoring of 'at risk' areas may prevent the need for prolonged hospital care or surgical repair.

Sexual function

Individuals with spina bifida may have neurological impairment of sexual functioning. The difficulties may include loss of normal sensation in both sexes. In females, pregnancy has been achieved on many occasions. However, there are a number of potential difficulties during pregnancy and confinement. These include urinary drainage difficulties, particularly in those women with ileal conduit urinary diversions and all the problems that one might associate with a person with a paralysed pelvic floor, e.g. prolapse, etc. The changes in the spinal column, associated with hormone changes in pregnancy, may also have an impact on the structural stability of the spine and perhaps neurological function. A number of problems have occurred at confinement, particularly to do with pelvic floor paralysis. In males the difficulties are if anything more complex. Relatively few have had children; difficulties range from impotence to retrograde ejaculation and sterility.

Education

Most children with spina bifida have a need for assistance at school. Difficulties with access, mobility and continence need to be overcome. Numbers of children with shunted hydrocephalus have specific learning problems. Varying degrees of difficulty with concentration span, attention control and fine motor and perceptual functioning have been noted.

However, the majority attend regular schools with the occasional assistance of therapists, aides and integration teachers.

Support for the child and family

This will be a major task. Any disorder requiring constant medical and surgical treatment will place severe strains on most families. A great deal of time and patience will be required by the team to provide the necessary emotional support. It is important that the financial implications of spina bifida are anticipated and that the various entitlements are obtained. Facilities such as kindergartens, schools and later, vocational training must be organized. Major emotional problems are frequent in spina bifida during adolescence; these problems need to be anticipated and properly managed as they arise. The general practitioner should be encouraged to be involved in the day-to-day care of children with spina bifida, remembering that these children experience the normal physical and emotional problems of any other child.

The young adult

Large numbers of individuals with spina bifida have now reached adult life. The transition from adolescence to adulthood provides major difficulties for those with chornic illness/disability and their families (see Ch. 66).

There is not yet a significant body of literature describing the medical, educational and social outcomes of spina bifida in adult life. There are likely to be on-going difficulties with urinary management, shunts and pressure sores. However, many young adults report great satisfaction with their lives.

PREVENTION OF NEURAL TUBE DEFECTS

Quite clearly, the ultimate management of neural tube defect is primary prevention. Recently, a great deal of interest has been taken in the possible impact of vitamin (in particular folic acid) supplements given prior to pregnancy and on the occurrence and recurrence of in-dividuals with neural tube defect in high-risk populations. Community-wide primary prevention is still not possible at this time.

Mass screening for neural tube defects by estimation of alphafetoprotein in maternal blood is currently under study. Amniocentesis, in the case of elevated serum alphafetoprotein levels is required for confirmation. If and when this screening is found to be reliable, major reductions in the incidence of neural tube defects should result.

Prenatal detection, with termination of pregnancy if the fetus is affected and family wish it, is available to high-risk families (those with a previous affected child). Amniocentesis and measurement of amniotic fluid alphafetoprotein will establish the diganosis of neural tube defects at 16–17 weeks gestation. (Alphafetoprotein is a glycoprotein synthesized by the fetal liver and yolk sac which enters the fetal circulation and thence the fetal urine and amniotic fluid; this can be assayed. In the presence of an open (not skin-covered) neural defect, excess amounts of alphafetoprotein enter the amniotic fluid; levels reach a maximum between 14 and 16 weeks gestation.) Although the technique is highly sensitive and reasonably specific, false positive results do occur in the presence of a number of situations. A major problem is contamination of the specimen by fetal blood. To minimize this, ultrasonography should always precede amniocentesis. Because of the risks of the procedure, amniocentesis cannot be performed on all pregnant mothers, but is a major priority in mothers who have previously given birth to an infant with a neural tube defect.

In the meantime the prevention of disability, both physical and emotional, in individuals who have spina bifida must be the principal goal of those involved in the management.

FURTHER READING

Anderson E M, Clark L 1982 Disability in adolescence. Methuen, London

Anderson E M, Spain B 1977 The child with spina bifida. Methuen, London

Minns R 1986 The management of children with spina bifida and associated hydrocephalus. In: Gordon N, MacKinlay I (eds) Neurologically handicapped children: treatment and management. Blackwell, Oxford

Minns R 1986 The treatment of the complications of spina bifida. In: Gordon N, MacKinlay I (eds) Neurologically sick children: treatment and management. Blackwell, Oxford

Shurtleff D B 1986 Myelodysplasias and extrophies: significance, prevention and treatment. Grune and Stratton, Orland

Fluid and electrolyte homeostasis. Renal disorders

SECTION X

Fluid and electrolyte

Renal disorders

51. Fluid and electrolyte physiology

H. R. Powell

WATER AND ELECTROLYTE DISTRIBUTION

Water accounts for 75% of the bodyweight at birth, but the proportion of water decreases throughout childhood to reach about 60% of the adult weight, the exact proportion depending on the amount of body fat. Body water exists in extracellular and intracellular compartments. Extracellular water comprises mainly the blood plasma and interstitial fluid bathing the cells in the tissues. Extracellular water represents 40% of the bodyweight at birth, 30% at 1 year of age, and 25% in adulthood. The proportion of intracellular water changes much less and is about one-third of bodyweight at all ages.

Blood volume remains fairly constant throughout life in relation to bodyweight, being approximately 80 ml/kg (or 8% of the bodyweight). Plasma volume is about 45 ml/kg of bodyweight if the haematocrit is normal. The distribution of body fluids is shown in Figure 51.1.

Disorders causing a change in the amount of water in the body, i.e. conditions of dehydration or overhydration, are associated mainly with changes in the volume of the extracellular fluid and many of the clinical signs of dehydration or overhydration depend on such changes in the extracellular fluid. Substantial intracellular volume changes occur only when marked osmotic abnormalities occur in the extracellular fluid leading to fluid shifts across cell membranes. Osmotic changes result from variations in the concentrations of electrolytes in the extracellular fluid. The electrolyte concentrations in the extracellular fluid are determined by measuring the concentrations in the plasma or serum. Serum electrolyte concentrations in childhood are generally similar to adult levels but, in the first few months of life, serum potassium and phosphorus concentrations tend to be higher than in older children and adults while pH, bicarbonate and calcium levels tend to be lower. The principle differences between intracellular and extracellular concentrations of electrolytes are that intracellular potassium, magnesium and phosphate are higher while sodium, chloride and bicarbonate are much lower than in serum (Table 51.1). These differences are important in catabolic states when intracellular fluid is released into the plasma.

WATER BALANCE

While growing infants are in detectable positive water balance, the bodyweight, and hence the volume of body fluid of older children and adults in caloric balance, is

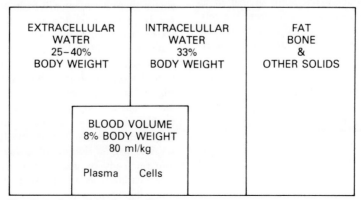

Fig. 51.1 Body fluid distribution.

Table 51.1 Representative electrolyte concentrations in extracellular and intracellular fluids (mmol/l)

Ion	ECF (serum)	ICF (skeletal muscle)
Na+	140	10
K+	4	160
Ca++	2.5	<1
Mg++	1	15
Cl–	100	3
HCO$_3$$^-$	25	10
P	1.5	60

remarkably stable from day to day. This stability implies that water input and output are balanced and the total water intake (ingested water plus water generated by metabolism of carbohydrate, fat and protein) equals the water excretion (in urine and faeces and by evaporation from the skin and lungs). Evaporative water loss from skin and lungs depends on body surface area and so water balance is most accurately described in terms of ml/m^2 of surface area at all ages. However, many clinicians prefer to calculate fluid requirements in terms of bodyweight. When this is done it is found that the daily water requirements per kilogram of bodyweight is high in infancy and gradually decreases throughout childhood (Table 51.2).

Each day orally fed infants require about 150 water/kg of bodyweight. If water is given only intravenously, 100–120/kg is required for daily maintenance as there is then no significant water loss in the faeces. Normal faecal water loss is relatively small and can generally be ignored in older children and adults.

The high water requirement of the infant is due to high insensible evaporative losses from a relatively large surface area of skin and lungs. While the weight of a newborn infant is less than one-twentieth of adult weight, surface area is about one-ninth of that of an adult. The cooling effect of evaporation from the relatively large surface area of the skin and lungs means that the infant needs a higher metabolic rate, or caloric re-

quirement, per kilogram of bodyweight than adults in order to maintain body temperature. The metabolic rate of infants is about 400 kJ/kg (100 Cal/kg or 1500 Cal/m^2) but adults take in, on average, only about 150 kJ/kg (35 Cal/kg or 1400 Cal/m^2). Note that the basal metabolic rate is almost constant throughout life when related to body surface area because the cooling effect of evaporative losses per unit of surface area remains relatively constant throughout life.

In the first few months of life an infant on oral feeds requires 150 ml/kg and 400 kJ/kg. This ratio of 400 kJ/150 ml is found in most milk formulae used to feed normal infants and is also present in breast milk.

Water balance for normal infants and children

A normal infant drinks about 150 ml/kg each day. In addition, metabolism of ingested sugar, fat and amino acids leads to the generation of water molecules at the rate of 10 ml/kg/day, leading to a total water intake of 160ml/kg/day. Water losses occur in urine, faeces and by evaporation. Evaporative loss varies greatly with body and environmental temperature and rises by 12% for every 1°C rise in body temperature. Urine water will be 80–100 ml/kg/day if isotonic urine is formed, but the kidneys vary the rate of water excretion over a wide range by concentrating or diluting urine, and thereby play a major role in maintaining water balance despite considerable variation in water intake. Faecal water losses in normal humans vary little throughout life and remain at 50–100 ml/day. The normal infant is in a state of net positive water balance so some water is retained in the body and accounts for much of the normal weight gain of growth.

Figure 51.2 shows the water balance of an infant fed totally intravenously (110 ml/kg/day) with no faecal losses. Metabolic water is generated by catabolism. If insensible evaporative loss and urine output are as shown then the infant will be in water balance, but will not be growing. If adequate nutrition is provided intravenously then growth will occur and a rather larger water intake will be tolerated, say 120–125 ml/kg/day.

For older children and adults it is usual to express water balance in terms of body surface area as shown in Figure 51.3. A 9-year-old child weighing 27 kg will have a surface area of about 1m^2. Insensible intake of metabolic water is 200 ml/m^2/day and the insensible evaporative losses are 500 ml/m^2/day leading to a net insensible loss of 300 ml/m^2 a day. Water incorporated into the body by growth can generally be ignored in older children as the proportional growth rate is so much less than in infants.

Table 51.2 Daily maintenance fluid requirements

Age (years)	Oral (ml/kg/day)	Intravenous (ml/kg/day)
0–1	150	100
1–5	80	80
5–10	60	60
10–15	50	50
15	40	40

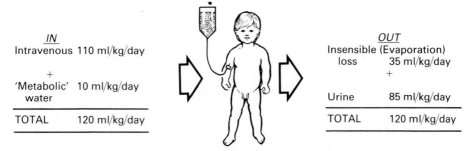

Fig. 51.2 Daily water balance in an infant fed by intravenous intake.

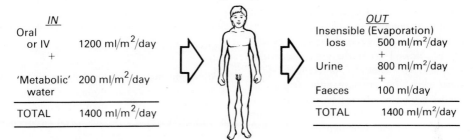

Fig. 51.3 Daily water balance in an older child and adult.

ELECTROLYTE BALANCE

Very efficient mechanisms exist within the body to keep plasma electrolyte concentrations constant despite wide variations in the amount of salt and potassium taken in the diet. These mechanisms operate by regulating urinary excretion of these ions to match the intake. Urinary sodium concentration can be decreased to near zero on a low sodium diet or increased to over 250 mmol/l on a high sodium diet. Hence a normal person will remain in salt balance despite a very wide range of dietary electrolyte intakes. An intake of 2 mmol/kg/day of sodium, potassium, chloride, and bicarbonate will meet normal maintenance requirements from infancy through to adulthood.

An example of the concentrations of sodium in the fluids entering and leaving a patient is shown in Figure 51.4. The urine sodium concentration is rather higher than the dietary concentration because of the loss of sodium-free water by evaporation. Note that the concentration of sodium in the diet and in the urine is less than that of plasma.

Control of water and electrolyte balance

Water intake is regulated by the sensation of thirst. Thirst is induced by small increases in the concentration

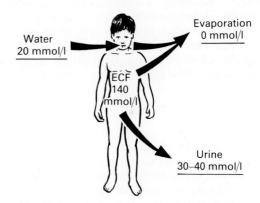

Fig. 51.4 Sodium concentrations in body fluids.

of osmolality of the plasma and also by small decreases in plasma volume. Such changes occur during mild dehydration. A normal person will then drink sufficient water to restore plasma volume and osmolality to their baseline level.

The rate of excretion of water in the urine is regulated by secretion of antidiuretic hormone (ADH) released by the pituitary gland in response to a rise in plasma osmolality or a fall in plasma volume, the same two stimuli which induce thirst. ADH produces water retention by increasing water permeability of the collecting ducts in the hypertonic renal medulla. The tubular fluid equilibrates with interstitial fluid and water diffuses out of the collecting ducts so that osmolality of the urine rises as its volume falls.

Following a water load the plasma becomes diluted with a fall in osmolality and an increase in volume which suppresses ADH release. The collecting ducts become impermeable to water and the normally hypotonic fluid leaving the distal tubule is passed as the final urine. Hence, a large volume of urine of low concentration is passed in response to a water load, restoring body water balance to normal.

There are several mechanisms and hormones which alter urine sodium excretion but one of the most important is aldosterone. This steroid is secreted by adrenal cortex in response to angiotensin, which is formed when the enzyme renin acts on a plasma α_2 globulin, angiotensinogen. Renin is released from the juxtaglomerular apparatus of the afferent arterioles in response to a decrease in renal perfusion pressure and changes in sodium flux in the region of the macula densa of the distal tubules. A small fall in plasma volume, as occurs in states of dehydration or salt depletion, leads to a fall in the afferent arteriolar pressure and consequent renin release from the juxtaglomerular apparatus. Renin then generates angiotensin which stimulates aldosterone production. Aldosterone causes avid sodium reabsorption in the distal tubule so that the urine contains a very low sodium concentration and the retained sodium, by its osmotic effect, helps to increase the volume of the depleted extracellular fluid.

FLUID AND ELECTROLYTE DISORDERS IN PAEDIATRICS

Many diseases lead to abnormal water balance in children and, depending on the relative effects of intake and loss, either dehydration or overhydration may occur. Children, especially infants, are more prone to dehydration than adults because of their relatively high water turnover relative to bodyweight.

Causes of abnormal water balance

Dehydration in children most often results from excessive loss of water, as in gastroenteritis, diabetes mellitus or diabetes insipidus, but also may occur when intake of water is reduced as in cases of bowel obstruction because of, for example, congenital pyloric stenosis. Overhydration most often occurs when water intake continues in the face of reduced output of urine, for example in oliguric renal failure or inappropriate secretion of ADH. Water retention also occurs in

hypoproteinaemic states and cardiac failure where high aldosterone secretion causes sodium, and consequenty water retention.

Clinical features of abnormal water balance

In the clinical assessment of water balance, the history will provide useful information regarding sites of fluid loss, the duration, nature and severity of the loss and urine output. Physical signs of dehydration or overhydration occur when the amount of water in the body changes sufficiently to alter the bodyweight by 5% or more. Clinical oedema occurs when an amount of fluid equal to at least 5% of the body weight is retained in the body. Clinical quantification of degree of dehydration can be made according to the following scale:

Bodyweight loss < 5%	– no clinical signs
Bodyweight loss 5–10%	– loss of skin turgor, sunken fontanelle, dry mucous membranes
Bodyweight loss > 10%	– peripheral circulatory failure (shock).

The fluid deficiency in dehydration is thus calculated as a percentage loss of bodyweight and the volume which this weight loss represents is used to calculate the volume of fluid to replace the deficit during treatment. When signs of dehydration are present (i.e. weight loss > 5%) intravenous rehydration will usually be required. Lesser degrees of dehydration, which are assumed to be present from the history rather than from physical signs, can often be corrected with oral fluids, particularly in gastroenteritis.

Types of dehydration

In dehydration, plasma may be isotonic, hypotonic or hypertonic. In hypotonic dehydration the loss of sodium is out of proportion to loss of water and the serum sodium concentration is low, whereas in hypertonic dehydration the water loss is proportionately greater and hypernatremia results. In most cases of hypernatraemic dehydration there is, however, still a total body deficit of salt even though the serum sodium is high. Hypernatraemic dehydration occurs most often in gastroenteritis but is also seen in diabetes insipidus. In these conditions the water lost in the faeces or urine has a sodium concentration less than that of plasma (diarrhoeal stool sodium concentration is usually 40–80 mmol/l) so that the body loses proportionately more water than sodium leading to hypernatraemia and dehydration. This tendency to hypernatraemia is countered by drinking water without salt, but if water intake is limited by vomiting hypernatraemia will occur.

In isotonic dehydration the major water deficit is in the extracellular fluid with less effect on the volume of intracellular fluid. Thus, when considering therapy, the volume of water calculated to replace the lost bodyweight can be given as an intravenous fluid with a sodium concentration similar to that of plasma.

In hypertonic dehydration the high osmolality of extracellular fluid leads to withdrawal of water from cells with depletion of intracellular water as well. Withdrawal of intracellular water into the extracellular space helps maintain the extracellular volume so that clinical signs in hypernatraemic dehydration tend to be rather less severe and weight loss may be underestimated. Generally the type of dehydration can be determined with certainty only by estimation of the serum sodium concentration. Occasionally, hypernatraemia may be suspected in a small infant when signs do not appear as severe as expected from the history of severe diarrhoea and vomiting. The skin of infants with hypertonic dehydration may have a doughy feel. Severe hypertonic dehydration may lead to venous thrombosis and long-term sequelae if cerebral veins are involved. Infants so afflicted develop convulsions and a full fontanelle may confuse the clinical picture of dehydration.

Electrolyte depletion

Assessment of electrolyte status requires an appraisal of degree of dehydration or overhydration and serum electrolyte levels together with a knowledge of the likely losses and shifts between extracellular and intracellular fluids in particular diseases as described later in this chapter.

In patients with a sodium deficit, the serum sodium can be used to calculate the approximate amount of sodium required to correct the deficit. Sodium is distributed throughout a volume greater than the extracellular fluid and the total exchangeable pool of sodium (at the concentration of plasma sodium) is about 0.6 litres per kilogram (60%) of bodyweight. Thus the amount of sodium required to restore the plasma concentration to normal (135 mmol/l) in a depleted patient can be calculated from the formula:

dNa^+ $= (135 - [Na^+] \times 0.6 \times b.w.$

Where, dNa^+ = deficit of sodium or amount required (mmol)

135 = the desired sodium concentration (mmol/l)

$[Na^+]$ = the observed sodium concentration (mmol/l)

b.w. = the bodyweight in kg

$0.6 \times b.w.$ = the sodium distribution volume (litres).

Problem: a 10 kg child presenting with mild dehydration has a serum $[Na^+]$ of 120 mmol/l. What is the total sodium deficit in this child?

The child has dehydration, so the low serum $[Na+]$ reflects a sodium deficit rather than haemodilution from overhydration. Therefore, the above formula can be applied. The sodium deficit per litre of plasma is $135 - 120 = 15$ mmol/l. This sodium is distributed through a volume of $0.6 \times 10 = 6$ litres. Therefore, the total serum deficit is $15 \times 6 = 90$ mmol.

Treatment of dehydration

When mild dehydration occurs with less than 5% of the bodyweight lost, oral replacement of the deficit will usually be possible. If physical signs of dehydration are present (> 5% b.w. loss) rehydration is best achieved by the intravenous route. A clinically dehydrated child requires urgent admission to hospital and an intravenous line established. The rate of administration and the total amount of water required is calculated by adding the following volumes:

1. Volume to replace the estimated deficit (calculated from the bodyweight and the estimated percentage weight loss).

2. Volume to provide for normal maintenance (see Table 51.2).

3. Volume to replace continuing abnormal losses during treatment.

The total volume of water required is usually calculated and given over about 24 hours. The type of intravenous fluid used depends on the deficit of salt, potassium and bicarbonate which in turn depends on the cause of the dehydration. Generally the volume deficit is replaced with a fluid containing an electrolyte content similar to extracellular fluid $[Na^+]$ i.e. about 140 mmol/l, the maintenance volume is given as fluid with a sodium concentration 20–40 mmol/l and the continuing losses are met with a fluid of electrolyte content similar to the estimated loss (e.g. diarrhoeal fluid contains 40–80 mmol/l of sodium). Replacement of continuing losses is most accurately achieved by measuring the volume and electrolyte concentration of the lost fluid but an estimate can usually be made of the likely volume of diarrhoeal stools without accurate assessment.

Problem: a 10 kg baby presents with gastroenteritis and physical signs suggesting 10% weight loss. Serum $[Na^+] = 140$ mmol/l. What is the volume and type of fluid required to correct the dehydration?

Fluid required to:

1. Correct volume deficit (10% of 10 kg = 1 litre of fluid with [Na^t] = 130 mmol/l.
2. Provide for maintenance (100 ml/kg/day) = 1 litre of fluid with [Na$^+$] = 20 mmol/l.
3. Replace continuing daily loss (estimated 400 ml = 0.4 litres of [Na$^+$] = 80 mmol/l.

The total volume required is 2.4 litres. The mean [Na$^+$] of the fluid required is 80 mmol/l. Therefore, the fluid used would contain [Na$^+$] = 80 mmol/l and would be infused at the rate of 100 ml/h over 24 hours.

Types of intravenous fluids

Table 51.3 shows some of the intravenous solutions in common use. Isotonic saline contains 9 g of sodium chloride per litre (0.9% saline), equivalent to 156 mmol/l, which is slightly above the normal plasma sodium level. Half-isotonic, quarter-isotonic, and fifth-isotonic saline solutions are made at least isotonic to plasma by the addition of glucose in varying concentration. 5% glucose solution is isotonic to plasma. 0.18% saline, which contains 30 mmol of sodium and chloride per litre, will provide slightly more than maintenance requirements of sodium (2 mmol/kg) if given at the maintenance rate of 100 ml/kg/day.

Potassium for addition to intravenous fluids is best used as the molar solution, i.e. 1 mmol/ml, although other preparations are available. Potassium is often added to intravenous fluids at a concentration of 20–40 mmol/l to meet the daily requirements of about 2 mmol/kg, but if a severe deficit requires urgent correction, the infusion rate should not exceed 0.5 mmol/kg an hour. Hyperkalaemic cardiac arrest may result from excessively rapid potassium infusion.

Sodium bicarbonate is available usually as an 8.4% solution which is molar (1 mmol/ml). Note that isotonic saline (0.9%) is about one-sixth molar (0.156 mol/l) but

Table 51.3 Intravenous solutions in common use

IV Solutions	Sodium (mmol/l)	Chloride (mmol/l)	Glucose (g/100 ml)
Isotonic saline (0.9%) ('Normal' saline)	156	156	0
0.45% saline ('Half-normal' saline)	78	78	2.5 or 5
0.22% saline ('Quarter-normal' saline)	39	39	5
0.18% saline ('Fifth-normal' saline)	30	30	4
5% dextrose	0	0	5

preparations of molar sodium chloride (6%) are available as well as solutions of 0.5 mol/l (3%) and 3.3 mol/l (20%) saline.

The fluid management of some common conditions

Gastroenteritis

The principles used to calculate the volume of fluid required to correct the deficit in a dehydrated patient have already been outlined. Fluid with a sodium concentration about 80 mmol/l is most suitable and, because there is usually a bicarbonate deficit as well, this fluid is prepared by adding 40 mmol of sodium bicarbonate to 1 litre of quarter-isotonic (0.22%) saline. Rehydration is achieved over 12–24 hours except in patients with hypernatraemia, in whom it is best to restore hydration over 36–48 hours to avoid sudden osmolality changes which could precipitate cerebral oedema and fitting.

Hypertrophic pyloric stenosis

This disease presents with vomiting in the first weeks of life leading to loss of water, hydrogen ion and chloride ion so that dehydration with hypochloraemia and metabolic alkalosis occur. Potassium depletion occurs because of diminished intake and renal wasting of potassium as the kidneys attempt to conserve hydrogen ion. Serum electrolyte assessment is mandatory in all patients with pyloric stenosis and most cases will need intravenous fluids before pyloromyotomy.

In the dehydrated baby with serious electrolyte disturbance the calculated volume deficit is replaced as isotonic (0.9%) saline and maintenance fluid requirement continued with quarter-isotonic (0.22%) saline until operation. Potassium chloride (30–40 mmol/l) is administered as soon as urine flow is established. In the less severely affected infant half-isotonic (0.45%) saline with potassium chloride will suffice to replace the fluid deficit. Thus, the chloride deficit is replaced as a mixture of sodium chloride and potassium chloride and the potassium given allows renal conservation of hydrogen ion to correct the alkalosis.

Problem: a 3 kg infant with pyloric stenosis has dehydration with signs of 10% bodyweight loss. Serum [Na$^+$] = 133 mmol/l, [K$^+$] 2.5 mmol/l, [Cl$^-$] 70 mmol/l, [HCO$_3^-$] 38 mmol/l. What is the appropriate fluid management?

The volume deficit of 10% or 3 kg, or 300 ml, is replaced with isotonic saline (with 40 mmol/l of potassium chloride once urine is passed) over the first 12 hours. As the baby has lost 10% of his weight he may be verging on shock so that the first 60 ml of the infusion is given rapidly followed by slow infusion to correct the deficit. The whole day's maintenance fluid requirement (300 ml) is then given as quarter-isotonic (0.22%) saline with 40 mmol/l of potassium chloride over the remainder of the first 24 hours.

Shock

Shock is a state of inadequate perfusion of vital organs and is characterized by a rapid weak pulse and hypotension. Poor skin perfusion leads to cold, clammy extremities.

Shock may result from hypovolaemia (e.g. dehydration, blood loss, plasma loss), from vasodilation with venous pooling (e.g. septicaemia, endotoxaemia, asphyxia, poisoning) or from impaired cardiac output (cardiogenic shock). Shock due to hypovolaemia or vasodilation requires rapid intravenous infusion to restore tissue perfusion and the type of fluid used depends on the cause, e.g. blood loss is replaced with whole blood, fluid loss from extensive burns is treated with plasma, and dehydration is corrected with saline solutions. It is essential that the fluids used for rapid infusion have an electrolyte composition similar to that of normal plasma.

The amount of fluid required will be determined by the immediate responses of the patient but about 20 ml/kg can be rapidly infused without risk to restore the circulation. This volume, 20 ml/kg, can be compared with the normal blood volume of 80 ml/kg.

Diabetes mellitus

See Chapter 57.

Acute oliguric renal failure

Acute oliguric renal failure is present when the kidneys are unable to excrete the water and electrolytes needed to keep the body content normal. In practice this occurs if the urine output is less than about 250 ml/m^2 a day. Acute oliguric renal failure may be the result of reduced renal perfusion from hypovolaemia due to shock (prerenal causes of renal failure), to renal parenchymal disease affecting glomeruli (e.g. poststreptococcal glomerulonephritis, haemolytic-uraemic syndrome) or tubules (acute tubular necrosis), or to obstruction to the flow of urine (postrenal causes of renal failure).

Causes of renal failure leading to poor renal perfusion clearly need treatment with urgent replacement of fluid as in the treatment of shock. Intravenous frusemide, 2 mg/kg, often helps restore the urine output. In other types of renal failure it is clearly necessary to restrict

water and electrolyte intake in order to prevent these accumulating in the patient. It is best to give no salt or potassium at all except in the rare patient who has a clear-cut deficiency at presentation. Water is restricted to no more than the net insensible loss of 300 ml/m^2/day plus the volume of any urine passed provided the patient is not oedematous and water overloaded. If water overload is present restriction of water intake to less than the daily losses will allow correction of the overload and the patient will lose weight.

Due to reduced caloric intake the oliguric patient is in a state of tissue catabolism, and intracellular fluid contents are released into the extracellular compartment resulting in a rise in serum concentrations of potassium, magnesium, phosphorus and hydrogen. Water released from cells produces haemodilution, with a fall in concentrations of serum sodium and calcium. Thus acute oliguric renal failure leads to hyperkalaemia and hyponatraemia largely as a result of tissue catabolism. These serum abnormalities are very likely to be present after 24 hours of anuria.

When hyperkalaemia of any degree occurs in a patient with established oliguric renal failure dialysis is indicated as, even if mild, the electrolyte disturbance is likely to worsen and more conservative measures to lower serum potassium are usually of only temporary benefit. However, if cardiac arrhythmia is present in a patient with hyperkalaemia then intravenous glucose, bicarbonate and calcium should be given urgently to allow time for dialysis to remove potassium and correct the hyperkalaemia. Dosages used are 2 ml/kg of 50% glucose, 2 mmol/kg of sodium bicarbonate and 0.5 ml/kg of 10% calcium gluconate. Peritoneal dialysis with potassium-free dialysate is then commenced.

Disorders of antidiuretic hormone secretion (diabetes insipidus and inappropriate secretion of ADH)

ADH causes water retention by rendering the collecting ducts permeable to water. Lack of ADH leads to water loss from the kidneys and the clinical condition is called diabetes insipidus. The loss of water is not accompanied by electrolyte loss as the urine is very dilute and, therefore, an increase in electrolyte concentration in plasma and extracellular fluids occurs. Thus diabetes insipidus is associated with dehydration and hypernatraemia. Treatment of diabetes insipidus caused by pituitary disease involves replacement of ADH, which is most conveniently given as intranasal desmopressin (DDAVP).

ADH is normally secreted in response to a low plasma volume or a high plasma osmolality. The volume receptors are in the left atrium and the osmoreceptors are in the hypothalamus. In certain diseases these receptors malfunction leading to inappropriate secretion of ADH which causes renal water retention, dilution of plasma sodium and, possibly, hypertension. This syndrome is seen commonly in meningitis and other intracranial disorders, but also is induced by drugs, e.g. vincristine or artificial ventilation, when the atrial volume receptors are affected by the abnormal intrathoracic pressure. The finding of hyponatraemia in a patient with one of these conditions should lead to a suspicion of inappropriate ADH secretion which is confirmed by finding an overhydrated patient with a high urine osmolality and urinary sodium concentration.

Restriction of water to submaintenance volumes is usually all that is required for the treatment of inappropriate ADH secretion but occasionally the condition causes cerebral oedema and convulsions. In this situation administration of frusemide and salt may be needed to rapidly correct the fluid overload.

Disturbance of acid-base balance

Disturbed hydrogen ion metabolism is very often associated with fluid and electrolyte imbalance. Acidosis implies that hydrogen ion is present in abnormally high quantities in the plasma and this is expressed as a low plasma pH. Acids are substances capable of ionizing to produce free hydrogen ion and, in physiological systems, two types of acid are of importance. These are carbonic acid, formed from carbon dioxide in water, and metabolic or non-volatile acids which are generated in metabolic pathways. Hence, two types of acidosis are recognized in pathological conditions – respiratory acidosis and metabolic acidosis.

Metabolic acidosis (pH <7.35,[HCO_3^-] <18 mmol/l, base excess negative)

In this condition hydrogen ions are partly buffered by combining with blood bases, particularly bicarbonate which becomes depleted so that low plasma bicarbonate concentration is characteristic of metabolic acidosis. The blood pCO_2 falls because of respiratory stimulation, thereby blowing off CO_2 and lowering the blood carbonic acid. This loss of carbonic acid tends to compensate for the accumulation of metabolic acid. Metabolic acidosis may result from increased production of metabolic acids as in diabetes mellitus and anoxic states, or from bicarbonate loss in diarrhoeal stools, or from failure of renal acid excretion.

Bicarbonate is not, however, the only buffer base in blood, as the basic forms of phosphate and protein also contribute to the ability of the blood to neutralize excess

hydrogen ion – that is, to buffer hydrogen. Thus the total base deficit is usually slightly greater than the depletion of plasma bicarbonate. The base deficit is expressed as a negative base excess.

A mild degree of metabolic acidosis needs no therapy as it undergoes spontaneous reversal once the concomitant fluid and electrolyte imbalance is corrected. In moderate and severe acidosis bicarbonate replacement will usually be necessary. The amount required can be calculated from the volume of the extracellular fluid (0.3 × bodyweight) and the base deficit in each litre of plasma. Thus:

$$\text{millimoles of bicarbonate required} =$$
$$0.3 \times \text{bodyweight in kg} \times \text{base deficit.}$$

This equation gives only approximate requirements and caution is advised, as often associated measures also aid correction of the acidosis, e.g. insulin or fluid replacement. To avoid lowering serum potassium it is suggested that no more than half the calculated amount be given immediately as molar (8.4%) sodium bicarbonate (1 mmol/ml) and the remainder infused slowly over several hours with careful monitoring of serum potassium levels.

Metabolic alkalosis (pH > 7.43,[HCO_3^-] 25 mmol/l, base excess positive)

This condition arises from excessive loss of hydrochloric acid as in pyloric stenosis or from potassium deficiency as in diuretic therapy. In potassium deficiency, hydrogen ion moves intracellularly to replace the potassium and is also lost in the urine because of distal tubular hydrogen secretion in exchange for reabsorbed sodium. Treatment of metabolic alkalosis involves correction of the dehydration with fluids containing adequate amounts of sodium chloride and, in addition, the provision of potassium chloride, so that distal tubules can secrete potassium and conserve hydrogen in exchange for reabsorbed sodium. Often 3–6 mmol of potassium per kg of bodyweight will be required over 24 hours.

Respiratory acidosis (pH < 7.35, pCO_2 raised)

Carbonic acid accumulates when pulmonary ventilation is inadequate. This is reflected in a high blood partial pressure of carbon dioxide (pCO_2) which occurs only in pulmonary alveolar hypoventilation. Thus a high pCO_2 causing an acidosis is referred to as a respiratory acidosis. The kidneys then attempt to correct the acidosis by retaining buffer base, in particular bicarbonate, which combines with and lowers the abnormally high hydrogen concentration. The high pCO_2 can only be corrected by improving alveolar ventilation by, for example, artificial respiration. As patients with respiratory acidosis often have associated hypoxia there is often a metabolic acidosis as well and these cases have a bicarbonate deficit with a negative base excess.

Respiratory alkalosis (pH >7.43, pCO_2 <35 mmHg)

Respiratory alkalosis arises from hyperventilation and consequent blowing off of carbon dioxide. It is seen in hysteria and stimulation of the respiratory centre by, for example, salicylate poisoning. Treatment is directed at the cause of the respiratory stimulation.

FURTHER READING

Robinson J T 1975 Fundamentals of acid-base regulation. Blackwell, Oxford

Smith H W 1962 Principles of renal physiology. Oxford University Press, New York

Winters R W 1973 The body fluids in pediatrics. Little Brown, Boston

52. Urinary tract malformations and infection

Andrew R. Rosenberg

Urinary tract malformations are often associated with urinary tract infection. While many malformations cause little trouble some lead to chronic renal failure in childhood and some have genetic implications.

ABNORMALITIES OF RENAL DEVELOPMENT

Renal agenesis

Bilateral renal agenesis (complete absence of kidneys) is rare. The diagnosis is often made by antenatal ultrasound. Babies with this condition have a characteristic facial appearance (beaked nose, misshapen and low-set ears) and positional defects of the extremities (talipes, dislocated hips). This is known as Potter's syndrome and is related to severe maternal oligohydramnios, which in turn is caused by a lack of fetal urine. There is also pulmonary hypoplasia and consequently severe respiratory distress is often present. Babies survive for only a few days.

Unilateral renal agenesis is much more common and, so long as the contralateral kidney is normal, is compatible with a normal life span. The diagnosis is often made incidentally and is sometimes first noted at postmortem. Children should probably avoid contact sports.

Renal dysplasia

Renal dysplasia is a developmental abnormality. Cysts of varying size are found in the kidney and there is abnormal tissue such as cartilage and smooth muscle. It may be associated with other anomalies of the urinary tract such as posterior urethral valves. If both kidneys are involved, chronic renal failure may develop.

Unilateral dysplastic kidneys may be very large and present in the newborn period as an abdominal mass (a multicystic dysplastic kidney). This is the single most common cystic disorder in the newborn. It is often visualized on antenatal ultrasound and may be difficult to distinguish from a hydronephrotic kidney. The contralateral kidney is usually normal.

Cystic renal disease

Only three of the many varieties of cystic disease will be discussed here.

Infantile polycystic kidney disease (Fig 52.1).

There is dilatation of collecting ducts to form sausage-shaped cysts. The disease is bilateral and, because its severity is variable, it may present at any time during

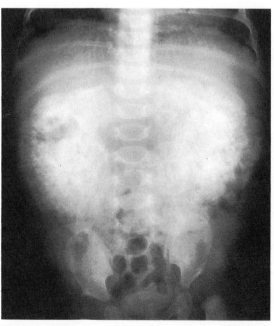

Fig. 52.1 Intravenous pyelogram in a neonate with infantile polycystic kidney disease. Note massively enlarged kidneys, palpable at birth, with characteristic 'streaky' appearance peripherally.

430

childhood. Children who are most severely affected present in the neonatal period with grossly enlarged kidneys and may die early because of respiratory distress related to pulmonary hypoplasia. Less severely affected children tend to develop hypertension in early childhood and often have slowly progressive chronic renal failure. Congenital hepatic fibrosis is always present and portal hypertension eventually develops in a small number. Infantile polycystic kidney disease is transmitted in an autosomal recessive fashion and subsequent children therefore are at a 1 in 4 risk of being affected.

Treatment includes antihypertensive therapy and management of progressive chronic renal failure. Dialysis and renal transplantation are often necessary in older children.

Adult polycystic kidney disease

This is a different disorder. It is inherited in an autosomal dominant fashion, is characterized by cysts not only in the kidneys but also in the liver and pancreas and characteristically leads to renal failure in middle age. However, it does sometimes present in childhood.

Medullary cystic diseases (also known as juvenile nephronophthisis)

Medullary cystic disease is usually inherited in an autosomal recessive fashion. It is one of the most common causes of end-stage renal failure in childhood. Presentation is between the ages of 3 and 7 years with growth failure, anaemia, polyuria and polydipsia. Characteristically the urinary sediment is normal and hypertension occurs late in the disease. Dialysis and transplantation are usually required by the age of 10 to 12 years.

Urinary tract obstruction

Congenital obstruction may occur at various sites along the urinary tract: at the junction of the renal pelvis and ureter, at the ureterovesical junction and at the level of the bladder outlet. Many of these abnormalities can be detected by antenatal ultrasound. Surgical intervention during fetal life, however, has generally not been successful and remains, at best, an experimental procedure.

Pelviureteric junction obstruction (Fig 52.2)

This obstruction is usually due to an area of aperistalsis secondary to an intrinsic abnormality of the muscle bundle at the junction of the pelvis and the ureter often associated with an overlying renal artery. It may be

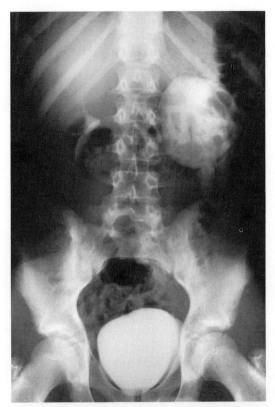

Fig. 52.2   Intravenous pyelogram in a child with left-sided pelviureteric junction obstruction. Note the dilated renal pelvis on the left. The right kidney is normal.

diagnosed in utero by antenatal ultrasound examination or may present in the newborn period as a palpable abdominal mass. In older children it may give rise to urinary infection or to haematuria and loin pain. The treatment is surgical correction (pyeloplasty).

Primary obstructive megaureter

This is less common. It is often diagnosed following urinary infection and the treatment is also surgical.

Posterior urethral valves (Fig. 52.3)

These are the most common cause of anatomical bladder outlet obstruction in boys. The kidneys are often affected by back pressure. Age at presentation is variable. Newborn babies may present with abdominal distension and dribbling or retention of urine. Older children often develop sepsis or failure to thrive. The diagnosis is made on micturating cystourethrography. The valves can be ablated surgically. Complex surgical reconstruction of the urinary tract is often necessary.

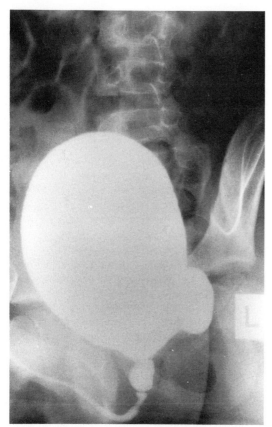

Fig. 52.3 Micturating cystourethrogram in an infant with posterior urethral valves. Note saccule of the bladder. There is dilatation of the urethra promixal to the valves. Vesicoureteric reflux is not present.

Neurogenic bladder

Neurogenic bladder is commonly found in association with spina bifida and myelomeningocele. The bladder is usually large and does not empty completely. The aim of current management is to keep the bladder drained and thereby prevent damage to the kidneys; this is usually done by intermittent catheterization.

Calculi in the urinary tract

These are rare in childhood and are usually radio-opaque. The most common cause is infection (particularly with Proteus organisms) associated with vesicoureteric reflux. The diagnosis of cystinuria should also be considered; this is an autosomal recessive disorder leading to the formation of calculi containing cystine. Treatment includes urinary alkalinization, high fluid intake and, rarely, the use of chelating agents such as d-penicil-

lamine. Other causes of calculi include hyperoxaluria and hyperparathyroidism, but these are very rare.

Children usually present with renal colic, loin pain, haematuria or urinary tract infection. The finding of a stone is an indication for full metabolic and radiological assessment.

The recent availability of lithotripsy (sound wave destruction of stones) has meant that not all children have to be subjected to surgery.

Duplication of the kidneys

Duplication of the kidneys can be total or incomplete and is not necessarily symptomatic. In total duplication there are two distinct ureters; the ureter from the upper pole of the kidney drains to a site distal to the drainage site of the ureter from the lower pole of the kidney. The upper pole ureter may drain to a site outside the bladder and give rise to incontinence or may be obstructed at its distal end (ureterocele). The lower pole ureter has an increased tendency to reflux.

Prune belly syndrome (Fig. 52.4)

This is rare, sporadic and occurs virtually only in boys. The syndrome comprises hypoplasia of the muscles of the anterior abdominal wall giving rise to laxity and a wrinkled, prune-like appearance, bilateral undescended testes and a variable degree of urinary tract dilatation which, in some cases, is very severe. Kidney failure may develop later in childhood.

URINARY TRACT INFECTION AND VESICOURETERIC REFLUX

There are few areas in clinical paediatrics as important as the proper diagnosis and management of children with urinary tract infection.

Clinical presentation

Urinary tract infection in childhood is frequently either missed or misdiagnosed because of a lack of appreciation of the symptomatology. Symptoms of urinary tract infection are often non-specific and the younger the child the more likely is this to be true. Neonates and infants may present with failure to thrive, poor feeding, vomiting, diarrhoea or even symptoms related to the central nervous system. Some neonates develop jaundice and septicaemia. Older children are more likely to have specific symptoms such as fever, loin pain and tenderness, dysuria and urinary frequency.

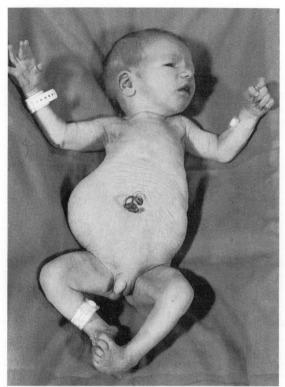

Fig. 52.4 Newborn boy with prune belly syndrome. Note the characteristic wrinkled appearance of the abdomen. Both testes are undescended.

Epidemiology

Normal bowel flora are responsible for most urinary tract infections with *Escherichia coli* causing 80%, followed by *Klebsiella*, *Pseudomonas* and other Gram-negative organisms. Gram-positive bacteria are not commonly found. Girls are much more likely to develop urinary tract infection than boys (at least 10:1); this applies throughout all ages except the newborn period, when the reverse is true. It is thought that, in most cases, urinary tract infection occurs as the result of bacteria gaining access to the bladder via the urethra. Only rarely, particularly in babies, is urinary tract infection thought to be blood borne.

Urinary tract infection is not at all uncommon in childhood. Approximately 5% of all girls have had at least one episode of bacteriuria by the age of 18 years.

Diagnosis

The diagnosis can only be made by bacteriological culture of a properly collected specimen of urine. It should be noted that routine dipstick urinalysis cannot diagnose urine infection even if proteinuria and haematuria are demonstrated. Similarly, urine microscopy alone is insufficient for the diagnosis. On the one hand, only 50% of children with urinary infection have pyuria, and on the other, pyuria does not necessarily indicate urinary infection.

Methods of urine collection

In most cases the vulval area should be cleaned with normal saline.

Midstream specimen. Bladder urine is normally sterile but can be contaminated by organisms present in the urethra. The first few millilitres of voided urine wash away these organisms so that a mid-stream specimen should not be contaminated by them. It is accepted that the presence of 100 000 bacteria/ml (or more) indicates urinary infection, so long as the growth is of a single organism. A mixed growth strongly suggests vulval contamination. A growth of 10 000 bacteria/ml (or less) indicates that the urine is sterile. Growth of an intermediate number of organisms (10 000 to 100 000/ml) should not be taken as evidence of infection but a further specimen of urine should be collected. In children who are continent and can void on request, a midstream specimen is ideal for diagnosing urinary infection. Even in children who are too young to void on request (under the age of 3 years) it is often possible to collect a mid-stream specimen by spreading the legs and waiting until spontaneous voiding occurs (clean catch specimen).

Bag urine specimens. Although used very commonly it should be noted that bag urine specimens are frequently contaminated. This technique is, therefore, suitable only for excluding urinary tract infection by the finding of a growth of less than 10 000 organisms/ml. If a colony count of more than 10 000 organisms/ml is obtained it is not possible to distinguish between contamination and true urinary infection.

Suprapubic aspiration of urine. This is the most accurate way of collecting urine for confirmation of infection in children aged less than 2 years; it is safe and relatively simple. It is performed when the child has not voided for at least 1 hour. After skin preparation, a 23 gauge needle attached to a syringe is inserted vertically just above the pubic symphysis with steady suction being applied until urine is obtained. Because bladder urine should be totally sterile, the presence of any organisms on culture indicates infection.

Catheter urine specimen. This technique is not recommended for routine use and should only be performed in rare cases where there has been failure to obtain urine by suprapubic aspiration.

The method of urine collection will depend upon the clinical situation. In children over 3 years, mid-stream collection will generally be used. In children under 3 years the clean catch method or suprapubic aspiration should be carried out, unless the clinical suspicion of urinary infection is low in which case a bag urine specimen can be collected. Should the bag urine specimen contain more than 10 000 organisms/ml, a suprapubic aspiration of urine or clean catch will usually be required. If, however, the child is toxic and ill, a suprapubic aspiration should be carried out before commencing antibiotic therapy.

In all cases the urine specimen should either be taken directly to the laboratory or refrigerated, as room temperature encourages the growth of organisms and makes subsequent interpretation impossible. The urine should be examined with a microscope; the identification of bacteria, while it does not necessarily distinguish significant infection from contamination, certainly suggests the former. The final proof must await the results of culture.

Treatment of urinary infection

Oral antibiotics are the treatment of choice for most children. Parenteral therapy is only indicated if the child is very sick or in infants. Amoxycillin or co-trimoxazole are commonly given for a week; sometimes the antibiotic has to be changed depending on the sensitivity of the cultured organism. In the case of children with their first episode of urinary infection, a low dose of an antibiotic such as co-trimoxazole should be given as prophylaxis against further infection until vesicoureteric reflux or some other urinary tract abnormality has been ruled out.

VESICOURETERIC REFLUX (Fig. 52.5)

This is the abnormal backflow of urine from the bladder into the ureter and the kidney, and should be suspected in all children who have suffered urinary tract infection. The major clinical concern regarding vesicoureteric reflux is the reflux of infected urine and its potential to cause scarring and destruction of the kidney (Fig 52.6). It is recognized that kidney damage, also known as reflux nephropathy, is most likely to occur in the first few years of life and that more than 10% of all patients with chronic kidney failure have reflux nephropathy. About 30% of children with urinary infection will be found to have vesicoureteric reflux, as will a significant number of their asymptomatic siblings.

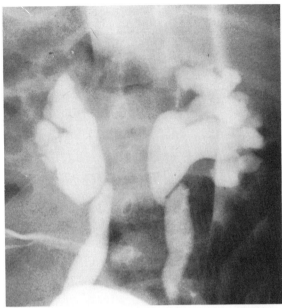

Fig. 52.5 Micturating cystourethrogram in a 12-month-old girl demonstrating bilateral grade 5 (gross) vesicoureteric reflux. Note the marked dilatation of ureters and pelvicalyceal systems.

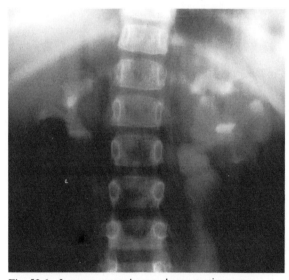

Fig. 52.6 Intravenous pyelogram demonstrating severe bilateral reflux nephropathy in a 3-year-old girl. There is marked dilatation and clubbing of all the calyces, with thinning of the overlying renal parenchyma (distance from calyx to edge of kidney). Only the left upper pole is relatively normal. The right kidney is smaller than the left. This patient might well progress to chronic renal failure in later childhood.

Investigation

All children with proven urinary infection should undergo investigation, not only to determine the presence of vesicoureteric reflux but also to determine whether there is some other abnormality such as pelviureteric junction obstruction, obstructive megaureter or duplication of the kidneys. There is no rationale for deferring investigation until the second infection.

Commonly used modalities of investigation are:

Micturating cystourethrogram (MCU)

The bladder is filled with either radiocontrast or radioisotope material via a urethral catheter. The diagnosis of vesicoureteric reflux is made by observing backflow of urine from the bladder into the ureter and kidney. The severity of vesicoureteric reflux is indicated by a reading system ranging from 1–5. Grade 1 is very mild, with reflux only into the lower end of the ureter, whereas grade 5 is very severe, with reflux all the way back to the kidney associated with gross distension and tortuosity of the ureter, as well as marked dilatation and clubbing of the calyces. The urethra is also delineated on MCU, and it is thus the ideal technique for diagnosing posterior urethral valves (see Fig. 52.3).

Intravenous pyelogram (IVP)

This technique (see Fig. 52.6) which outlines the kidneys and ureters, is used to determine whether there is reflux nephropathy or other abnormalities of the renal tract.

Renal isotope scan

The renal parenchyma can be outlined very accurately with certain radioisotopes (Fig. 52.7). Even small scars can be detected in this way.

Renal ultrasound

This technique has the advantage of being non- invasive and simple. It is sensitive in the detection of pelvicalyceal dilatation but is not as reliable as other techniques in the diagnosis of vesicoureteric reflux or reflux nephropathy.

The choice of investigations in the child with urinary tract infection will depend on the age of the child and the local expertise available. A commonly accepted procedure is to perform micturating cystography a few weeks after the episode of infection. If no vesicoureteric

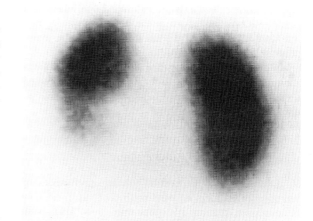

Fig. 52.7 Renal radioisotope (DMSA) scan showing obvious scar at lower pole of right kidney. The left kidney is normal.

reflux is found, a renal ultrasound is carried out; if reflux is present, an IVP is done. Isotope scan is usually reserved for subsequent investigation in complex cases.

Management

Children with normal kidneys and no vesicoureteric reflux do not require further treatment although about a quarter of them will develop further episodes of urinary infection. The infection, however, being confined to the bladder, will not cause any renal damage.

When vesicoureteric reflux is present, the aim of management is to control infection until reflux ceases, either spontaneously or with surgery. About 70% of children will spontaneously stop refluxing over a period of years; this is particularly relevant to mild and moderate reflux (grades 1–3), and is less true for severe reflux (grades 4 and 5). There is continuing dispute over the benefits of surgery, and it is usually reserved for these latter cases.

Non-surgical management is appropriate for the majority of children with vesicoureteric reflux. Prophylactic antibiotics are given long term until reflux ceases. Commonly used antibiotics are co-trimoxazole, nitrofurantoin and nalidixic acid. They are given once nightly in low dose, achieve high concentrations in the urine and do not affect bacterial growth in the gut. Their complication rate is low but possible side effects should be borne in mind. These include skin rashes and Stevens-Johnson syndrome with co-trimoxazole, nausea and vomiting with nitrofurantoin and photosensitivity and benign intracranial hypertension with nalidixic acid.

Regular urine cultures should be carried out, and a high index of suspicion for the presence of a urinary tract infection whenever the child is unwell should be maintained.

Children whose kidneys are not extensively scarred are not at risk of kidney failure but do have an increased incidence of hypertension. Therefore, long-term follow-up should be maintained with blood pressure measurements every 6–12 months.

RENAL TUBULAR DISORDERS

In these disorders the normal tubular mechanisms of secretion and absorption are disturbed. Thus, there may be excessive sodium and potassium loss, leading to hyponatraemia and hypokalaemia, failure of normal renal acidification leading to a metabolic acidosis, failure of phosphate reabsorption leading to hypophosphataemia and rickets, or lack of the normal tubular concentrating mechanism leading to the production of an inappropriately dilute urine. These defects may be isolated or combined, and can be secondary to conditions such as polycystic kidney disease, reflux nephropathy or obstruction of the urinary tract.

A number of conditions with primary abnormalities of renal tubular function are also recognized.

Fanconi syndrome

This is a generalized disorder of renal tubular transport leading to glycosuria, generalized aminoaciduria, phosphaturia and metabolic acidosis. The clinical manifestations are polyuria, rickets and growth failure.

Cystinosis

This rare condition, which is inherited in an autosomal recessive fashion, is characterized by the deposition of cystine in various organs, including renal tubular cells. Usually children present in the first year of life with Fanconi syndrome, and there is progression to renal failure during childhood. A drug called cysteamine may slow the progression of the disease.

Renal tubular acidosis

A number of the varieties of renal tubular acidosis exist, depending on whether the defect is in the proximal or distal tubule. Infants usually present with failure to thrive and episodes of vomiting. Oral bicarbonate replacement is the therapy of choice.

Nephrogenic diabetes insipidus

In this condition there is a lack of renal concentrating ability due to failure of the collecting duct to respond to circulating antidiuretic hormone. The infant commonly presents with polyuria, polydipsia and growth retardation and is found to have hypernatraemia with inappropriately dilute urine. The disease is usually inherited in a sex-linked dominant manner and is thus more severe in boys. Treatment includes a low solute diet, chlorothiazide and prostaglandin synthetase inhibitors such as indomethacin.

Primary hypophosphataemic rickets

Children with this condition present at about the age of one year with growth retardation and rickets. The condition is characterized by reduced tubular reabsorption of phosphate and is inherited as a sex-linked dominant. The treatment includes large doses of inorganic phosphate and vitamin D.

FURTHER READING

Burns M W, Burns J L, Krieger J N 1987 Paediatric urinary tract infection. The Pediatric Clinics of North America 34 (5): 1111–1120
Holliday M A, Barratt T M, Vernier R L (eds) 1987 Paediatric nephrology. Williams & Wilkins, Baltimore
Lerner G R, Fleischmann L E, Perlmutter A D 1987 Reflux nephropathy. The Pediatric Clinics of North America 34 (3): 747–770

53. Glomerulonephritis and related diseases Hypertension

John Burke

Glomerulonephritis presents with various clinical manifestations – nephrotic syndrome, acute nephritis, recurrent haematuria, isolated proteinuria or chronic renal failure. Most forms of glomerulonephritis result from an immunological mediated injury involving either deposition of circulating immune complexes in the glomerulus or a specific antibody to the glomerular basement membrane. The common form of nephrotic syndrome in children does not result from these pathogenic mechanisms but is now believed to result from an abnormality in cell-mediated immunity.

NEPHROTIC SYNDROME

Nephrotic syndrome is defined as oedema, proteinuria, hypoalbuminaemia and hyperlipidaemia. The annual incidence in children is approximately 2–4:100 000. The major pathological lesions in primary nephrotic syndrome are given in Example 53.1.

Example 53.1 Classification of primary nephrotic syndrome

Minimal change
Focal segmental glomerulosclerosis
Mesangial proliferative glomerulonephritis
Membrano-proliferative glomerulonephritis
Membranous glomerulopathy
Congenital nephrotic syndrome.

Minimal change nephrotic syndrome

Evidence now suggests the aetiology of minimal change nephrotic syndrome is caused by an alteration in the glomerular anionic status. Sensitized lymphocytes secrete a number of lymphokines that alter the normal negatively charged sialoproteins on the glomerular basement membrane. Loss of membrane negative change allows anionic proteins to leak across the basement membrane into Bowman's space. Light microscopy

shows normal glomeruli but in some cases a mild increase in mesangial cells and mesangial matrix may occur. Immunofluorescence is negative and electron microscopy shows fusion of foot processes.

Generalized oedema is the usual presenting symptom (Fig. 53.1). Minimal change lesion comprises 80% of

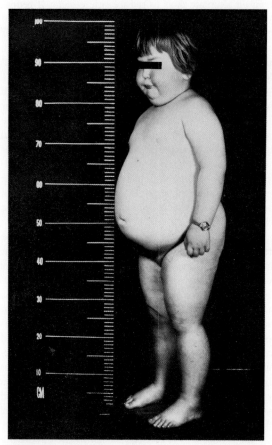

Fig. 53.1 Child with gross generalized oedema due to the nephrotic syndrome. Cushingoid features are obvious which suggests this child has steroid-resistant nephrotic syndrome.

437

cases of nephrotic syndrome without significant constitutional disturbance in childhood and is more frequent in males than females, the majority presenting between 1–4 years. Macroscopic haematuria is rare although 30% have microscopic haematuria. Blood pressure is normal and a renal biopsy is not indicated initially in a child presenting with nephrotic syndrome with normal renal function, normal blood pressure, absence of macroscopic haematuria, normal complement activity and a selective index showing a low molecular weight urinary protein loss.

Unless large pleural effusions, gross ascites, or severe genital oedema are present, strict bed rest is not necessary and the child should be allowed normal ward activity. A high protein, low salt diet is encouraged. Fluid intake should not be restricted because of the risk of hypovolaemia and a free intake is encouraged. Prednisolone 2 mg/kg/day or 60 mg/m^2/day induces a remission in 90% of cases. The prednisolone dose is then reduced over 2–3 months, with later doses being given on alternate days to reduce side effects. If remission, as defined by complete loss of proteinuria, has not occurred by four weeks, the nephrotic syndrome is steroid resistant and a renal biopsy is then indicated to exclude other pathology, particularly focal segmental glomerulosclerosis.

Approximately 70% of children have relapses which are more likely to occur in association with viral upper respiratory tract infections. These relapses may be prevented by prophylactic prednisolone 5mg given on alternate days. Cyclophosphamide 2.5–3 mg/kg/day for 8 weeks is indicated when steroid side effects with multiple relapses become significant. 50% of children given cyclophosphamide have no further relapses and most of the rest have substantially fewer episodes of nephrotic relapse.

The major complications of the nephrotic syndrome are infections, hypovolaemia, and thromboembolism. Both Gram-positive and negative organisms cause peritonitis and septicaemia. The susceptibility to infections is related to loss of opsonins and immunoglobulins in the urine. If the patient develops a serious infection, the initial antibiotic treatment should cover both Gram-positive and negative organisms until cultures and sensitivity results are available. Hypovolaemia which occurs in 5% should be suspected if such a child develops oliguria (100 ml per day), abdominal pain, tachycardia or postural hypotension. This complication is confirmed by a high haematocrit and a low urine sodium (< 10 mmol/l). Hypovolaemia is due to loss of plasma water into the tissues with a consequent fall in the circulating blood volume. The preferred treatment is intravenous 25% albumin (1 g/kg over 3–6 hours). Albumin infusion

may need to be repeated according to response. At the end of each infusion intravenous frusemide (2 mg/kg) is given.

A hypercoagulable state exists for a number of reasons. These include haemoconcentration and loss of anti-thrombin III in the urine. Renal vein thrombosis and pulmonary embolism are relatively rare occurrences which require prompt treatment with anticoagulants. The avoidance of bed rest and treatment of hypovolaemia probably accounts for the decreasing incidence of this complication.

Approximately 90% of children with relapsing nephrotic syndrome cease relapsing by 16 years of age. Even those children who continue to relapse into adult life usually remain steroid sensitive. It is very rare for a child with steroid-sensitive minimal change lesion to progress to chronic renal failure. The 20-year mortality has now decreased from 60% to less than 5% since the introduction of antibiotics and corticosteroids. The morbidity and mortality should continue to decrease with adequate management of complications and avoidance of excess immunosuppression.

Focal segmental glomerulosclerosis

This glomerulopathy comprises 5–10% of children with nephrotic syndrome. The presentation is often similar to a minimal change lesion but with steroid resistance. Renal biopsy (Fig 53.2) shows segmental sclerosis or hyalinosis with other glomeruli completely sclerosed or normal. Immunofluorescence shows IgM and IgG in the affected segmental lesions.

As the majority of children are resistant to steroids and cyclophosphamide, cyclosporin is now being evaluated for this condition. Those children who remain nephrotic require treatment with diuretics (frusemide and spironolactone), mild fluid restriction and a low salt diet. Approximately 60% progress to end-stage renal failure over 10 years. This glomerulopathy has a 30% recurrence risk in a transplanted kidney.

Congenital nephrotic syndrome

Nephrotic syndrome in the first three months of life is most common in Finland where the pathology is described as microcystic disease. Other types with minimal lesion histology, diffuse mesangial sclerosis, or congenital syphilis are occasionally seen. The Finnish types are now seen in descendants of other European communities and the condition is inherited in an autosomal recessive fashion. Oedema is noted in the first weeks of life with placentomegaly and prematurity being common precursors. There is no specific treatment but

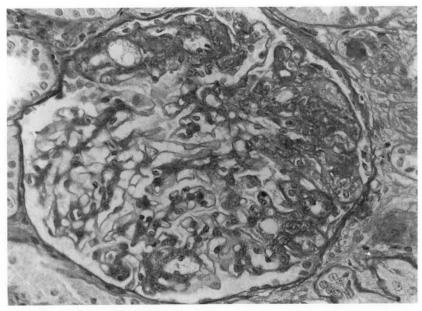

Fig. 53.2 Segmental sclerosis (PAS × 42)

transplantation can be considered if survival is longer than 18 months to 2 years. Elevated amniotic fluid alphafetoprotein, if the fetus is affected, allows prenatal diagnosis.

GLOMERULONEPHRITIS

Acute glomerulonephritis is defined as haematuria, proteinuria, oedema, hypertension and renal insufficiency. This acute onset is usually seen in post-streptococcal glomerulonephritis. Other forms of glomerulonephritis (Example 53.2) in childhood have a less severe onset.

Example 53.2 Causes of acute nephritis

Post-infectious glomerulonephritis
Henloch-Schönlein purpura
IgA nephropathy
Alport's syndrome
Lupus erythematosus

Post-streptococcal glomerulonephritis

This disorder follows 2–3 weeks after Group A haemolytic streptococcal throat or skin infection. Circulating antigen-antibody complexes form in the blood and deposit in glomeruli with activation of the complement system. The pathological appearance consists of proliferation of mesangial and endothelial cells with neutrophil infiltration. Crescents may be present. Immunofluoresence shows IgA and C3 and electron dense deposits are demonstrated by electron microscopy (Fig. 53.3).

The usual presentation is a child usually of school age, with macroscopic haematuria, oedema or headache caused by hypertension. Lassitude, fever and loin pain may also be present. Physical examination may reveal hypertension, papilloedema, facial and leg oedema. On laboratory investigation urinalysis shows red blood cell casts and dysmorphic red cells. Serum urea, creatinine and potassium are often elevated. Mild normocytic normochromic anaemia is common and indicates haemodilution is present.

The anti-streptolysin O titre (ASOT) and anti-streptococcal DNase B are elevated in 90% of cases. Serum levels of C3 complement are low and return to normal within 6–12 weeks. Complement C4 is low in the early stages of the disease.

Careful management of the acute renal failure and especially of the hypertension is the basis of treatment in this condition. Salt and water accumulation, with suppression of plasma renin, is the major cause of hypertension. Mild hypertension is best managed with frusemide 2–4 mg/kg/day and fluid restriction. Moderate to severe hypertension requires management with sublingual nifedipine, or oral prazosin. Parenteral hydralazine and diazoxide are rarely required. Beta-blockers should be avoided in the presence of

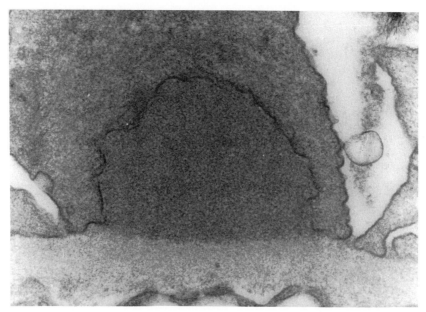

Fig. 53.3 EM demonstrating subepithelial hump in post-streptococcal glomerulonephritis (1 × 9 900).

pulmonary oedema. Bed rest is necessary only when the blood pressure is elevated. A course of oral penicillin for 5–7 days eradicates any existing streptococcal infection but does not alter the natural history of this condition. When renal insufficiency is present the diet consists of restricted protein (1 g/kg/day), low salt and potassium intake.

The major complications of acute post-streptococcal glomerulonephritis are hypertensive encephalopathy, left ventricular failure and acute renal failure. Hypertensive convulsions are often associated with papilloedema and a temporary cortical blindness. This complication is best treated by parenteral diazoxide 2–5 mg/kg followed by oral medication.

Acute heart failure is related to hypertension and fluid overload. Severe fluid restriction, high dose frusemide administration and adequate control of hypertension are then necessary.

The period of oliguria lasts up to 10 days and dialysis is indicated in cases where the blood urea rises above 50–60 mmol/l, or when hyperkalaemia or pulmonary oedema are not controlled by intravenous frusemide and fluid restriction. Dialysis should be performed only in a centre with the appropriate expertise. The long-term prognosis is excellent with only 1% developing chronic renal failure. Microscopic haematuria may continue for two years but proteinuria should clear within six months. Renal biopsy is not indicated unless there is uncertainty of diagnosis with the initial investigations or the period of oliguria lasts longer than three weeks.

Other infectious agents including viral and bacterial organisms can rarely produce an illness similar to post-streptococcal nephritis. These organisms include staphylococcus and pneumonococcus, echo-, Coxsackie- and Epstein-Barr viruses.

Henoch-Schönlein purpura

This disease presents with a petechial or purpuric rash, abdominal pain and arthritis. A mild nephritis is seen in 50–70% of cases, manifest usually by microscopic haematuria and proteinuria. Rarely blood pressure and serum creatinine are elevated. Renal histology shows a proliferative glomerulonephritis with IgA in the mesangium. The prognosis is good with only 1% developing chronic renal failure.

IgA disease (Berger's)

This glomerulopathy is present in 50% of children who have recurrent episodes of macroscopic haematuria. The episodes of haematuria often occur simultaneously with intercurrent viral infections and flank pain. Other presentations include abnormal urinalysis on medical examination and rarely chronic renal failure in childhood. The histology of focal proliferative glomerulonephritis with IgA in the mesangium is similar to that of Henoch-Schönlein purpura. In children very few develop chronic renal failure but this is more common in adults.

Alport's syndrome

This is a familial disorder inherited as an X-linked dominant or autosomal dominant. Males are more severely affected than females. In males this disorder presents in the first ten years of life with haematuria and proteinuria. Renal histology shows a proliferative glomerulonephritis with typical changes on electron microscopy. Renal failure develops in the teenage years. High tone nerve deafness and eye abnormalities are the other features of the syndrome.

Lupus erythematosus

Systemic lupus erythematosus in childhood is seen more in females in the later childhood years. Facial rash, arthritis and fever are common presenting symptoms. Renal biopsy is indicated if haematuria and proteinuria are present. Serum C3 complement is usually low. This disorder is discussed further in Chapter 73. The type of glomerulonephritis in SLE can vary from a mild focal proliferative glomerulonephritis to a diffuse crescentic glomerulonephritis with associated membranous features. The treatment includes prednisolone, azathioprine, cyclophosphamide and plasmapheresis and the amount of immunosuppression is dependent on severity of renal impairment, proteinuria and type of renal histology.

Benign microscopic haematuria

One in 200 children have intermittent microscopic haematuria as an incidental finding on urinalysis. This condition is usually benign providing there is no infection or proteinuria, renal function is normal and no structural abnormality is present on ultrasonography. Often inheritance is in an autosomal dominant fashion.

Postural proteinuria

Intermittent or orthostatic proteinuria occurs in 10% of children. Testing with albustix or timed 12-hourly urine collections shows a normal amount of urinary protein in the early morning and increased protein during the day. The 24-hour protein estimation can sometimes be as high as 300–400 mg/day. This phenomenon is benign but proteinuria in an overnight urine specimen will usually require biopsy to determine the cause.

Haemolytic uraemic syndrome (HUS)

This is an uncommon disorder being most common under the age of 3 years. Usually it follows a mild gastroenteritis but the diarrhoea is often blood stained.

Over the next few days the child becomes pale and oliguric and unwell. Examination of the blood film shows fragmented red blood cells and thrombocytopenia. Urinalysis reveals haematuria and proteinuria. The serum creatinine is usually elevated and hypertension is often severe.

The primary injury of HUS appears to be swelling of endothelial cells in arterioles and widening of the subendothelial space with fibrin deposition. The cause is unknown but recent evidence suggests a role for infection by verocytoxin-producing *Escherichia coli*, and reduced prostacyclin production.

Dialysis is often necessary in the management of acute renal failure. Management is complex and should only be undertaken by an expert in paediatric renal disease. 90% of children make a complete recovery. Bad prognostic signs are oliguria lasting over two weeks, cerebral involvement and age of onset over five years.

CHRONIC RENAL FAILURE

The incidence of chronic renal failure in children is 2–4 per million of total population per year. The commonest causes include chronic glomerulonephritis, reflux nephropathy, obstructive uropathy and medullary cystic disease. Identification of structural renal abnormalities by obstetric ultrasound and early investigation of urinary tract infections may decrease the incidence of renal failure in the future.

The principles of management are:

1. Control of hypertension (see page 442).
2. Adequate nutrition. Growth becomes impaired when glomerular filtration rate is less than 25% of normal/1.73 m^2. With this degree of renal impairment, hyperfiltration from a high solute intake can produce further sclerosis to the remaining functioning glomeruli. A low protein diet (1.2 g/kg/day) with low phosphate and adequate calorie intake may delay the progression of renal failure. Salt and fluid intake will vary with type of renal disease.
3. Prevention of renal osteodystrophy. Hyperphosphataemia should be vigorously treated with low phosphate diet and dietary phosphate binders (calcium carbonate or aluminium hydroxide), in an attempt to prevent secondary hyperparathyroidism. Vitamin D supplementation with calcitriol (1,25 dihydroxycholecalciferol) is now given in early renal failure.
4. Administration of alkali to control acidosis (2–3 mmol/kg/day).

Dialysis and transplantation are normally considered for children over two years of age with end-stage renal failure. Under this age there are considerable technical, ethical and psychological problems. Young children tolerate continuous ambulatory peritoneal dialysis (CAPD) better than haemodialysis. Both cadaver and live related transplants are performed in children with good results. Approximately 90% of children survive for at least five to ten years after entering dialysis-transplant programmes.

HYPERTENSION

The recording of blood pressure should be part of the normal examination in children. The blood pressure cuff should cover two-thirds of the upper arm as a smaller cuff will often lead to a falsely high reading. The child should be still and not crying. Using sphygmomanometry the diastolic component is probably best recorded by the 5th Korotkoff sound, but if difficulties arise in obtaining an accurate recording a machine using oscillometric techniques should be used.

Normal blood pressure for children varies with age (Fig. 53.4). A child should not be regarded as being hypertensive unless three recordings give levels above 95th percentile for that age group.

The major causes of hypertension are given in Example 53.3. Renal disease accounts for approximately 80% of cases.

The investigation of hypertension should commence with a good history and examination. Symptoms of

---

Example 53.3 Causes of hypertension

Renal
  1. Acute glomerulonephritis
  2. Chronic glomerulonephritis
  3. Reflux nephropathy
  4. Obstructive uropathy
  5. Haemolytic uraemic syndrome
  6. Polycystic kidneys
Coarctation of aorta
Renal artery stenosis
Phaeochromocytoma
Adrenogenital syndrome
Essential.

---

chronic renal disease include polyuria and polydipsia, enuresis and headaches. Hypertension in a parent or an early stroke in a relative may be a pointer to essential hypertension. Physical examination may assist in making a specific diagnosis – e.g. palpable renal mass, pigmentation, delayed femoral pulses and renal artery bruit.

Initial screening investigations will include examination of the urine for erythrocytes, proteinuria, infection, and estimation of serum creatinine and electrolyte levels. An ultrasound and DMSA (Tc-dimercaptosuccinic acid) scan of the kidneys will reveal scarring from reflux nephropathy. A DTPA (Tc-diethylene-triaminepentaacetic acid) renal scan will exclude an obstructive uropathy and is useful in renal artery stenosis. If renal artery stenosis is suspected further investigations with renal angiograms and renal vein renin ratio are necessary. In acute nephritis elevated ASOT and depressed C3 complement levels will establish a diagnosis of acute post-streptococcal glomerulonephritis. Estimation of urinary and plasma catecholamines could be a delayed investigation unless a phaeochromocytoma or neuroblastoma is suspected clinically as the incidence of phaeochromocytoma in childhood hypertension is only 1%. If a rare form of adrenogenital syndrome (11-hydroxylase or 17-hydroxylase deficiency) is suspected plasma and urine analyses are performed.

Treatment of hypertension depends on the severity, presence of symptoms and underlying cause. Severe hypertension is present if examination of the fundi, or chest radiograph and electrocardiograph are abnormal. In the acute hypertensive emergency situation, drugs with a rapid onset of action are needed (Example 53.4).

In essential hypertension observation only is indicated unless the diastolic blood pressure is 95 mmHg or more. Advice on a low salt diet, weight reduction and exercise may assist reduction in blood pressure. Intervention techniques such as transluminal angioplasty for renal

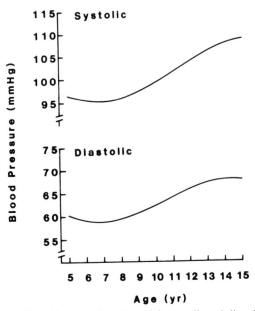

Fig. 53.4 Normal values (means) for systolic and diastolic blood pressure in children from 5 to 15 years.

Example 53.4 Drug therapy of hypertensive emergency	
Nifedipine	5–10 mg sublingual
Hydralazine	0.1–0.5 mg/kg IV or IM
Diazoxide	2–5 mg/kg IV
Minoxidil	2.5–5 mg oral
Sodium nitroprusside	0.5–10 mcg/kg/min IV
Frusemide	2 mg/kg IV
Labetolol	1–3 mg/kg/hr IV

artery stenosis, resection of coarctation of aorta, and nephrectomy for a small scarred kidney may cure a small percentage of children.

The drug treatment of chronic hypertension is similar to that of adult patients – drugs used include diuretics (chlorothiazide or frusemide), beta-adrenergic blockers (atenolol, metoprolol), vasodilators (hydralazine, prazosin), calcium channel inhibitors (nifedipine) and converting enzyme inhibitors (captopril, enalapril).

FURTHER READING

Cameron J S, Turner D R, Ogg C S et al 1980 The long term prognosis of patients with focal segmental glomerulosclerosis. Clinical Nephrology 10: 213–218

Niaudet P, Habib R, Tete M et al 1987 Cyclosporin in the treatment of idiopathic nephrotic syndrome in children. Paediatric Nephrology 1: 566–573

Nissenson A R, Mayor-White R, Potter E V et al 1979 Continued absence of clinical renal disease 7 to 12 years after post-streptococcal acute glomerulonephritis in Trinidad. American Journal of Medicine 67: 255

Postlethwaite R D (ed) 1986 Clinical Paediatric Nephrology. Wright, Bristol

Powell H R 1987 Haemolytic uraemic syndrome: new perspectives. Australian Paediatric Journal 23: 213–214

Roy L P, Tiller D J, Jones D L 1984 The range of blood pressures in Australian children. Medical Journal of Australia 141: 9–12

Task force on blood pressure control in children. Report on the second task force on blood pressure control in children – 1987. Paediatrics 79: 1–25

Trompeter R S, Hicks J, Lloyd B W et al 1985 Long term outcome for children with minimal change nephrotic syndrome. Lancet 1: 368–370

Endocrinology and metabolism

54. Growth

James Penfold

From the viewpoint of a casual observer, growth is seen as a natural increase in body size with age which usually reaches completion in late teenage years.

In reality the normal growth of a child is a highly complex phenomenon and involves the multiplication and differentiation of individual cells, which organize into specific organs, the integration of which results in the healthy human body. It is estimated that there are approximately 10^{14} cells present in the mature adult, each cell in many respects being a unique self-contained metabolic factory, often with widely differing functions, yet usually working in perfect harmony with its neighbours. Study of growth not only emcompasses study of change in body size, but also the study of change in function and maturation of tissues with age – so-called development.

Normal and abnormal physical growth may readily be recognized by simple comparisons of height and weight with known standards for age and sex. The study of normal and abnormal growth is facilitated by a knowledge of the effects of physiological and pathological processes on growth and development at three periods of life: (a) at conception with the formation of the genome; (b) in utero with its strong maternal influence and, finally, (c) during postnatal existence when the child is exposed to the external environment with its potential hazards.

Genetic influences

With the fusion of the nuclei of the sperm and ovum the genome contains genetic material from each parent and the blueprint for the future growth pattern of the child.

Although children's heights at maturity resemble those of their parents, little is known about the exact location of the individual height-controlling genes on the chromosomes, exactly how many genes are involved, or how they direct cellular growth. A gross disturbance of genetic complement, particularly when it involves the sex chromosomes, is often reflected in abnormal growth patterns, e.g with loss of a sex chromosome in 45XO Turner's syndrome, as shown in Figure 54.1, adult stature is severely compromised, while the addition of an extra sex chromosome in the XXY (Klinefelter), XYY and XXX syndromes frequently leads to adult height above that anticipated from the family pattern (Fig. 54.2).

Apparent single gene aberrations, either the result of direct inheritance or mutation, can result in unusual

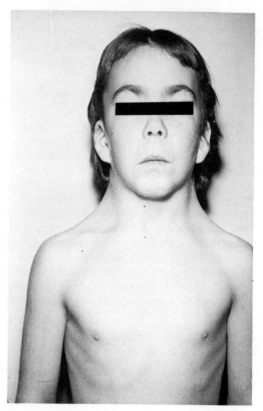

Fig. 54.1 Turner's syndrome. Note webbing of the neck.

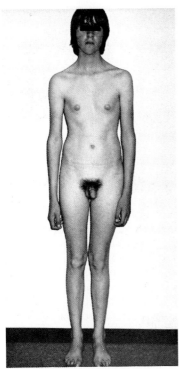

Fig. 54.2   Klinefelter syndrome. Note eunuchoid build and gynaecomastia.

growth disturbances, e.g the disproportionate short stature seen in achondroplasia, where the limbs are relatively shorter than the trunk. This is to be contrasted with the phenotype of Marfan's syndrome, also probably the result of a single gene abnormality, which is associated with disproportionate tall stature and an asthenic body build, the limbs being relatively longer than the trunk.

The reasons for the wide variations in stature within the normal population are unknown. There is some evidence that short children may produce less growth hormone than tall children (see Hormonal control of postnatal growth) but genetically transmitted variations in tissue response to hormonal stimuli probably also account for some of the extreme variations encountered e.g. the difference between the African pygmy and the unusually tall Masai tribesman.

Intrauterine influence on growth

In utero, the genome must be transcribed according to a strictly co-ordinated programme, the individual cells must be surrounded by the correct microenvironment, which is, in turn, dependent upon the close communication between the maternal and fetal circulation via the placenta.   Growth   promoting   hormones,   fetal somatomedins, and tissue inducers must be present at the correct concentrations and at exactly the right times during gestation and, finally, the individual cells must be responsive to these signals. No aspect of prenatal growth and development is better understood than the area of sex discrimination and differentiation. The general principles, which have been carefully worked out in this field, probably also apply to the growth and differentiation of other fetal tissues.

Usually, disturbances in utero lead to growth retardation, e.g. low birthweight babies are associated with congenital rubella infection, but occasionally there may be overgrowth of tissues resulting in macrosomia as seen in the fetus of a mother with poorly controlled diabetes mellitus. There is much evidence to suggest that the growth factors and hormones controlling fetal growth are unique to this period of life. At or around birth it is likely that fetal growth hormone, thyroid hormone, and postnatal somatomedins start to take control. It has been recognized for some time that infants born with prenatal growth hormone or thyroid hormone deficiency are not growth retarded at birth, a fact suggesting that these two hormones are not essential for normal fetal growth.

A list of factors which can lead to intrauterine growth retardation is given in Example 54.1. Some of these are discussed in more detail in Chapter 20 as they are frequent causes of growth failure in the first two years of life. In some children intrauterine growth failure may be irreversible, with failure of postnatal catch-up growth resulting in short adult stature.

Example 54.1 Causes of intrauterine growth retardation

Maternal malnutrition
Heavy smoking
Excess alcohol consumption
Caffeine ingestion
High altitude
Intrauterine infection (STORCH syndrome)
Chromosomal defects, e.g. trisomy 13–15
Dysmorphic syndromes of unknown aetiology, e.g.
    Russell-Silver dwarfism

Postnatal influences on growth

After birth, cellular growth depends primarily on the correct quantity and balance of food nutrients eaten, digested and absorbed from the gastrointestinal tract and transported via the circulation to the individual cell. The local cellular microenvironment must be maintained at the correct electrolyte concentration, pH, pO_2 and pCO$_2$ and the waste products of metabolism must be removed quickly before they build up to toxic levels. Thus, optimal postnatal growth depends on a normal diet and adequate function of the major systems including the gastrointestinal, cardiovascular, respiratory and renal. Postnatal control of growth appears to be through hormone signals which include growth hormone, thyroid hormone, insulin and polypeptide growth factors called somatomedins/insulin-like growth factors, which are partially under control of growth hormone.

HORMONAL CONTROL OF POSTNATAL GROWTH

Growth hormone

It has been known since 1920 that anterior pituitary lobe extracts contained a growth promoting factor. Subsequently, this 'growth hormone' (GH) has been shown to be a mixture of polypeptides in which the major physiological component is a single chain polypeptide of 191 residues with a molecular weight of 22kDa. Recently, GH has been synthesized in *Escherichia coli* bacteria and in mammalian cell lines, using recombinant DNA technology. This major breakthrough offers the promise of a relatively unlimited supply for treatment of children with GH deficiency.

Control of growth hormone secretion (Fig 54.3)

Although GH is the most abundant hormone in the human pituitary gland and its primacy in controlling postnatal somatic growth is unquestioned, there remain many unresolved questions concerning its physiological control and mechanism of action. Growth hormone is normally secreted in a pulsatile manner in response to hypothalamic releasing and inhibiting hormones, which reach the somatotrophes (GH secreting cells) via a portal circulation adjacent to the pituitary stalk. In normal children serum GH levels of greater than 20 μu/ml are found during sleep and following vigorous exercise and these observations have formed the basis of physiological tests for GH deficiency.

A positive correlation between a child's growth velocity and the sum of its serum GH peaks determined over a 24-hour period by blood sampling at 20-minute intervals has been noted. In other words, short children, who have become short by growing relatively slowly over a period of time, have a daily production of growth

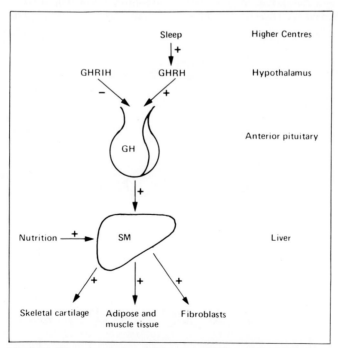

Fig. 54.3 The control of growth hormone (GH) secretion and its indirect mechanism of action on skeletal cartilage and other tissues through circulating somatomedin (SM) produced in the liver. (GHRH = GH releasing hormone; GHRIH = GH release inhibiting hormone, also known as somastatin.)

hormone which is less than that of average sized children who, in turn, are producing less GH than tall children. Clinical trials are underway at present to determine if normal short children (in contrast to GH deficient children) will improve their growth velocity if given parenteral GH therapy. There is now evidence that cartilage growth may be controlled both by circulating SM/IGFs (endocrine effects) and by locally produced SM/IGFs (autocrine and paracrine effects).

Mechanisms of growth hormone action – somatomedins/insulin-like growth factors (see Figs 54.3 and 54.4)

Longitudinal growth is mainly the result of differentiation and proliferation of cartilage cells situated in the epiphyseal growth plates at the ends of the lower limb long bones and in the vertebral bodies.

1. Endocrine SM/IGF control of cartilage growth – indirect GH effect (see Fig. 54.4). In vitro experiments with cartilage 30 years ago suggested that GH had little effect on the incorporation of sulphate into the ground substance of cartilage or on the incorporation of thymidine into DNA. Normal serum, however, was found to be quite active in promoting sulphate and thymidine uptake whereas serum obtained from GH deficient patients had limited effect. This GH dependent serum factor was initially called sulphation/thymidine factor and later designated somatomedin (SM).

A family of somatomedins was identified and in addition to their growth effects on cartilage they were shown to have potent insulin-like effects in non-skeletal tissues, such as muscle and adipose tissue. Also, a member of the SM family appeared to have multiplication stimulating properties when added to fibroblasts in tissue culture.

Fortunately after many years of confusion the structural analysis of these growth factors has led to clarification. It now appears that there are two major somatomedin/insulin-like growth factors. Somatomedin C (SMC) is identical to insulin-like growth factor-1 (IGF-1). Insulin-like growth factor-2 (IGF-2) is structurally different to IGF-1 and is identical to one form of multiplication stimulating activity (MSA).

Somatomedin A was identified as a deamidated form of SMC/IGF-1 and somatomedin B was found to be an artefact and is no longer classified as a somatomedin.

The two somatomedins SMC/IGF-1 and IGF-2/MSA are structurally related to proinsulin, the precursor of insulin. In contrast to insulin the SM/IGFs circulate in the blood bound to binding proteins which probably prevents them from exhibiting strong insulin hypoglycaemic action in vivo.

SMC/IGF-1 is strongly GH dependent and its con-

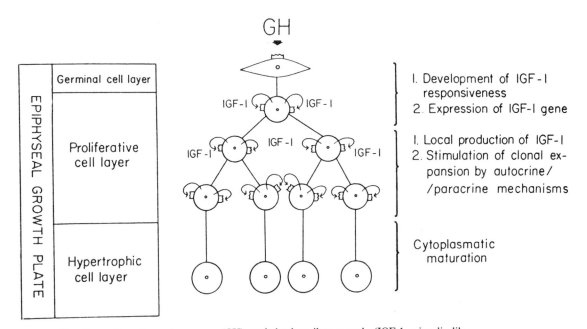

Fig. 54.4 The direct effect of growth hormone (GH) on skeletal cartilage growth. (IGF-1 = insulin-like growth factor-1 which is structurally identical to somatomedin C (SMC).)

centration is low in the serum of children with GH deficiency and elevated in the serum of patients with pituitary gigantism/acromegaly. IGF-2, on the other hand, has limited GH dependence and is only moderately reduced in GH deficiency and not elevated in pituitary gigantism/acromegaly.

It appears that the major source of circulating SM-IGFs is the liver (see Fig. 54.3).

Serum SMC/IGF-1 levels vary with age and the nutritional state of the patient, being low in infants and young children and in patients with nutritional deficiency, such as kwashiorkor. Therefore, it should be noted that low levels of serum SMC/IGF-1 are compatible with, but not diagnostic of, GH deficiency.

2. Paracrine and autocrine SM/IGF control of cartilage growth – direct GH effect (see Fig. 54.4). Contrary to the long-standing hypothesis that GH only acts indirectly on cartilage through circulating SMC/IGF-1 (endocrine effect), some recent elegant in vivo and in vitro research has shown that GH may indeed act directly on cartilage cells (see Fig. 54.4).

This work suggests that GH stimulates the differentiation of prechondrocytes in the germinal cell layer. During the process of cell differentiation the cells become responsive to IGF-1 and genes coding for IGF-1 are expressed. As a result, IGF-1 is produced by the differentiating chondrocytes themselves. Locally produced IGF-1 stimulates the clonal expansion of cells that have recently become susceptible to IGF-1 effects. IGF-1 may act on the same cell from which it is produced (autocrine effect) or on adjacent cells (paracrine effect). The relative importance of the endocrine versus the autocrine/paracrine effects of SM/IGFs remains to be clarified.

Thyroid hormone

Thyroid hormone is important in postnatal growth, as evidenced by the poor growth of children with untreated hypothyroidism. Thyroid hormone also has a profound effect on brain development in the first year or so of life and bone maturation at all ages. Thyroid hormone probably has its major growth effect by direct action at the tissue level, but it also exerts some effect indirectly at the pituitary level by facilitating the synthesis and secretion of growth hormone. Some, but not all, children with hypothyroidism show a reduced secretion of GH to pharmacological stimuli such as insulin hypoglycaemia. Fortunately, the postnatal retarded growth and intellectual development associated with neonatal hypothyroidism is rarely seen these days in countries which have a well-developed neonatal thyroid

screening programme, but late onset hypothyroidism is seen not infrequently as a cause of short stature.

Steroid hormones

Glucocorticoids

Cortisol, particularly in large doses, tends to inhibit growth. It appears to do this at several levels. It can decrease the secretion of GH from the pituitary and decrease the production of SMC/IGF-1 by the liver, but probably its most significant effect is directed at the periphery. High doses of cortisol lead to osteoporosis and retarded bone maturation.

Testosterone and adrenal androgens

These are anabolic and promote growth. In boys, testosterone and growth hormone act synergistically to promote the adolescent growth spurt. Testosterone in pharmacological doses advances bone age rapidly, hastens closure of the epiphyses, and will compromise adult height if given for any length of time.

Oestrogens

In large doses, oestrogens tend to inhibit growth and promote early fusion of the bony epiphyses. This effect is associated with a fall in SMC/IGF-1 levels. Use is made of this in the treatment of tall girls with high-dose oestrogens to reduce their adult height potential. Recently it has been shown that low doses of oestrogen may, in fact, stimulate growth and have been used for this purpose in the treatment of girls with Turner's syndrome.

CLINICAL ASSESSMENT

Percentile charts

The physician dealing with children must have a working knowledge of normal variations in growth and development and be able to use percentile charts.

Australian percentile charts are available for height and weight (mass) of children between the ages of birth and 18 years. These are based on cross-sectional studies of New South Wales children between 1970 and 1972. Because children enter puberty at different ages and, therefore, will have their adolescent growth spurts at different ages, cross-sectional data based on average heights and weights at each age will tend to mask the individual growth acceleration pattern during this period. For this reason, an individual child plotted on

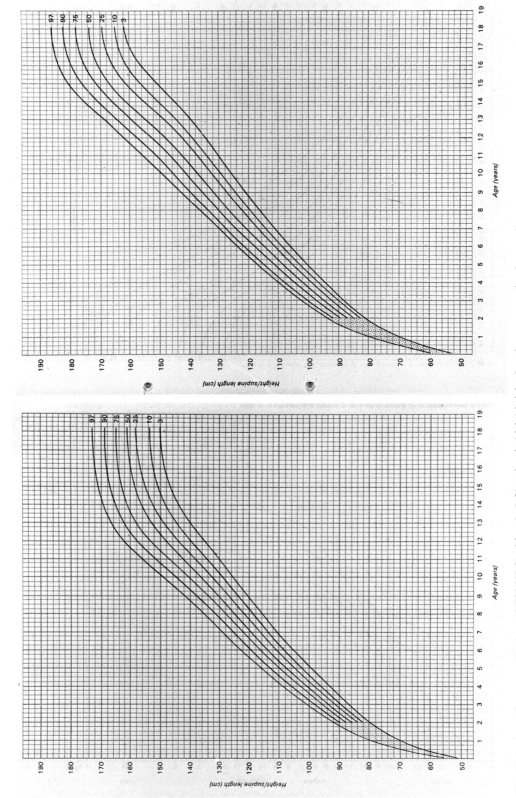

Fig. 54.5 Australian percentile charts (NH&MRC) of female (left) and male (right) heights based on cross-sectional survey by the New South Wales Department of Health 1970 to 1972.

cross-sectionally derived growth charts will appear to deviate from his prepubertal percentile channel at puberty only to re-enter this channel at maturity. This is purely an artefact and the result of the method of chart construction (Fig. 54.5).

Tanner & Whitehouse (1976) have devised percentile charts for English children which are based on mixed cross-sectional and longitudinal data and show more clearly the individual type of pubertal growth pattern (Fig. 54.6) but sufficient longitudinal growth studies have not been carried out in Australia for such charts to be constructed.

The most rapid growth postnatally occurs in the first two years of life, with a second growth spurt at puberty. The most rapid period of growth during the whole of life is in utero when the fetus grows 50 cm in nine months, or an impressive 67 cm per year, about three times the maximum rate seen in postnatal life.

Children who fall outside the 3rd to 97th percentile range for height or weight should be regarded with suspicion as having a growth problem, and the further they are away from these percentiles the more likely is this to be so. However, it must be realized that there will be 3 normal children in every 100 who will be at

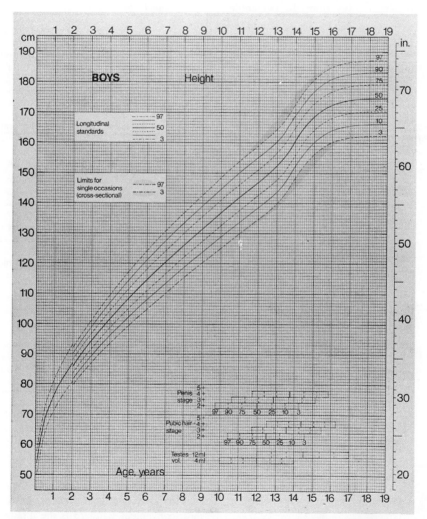

Fig. 54.6 English percentile chart (Tanner & Whitehouse 1976) based on mixed cross-sectional and longitudinal data. Note the similarity of prepubertal and final mature heights between Australian and English boys but the difference in slopes of height velocity of peak pubertal growth spurt (13 to 15 years) with the English chart giving a better indication of the individual growth pattern.

or below the 3rd percentile and 3 in every 100 who will be at or above the 97th percentile. Of far greater clinical significance than single measurements of height and weight is the assessment of growth velocity based on sequential measurements taken over a minimum period of three months and preferably over 6–12-monthly intervals. Longer periods of observation will minimize errors in measuring techniques as well as seasonal and other normal variations in growth velocity.

When plotted over a reasonable period of time, the normal child will tend to follow the same percentile channel with the exception of the pubertal period as outlined above. The child with an organic or endocrine disease will tend to deviate away from the percentile channels.

The use of reliable equipment and standardized measuring technique are absolutely essential in the assessment of growth (see Fig. 54.7).

Puberty

Growth must always be considered not only with respect to age but also in relation to the pubertal development of the child.

Pubertal stages for boys and girls are summarized

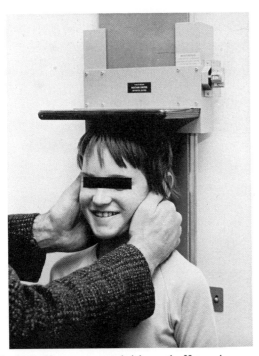

Fig. 54.7 How to measure height on the Harpenden stadiometer – head level and gentle traction under both mastoid processes.

Example 54.2 Pubertal stages of development (from Tanner 1962)

Girls: breast development
Stage 1. Pre-adolescent: elevation of papilla only.
Stage 2. Breast bud stage: elevation of breast and papilla as small mound. Enlargement of areola diameter.
Stage 3. Further enlargement and elevation of breast and areola, with no separation of their contours.
Stage 4. Projection of areola and papilla to form a secondary mound above the level of the breast.
Stage 5. Mature stage: projection of papilla only, due to recession of the areola to the general contour of the breast.

Boys: genital (penis) development
Stage 1. Pre-adolescent, testes, scrotum and penis are of about the same size and proportion as in early childhood.
Stage 2. Enlargement of scrotum and testes. Skin of scrotum reddens and changes in texture. Little or no enlargement of penis at this stage.
Stage 3. Enlargement of penis, which occurs at first mainly in length. Further growth of testes and scrotum.
Stage 4. Increased size of penis with growth in breadth and development of glans. Testes and scrotum larger; scrotal skin darkened.
Stage 5. Genitalia adult in size and shape.

Both sexes: pubic hair
Stage 1. Pre-adolescent. The vellus over the pubes is not further developed than that over the abdominal wall, i.e. no pubic hair.
Stage 2. Sparse growth of long, slightly pigmented downy hair, straight or slightly curled, chiefly at the base of the penis or along labia.
Stage 3. Considerably darker, coarser and more curled. The hair spreads sparsely over the junction of the pubes.
Stage 4. Hair now adult in type, but area covered is still considerably smaller than in the adult. No spread to the medial surface of thighs.
Stage 5. Adult in quantity and type with distribution of the horizontal (or classically 'feminine') pattern. Spread to medial surface of thighs but not up linea alba or elsewhere above the base of the inverse triangle (spread up linea alba occurs late and is rated stage 6).

(Example 54.2). These stages are based on the work of Tanner in English children. Some studies around the world suggest that they may be advanced by about 6 months in development compared to their English counterparts.

The size of the testis can be estimated clinically by comparing it with standards of known volume. The most convenient standard is the 'Prader orchidometer', which is a series of wooden or plastic ovoids mounted on a string and numbered according to their volume in millilitres (Fig. 54.8). The testis volume of greater than 3 ml before puberty is unusual and a testis of less than

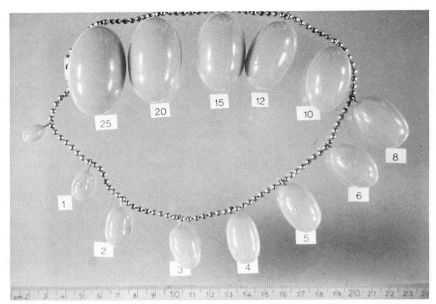

Fig. 54.8   The Prader orchidometer.

1 ml volume is considered small. The volume of the adult testis varies between 12 and 25 ml.

Bone age

Bone age, or skeletal maturity, can be estimated by the time of appearance of different epiphyseal centres or, when all are present, by their stage of maturity. This is done by comparison of a radiograph of the left hand and wrist with a series of radiographic standards. If a child has a bone age which is retarded, this means that less of the potential final adult height has been achieved than a child who has a normal or advanced bone age. Tables are available which allow estimation of the child's final adult height knowing his or her actual height and bone age. Thyroid hormone, growth hormone and androgens have significant accelerating effects on bone maturation, and chronic severe illness tend to cause retardation of bone age. However, variations in bone age do not necessarily mean that a child has an endocrine or organic disease any more than variations in growth percentiles necessarily reflect an ongoing disease process. The whole clinical situation must be taken into account when assessing the relevance of the bone age.

Dental age

As a useful clinical guide it has been found that the dental age is a rough indicator of skeletal maturity. For example, a child of 14 years whose 12-year-old molar teeth have not yet erupted is likely to have a bone age two or more years retarded.

GROWTH DISORDERS; THE SHORT CHILD

Short stature may not only be a sign of disease but it can be a disability and a cause of distress in itself. Treatment, if appropriate, must be started well before the epiphyses fuse and, where no specific treatment is available, an informed prognosis at an early age may allay anxiety and enable the right advice and support to be given.

Definition

There is no clear demarcation between normal and short stature. As a general rule, any child whose height falls below the 3rd percentile (equivalent to approximately 2 s.ds below the mean for the community) should be considered short. However, occasionally a child whose height is above the 3rd percentile may be considered short in relation to the family pattern. It is of value to mark the parents' percentiles to the right of the child's growth chart. All but 5% of normal children will have a final height within 8.5 cm on either side of the midparental centile, the midpoint between the mother's and father's centile positions.

Causes of short stature

Normal variants: genetic short stature and constitutional delay in puberty

Most short children will be simply variations of normal

and there will be 30 in every 1000 normal children at or below the 3rd percentile in each age group. Most of these otherwise healthy children will not present to a doctor, because their stature is recognized to have a genetic basis by their parents.

Often a child is short because of a general delay in body maturation, which is reflected by a delay in bone maturation. These children will have a delayed onset of puberty (> 13 years in girls and > 14 years in boys) but eventually reach their genetic height potential at a significantly older age than most of their peers. If a child is destined to be a short adult (< 3rd percentile) for genetic reasons, and also has a delay in maturation and puberty, he or she will be a very short child before puberty.

Most children with genetic short stature, constitutional delayed puberty, or a combination thereof, will have a normal growth velocity after 2–3 years of age, i.e. they will remain below but parellel to the 3rd percentile in mid-childhood. Those with delayed onset of puberty will appear to deviate away from the percentiles when their peers begin their adolescent growth spurt at the normal age. However, they will eventually undergo their adolescent growth spurt and climb back into their genetically predetermined percentile range.

Low birthweight babies

These children will have been 'small for dates' infants as opposed to true premature babies with appropriate weight for gestational period. Many of the growth-retarded children in this group will be lean in build, and a history of an infective or toxic insult in utero may be obtained (see Example 54.1). The effects on the growth pattern postnatally will depend on the timing, duration and severity of the insult during pregnancy.

Nutritional disorders

Impaired growth is a feature of children who are undernourished, whatever the cause. Varying degrees of undernutrition and malnutrition affect up to 50% of children in the developing world. Poor growth in emotionally deprived children (psychosocial dwarfism) may be related to disturbances in the hypothalamic-pituitary axis with GH deficiency that is reversible when the child is placed in a caring environment. However, some of the growth failure may be due to anorexia and reduced calorie intake, particularly in younger infants. Regional ileitis (Crohn's disease) and coeliac disease may present as short stature as a result of malabsorption and anorexia. It is now becoming clear that at least part of the growth failure seen in other major system diseases (e.g. renal, cardiac, pulmonary) is directly related to in-adequate caloric intake because of anorexia, vomiting and an inability to meet the body's increased metabolic demands.

Diseases of major systems

In addition to impairment of appetite and vomiting, which may limit caloric intake as mentioned above, chronic severe disorders of the major systems, e.g. cyanotic heart disease and chronic renal failure, may lead to a suboptimal cellular milieu which can depress cellular growth. Recently it has been shown that, in many such children, if sufficient calories can be transferred to the circulation by either intravenous alimentation or prolonged intragastric feedings, growth can be improved despite quite severe metabolic disturbances being present.

Skeletal disorders

Possibly the most widely recognized skeletal cause of short stature is achondroplasia. There are over 50 varieties of skeletal disorders associated with short stature and they are most commonly recognized by a disproportion between limbs and trunk (Ch. 7).

Dysmorphic syndromes

Many of the syndromes associated with short statures have common features of low birthweight and intellectual retardation, e.g. Down syndrome, trisomy 13–15 and 16–18. In any unusual looking child with short stature diagnostic help can often be obtained by reference to textbooks of dysmorphology (see Ch. 7).

It is important to consider the diagnosis of Turner's syndrome in any very short girl, even in the absence of the classical features of neck webbing, shield chest, increased cubitus valgus, etc. Mosaic Turner's syndrome (e.g. XO/XX) patients frequently present with short stature only and, since this diagnosis may be missed by buccal smear examination, it is essential to carry out a full blood karyotype in all suspected children.

Endocrine disorders

Although only a relatively small percentage of short children will have an endocrine disorder, they are an important group as effective treatment for them is possible.

1. Late onset of hypothyroidism can be insidious and affected children (Fig. 54.9) may present only with short stature. However, if examined closely they will show evidence of hypometabolism, such as poor peripheral

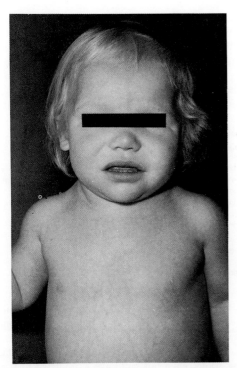

Fig. 54.9 Hypothyroidism in an infant aged 3 years and 4 months.

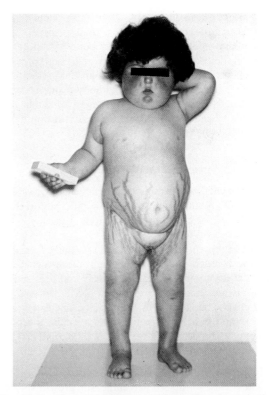

Fig. 54.10 Marked Cushing's syndrome. Note the typically moon-faced appearance, obesity and striae.

circulation with cool hands and feet and delayed tendon jerks.

2. Corticosteroid excess (Cushings's syndrome). It is usually iatrogenic and although oral steroids are occasionally necessary to control a life-threatening disease process, care should be taken to give the minimum dose necessary to obtain the desired effect. Growth failure is a prominent feature of childhood Cushing's syndrome (Fig. 54.10).

3. Growth hormone deficiency may result in a characteristic appearance with a short plump build and a round immature face (so-called 'doll-like appearance').

In all of the endocrine causes of short stature mentioned above, growth failure develops postnatally, with the birthweight and length being normal. In distinction to children with genetic short stature and constitutional delay in growth and puberty, children with endocrinopathies tend to deviate further away from the percentiles with time, i.e. they have a slow growth velocity.

Approach to diagnosis

Routine careful measurement of all children and determination of their percentiles will allow confirmation of short stature and recognition of a growth problem when this may not be specifically mentioned by the child or family. A series of such measurements will allow the child's growth velocity pattern to be determined. This is a most valuable clue in sorting out normal short stature variants (normal velocity) from organic causes of short stature (slow velocity).

History

This will include details of pregnancy, birthweight and length, specific symptoms, appetite, sleep, energy and whether abnormal bowel or micturition patterns are present.

Social history will include birth order of the child, evidence of marital or financial instability, emotional, sexual, physical or drug abuse.

The family heights and maturational patterns are obtained.

Examination

All short children should have a full physical examination with particular emphasis on the following: limb proportions determined by span and upper segment/lower segment ratios, head shape and circumference, assessment of body build – lean or fat, pubertal development, teeth as a reflection of bone maturation, blood pressure, fundal and visual field examination. Dysmorphic facial and body features should be noted, together with an assessment of intellectual function. Chemical and microscopic examination of the urine should be routine.

Indications for immediate further investigation

1. The child is extremely short for the family pattern; this usually means height well below the 3rd percentile (equivalent to 2 s.ds from the mean) and usually below 3 s.ds.

2. The presence of symptoms or signs suggest a chronic disorder, e.g. diarrhoea might mean coeliac disease and malabsorption; lack of energy and proteinuria, renal disease, etc.

3. A slow rate of growth. This can be calculated from present and past measurements. As a guide, a growth velocity of less than 5 cm per year in mid-childhood can be considered slow.

Immediate investigation is not usually necessary if the height is close to the 3rd percentile, the growth velocity (if available) is normal, there is a family history of short stature and/or delayed puberty and the child is generally well and energetic. In certain cases it may be deemed appropriate to carry out a bone age and estimate the child's final adult height. In all cases sympathetic reassurance is essential and attention given to psychological problems possibly related to their small size. It is of value to follow all short children for at least 12 months to confirm that their growth velocity is normal.

When indicated, investigations which have proved of value in determining the cause of short stature include:

1. Radiographs of skull and bone age estimation
2. Karyotype on all very short girls
3. Renal function studies
4. Thyroid function
5. Haemoglobin, blood folate and ESR
6. Jejunal biopsy
7. Hypothalamic-pituitary studies including growth hormone estimation.

THE TALL CHILD

In contrast to children with short stature, where not infrequently an organic or psychosocial problem will be uncovered, very few unusually tall children will have an ongoing disease process. The great majority will be tall on a genetic basis. Girls will often be concerned if their final height is likely to be in excess of 70 inches (178 cm), whereas there seems to be less concern about boys becoming tall men. It is quite common for a tall mother to request treatment for her daughter stating that she does not wish her daughter to go through the psychological trauma that she went through herself in adolescence, and possibly still suffers as an adult, because of her height.

Definition

As with short stature, there is no clear demarcation between normal and tall stature, since this is somewhat subjective. As a general rule a child whose height is above the 97th percentile for the community should be considered tall.

Causes of tall stature

Normal variants

Most tall children are normal in all other respects and their height is genetically determined. Some children with early, but otherwise normal, pubertal development, between 8 and 10 years in girls and 10 and 12 years in boys, will appear tall in relation to their peers and family during adolescence but will have a predicted final adult height within the accepted normal range. These early developers have an advanced bone age and are at the opposite end of the spectrum to the short children with delayed maturation, who have delayed puberty, but who will also reach a normal adult height commensurate with their mid-parent percentile.

Precocious puberty

In our community puberty is regarded as precocious if it occurs before 8 years of age in girls and before 10 years of age in boys. Because of rapid acceleration of bone maturation and early epiphyseal closure, many of these children will be excessively tall in early to mid-childhood, but finish up as relatively short adults. It is important to determine if the pubertal development is due to premature activation of the hypothalamic-pituitary-gonadal axis, or if there is an aberrant source of androgen or oestrogen, such as an adrenal or ovarian tumour. Occasionally, one encounters a type of precocious pseudopuberty due to iatrogenic causes such as oestrogen cream application, or excessive administration of anabolic steroids given to improve appetite and growth.

Large babies and infant giants

Unduly large size is seen in the newborn period among the offspring of diabetic mothers, with tall parents, and in certain uncommon syndromes such as cerebral gigantism of Sotos and the Beckwith-Wiedemann syndrome. In the Sotos syndrome, large size is associated with a dilated ventricular system, developmental retardation, clumsiness and rapid growth which usually slows by school age. In the Beckwith syndrome macroglossia, umbilical hernia and visceromegaly are likely to be associated with hypoglycaemic episodes (due to pancreatic B cell hyperplasia) but not with prolonged rapid growth after infancy.

Syndromes

Marfan's syndrome, if it presents with the classical picture of asthenia, arachnodactyly, ligamentous laxity, chest deformity, cardiac abnormalities, high arched palate and subluxation of the lenses, is readily diagnosed, but often one sees tall thin children with some marfanoid features who are difficult to classify, as there is no definitive diagnostic test for this condition.

Children with homocystinuria have a Marfan's phenotype but are intellectually retarded. This may be diagnosed by study of urinary and serum amino acids.

Tall girls with intellectual retardation should also be screened for the XXX syndrome and tall boys, particularly with aggressive antisocial behaviour, for the XYY syndrome. Tall boys with Klinefelter syndrome (XXY) may show evidence of hypogonadism with relatively small testes and gynaecomastia. They also tend to have relatively long limbs and may be intellectually retarded.

Endocrine

Endocrine causes of tall stature, other than precocious puberty, include hyperthyroidism and true pituitary gigantism.

Hyperthyroidism is uncommon in childhood. As the presentation varies, diagnosis is frequently delayed. It occurs more frequently in girls having an insidious onset of behavioural problems, poor school performance and accelerated growth. At the time appetite is often voracious so that weight may not be lost. On physical examination the child is usually tall and thin and exophthalmos is frequent but by no means the rule. Tachycardia, sweating and a fine tremor of the hands may also be observed. The thyroid gland is usually diffusely enlarged with a murmur audible over its surface.

True pituitary gigantism is very rare but should be suspected if there are any other signs to suggest pituitary involvement including visual disturbance and headaches. True acromegaly is not seen before adulthood, but often children with a growth hormone-producing tumour have rather heavy facial features with large hands and feet. Their appetite and thirst are often prodigious and their growth velocity is markedly increased compared with that seen in the normal variant genetically tall child who normally runs above, but parallel to the 97th percentile (see Case 3 page 463).

Approach to diagnosis

History

Time of onset of tall stature is relevant in order to differentiate the perinatal disorders of Beckwith-Wiedemann and Sotos syndrome from those disorders associated with later onset of tall stature in childhood including hyperthyroidism, true pituitary gigantism and precocious puberty.

Family heights and pubertal patterns are noted. Developmental delay, clumsiness and behaviour disorders will suggest one of the chromosomal disorders (XXX, XXY or XYY) homocystinuria or Sotos syndrome.

Examination

A full physical examination is essential with emphasis on accurate height measurement, body build, limb proportions as assessed by span and upper segment/lower segment ratios and pubertal status.

Neurological assessment should include fundoscopy, assessment of visual fields and intellectual function. Proptosis and other eye signs, together with evidence of hypermetabolic state will suggest hyperthyroidism (Graves disease).

Indications for further investigation

In most instances the tall child will be a girl who comes from a tall family, has no symptoms suggestive of an organic problem, and if previous measurements are available, will be found to be running above but parallel to the 97th percentile, i.e. has a normal growth velocity. An accurate height measurement and bone age assessment by someone experienced in this procedure will enable an adult height prediction to be made relatively accurately. Frequently this is found to be at or below 70 in (178 cm) and no further action is necessary. If the height prediction is above 70 in, the girl is best referred to a specialist centre experienced in high-dosage oestrogen therapy if treatment is contemplated. An explanation of the risks involved and likely duration of the treatment can be given.

In general, referral for oestrogen therapy is not necessary before the girl has reached 66 in (168 cm) in height;

HEIGHT (LENGTHS) OF FEMALES   2 to 18 YEARS

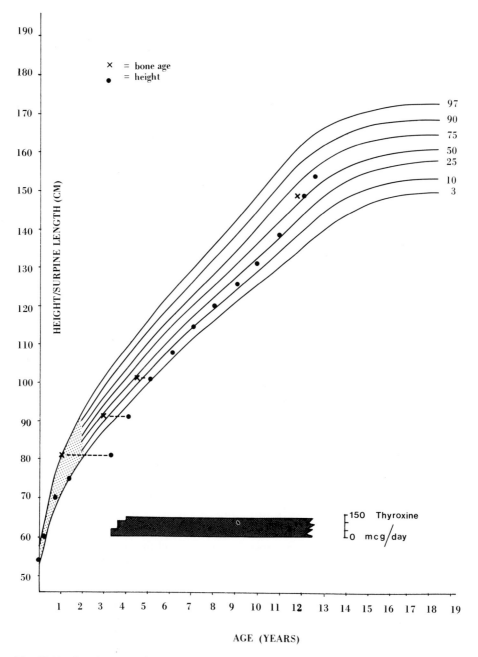

Fig. 54.11 Growth chart before and after treatment of hypothyroidism.

however, this is indicated by the individual problem and family anxieties. The earlier the treatment is begun, the greater the height reduction achieved. Other indications for further investigation and/or referral to a specialist centre, will include children with suspected pituitary gigantism, precocious puberty, hyperthyroidism and the chromosomal and other metabolic disorders associated with tall stature. An unusually rapid growth velocity, i.e. progressive deviation away from the 97th percentile, will usually mean a pathological cause for the tall stature, and requires further investigation.

Management

It has been shown that high-dosage oestrogen therapy is effective in significantly reducing final adult height if started early enough in tall girls. Ethinyloestradiol is given with a short course of norethisterone each month to hasten epiphyseal fusion. This therapy is continued until growth has ceased and takes about two years if started when the height is round 66 in (168 cm). The family should be counselled on the potential side effects which include nausea, nipple pigmentation, possible excessive weight gain, thromboembolic phenomena, ovarian cyst development and possible problems with fertility. They should also be warned about the unknown, but possible long-term, carcinogenic effects of oestrogen therapy. If they (and particularly the patient concerned) wish to go ahead with treatment this should be done under careful supervision. Wettenhall and colleagues (1975) studied a 15-year follow-up of a group of 168 girls so treated and reported minimal side effects and no apparent interference with fertility.

Tall boys can be similarly managed by the use of high dosage testosterone therapy. Boys with Marfan's syndrome tend to benefit from this therapy as it also causes an increase in muscle bulk and improves their general appearance and self-confidence. Testicular volume may decrease during therapy but rapidly returns to normal when it is ceased. Sperm counts are not affected in the long term. Again caution is necessary with regard to possible unknown long-term effects, e.g. prostatic carcinoma.

CASE HISTORIES

The following case histories illustrate some problems of growth, their diagnosis and treatment.

Case 1: Short stature: hypothyroidism

This girl (see Fig. 54.9) presented at 3 years and 4 months with constipation and rectal prolapse. It was noted that she

had rather puffy features, biggish tongue, hoarse cry, mottled skin and cool extremities.

Examination of old records showed that she had grown and developed normally until almost 12 months of age (Fig. 54.11), but then began to fall through the percentiles so that at 3 years and 4 months she was well below the 3rd percentile for height. Her bone age was equivalent to that of a normal infant of 12 months of age. Primary hypothyroidism was demonstrated by a low total thyroxine level of 2.9 μg/dl (N 6.4 to 13) and elevated TSH to 451 μu/ml (N < 10). A ^{99}Tc sodium pertechnate scan showed no evidence of thyroid tissue. Thyroglobulin and microsomal antibodies were negative.

Rapid catch-up in growth and bone maturation was achieved with thyroxine therapy.

At 12 years of age she appears physically and intellectually normal. This supports the belief that thyroid hormone is of less importance in neurological development after the first year of life. Presumably she had a small but adequate amount of functioning thyroid tissue during early infancy which rapidly disappeared after 12 months of age. It is to be noted, however, that a negative Tc scan does not completely exclude a small amount of ectopic thyroid tissue.

Case 2: Craniopharyngioma – panhypopituitarism

This girl (Fig. 54.12) demonstrates the remarkable 'catch-

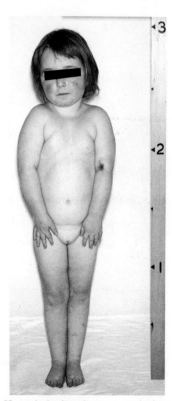

Fig. 54.12 Hypopituitarism due to a craniopharyngioma. This photograph was taken before the introduction of growth hormone.

HEIGHTS (LENGTHS) OF FEMALES 2 to 18 YEARS

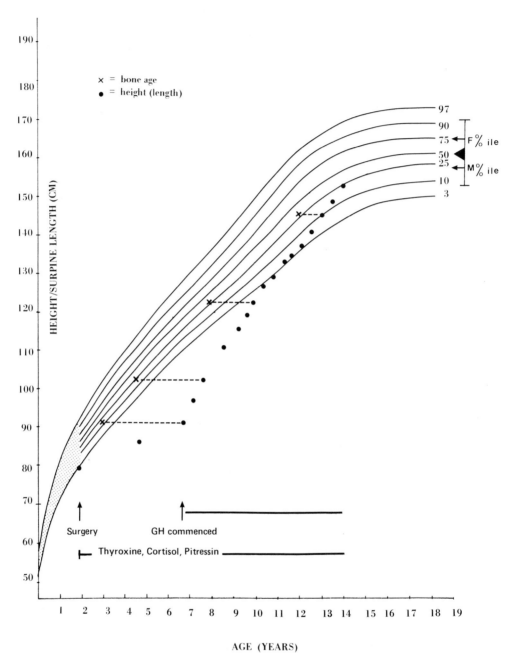

Fig. 54.13 Growth chart after surgery and replacement hormonal treatment after removal of craniopharyngioma.

up' growth that can occur in children with growth hormone deficiency if growth hormone therapy is started at a relatively young age. She initially presented in a comatose state from raised intracranial pressure at 22 months of age. A suprasellar craniopharyngioma was removed and she was left with some visual loss and panhypopituitarism. Growth velocity was then slow (2 cm per year) on thyroxine, cortisone and Pitressin replacement therapy (Fig. 54.13) but increased markedly after introduction of human pituitary growth hormone at 6 years and 8 months. Prior to therapy she had the typical immature, chubby, doll-like appearance often associated with growth hormone deficiency. Her bone age was then almost 4 years retarded and has gradually caught up to her chronological age so that at 14 years of age her bone age was 12 years. She will require either gonadotrophin or oestrogen therapy for development of her secondary sexual characteristics and for menstruation to occur. Her adult height should be well within that expected from her mid-parent percentile.

Case 3: Pituitary gigantism

This girl (Fig. 54.14) presented at 3.5 years of age with tall stature. There was no evidence of precocious sexual

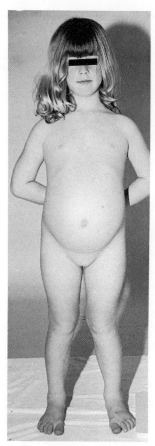

Fig. 54.14 Pituitary gigantism in a child of 3.5 years. Height at this age was 124.8 cm and weight 34.2 kg.

development. Her birth length (53 cm) and weight (3.84 kg) were normal and it appears that acceleration of her growth began in the first 3 months of life.

At 3.5 years she measured 127 cm - approximately 22 cm greater than the 97th percentile and equivalent to a height age of 8.5 years, i.e. 50th percentile for a normal 8.5–year-old girl. Her weight of 37.2 kg was 18 kg above the 97th percentile and equivalent to a weight age of 10.5 years. Her bone age approximated her chronological age. She had large hands and feet, widely spaced teeth, and normal intelligence. Basal serum growth hormone and prolactin levels were elevated and growth hormone was not suppressed by glucose. SMC-RIA was markedly elevated.

A mixed growth hormone/prolactin secretory pituitary adenoma was demonstrated radiologically and removed by transsphenoidal hypophysectomy, but because it had intimately involved the compressed normal pituitary gland this had to be removed at the time. GH and PRL fell to zero and SMC-RIA to hypopituitary levels.

On replacement (thyroid, cortisone and Pitressin DDAVP) therapy she has remained well with no evidence of recurrence. Her growth velocity has been virtually zero (Fig. 54.15) so that at 8 years of age she is around the 50th percentile for height and consideration is being given to commencing human pituitary growth hormone in physiological dosage so that she can achieve a normal adult height. Gonadotrophin or oestrogen therapy will be necessary at pubertal age to achieve normal female secondary sexual characteristics.

Case 4: Marfan's syndrome

This boy presented at 8 years and 8 months with tall stature and learning problems.

On examination he was very tall, being 16 cm above the 97th percentile for age. He has a very lean build and marked arachnodactyly. His span was 7 cm greater than his height. Pectus carinatum and a high arched palate were noted. There was no evidence of lens dislocation. Blood pressure was 90/60. There were no cardiac bruits.

Blood and urinary amino acids showed no evidence of homocystinuria.

At 10 years and 3 months of age his bone age was advanced at 12 years and 6 months. On this basis his estimated final height was 203 cm (6 ft 8 in) (Fig. 54.16). He elected to undergo high dosage androgen therapy in an attempt to limit his final adult height and was commenced on testosterone oenanthate 250 mg IM every 2 weeks.

His height velocity initially accelerated and then slowed down from 12 years of age. His weight increased rapidly and his severely asthenic appearance improved by increased muscular development. At the start of therapy he was prepubertal and on therapy he showed rapid genital and pubic hair development but his testes increased only slightly from 2 to 5 ml in volume.

Testosterone therapy was ceased at 13 years and 5 months when his height was 193.8 cm (6 ft 4.5 in). His bone age had advanced to 17 years, and on this basis his final adult height was estimated at 195 cm (6 ft 5 in). It would appear that a significant height reduction of approximately 8 cm (3 in) has been gained by use of high dosage androgen therapy. Other workers have shown that there are no permanent effects on testicular function in the long term with this form of therapy.

HEIGHTS (LENGTHS) OF FEMALES 2 to 18 YEARS

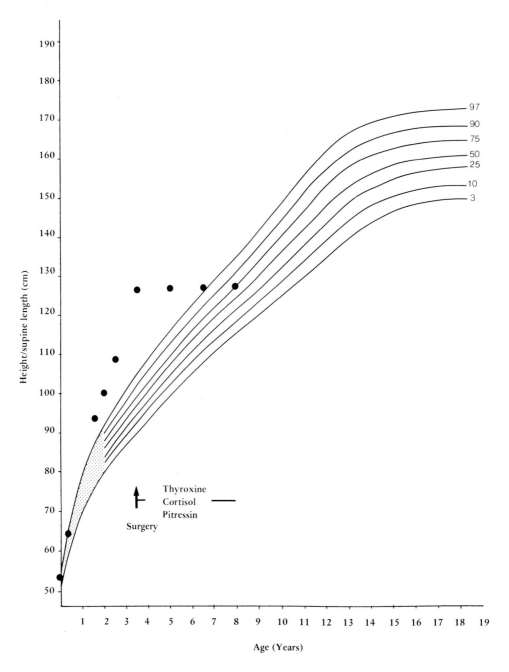

Fig. 54.15 Growth chart before and after surgery and replacement therapy after removal of pituitary adenoma.

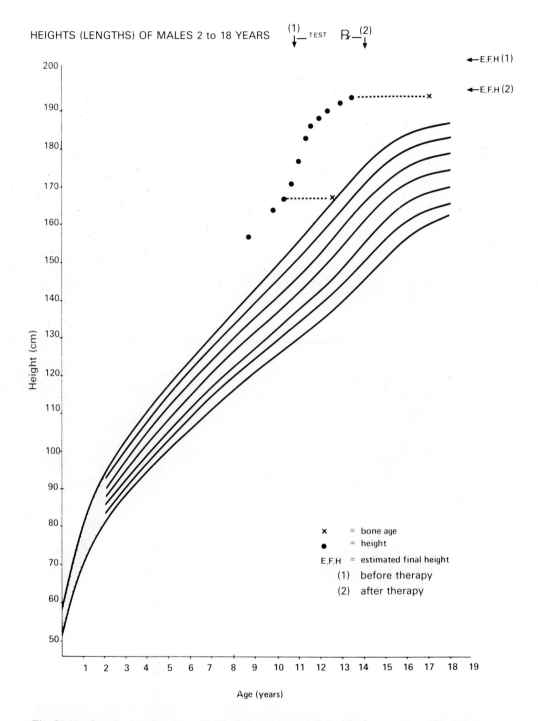

Fig. 54.16 Growth chart in a boy with Marfan's syndrome before and after treatment with androgens to reduce final height.

FURTHER READING

Brook G D (ed) 1981 Clinical paediatric endocrinology. Blackwell Scientific Publications, Oxford

Isaksson O 1987 Growth hormone. Basic and clinical aspects. Nordisk Insulin Symposium No. 1. International Congress Series 748. Excerpta Medica

Penfold J L, Boulton T J C, Thomsett M J et al 1980 Hormonal profile of puberty in South Australian children. Australian Paediatric Journal 16: 9–16

Tanner J M 1962 Growth at adolescence. Blackwell Scientific Publications, Oxford

Tanner J M, Whitehouse R H 1976 Clinical longitudinal standards for height, weight, weight velocity and stages of puberty. Archives of Diseases of Childhood 51: 170–179

Transactions of the First Karolinska Institute Nobel Conference 1981 The biology of normal human growth. Raven Press, New York

Wettenhall H N B, Cahill C, Roche A F 1975 Tall girls. A survey of 15 years of management and treatment. The Journal of Paediatrics 86: 602–610

Zachmann M, Ferrandez A, Maseet G, Gnehm H E, Prader A 1976 Testosterone treatment of excessively tall boys. The Journal of Paediatrics 88: 116–123

55. Thyroid disorders in children

George Werther

Thyroid hormone plays a central role in growth and development, as well as in the maintenance of most physiological systems from fetal to adult life. The actions of thyroid hormone are on growth and maturation as well as on metabolism especially via the sympathetic (adrenergic) nervous system. Disorders of the thyroid gland, or of its regulation, often result in abnormal circulating levels of thyroid hormone leading to profound effects on many body systems, especially the developing brain and skeleton. Some 1–2% of all children will have a thyroid gland disorder at some time, possibly associated with disturbed thyroid function.

THYROID PHYSIOLOGY

Development and secretion of the thyroid gland

The thyroid gland is first active in the embryo at eight weeks. Its growth is regulated by thyroid-stimulating hormone (TSH) from the anterior pituitary gland, which is in turn regulated by thyrotropin-regulating hormone (TRH) from the hypothalamus (see Fig. 55.1). These regulating hormones will continue to stimulate thyroid hormone production throughout life, and are in turn regulated in a negative feedback fashion by tri-iodothyronine (T_3), the active metabolite of the major thyroid hormone thyroxine (T_4).

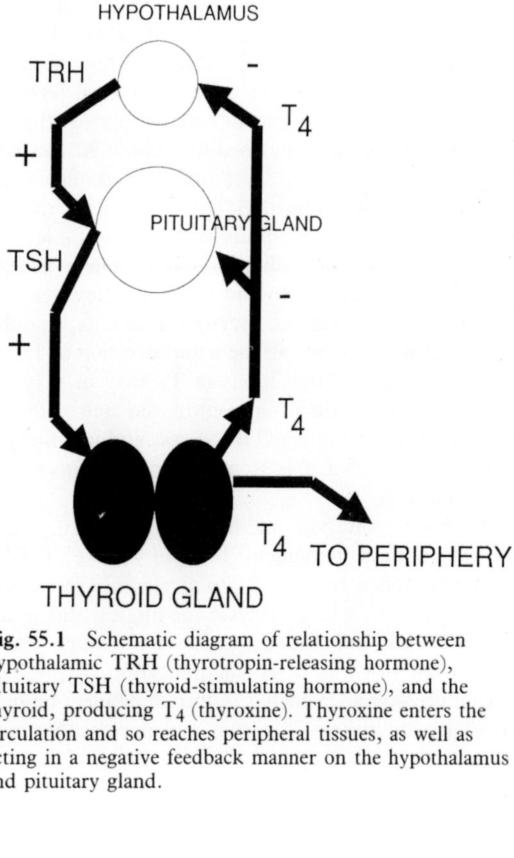

Thyroid hormone in fetal life, infancy and beyond

Thyroxine (T_4) is derived from a complex series of steps from iodinated thyroxine molecules to the large molecule thyroglobulin. Iodine plays a central role in the synthesis of thyroxine, and its incorporation into the final product involves adequate dietary iodine. Endemic dietary iodine deficiency is still seen in many parts of the world, usually because of soil leaching, but it is now rare in Australia because of food supplementation, e.g. iodination of table salt, infant milks and from sea foods. Absorbed iodine must be trapped, and transported into

Fig. 55.1 Schematic diagram of relationship between hypothalamic TRH (thyrotropin-releasing hormone), pituitary TSH (thyroid-stimulating hormone), and the thyroid, producing T_4 (thyroxine). Thyroxine enters the circulation and so reaches peripheral tissues, as well as acting in a negative feedback manner on the hypothalamus and pituitary gland.

the thyroid gland, organified and incorporated into thyroglobulin. Each of these and subsequent steps in the synthesis of thyroxine involve specific enzymes.

Secreted thyroxine is transported into the blood stream mostly in a bound form. The binding proteins are thyroid-binding globulin (TBG), prealbumin, and albumin. Less than 0.1% of thyroxine (T_4) and 0.5% of tri-iodothyronine (T_3) are in a free form in the circulation, so that measurements of serum thyroxine are measuring mostly bound T_4. There are a number of indirect and direct means of measuring 'free' or available thyroxine in serum.

Most of the actions of thyroid hormone are via the active metabolite T_3 formed by peripheral conversion in tissue sites of action around the body. This is even so in the hypothalamus-pituitary gland where T_3 is the active feedback agent. Thyroid hormone acts by binding to specific intracellular receptors after passing through the cell membrane.

Thyroid function tests and their interpretation

The most commonly performed thyroid function tests in infants and children are the measurement of total T_4 and thyroid-stimulating hormone (TSH) in blood. The absolute level of T_4 normally falls through infancy following a peak in the first week. A normal level for age will usually be sufficient to confirm normal thyroid function, and is commonly used to exclude 90% of normal babies in neonatal screening programmes for congenital hypothyroidism. A low level of T_4 may or may not indicate hypothyroidism as a low T_4 level is seen in a number of euthyroid states. These include prematurity, the sick euthyroid syndrome (low total T_4 due to systemic disease), hypoproteinaemia, familial TBG deficiency and during the administration of Dilantin and androgens. High levels of T_4 may or may not indicate hyperthyroidism, since euthyroid states can lead to high total T_4 in familial TBG excess and in oestrogen excess. 'Free' or available thyroxine may be normal in these conditions.

The most common method of measuring free thyroxine is measurement of T_3 resin uptake (T_3RU). This is multiplied by total T_4 to give a calculated 'free thyroxine index', which corrects for modest disturbances of thyroid-binding proteins. The other major measurement used is TSH, an indication of pituitary drive on the thyroid, which is in turn dependent on both hypothalamic-pituitary integrity, and normal thyroxine feedback.

HYPOTHYROIDISM IN THE NEWBORN

A deficiency of thyroid hormone in early life may result in irreversible consequences for brain development, intellectual functioning and a multiplicity of body functions. Congenital hypothyroidism is the most common cause while acquired hypothyroidism is unusual and usually transient.

Congenital hypothyroidism

Based on newborn screening programmes congenital hypothyroidism has an incidence of 1 in 3500 to 1 in 4500. Usually it is not clinically evident at the time of screening, with only minor signs elicited in many babies, often only in retrospect. The likelihood of fullblown hypothyroidism presenting clinically in the newborn baby is determined both by the degree of the underlying defect, and the time of its onset. An underfunctioning thyroid gland may suffice for a small fetus in late intra-uterine life and the early extra-uterine period. However, as the baby grows rapidly, it may 'outgrow' any residual functioning thyroid gland, and overt hypothyroidism may appear. Fortunately, in most babies, hypothyroidism is diagnosed biochemically on screening programmes before the baby is overtly hypothyroid.

Causes of congenital hypothyroidism

The major causes of congenital hypothyroidism are:

1. Primary hypothyroidism (defects of the gland itself) including: congenital absence of the gland; ectopic gland; enzyme defect (dyshormonogenesis).
2. Secondary or tertiary hypothyroidism: these imply defects of the pituitary gland or hypothalamus, respectively.

The commonest abnormal positions of the thyroid include the lateral neck or at the base of the tongue (lingual thyroid) due to failure or abnormal descent from the pharyngeal arch. Under these circumstances the thyroid gland is usually impalpable.

Enzyme defects (dyshormonogenesis) are rare, usually being familial and inherited in an autosomal recessive manner. The commonest of these is Pendred's syndrome, which is variably associated with nerve deafness. Almost all enzyme defects are associated with large goitres, in contrast to the commoner congenital absence and ectopic glands.

Acquired (transient) hypothyroidism in the newborn and infant

Hypothyroidism may occur secondarily to the transplacental passage of iodine, to antithyroid antibodies or to blockers of thyroxine synthesis, such as carbimazole used in the treatment of thyrotoxicosis. Usually these conditions are associated with a significant goitre in the infant. Occasionally topical or systemic iodine containing agents, such as betadine washes to prevent wound sepsis, may result in transient hypothyroidism.

Clinical features of hypothyroidism in the newborn and infant

Full-blown 'cretinism' with all of the classical features of hypothyroidism is now rarely seen in infants and children in developed countries, with the development and success of newborn screening programmes. However, infants may be born with some or many of the clinical features already evident, especially if the deficiency is severe and developed early in fetal life.

Sluggishness of body systems is the characteristic of hypothyroidism in the newborn and in infancy so that affected babies may have some of the features listed in Example 55.1.

Example 55.1 Clinical features of hypothyroidism in the newborn and in infancy

failure to thrive
listlessness
lack in movement
dry skin
hoarse cry
puffy face and large tongue
constipation
hypothermia
bradycardia
peripheral reflexes slow relaxation.

Delayed bone maturation is a feature and is reflected in large anterior fontanelle, an obviously palpable posterior fontanelle and an absent lower femoral epiphysis, the latter being normally present at birth.

Liver enzyme systems are impaired frequently leading to prolonged primarily unconjugated hyperbilirubinaemia.

Screening for hypothyroidism in the newborn

This has been in place in most developed countries for 5–15 years and has proven to be one of the most effective preventive health programmes. Screening has largely eradicated the brain damaged 'cretin'.

The procedure adopted generally is to combine screening with that for phenylketonuria using heel-prick blood collected about the third day of life on to filter paper. In Australia screening is performed by an assay of T_4. Samples with T_4 values reading below the normal range are then reassayed for TSH which will be elevated in hypothyroidism.

In many countries TSH is the initial screening test. If it is elevated, full thyroid function tests including T_4 and T_3 resin uptake are then arranged. Should thyroid screening indicate hypothyroidism, thyroid hormone replacement therapy is instituted without delay.

There are a number of confounding situations in thyroid screening. The following situations may lead to low T_4 which is not associated with an elevated TSH:

– thyroid-binding globulin (TBG) deficiency
– prematurity or 'sick euthyroid' syndrome
– secondary or tertiary hypothyroidism.

For further details of these disorders the reader is referred to the references in 'Further Reading'.

Outcome of neonatal screening programmes

This has included the following:

1. A precise figure for the incidence of neonatal hypothyroidism (1 in 4000 live births in Victoria, Australia).
2. A better understanding of defects mimicking hypothyroidism.
3. Primarily, earlier diagnosis and treatment of neonatal hypothyroidism.

Management of newborn and infant hypothyroidism

Confirmation of thyroid screening or a clinical diagnosis – particularly in an infant who missed neonatal screening – involves thyroid function studies. In primary hypothyroidism these will indicate low T_4, low or normal T_3RU, low calculated FTI and elevated TSH. A thyroid scan is useful in order to determine whether there is complete absence of the thyroid gland or an ectopic dysgenetic gland.

Treatment

The early administration of oral thyroxine (T_4) is essential, usually in a dose of 25–50 μg daily. In transient hypothyroidism due to exogenous iodine or some other agent, therapy may not be necessary or only required for several weeks or months.

Follow-up and prognosis of newborn hypothyroidism

In children diagnosed as hypothyroid on neonatal screening and treated appropriately, all have been completely normal intellectually and exhibiting normal growth and bone development. Only in cases where treatment has been delayed beyond 1–2 months have there been suggestions of development delay. Close follow-up is essential with frequent monitoring of the child's wellbeing, observing for symptoms of hypo- or hyperthyroidism (under or over treatment), linear growth, bone age, and biochemical thyroid status. Thyroid hormone dosage will vary according to bodyweight and rate of growth.

HYPOTHYROIDISM IN THE CHILD AND ADOLESCENT

This is less common in children than in adults especially beyond the neonatal period. The causes in order of frequency are:

1. Primary hypothyroidism: chronic lymphocytic (Hashimoto's) thyroiditis; congenital – late appearing ectopic gland and enzyme defects; exogenous agents, e.g. iodine, irradiation; miscellaneous, including enzyme defects.
2. Secondary or tertiary hypothyroidism: these include congenital or acquired defects and intracranial lesions including pituitary and suprasellar tumours and irradiation.

The clinical features in these age groups are similar to those in the infant in that the common feature is sluggishness of most body systems. The triad of short stature, obesity, and mental dullness points to hypothyroidism or other endocrine syndrome until proven otherwise. Other features are dry hair and skin, facial puffiness, constipation, hypothermia, bradycardia, slow reflex relaxation and dental delay. Goitre is common. A typical case is illustrated in Example 55.2.

Example 55.2 Hypothyroidism in a 13-year-old girl

A girl aged 13, presented to the school medical officer with short stature and some gradual fall off in school performance. She was noted to be rather quiet in class, having been more active and involved in previous years. She had become somewhat obese. On further questioning she admitted to constipation for 2 years as well as a preference for warm weather – in summer she required more clothes than her siblings. Hair and skin had been rather dry in spite of various lotions. She still had many primary teeth. On examination, she was short, moderately obese, with a height below the 3rd percentile. She was pale with a puffy face and dry hair and skin. The voice was hoarse and she moved slowly. The hands were cool and the pulse only 55 per minute. Ankle jerks showed a markedly delayed relaxation phase. The thyroid gland was diffusely enlarged, firm and non-tender.

Provisional diagnosis – primary hypothyroidism due to chronic lymphocytic (Hashimoto's) thyroiditis.
Investigations – T_4 35 (low), TSH 100 (high).
Thyroid microsomal antibodies – positive.
Bone age 8 years.
Treatment – thyroxine 100 μg daily.

In childhood hypothyroidism slow mental functioning may not be immediately obvious because of its gradual onset. In fact, some children with undiagnosed hypothyroidism perform quite well in class, having an apparently improved ability to 'focus' on a particular object. Teachers often regard them as quiet, conscientious 'model' students. This results from a reduced awareness of extraneous stimuli so that they may excel in narrow specific tasks. Ironically, once treated and made euthyroid, these children may have considerable difficulty adapting to the increased range of environmental stimuli apparently available to them.

Management of hypothyroidism in children and adolescents

The following investigations are appropriate:

1. Thyroid function tests T_4 (low), T_3RU (low), FTI (low), TSH (usually high)
2. Bone age (index of bony maturation) is delayed in long-standing hypothyroidism
3. Thyroid autoantibodies (positive in Hashimoto's thyroiditis)
4. Thyroid scan (patchy uptake in Hashimoto's thyroiditis)
5. Other: free T_4, cranial CT scan (if secondary or tertiary hypothyroidism is suspected).

Treatment

Thyroid hormone replacement therapy is always indicated if thyroid function is impaired. A starting dose of thyroxine of 50–100 μg daily is appropriate, depending on age and body weight. The aim is to bring the T_4 level back into the normal range, and to suppress TSH to normal.

Follow-up and prognosis of hypothyroidism in children and adolescents

As well as assessing clinical symptoms and signs and especially linear growth, thyroid function should be checked each few months, and bone age determined annually. Severely hypothyroid children show dramatic changes with treatment. These include weight loss, rapid growth, loss of primary teeth, increased energy and interest.

The long-term outcome of hypothyroidism presenting in childhood or adolescence is usually very good, since the rapid growth phase of the brain in the first two years of life has usually been protected.

GOITRES IN CHILDREN AND ADOLESCENTS

'Goitre' means diffuse enlargement of the thyroid gland, which occurs in approximately 4–5% of all children. Goitres are more common in girls during puberty, but are often not detected as they are usually not associated with disturbed thyroid function. The commonest cause of goitre in childhood and adolescence is chronic lymphocytic (Hashimoto's) thyroiditis. The entity known previously as 'goitre of puberty' is most commonly Hashimoto's thyroiditis, but could include mild enzyme defects. The major causes in order of frequency are:

1. Chronic lymphocytic (Hashimoto's) thyroiditis
2. Thyrotoxicosis
3. Enzyme defect or familial goitre
4. Tumour (benign and malignant)
5. Acute and subacute thyroiditis.

Clinical features of goitres in children and adolescents

The clinical questions to be answered are as follows:

– Is this child euthyroid?
– Is the goitre diffuse or localized?
– Is the goitre tender?
– Are there other systemic signs?

Chronic lymphocytic thyroiditis (otherwise known as Hashimoto's thyroiditis)

This is a relatively common autoimmune inflammatory disorder mainly seen in adolescent girls and young women. Although not usually associated with disturbed thyroid function, it is still the commonest cause of hypothyroidism in the older child and adolescent. Hashimoto's thyroiditis is often a self-limiting disease, and may remit spontaneously. The pathology involves an autoimmune infiltration of lymphocytes with consequent destruction of thyroid tissue. The disorder presents as a painless diffuse film enlargement of the thyroid gland, which has a slightly irregular consistency. Clinical features of hypothyroidism may be seen at presentation. Occasionally, the presenting features are consistent with hyperthyroidism, which is transient and possibly due to release of excess thyroid hormone secondary to gland destruction. These are associations with other autoimmune diseases such as type 1 diabetes, Addison's disease, vitiligo and pernicious anaemia.

Thyroid function tests are either normal, or may simply show an elevated TSH with a normal T_4 indicating a failing thyroid gland requiring greater TSH drive. When hypothyroidism is fully established the T_4 level falls. Thyroid autoantibodies (microsomal) are usually, but not invariably detected.

The clinical picture and findings described are usually sufficient to make the diagnosis, and further investigation is normally not indicated. If there is doubt, a thyroid scan, ultrasound examination and TSH receptor antibodies (positive in Graves' disease) will be required. Occasionally, a needle or open biopsy may be necessary, especially if there is a possibility of a tumorous nodule.

Therapy is indicated in Hashimoto's thyroiditis associated with hypothyroidism and in cases without overt hypothyroidism but with elevated TSH, as the gland is failing. Returning the TSH level to normal may also reduce the size of the gland by removing hyperstimulation of remaining thyroid cells by TSH.

Management of goitres in children and adolescents

In the presence of a goitre the following investigations are indicated:

1. Thyroid function studies – these are usually normal
2. Thyroid antibody screen – positive in Hashimoto's disease
3. Thyroid scan – occasionally but not always necessary
4. Other tests, e.g. full blood examination, ESR
5. A biopsy is rarely required.

Treatment

If thyroid function is disturbed this should be treated. Most euthyroid goitres will require no treatment but should be followed carefully as they may become hypothyroid, especially in the case of Hashimoto's thyroiditis. Thyroxine replacement will be indicated if the TSH is elevated. Tumours will require biopsy and definitive treatment (see below).

HYPERTHYROIDISM

Thyrotoxicosis is not common in childhood, occurring more frequently in adolescence, particularly in females.

The major causes in order of frequency are:

1. Graves' disease
2. Acute toxic Hashimoto's thyroiditis
3. A toxic nodule (rare).

Clinical features (see Example 55.3)

These are mostly due to a hypermetabolic state, with

Example 55.3 Clinical features of hyperthyroidism

tiredness
restlessness
tremor/involuntary movements
sweats/heat intolerance
diarrhoea
amenorrhoea
weight loss with good appetite
accelerated growth
tachycardia
a brisk relaxation phase of tendon reflexes
goitre (see Fig. 55.2).
eye signs – lid retraction, 'stare', proptosis
proximal muscle weakness (rare in childhood).

All of these features are rarely combined in the one patient.

---

over-activity of various systems through increased sympathetic drive.

The differential diagnosis of thyrotoxicosis includes anxiety states, sepsis, other causes of diarrhoea, eating disorders and some neurological disorders associated with choreiform movements.

Graves' disease

This, the commonest cause of hyperthyroidism at all ages, is an autoimmune disease, with some genetic predisposition, and therefore often familial. It is more common in females. The primary defect is a stimulating antibody to the receptor for TSH on thyroid cells (so mimicking TSH). This leads to both excess thyroid growth (goitre) and excess thyroid hormone production. There is often associated ophthalmopathy, due to deposition of proteoglycans in the extra-ocular muscles and retro-orbital space. This is distinct from the stare and lid retraction due to sympathetic over-activity.

Investigations indicated when hyperthyroidism is suspected are:

– thyroid function tests – elevated T_4 and T_3RU and FTI
– thyroid autoantibodies
– TSH receptor antibodies (positive in Graves' disease)
– bone age (often advanced).

Treatment

The following are three treatment options available for thyrotoxicosis:

– drug therapy (blockage of thyroid hormone synthesis)

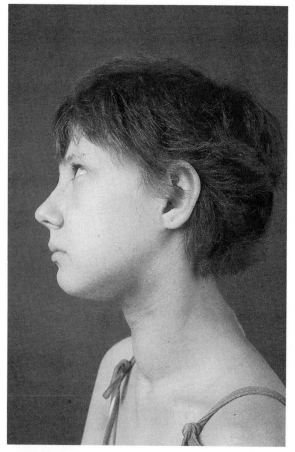

Fig. 55.2 Thyroid enlargement in a young girl with hyperthyroidism.

– surgery (partial thyroidectomy)
– radioactive iodine (partial destruction of the thyroid gland, which traps iodine).

The favoured option is drug therapy, using either Neo-Mercazole or propylthiouracil, both of which block organification in the thyroid. Also, they may influence the natural history by dampening the autoimmune process. Beta-blockers, adrenergic blocking agents e.g. propanolol, are useful in the acute phase in blocking the effects of sympathetic over-activity.

Treatment with organification-blocking drugs is continued for two years, by which time about 50% of children will have spontaneously remitted and therapy can be ceased. A reduced level of TSH receptor antibodies and reduced goitre size are both indicative of remission. If relapse occurs, drug therapy can safely be reinstated long term. Surgery and radio-active iodine are both definitive therapies useful in adults.

THYROID NODULES IN CHILDREN

In the assessment of a thyroid nodule the clinical questions to be asked are all designed to exclude possible malignancy. In the history they are the following:

1. Is there a family history of neck irradiation?
2. Is there a family history of multiple endocrine adenomatosis? (MEA – familial tumours of thyroid, pancreas, and phaeochromocytoma).
3. Have goitrogens or iodine deficiency been excluded (against malignancy)?
4. Is there a history of thyrotoxicosis (against malignancy)?

Important questions to be answered on examination are:

1. Is the nodule hard and attached to skin or muscle?
2. Is there dysphagia?
3. Are there features of the MEA syndrome? (Marfan-like habitus and bumpy lips).
4. Are there multiple nodules? (against malignancy)
5. Is the nodule tender? (against malignancy)

Investigations are designed to exclude malignancy; these are:

– thyroid function tests (if disturbed, against malignancy)
– thyroid autoantibody screen (if positive, against malignancy)
– Blood calcitonin (elevated in MEA with medullary carcinoma)

– thyroid scan (a cold nodule suggests malignancy or cyst)
– ultrasound (distinguishes a cyst from a solid cold nodule)
– needle aspiration (not widely used in children)

A decision concerning excision biopsy is then made based on the above findings. If there is doubt it is better to biopsy.

Treatment

Treatment of a benign nodule will depend on its size. Thyroid cancer (mostly 'papillary') is treated by total thyroidectomy and most are permanently eradicated and cured by surgery alone. Radioactive iodine therapy is only rarely required, namely, when metastases have occurred.

FURTHER READING

Fisher D A 1987 Effectiveness of newborn screening programmes for congenital hypothyroidism: prevalence of missed cases. The Pediatric Clinics of North America 34 (4) 881–890
Fisher D A, Pandian M R, Carlton E 1987 Autoimmune thyroid disease: an expanding spectrum. Pediatric Clinics of North America 34 (4) 907–918
Mahoney C P 1987 Differential diagnosis of goitre. The Pediatric Clinics of North America 34 (4) 891–905
Lifshitz F (ed) 1985 Pediatric endocrinology – a clinical guide. Marcel Dekker, New York

56. The child with ambiguous genitalia

Garry L. Warne

AMBIGUOUS GENITALIA

Immediately an infant is born, its genitalia are examined so that the parents (with father frequently in attendance) can be informed of the sex. Major problems arise when the genitalia are malformed to the extent where the gender cannot readily be identified. Not only do the parents have to contend with the physical malformation, but they also face a dilemma in deciding what to tell their other children, relatives and friends, and how to announce the birth in the newpapers. They commonly feel very isolated. The psychological effects of such an experience on the parents can be devastating and may affect their relationship with the child for years to come. The problem will be compounded if an incorrect announcement is made about the child's sex and so recorded on the official birth certificate.

Ambiguity of the genitalia is an important anomaly, not only because of the psychological problems that are caused, but also because of the very real possibility that the infant could have a life-threatening internal disorder.

Congenital adrenal hyperplasia (CAH)

Also know as the adrenogenital syndrome, this is a common cause of ambiguous genitalia. In most cases, the underlying defect is a deficiency in the adrenal cortex of the enzyme 21-hydroxylase. This results in a partial block in the biosynthesis of both cortisol and aldosterone. Because of the lack of cortisol, ACTH-mediated adrenal hypertrophy occurs, but the glands are incapable of secreting large quantities of any steroids other than androgens. In a female, these androgens are sufficient to cause clitoral enlargement and fusion of the labia. In some cases, the genitalia may resemble those of a male with undescended testes. More importantly, however, the child is at risk from sudden death due to salt-loss, hypoglycaemia and susceptibility to infection. Unless the correct diagnosis is made and

treatment (with both a glucocorticoid and a mineralocorticoid) started, the infant will die.

Thus, in each patient with ambiguous genitalia, three aspects of management must be considered:

1. How to minimize psychological stress in the parents
2. Diagnosis of life-threatening diseases
3. Surgical correction of anatomical defect.

Sexual differentiation and its regulation

In man, the process of primary sexual differentiation is androgen-dependent; oestrogens play no role in it. In the first 4–6 weeks of fetal life, male and female genitalia have an identical appearance. In each, a genital tubercle occupies the position of the phallus, at the apex of the two labioscrotal folds. Between these folds is the urogenital cleft (Fig. 56.1).

Internally, two pairs of tubular structures, called the Wolffian and Mullerian ducts, run in parallel down each side of the posterior abdominal wall. The Wolffian ducts are testosterone-dependent, and develop, in the male, into the vasa deferentia, the epididymis, the seminal vesicles, and the ejaculatory duct. The Mullerian ducts develop in the female into the Fallopian tubes, the uterus, and the upper third of the vagina.

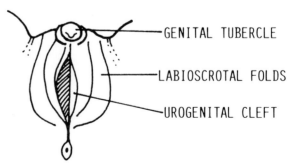

Fig. 56.1 Male and female genitalia in the first 4–6 weeks of fetal life.

The testes of the male fetus secrete two hormones: testosterone (a steroid), and Mullerian inhibitory substance (MIS), a polypeptide. Testosterone undergoes peripheral conversion to a more potent androgen, dihydrotestosterone (DHT), by the tissue enzyme, 5α-reductase.

The functions of testosterone, dihydrotestosterone and MIS with regard to sexual differentiation are summarized in Table 56.1.

Table 56.1 Embryological roles of testosterone, dihydrotestosterone, and Mullerian inhibitory substance (MIS)

Hormone	Embryological function
Testosterone	Stimulates ipsilateral Wolffian duct differentiation into vas deferens, prostate, seminal vesicle and ejaculatory duct
Dihydrotestosterone (formed from testosterone by 5α-reductase activity)	Promotes phallic growth, fusion of the labioscrotal folds, and enclosure of the penile urethra
Mullerian inhibitory substance	Induces ipsilateral regression of the Mullerian ducts, thus preventing development of Fallopian tubes, uterus or upper vagina

Aberrant genital differentiation in the female

The fetus may be exposed to testosterone as a result of:

1. Possessing testes
2. Aberrant adrenal activity (e.g. CAH)
3. A virilizing disease in the mother
4. The transplacental passage of virilizing drugs ingested by the mother.

Therefore, a genotypic female could be exposed to androgens for any of the latter three reasons, and would show masculinization of the external genitalia. The internal ducts, however, respond only to the high local concentration of testosterone that occur adjacent to the testis, and their development is not affected by the relatively low circulating levels of androgen.

Female pseudohermaphroditism

Genotypic females with masculinized external genitalia are sometimes called 'female pseudohermaphrodites'. This is a poor term, because it lacks diagnostic specificity.

It is more constructive to think of such infants simply as virilized females and then to set about finding why they are virilized. Congenital adrenal hyperplasia, due

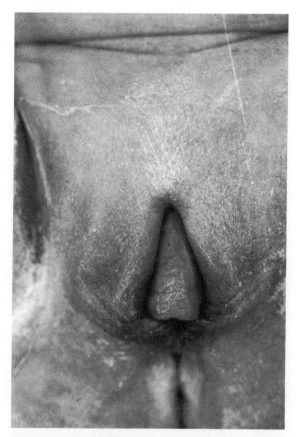

Fig. 56.2 External genitalia of female infant with Congenital adrenal hyperplasia

to either 21- or 11-hydroxylase deficiency, is by far the most important cause of virilization in female infants (Fig. 56.2).

Aberrant genital differentiation in the male

The normal development of the male reproductive system requires the following processes to occur:

1. Normal differentiation of the testes.
2. Normal testicular secretion of both testosterone and MIS.
3. Normal DHT production from testosterone in the genital tissues (i.e. normal 5α-reductase activity).
4. Normal tissue responses to both testosterone and DHT.

Each of the above steps can fail. The anatomical results of specific defects in the sequence are summarized in Table 56.2.

Table 56.2 Summary of the known causes of male
pseudohermaphroditism

Defect	Hormone deficit	Anatomical and functional results
Dysgenesis of the testes	No testosterone, DHT or MIS	Female or ambiguous phenotype, persistence of Mullerian structures (uterus and tubes). Infertility. No pubertal development
Isolated MIS deficiency	No MIS	Male phenotype, uterus and tubes present. Masculinize at puberty. Occasionally fertile.
Enzyme defect in testosterone biosynthesis	Reduced testosterone, normal MIS. Adrenal steroids may also be deficient	Ambiguous phenotype, no uterus. Do not masculinize at puberty. Infertile
5α-reductase deficiency	Abnormal ratio of testosterone: DHT	Ambiguous phenotype; no uterus. Undergo marked pubertal virilization. Infertile.
Androgen receptor deficiency (= syndrome of testicular feminization)	None: testosterone levels may be above normal. Ratio of T: DHT normal	Ambiguous or female phenotype, no uterus. At puberty breasts develop, but pubic hair may not. Shallow vagina. Testes may undergo malignant change. Infertile.

Male pseudohermaphroditism

'Male pseudohermaphroditism' is the term used for genotypic males who are born with phenotypic female or ambiguous genitalia. The adjectives 'complete' or 'incomplete' are used to indicate the extent to which the genitalia have retained the female phenotype. The term is still used quite commonly, because in many cases, it is impossible to arrive at a complete aetiological diagnosis, and hence a generic term is needed.

True hermaphroditism

'True hermaphroditism' is the term used for patients whose gonads contain both ovarian and testicular elements. Sometimes the ovotestis is unilateral. It can be regarded as a variant form of gonadal dysgenesis. Of patients with this condition, 75% have a 46XX karyotype, but chromosomal mosaicism (e.g. XX/XY) may also be present. Sterility is almost inevitable, and the external genitalia are usually ambiguous.

Other forms of gonadal dysgenesis

Turner's syndrome (45XO) is associated with streak gonads, but the external genitalia are unambiguously female. Occasionally, genotypic males (46XY) are encountered with either two streak gonads, or with a streak on one side and a testis on the other. They may be phenotypically female or have ambiguous genitalia, depending on how much testosterone secretion has occurred. Other karyotypes (e.g. XO/XY mosaicism may also be found in individuals with this syndrome of 'mixed gonadal dysgenesis'. There is an unacceptably high risk (approximately 30%) of malignant tumour development in the dysgenetic gonads when a Y chromosome is present and it is mandatory to remove them as soon as possible after diagnosis.

Defects in the biosynthesis of testosterone

A number of genetic enzyme defects have been described in the biosynthetic pathway for testosterone. All are transmitted as autosomal recessive traits. The adrenal cortex, as well as the testis, may be affected, so that there may be a significant risk of adrenal insufficiency. Each of the enzyme defects is very rare and, for a detailed description, the reader is referred to a comprehensive textbook of endocrinology. In a patient with an enzyme defect, one would find:

1. Normal testicular histology.
2. Low basal serum testosterone levels, with little or no testosterone response to human chorionic gonadotrophin (hCG).
3. Elevated levels of the steroid precursors proximal to the enzyme block.
4. A subnormal cortisol response to injected ACTH (but only in some enzyme defects).

Androgen insensitivity

The situation may arise where a phenotypic female, or an infant with ambiguous genitalia, is found to have histologically normal testes which show a normal testosterone response to hCG. The testes may be found unexpectedly during surgery for inguinal herniae in a phenotypic girl, or be noticed as swellings in the inguinal region or labia. (It should be noted, however, that ovaries may prolapse into the inguinal herniae.) In addition, such individuals usually lack a uterus, although a short vagina is usually present. The karyotype is 46XY. Other family members may be affected.

The explanation for these abnormalities is androgen insensitivity, which may be due to either a deficiency in the target tissues of the nuclear androgen receptor (a protein regulated by an X-linked gene), or a tissue deficiency in the cytoplasmic enzyme, 5α-reductase, which is controlled by an autosomal gene.

In girls with androgen insensitivity due to androgen receptor deficiency (a disorder formerly called 'testicular feminization'), breast development occurs at puberty due to the peripheral aromatization of testosterone to oestrogens, but pubic hair is either absent or sparse. Women with this disorder are at an increased risk of gonadal malignancy, and removal of both gonads followed by oestrogen replacement is generally recommended before patients reach adulthood. Spontaneous pubertal breast development does not occur in 5α-reductase deficiency – in fact, quite remarkable pubertal virilization may occur. Pubertal virilization, to a limited extent, is also possible in cases of partial androgen receptor deficiency, where the genitalia will be ambiguous. In these children, the gonads should always be removed at an early age.

It is possible to measure androgen receptor and 5α-reductase levels in cultured genital skin fibroblasts.

MANAGEMENT OF THE INFANT WITH AMBIGUOUS GENITALIA

Minimization of psychological distress in the parents

The parents should be shown the infant's genitalia so they may see for themselves that there is a problem in gender assignment. They should at the same time be told that, despite the confusing external appearance, their child will prove to be either a boy or a girl, and not something 'in between'. The genital malformation should be placed in the context of other congenital malformations and parents should be reassured that urgent investigations will be initiated to establish the true gender. A decision will be promised within two or three days, a promise which must be kept. The birth certificate should not be completed, or the infant named, until the final decision on the sex of rearing has been reached.

Diagnosis

An accurate family history, and a full history of the mother's drug ingestion during pregnancy, are essential.

From the physical examination, the following information should be gathered:

1. The infant's general conditon (hydration, colour, temperature, etc.).
2. Whether or not hyperpigmentation of the skin (suggestive of CAH) is present.
3. Whether or not gonads are palpable.
4. Whether or not (on rectal examination) a uterus can be palpated.

An infant who has ambiguous genitalia, impalpable gonads, increased pigmentation of the skin, and a palpable uterus, is a female with CAH until proved otherwise.

When CAH is suspected

The following procedure is essential:

1. Monitor the serum electrolytes (in the salt-losing form of CAH, the serum sodium will fall and the potassium will rise).
2. Monitor the blood glucose level (hypoglycaemia may occur).
3. Take blood urgently for a serum 17-hydroxyprogesterone assay (the result, under optimal circumstances, should be available the same day).
4. Collect a 24-hour urine specimen for steroid analysis by gas-liquid chromatography (GLC). The GLC profile provides useful information as to the nature of the enzyme block.
5. Request that chromosome karyotyping be done urgently.

When CAH has been diagnosed management is as follows:

1. Intravenous electrolyte replacement.
2. Maintenance of blood glucose levels.
3. Hydrocortisone or cortisone acetate.
4. 9α-fluorohydrocortisone, if the child proves to be a salt-loser.
Note: These steroids will be required for life.
5. Referral to an experienced paediatric surgeon for the planning of genital surgery. Radiological or endoscopic investigations may form part of the assessment of the lower genital tract. Females with virilization due to

CAH should always be raised as females because they have normal reproductive potential.

6. Genetic counselling. CAH is inherited as an autosomal recessive defect.

When CAH has been excluded

It should be possible to know within 24 hours whether or not the infant has 21-hydroxylase deficiency. In some cases, this diagnosis will have been eliminated on clinical grounds.

Laparotomy with gonadal biopsy is the most expedient approach to a working diagnosis in patients shown not to have CAH. Surgery is contraindicated, however, where there is still a possibility of CAH, because of the grave risk that adrenal insufficiency could be precipitated. If in doubt, glucocorticoid cover should be given.

The purpose of the laparotomy is to discover whether or not a uterus is present (indicating lack of MIS activity) and to identify patients with gonadal dysgenesis. Some information regarding the presence of the uterus could be gained by other means (e.g. ultrasound, laparoscopy or a urogenital sinugram), but surgery is, generally, the only practicable means of obtaining gonadal tissue for microscopic examination.

Information about the endocrine function of the gonads can be obtained by studying the serum testosterone response to the intramuscular injection of human chorionic gonadotrophin (hCG). For this test, blood is taken before, and 72 hours after, a single intramuscular injection of hCG (2000 iu)

By the time the infant is 2–3 days old, the following information should be available:

1. Whether or not the infant has CAH
2. Whether or not the gonads are dysgenetic
3. Whether or not there is a uterus.

This is sufficient information to permit a decision on the sex of rearing to be made; a longer delay will have a detrimental effect upon the parents' emotional state.

Further investigations are necessary to provide a sound basis for genetic counselling. Androgen receptor deficiency, 5α-reductase deficiency, and the various enzyme defects in steroidogenesis (including CAH) are all genetically transmissable disorders which could affect future generations.

Table 56.3 summarizes the major clinical features and diagnostic test results of the main disorders causing ambiguity of the external genitalia.

Deciding on the sex of rearing

When there is serious doubt as to what the sex of rearing should be, it should be remembered that the female sex of rearing is generally the more practicable and successful one to select. This is because it is virtually impossible to create an adequate penis surgically if the phallus is very small and contains little erectile tissue. It is quite feasible, on the other hand, to create a cosmetically acceptable vulva and a functional vagina in all cases. One should also consider that recent advances in the field of in vitro fertilization using donor ova may make it possible for patients who have a uterus and a

Table 56.3 Comparison of the major causes of ambiguous genitalia with regard to clinical and laboratory features

	Testes usually palpable	Uterus palpable	Pigmentation	Salt depletion	Karyotype	hCG stimulation test	Other tests required
Gonadal dysgenesis	−	+	−	−	XO/XY XY	No T	Laparotomy Gonadal biopsy
Defective testosterone biosynthesis	+	−	±	±*	46 XY	No T	Measure testosterone precursors
Androgen insensitivity Receptor deficiency	+	−	−	−	46 XY	T, DHT	Fibroblast AR assay on genital skin
5α-reductase deficiency	+	−	−	−	46 XY	T, no DHT	Fibroblast 5α-reductase assay on genital skin
CAH (21-hydroxylase deficiency)	−	+	+	+	46 XX	Not necessary	Serum 17 OHP Urinary pregnanetriol

*3β-hydroxysteroid dehydrogenase, 20–22 desmolase deficiencies. *Abbreviations:* T = testosterone; OHT = dihydrotestosterone; AR = androgen receptor.

vagina, but no gonads, to become pregnant, even, theoretically, if the karyotype were 46XY!

The only patients born with ambiguous genitalia who are likely to be fertile are those with CAH and those who simply have a severe degree of penile hypospadias. Normal spermatogenesis, coupled to an intact ejaculatory duct system and an adequate erectile penis, is hardly ever found in individuals with ambiguous genitalia. The onus is, therefore, on the physician to demonstrate that the patient could function successfully as a male, if reared as such. Two questions are relevant to this issue:

1. Will the child be able to micturate standing up, as other boys do?
2. Will he be able to perform satisfactory sexual intercourse in the male role?

If the male sex of rearing is decided upon, it may be useful to carry out an immediate therapeutic low-dose trial of testosterone, to measure the extent of the penile response to this hormone. If there is little or no response, the decision to raise the child as a male should be seriously questioned, as pubertal virilization may not be possible. The possible outcome of the test should be fully discussed with the parents before it is begun.

Counselling the parents

Most parents are capable of accepting the nature of the child's defect if the information is given sensitively and in a manner they can understand. It is stressed that the physician who performs this task must have both the necessary expertise and compassion. Parents must be very positively informed that the child is not somewhere 'in between', but definitely male or definitely female.

Fears that the child may become homosexual should be anticipated and openly discussed. These fears have no factual basis.

The parents should be encouraged to refer to the child as 'he' or 'she', and never as 'it', as must the doctor and nurses. The choice of sexually ambiguous given names is to be discouraged.

While the mother is still in hospital, it is important that the staff involved in her care communicate well with one another, to avoid presenting her with conflicting ideas.

Later issues for the patient

Since most patients with ambiguous genitalia (excluding those with CAH and those with simple hypospadias) will be sterile and will need sex hormone replacement to induce pubertal development, they will need at some stage to be given an explanation of their problem. The explanation can be given gradually, beginning at around the age of 8–9 years. It should never contain information that would shake the child's confidence in his or her gender-identity. If a child with a 46XY karyotype had been raised as a female, for example, the presence of a 'male' genotype should probably not be revealed to her. Such information, apart from being likely to have a shattering effect on the girl, is irrelevant, because the child's gender is, in fact, the one that she perceives as her own, and the one in which she functions.

Can genital ambiguity be prevented?

Where a mother has previously given birth to a child with CAH, an option which may be considered is to offer her treatment with dexamethasone during subsequent pregnancies. The purpose of this is to suppress the adrenal glands of the fetus. To be effective, treatment has to be started as soon as the pregnancy has been confirmed, and be continued throughout the pregnancy. An amniocentesis at 15 weeks' gestation would show (through sex chromosome, HLA typing and hormone assays) the sex of the fetus and its CAH status, and treatment could be stopped if the fetus was either unaffected, or male. Early experience with this treatment has given promising results.

FURTHER READING

Miller W L, Levine L S 1987 Molecular and clinical advances in congenital adrenal hyperplasia. Journal of Pediatrics 111: 1–17
Saenger P 1984 Abnormal sexual differentiation. Journal of Pediatrics 104: 1–17
Warne G L, Gyorki S, Risbridger G P, Khalid B A K, Funder J W 1983 Correlations between fibroblast androgen receptor levels and clinical features in abnormal male sexual differentiation and infertility. Australian and New Zealand Journal of Medicine 13: 335–344

57. Childhood diabetes and hypoglycaemia

Martin Silink

DIABETES MELLITUS

Diabetes mellitus is a complex metabolic disorder caused by insufficient insulin action. In childhood, 98% of diabetes is type 1 or insulin-dependent diabetes mellitus (IDDM) and 1% is secondary to pancreatic fibrosis (following cystic fibrosis, or haemosiderosis). These conditions are associated with a true deficiency of insulin. Approximately 1% of children have type 2 or non-insulin-dependent diabetes mellitus (NIDDM) which is due to a peripheral resistance to the action of insulin. Apart from the avoidance of sugar and the prevention of obesity, no further therapy is required for children with NIDDM and it will not be discussed further.

The prevalence of type 1 diabetes mellitus in Australia is approximately 1 in 750 for children under the age of 19 years with an annual incidence rate of 16 per 100 000 population. This is similar to New Zealand, USA and Britain. In parts of Scandinavia the incidence rate exceeds 30 per 100 000. The reasons for these variations are not known.

Aetiology

The causes of type 1 diabetes are multifactorial (Fig. 57.1). The vast body of scientific opinion suggests that an autoimmune process is directed against the pancreatic beta cell in genetically predisposed individuals following an environmental trigger. The evidence for the genetic predisposition resides in the familial tendency to type 1 diabetes and in the demonstration that over 90% of patients have tissue types which contain the HLA DR3, and/or HLA DR4 antigens.

The evidence for the autoimmune process is the histological demonstration of insulinitis (lymphocytic infiltrations of the islets of Langerhans) and the presence of islet cell antibodies and lymphocytotoxicity directed against islet cells.

The environmental trigger may be either a viral in-

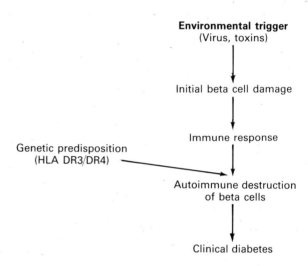

Fig. 57.1 The aetiology of diabetes mellitus.

fection (most of the evidence so far points to the Coxsackie group), a naturally occurring beta cell toxin (nitrosamines and others) or certain chemicals.

The autoimmune destruction of the beta cell proceeds relentlessly and clinical diabetes occurs when less than 10% of the beta cell mass remains. This process may take months or years. (In a small group of patients in whom there is no evidence of autoimmune destruction, the cause of diabetes may be direct damage of the beta cells by the viral disorder.)

Pathogenesis

Insulin is the hormone of energy storage and anabolism. It allows glucose to enter cells and be stored as glycogen (in liver and muscle) and as triglyceride (in fat). Insulin deficiency prevents glycogen and triglyceride storage and promotes their breakdown as well as that of protein. In addition, hepatic gluconeogenesis is promoted. The combined effects of glycogen breakdown, gluconeogenesis and failure of glucose entry into cells results in the blood glucose rising. When the blood glucose exceeds 10 mmol/l, the renal threshold is exceeded and glycosuria occurs. The osmotic effect of the glycosuria causes polyuria and dehydration. In severe cases over a kilogram of glucose can be excreted in the urine daily. The breakdown of triglyceride (lipolysis) releases free fatty acids into the circulation. In the liver these are converted to ketoacids (ketogenesis). In insulin deficiency, ketogenesis is marked and peripheral use of the ketoacids is diminished. This results in a rapid accumulation of these organic acids with eventual development of ketoacidosis.

The weight loss is initially caused by the breakdown of fat and muscle (due to insulin deficiency per se and the loss of many kilojoules as glucose in the urine) and subsequently by dehydration.

Course

IDDM is characterized by several phases. The first is the phase of autoimmune destruction of the beta cells of the pancreas. There are no clinical clues to the presence of this process and the child feels well. As the destruction approaches 90% of the beta cell mass, episodic glycosuria may occur, especially if there is a stress factor such as infection, acute asthma etc. The second phase is the sudden onset of clinical diabetes when the blood glucose has risen to levels high enough to exceed the renal threshold and glycosuria occurs. As the insulin deficiency proceeds diabetic ketoacidosis supervenes and, if not treated, would result in death.

Phase three occurs in about 50% of children, soon after insulin therapy has been started. Within days to weeks of treatment being started, some recovery of the remaining beta cells occurs. During this period of partial remission (also known as the 'honeymoon' phase), insulin requirements may diminish. This phase may last for weeks or months, but as the underlying autoimmune destruction of beta cells is still in progress, more complete insulin deficiency occurs so that blood glucose levels gradually rise and phase four is entered. This is the chronic phase of insulin deficiency and life-long dependence on administered insulin.

Clinical features

The sex ratio in type 1 diabetes is equal. Diabetes is uncommon in infancy. In childhood the incidence shows two peaks, 4–6 years and 10–14 years. In colder climates, clustering of newly diagnosed cases occurs in winter. This is seen in Melbourne but not in Sydney.

Symptoms are usually present 4–6 weeks before the diagnosis is made. In about 5% of cases the onset is more gradual, with clinical features being present for several months before diagnosis. In a further 5% the onset is catastrophic with progression from first symptoms to life-threatening ketoacidosis within a few days. The most frequent early clinical features are polyuria and polydipsia, nocturia, lethargy, irritability, rapid weight loss, secondary enuresis, recurrent skin infections (staphylococcal) and perineal *Candida albicans* infections (thrush). Most of these early features can be explained by the hyperglycaemia, the resulting osmotic diuresis and the increased liability to infection in hyperglycaemic individuals. As the insulin deficiency becomes more profound, more serious metabolic disturbances occur. Metabolic acidosis results from the overproduction of ketoacids (β-hydroxybutyric acid and acetoacetic acid). When the arterial pH falls below 7.2 rapid deep breathing (Kussmaul respiration) becomes clinically evident. This is an attempt by the body to compensate for the metabolic acidosis by inducing a respiratory alkalosis (breathing off carbon dioxide). Chemical breakdown of acetoacetic acid in the body yields acetone which, because of its volatility, can be detected on the patient's breath. Weight loss becomes more dramatic with breakdown of fat and protein, and dehydration all contributing. Abdominal pain, mimicking an acute surgical abdomen may occur. Acute decompensation occurs when the child starts to vomit and life-threatening dehydration (shock) occurs because of continuing massive urinary losses (caused by the osmotic diuresis). The acidosis, dehydration, and changes in plasma osmolality all contribute to central nervous dysfunction and cause initial precoma (confusion and obtundation) and eventual coma. Because immune function becomes compromised in diabetes the possibility of serious infection should always be considered.

Diagnosis

The diagnosis of IDDM in childhood is usually not difficult providing the physician is aware that this condition does occur even in the very young. The most common misdiagnoses are to call the polyuria a urinary tract infection and the overbreathing of metabolic acidosis, a respiratory tract infection or asthma.

The diagnosis of diabetes is made by:

1. History.
2. Urinalysis (glycosuria and ketonuria).
3. Estimation of blood glucose (levels over 15 mmol/l are diagnostic). It is not necessary to perform glucose tolerance tests for diagnosis.

The initial laboratory assessment in the seriously ill

patients should also include serum electrolytes, blood gases and pH (preferably arterial). Evidence of infection (urine, respiratory tract, skin and septicaemia) should be looked for.

Treatment of diabetic ketoacidosis

Therapy is directed at:

1. Emergency fluid replacement (using volume expanders such as albumin) if shock is present so the circulation is restored.
2. Correction of dehydration over 24 hours.
3. Replacement of electrolyte loss (due to vomiting and to urinary losses occurring with osmotic diuresis and acidosis).
4. Reversal of the metabolic acidosis (if pH is less than 7.1) with intravenous bicarbonate (alkali).
5. Correction of the insulin deficiency (and consequently the hyperglycaemia and metabolic acidosis).

Treatment should be undertaken only in a centre equipped with intensive care facilities; the child may need to be transported there by an expert retrieval team. Frequent biochemical monitoring of the blood glucose, electrolytes and blood gases is important in the emergency treatment. Following the treatment of shock, if present, the usual intravenous fluid used is normal saline (i.e. isotonic or 0.9%) to which potassium is added. This replaces both the fluid (volume) and electrolyte losses. Because total body potassium deficits may be major (e.g. 8–10 mmol K^+ per kg body weight) intravenous fluids with supplemental posassium to levels of 40–60 mmol/l are frequently required. The volume of intravenous fluids should be such as to repair the dehydration over 24 hours, and provide for maintenance requirements and insensible losses. Because the glycosuria causes an osmotic diuresis, continuing urinary losses may be large and a meticulous fluid balance needs to be kept.

Correction of the metabolic acidosis with intravenous bicarbonate may be necessary if the pH is less than 7.1 and the patient is very sick. This is a potentially dangerous manoeuvre, as it can drive potassium out of the extracellular fluid into cells and cause life-threatening hypokalaemic cardiac rhythm changes. If bicarbonate needs to be given, then the following guidelines should be observed: replacement should be given as a slow infusion over 1–2 hours; only a quarter of the calculated losses be given at any one time (base deficit figures are derived from blood gas measurements); potassium replacement should be ongoing; ECG monitoring should be continuous.

Insulin replacement is best given by a continuous intravenous infusion of quick-acting (soluble) insulin. The initial rate of 0.1 unit/kg/hr is adjusted to produce a fall in the blood glucose level of 5 mmol/l/hr. More rapid reductions in the blood glucose level alter the plasma osmolality too quickly and increase the risks of life-threatening cerebral oedema. As soon as the blood glucose falls to below 10 mmol/l, the intravenous fluids are changed to 2.5% dextrose in 0.45% saline and the insulin infusion is adjusted to maintain blood glucose levels between 4 and 10 mmol/l. Usually this regime takes 24 hours to restore homeostasis. When the urinary ketones disappear, oral fluids are allowed and if tolerated, a diabetic diet is commenced. Continuing insulin therapy is graded to 6-hourly doses of subcutaneous quick-acting insulin and finally to twice-daily injections of the appropriate combination of short- and intermediate-acting insulin.

Aims of management

IDDM is a lifelong disorder. By definition insulin treatment is necessary and at present can only be given by injection. The aims of management are to achieve the following short- and long-term aims.

1. The short-term aims are for the child to have good health (with avoidance of hypoglycaemia), normal growth and pubertal development, a normal school-life and normal psychological growth and development.
2. The long-term aims are the avoidance of long-term diabetic complications (nephropathy, neuropathy, retinopathy, microvascular and macrovascular disease) and the fulfillment of the patient's aspirations for employment and family life.

Management principles

The attainment of these aims is largely dependent on maintaining good diabetic control. This is difficult to achieve and especially difficult in the under 5-year-age group and the adolescent. Basically the aim is to keep the blood glucose levels between 4 and 10 mmol/l pre- and postprandially. To measure the blood glucose the patient uses a spring-loaded lancet to prick a finger and obtain a drop of blood which is placed on a reagent strip impregnated with glucose oxidase and a dye. Hydrogen peroxide generated as a by-product of the reaction catalysed by glucose oxidase alters the colour of the dye. This change can be accurately quantitated by a reflectance meter. Most children measure their blood glucose two to three times a day. The key elements in achieving stability in the blood glucose levels are:

1. Diet

2. Insulin
3. Exercise.

Diet

The effect of food is to raise the blood glucose level and this must be balanced by the glucose lowering effect of insulin and exercise. This delicate balancing act is best achieved by having the diabetic diet supply the same quantity of carbohydrate each day and for the carbohydrate to be distributed as three major meals (breakfast, lunch, evening meal) and three snacks (morning tea, afternoon tea and supper). The diabetic diet is basically free of simple carbohydrates (sugar), low in saturated fats, and provides 50–55% of the kilojoules as complex carbohydrate, 30–35% as fat and 15% as protein. The diet must be nutritionally adequate (including vitamins, iron, calcium) to allow the child to grow normally and satisfying to the child. Frequent review by an experienced dietitian is necessary to cope with changing requirements as the child grows. Extra food needs to be taken before and during exercise to prevent the occurrence of hypoglycaemia.

Insulin

Because the child grows, insulin therapy has to be adjusted frequently. Insulin therapy has to be individualized and usually the children require less than 1 unit per kg body weight per day given as one, or more commonly, two subcutaneous injections daily. Approximately two-thirds of the total dose is given before breakfast and one-third before the evening meal, in a combination of rapid-acting (e.g. Actrapid, Velosulin or Humulin R) and intermediate-acting insulin (Protaphane, Insulatard or Humulin NPH).

The dose of insulin is adjusted according to blood sugar measurements which are done several times daily at home. The ability to perform home blood glucose monitoring (using reagent sticks and reflectance meters) has introduced a great measure of safety in the control of diabetes.

Exercise

Exercise is the third major component of diabetes management after insulin and diet. Exercise increases cellular uptake of glucose by the exercising muscles and lowers the blood glucose level. This effect is only seen if the diabetes is in good control and adequate serum levels of insulin are present (exercise undertaken during poor control and low circulating insulin levels may paradoxically raise the blood glucose levels). To combat the usual blood glucose lowering effect of exercise, the child should eat extra food which should contain both rapidly absorbed carbohydrate (e.g. simple sugar) and more complex carbohydrate (e.g. starches as present in bread and cereals) for more prolonged absorption. Exercise should be encouraged in all diabetic patients and should be done on a regular (preferably daily) basis.

Outpatient management

For most children with diabetes, their initial hospitalization at diagnosis is their only hospital admission because of their diabetes. Medical follow-up visits are usually every three months and at each visit the following clinical points are assessed:

– General wellbeing
– Occurrence of hypoglycaemic episodes
– School absenteeism
– Height
– Weight
– Pubertal stage
– Injection sites
– Presence of hepatomegaly
– Presence of skin infections
– Evidence of diabetic complications.

The blood glucose profile is examined in the logbook kept by the patient and the adequacy of the dietary and insulin regime assessed.

In addition to the blood glucose logbook, the physician also has at his disposal several other biochemical parameters that indicate the degree of glycaemic control. The serum fructosamine measures the extent of non-enzymatic glycosylation of serum proteins whilst the glycosylated haemoglobin (also called HbA_{1C} or fast haemoglobin) measures the degree of glycosylation of the haemoglobin. These parameters thus give an indication of the glycaemic control over the life span of the serum proteins (3 weeks) and the red cells (120 days).

With the combined efforts of the parents, the child with diabetes and the diabetes management team (physician, dietitian, diabetes educator, social worker and psychologist) most children grow and develop normally, achieve their educational potential and have a satisfying childhood.

Special problems in management

Hypoglycaemia

To the parents the occurrence of severe hypoglycaemia in their child is one of the most distressing and worrying aspects of diabetes management. In the vast majority of cases no long-term harmful effects result from the occasional severe hypoglycaemic episode; however, the underlying concern of possible brain damage remains. Minor hypoglycaemic episodes are very frequent and reflect the difficulties in achieving good control. The best treatment is prevention. All patients with IDDM should carry some rapidly absorbable carbohydrate for immediate treatment of hypoglycaemia symptoms.

Hypoglycaemia may occur if the insulin dose is excessive, insufficient food eaten or extra exercise undertaken. The clinical features of hypoglycaemia can be divided into:

a. Stimulation of the sympathetic nervous system (anxiety, palpitation, tachycardia, pallor, perspiration)

b. Effects on the central nervous system (lethargy, dizziness, ataxia, weakness, confusion, personality changes, visual disturbances, unconsciousness, localized and generalized seizures)

c. Bodily symptoms of headaches and abdominal pains.

These clinical features appear rapidly (less than 30 minutes), in a previously well child, and there is no difficulty in differentiating hypoglycaemic coma from the coma of diabetic ketoacidosis.

The emergency treatment in the unconscious child is either the intramuscular injection of glucagon (half unit for children under five years of age and 1 unit for older children and adults) or the use of intravenous glucose (1 ml of 50% dextrose per kg body weight). All families with a diabetic child should have glucagon at home and be able to give it intramuscularly. Response to therapy is rapid (in minutes). For the less severely affected, hypoglycaemia can be treated with oral glucose (e.g. half glass sweet lemonade or 7 jelly beans). On improvement after the emergency treatment, the child should receive some food containing complex carbohydrate (e.g. starch) to ensure glucose levels are maintained by slow release of carbohydrate.

Management of sick days

Children with well-controlled diabetes are no more prone to infections than the non-diabetic child. When these occur, however, special problems arise. The stress of the infection, especially if associated with fever, causes a temporary insulin resistance and more insulin is required. The blood glucose tends to rise despite anorexia and a poor intake. Ketonuria may occur. This is a sign of significant insulin deficiency allowing fat to be broken down and converted into ketoacids. If untreated, diabetic ketoacidosis could develop. Parents are taught to measure blood glucose levels frequently,

monitor the presence of ketonuria (with reagent strips) and give frequent small doses (10–20% of daily requirements) of short-acting insulin every 3 to 4 hours until the diabetes is stabilized again.

Growth

Because insulin is the principal hormone of energy storage and anabolism, growth disturbances occur if diabetes control is not satisfactory. The growth velocity decreases and short stature may result from prolonged poor control. The Mauriac syndrome is an extreme example of this (shortness, hepatic enlargement due to fat-infiltrated liver). The growth of a diabetic child should be formally charted on a growth curve at each clinic visit.

Delayed puberty

Similarly, chronic poor control delays entry into puberty. The combined effects of short stature, and delayed sexual maturation may lead to significant psychological and emotional stresses.

Psychological stresses

Major problems arise with diabetic control in the presence of psychological stresses. Blood glucose levels tend to rise quickly and insulin therapy cannot cope to maintain diabetic balance. Easily identifiable stresses such as school examinations usually do not cause major problems. Family conflicts, parental separation, teenage rebellion and other emotional problems may cause a more profound instability and psychological counselling or formal psychotherapy may be required by the child and the whole family. The relevance of psychological and emotional wellbeing to good diabetes control is of such importance that the social worker or psychologist is an integral part of the management team.

Compliance

Good diabetes control is difficult in the best of circumstances. It becomes impossible when the child alone or the family as a whole become non-compliant with diet, monitoring or injections of insulin. Refusal to perform blood tests and to conform to the prescribed diet are not unusual periodically and represent a rebellion against the never-ending discipline that characterizes diabetic management. Patience, counselling and empathy are necessary, especially in adolescence, when the burden of having diabetes is particularly heavy to bear.

Future directions

Much research is in progress. New insulin analogues will soon be available to provide a better range of short-, intermediate- and long-acting insulins. Experimental trials of alternate ways of insulin administration (nasal, inhalational and oral) are under way but all suffer the problems of inconsistent absorption. Immunomodulation of the autoimmune process is being tried with some success in newly diagnosed patients who have some insulin secretion remaining. So far the dangers of the immunomodulation therapy outweigh the risks of having diabetes. Pancreatic transplantation of segments of the whole pancreas has been successfully undertaken. However, the operation is hazardous, prevention of rejection of the transplant requires lifelong immunosuppression and donors of the pancreatic graft are hard to find. The use of fetal pancreatic tissue to cure diabetes has not been successful in humans and major ethical issues have to be resolved for continued experimentation to occur. Artificial insulin delivery systems (external and internal pumps) are under trial. The long-term aim is to devise an implantable blood glucose sensor that could be linked with an internal insulin pump (i.e. an artificial pancreas). It is likely that by the turn of the century, many of these therapeutic options will be a reality.

HYPOGLYCAEMIA

The definition of hypoglycaemia is a plasma glucose level of less than 2.2 mmol/l (40 mg%). The level of blood glucose depends on the balance of glucose entering the blood stream (from food, hepatic glycogen breakdown and hepatic gluconeogenesis) and glucose leaving the circulation (for use as an energy substrate and for storage in fat and glycogen depots) (Fig. 57.2). Hepatic glycogen breakdown, gluconeogenesis and the storage of glucose as fat or glycogen are all under the control of the hormonal system which modulates the activity of key enzymatic steps. This balance is finely

tuned, especially in the neonatal period and the very young. All children can become hypoglycaemic if stressed sufficiently (e.g. prolonged fasting and high metabolic demands due to infection, fever, tachycardia and increased respiratory efforts). The measurement of the blood glucose level should be part of the clinical evaluation of any sick child. This section will not deal further with the occasional hypoglycaemia occurring in the very sick child, but will concentrate on the causes of recurrent hypoglycaemia (see Example 57.1).

Example 57.1 Causes of hypoglycaemia

1. **Endocrine**
   Hyperinsulinism
   infant of diabetic mother
   Rh incompatibility
   Beckwith-Wiedemann syndrome
   nesidioblastosis
   islet cell adenoma

   Growth hormone deficiency
   isolated GH deficiency
   panhypopituitarism

   Adrenocortical deficiency
   Addison's disease
   congenital adrenal hyperplasia
   secondary to ACTH deficiency (hypopituitarism)

2. **Hepatic**
   Immaturity
   Liver disease
   hepatitis
   anoxic liver disease
   drugs, toxins (alcohol, aspirin)
   Reye's syndrome
   Galactosaemia
   Hereditary fructose intolerance
   Glycogen synthase deficiency
   Glycogen storage disorders
   Gluconeogenic enzyme deficiencies
   Other enzyme deficiencies (protein, lipid metabolism)

3. **Increased use**
   Fever
   Infection
   Hypothermia
   Exercise

Clinical features

The main features of hypoglycaemia have been outlined in the section dealing with hypoglycaemia as a complication of the management of insulin-dependent diabetes mellitus. In the neonate in whom hypoglycaemia is most likely to occur, additional clinical features are jitteriness, recurrent apnoea, hypotonia, hypothermia, irritability or apathy. In the older infant and child, the clinical features are more readily recognized as being due to sympathetic nerve stimulation (tachycardia, palpitation,

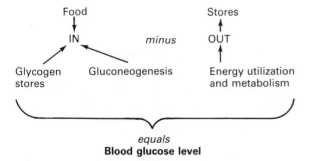

Fig. 57.2 Normal glucose homeostasis.

pallor, perspiration, tremor), disturbed CNS function (confusion, mood changes, ataxia, convulsions, coma) and some general symptoms such as headaches and abdominal pains.

Therapy

The emergency treatment of hypoglycaemia is the provision of glucose orally or intravenously if the patient is unconscious (see diabetes section). Glucagon will not be effective if hepatic glycogen stores are depleted and hence is not used routinely.

Recurrent hypoglycaemia

Recurrent hypoglycaemia can occur during fasting or in the immediate postprandial period (reactive hypoglycaemia). In childhood, reactive hypoglycaemia is rare. Causes of reactive hypoglycaemia include hyperinsulinism and inadequate hepatic glycogen breakdown. These are also associated with fasting hypoglycaemia and hence the remainder of this section will deal with the evaluation of fasting hypoglycaemia.

Causes of recurrent hypoglycaemia

Endocrine. By far the most important hormone in the regulation of glucose metabolism is insulin. If insulin is present in excessive amounts not only does hypoglycaemia occur, but fat breakdown is prevented and the cells are deprived of their three main energy substrates (glucose, free fatty acids and ketone acids). The hypoglycaemia of hyperinsulinism is the most severe of all the causes and the most likely to cause cerebral injury.

Growth hormone and hydrocortisone are important in maintaining the enzyme systems that promote hepatic glycogen synthesis and gluconeogenesis. Deficiencies of these hormones thus lead to inadequate glycogen stores and gluconeogenesis. The stress of fasting will, therefore, uncover the tendency to hypoglycaemia in hypopituitarism and in primary adrenal insufficiency. A fasting study in these hormone deficiencies will reveal suppressed serum insulin levels associated with progressively more elevated free fatty acid and ketoacid levels as the body tries to conserve its glucose stores by changing to a fat-energy metabolism. Most of the examples of fasting hypoglycaemia due to inadequate glycogen stores and insufficient gluconeogenic activity of the liver are associated with elevated serum ketoacid levels. Treatment of the hormone deficiency by the appropriate hormone replacement rapidly corrects the tendency to hypoglycaemia.

Enzymatic. The complex hepatic enzyme systems of the liver are not mature till full gestation. Premature infants are especially prone to hypoglycaemia due to hepatic immaturity and poor glycogen stores.

A large number of inherited primary deficiencies of glycogen formation (glycogen synthase deficiency) and breakdown (glycogen storage disorders) have been elucidated. They are rare and usually inherited in an autosomal recessive manner. Primary deficiencies of key gluconeogenic enzymes are also known. In addition, secondary enzyme defects may occur in widespread liver disease (hepatitis, anoxic liver injury), and deficiencies of certain protein and lipid enzyme systems (e.g. methyl malonic aciduria) and in deficiencies affecting the metabolism of certain carbohydrates (galactosaemia and hereditary fructose intolerance).

Stresses to energy homeostasis. Because the maintenance of a normal blood glucose is dependent on so many factors, minor problems in glucose homeostasis will be brought out if glucose is used at a faster than normal rate as a metabolic fuel. This is especially so if the patient is fasting and totally reliant on glycogen stores (which may be limited) and gluconeogenesis to maintain glucose levels. The causes of increased metabolic demands are exercise, infection, fever and increased muscular activity of respiratory distress and hypothermia. Frequently they occur in combination, especially in the neonatal group.

Investigation

The evaluation of fasting hypoglycaemia depends on the accurate measurement in the serum of glucose, insulin, free fatty acids and ketoacids during a monitored fast. Adrenocortical insufficiency is excluded by an ACTH stimulation test. Growth hormone deficiency is excluded by pharmacological stimulation of the anterior pituitary. These tests will provide the answer whether the cause is hormonal or whether the problem is primarily a metabolic one. More detailed evaluation of a metabolic defect will be dependent on the search for associated biochemical clues, e.g. lactic acidosis, organic aciduria, aminoaciduria, galactosuria (see Ch. 28).

Clinical conditions and management

Recurrent hypoglycaemia has many and varied causes but some causes are more common in certain age groups.

Neonatal

Recurrent hypoglycaemia occurring in the neonatal period is discussed in Chapter 24.

1 month to 18 months

Nesidioblastosis (hyperplasia of primitive beta cells) is the most serious cause of recurrent fasting hypoglycaemia in this age group. While the milder cases of nesidioblastosis may be managed with medical therapy using diazoxide, partial pancreatectomy may be required if the hyperinsulinism persists. With time, many patients with nesidioblastosis grow out of their hyperinsulinism. It is emphasized that in this group therapy must be aggressive to prevent brain damage.

Less complete enzyme defects and deficiencies of growth hormone and hydrocortisone may present for the first time in this age group as the developing child is expected to feed less frequently and, therefore, endure increasing periods of fasting. Therapy in this age is obviously to replace the hormone that is deficient.

The treatment of hypoglycaemia associated with hepatic enzyme deficiencies is more complex. For example, in galactosaemia and hereditary fructose intolerance the treatment is the total avoidance of these sugars in the diet. For primary defects in hepatic glycogen synthesis or breakdown (glycogen storage disorders), the main stay of therapy is frequent carbohydrate feeds. At times continuous nasogastric feeding throughout the night may be necessary.

18 months to 8 years

The most frequent cause in this age group is a condition known as ketotic hypoglycaemia. In this disorder the child (usually thin) has inadequate glycogen stores and cannot make enough glucose (gluconeogenesis) from amino acid precursors to cope with the fasting associated with longer periods of sleep. Episodes of poor intake or excess activity during the preceding day seem predisposing factors in these children who outgrow this tendency usually without sequelae. At the time of hypoglycaemia children in this group are ketotic. Urinalysis reveals ketonuria but no glycosuria. Plasma levels of alanine, the main gluconeogenic amino acid precursor are low which suggests that the cause of the hypoglycaemia is a deficiency of gluconeogenic substrates. This is not a uniform finding. Treatment is simple – avoid prolonged fasting. If clinically indicated, growth hormone or hydrocortisone deficiency should be excluded as they too can cause hypoglycaemia with ketosis. It should also be mentioned that all the previous causes of hypoglycaemia mentioned above may also occur in this age group.

FURTHER READING

Aynsley-Green A, Soltesz G 1985 Hypoglycaemia in infancy and childhood. Churchill Livingstone, Edinburgh

Drash A L 1986 Clinical care of the diabetic child. Year Book of Medical Publishers, Chicago

58. Disorders of calcium metabolism and bone

D. A. McCredie

CALCIUM

Calcium is of major importance in the body, both as a physiological ion and, together with phosphate, as the major structural component of bone mineral. The newborn infant contains approximately 750 mmol (30 g) of calcium, largely in the form of bone crystal or hydroxyapatite, and this increases to something of the order of 25 mol (1 kg) in the mature adult. The organization of much of the bony skeleton into a lamellar structure not only confers strength on the skeleton, but also ensures that the surface area of bone crystals is very large. Thus ionic exchange can readily occur between extracellular fluid and bone crystal surface. This enables ready mobilization of calcium from bone and also enables bone to act as a detoxifier under certain circumstances, e.g. the taking up of heavy metals as in lead poisoning.

Calcium in extracellular fluid comprises rather less than 1% of total body calcium but its ionic activity is maintained constant between narrow limits. Plasma calcium is normally maintained between 2.1 and 2.7 mmol/l. Approximately half of this is ionized and responsible for its physiological effects, the remainder being bound to plasma proteins or in complex formation with anions such as phosphate. Constancy of extracellular ion activity is maintained in the short term by equilibrium with bone mineral, and in the long term by changes in intestinal absorption and urinary excretion. Such changes are controlled largely by the activity of calcitriol and parathormone.

Intracellular calcium concentrations are much smaller again – nanomolar in the resting state. Despite such relatively minute concentrations, intracellular calcium is of extreme importance for many cell functions and concentration increases considerably on stimulation, to micromolar levels. Calcium thus acts as one component of an intracellular messenger system which regulates a large number of physiological processes. Hormone secretion, muscle contraction and many metabolic processes are closely regulated by this system.

Factors influencing plasma calcium levels

Plasma calcium levels will be affected by changes in serum proteins so that plasma calcium will fall by approximately 0.02 mmol/l for each g/l fall in plasma albumin. Calcium ion activity will not be appreciably affected by such changes, but will be affected by changes in hydrogen ion activity. Acidosis will lead to an increased ionized fraction, and alkalosis (e.g. induced by over-breathing) will tend to reduce ionized calcium levels. Calcium and phosphate ions are in equilibrium with bone crystal (hydroxyapatite) and, under normal circumstances, are present in a supersaturated solution. A rise in plasma phosphate will lead to the deposition of more calcium phosphate into bone, and hence hypocalcaemia.

Calcium ion activity in plasma is under the control of the hormones parathormone and calcitriol. Parathormone is produced by the parathyroid gland in response to reduced calcium ion activity. This hormone then acts on bone to increase calcium release, and on the kidney to increase tubular reabsorption of calcium and renal excretion of phosphate. It also activates the vitamin D-1-hydroxylase mechanism in the kidney leading to the synthesis of the other important calcium hormone – calcitriol (1α,25 dihydroxycholecalciferol).

Calcitriol (Fig. 58.1) acts on the intestine to enhance intestinal absorption of calcium and is important in regulating bone remodelling. Calcitriol arises from two sources in the body. The natural source is by irradiation of 7-dehydrocholesterol in the skin by sunlight. This breaks the B ring of the sterol to produce cholecalciferol (vitamin D_3) which then requires two further hydroxylations, by 25-hydroxylase in the liver and 1-hydroxylase in the kidney to produce the active hormone calcitriol. 1-hydroxylase, and hence vitamin D activation, is

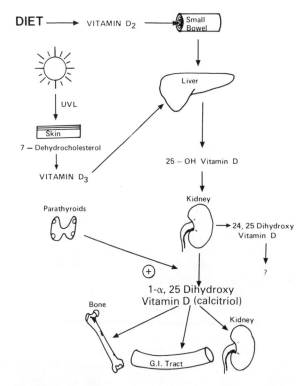

DIET ⟶ VITAMIN D₂ ⟶ Small Bowel

Liver

UVL

Skin

7 – Dehydrocholesterol

VITAMIN D₃

25 – OH Vitamin D

Kidney

Parathyroids

24, 25 Dihydroxy Vitamin D

(+)

?

1-α, 25 Dihydroxy Vitamin D (calcitriol)

Bone

Kidney

G.I. Tract

Fig. 58.1 The origins and activity of calcitriol.

stimulated by both calcium and phosphate depletion as well as parathormone. A 24-hydroxylase enzyme is also present in the kidney producing 24,25 dihydroxycholecalciferol which is not thought to be important physiologically. Alternatively, ergocalciferol (vitamin D_2) obtained in foodstuffs, particularly in cereal, results in the production of 1,25 dihydroxy ergocalciferol which has similar biological activity to calcitriol. Recent studies have shown calcitriol receptors in a number of cells, particularly those derived from bone marrow, and there is evidence that calcitriol may play a role in the regulation of the immune system.

A third hormone, calcitonin, is produced by the medullary cells of the thyroid gland and inhibits bone resorption, but its physiological significance is uncertain. It does not appear to play an important role in the maintenance of calcium homeostasis in the physiological state, at least in postnatal life.

Hypercalcaemia

Plasma calcium levels greater than 2.7 mmol/l are abnormal. Causes are outlined in Example 58.1.

Example 58.1 Causes of hypercalcaemia

Vitamin D associated
  Hypervitaminosis D
  Extrarenal-hydroxylation of vitamin D. May occur in sarcoidosis, tuberculosis, lymphoma, leukaemia.
  Increased sensitivity to vitamin D, e.g. idiopathic hypercalcaemia of infancy.
  Decreased metabolism of vitamin D, e.g. hypothyroidism

PTH associated
  Hyperparathyroidism
  Neoplasm secreting PTH or PTH-related compound

Other
  Bone disease and trauma
  Immobilization
  Thyrotoxicosis
  Prostaglandin excess
  Therapeutic, e.g. thiazides, milk-akali syndrome

Hypercalcaemia may be due to increased vitamin D levels or increased sensitivity to vitamin D, increased parathormone production, whether by parathyroid adenoma or by neoplasm secreting PTH, or other mechanisms as outlined. Most of these conditions are quite uncommon in childhood. Malignant tumours may produce hypercalcaemia, also from bone destruction or by production of substances such as prostaglandins, which may increase bone resorption. Such hypercalcaemia may be quite severe. Other causes of hypercalcaemia are usually relatively mild.

Symptoms of hypercalcaemia are nausea and vomiting, thirst and polyuria, redness of the conjunctiva and, in severe cases, drowsiness, and disorientation. Renal calcification and urinary calculi may occur. Treatment consists of correcting the cause where possible and ensuring a good fluid intake and urinary output. Where symptoms are severe phosphate supplements may be indicated.

Hypocalcaemia

In the presence of normal serum proteins, values of plasma calcium less than 2.1 mmol/l constitute hypocalcaemia. Causes are listed in Example 58.2 and, in the great majority of cases are either PTH related, or result from increased plasma phosphate levels.

Primary idiopathic hypoparathyroidism is rare and may be part of a more general disorder in which chronic candidal infection, steatorrhoea and adrenocortical insufficiency may also be present. The child most commonly presents with tetany or convulsions. Calcitriol (0.25–1.0 μg daily) may be adequate to control

Example 58.2 Causes of hypocalcaemia

Pseudohypocalcaemia
   Low serum albumin

Hypoparathyroidism
   Idiopathic
   Neonatal
   Hypomagnesaemia
   Multiple endocrinopathy
   Di George syndrome
   Rickets

Pseudohypoparathyroidism

Hyperphosphataemia
   Renal failure
   Excess phosphate administration
   Excess cell breakdown

Other
   Pancreatitis

citability leading to twitching, tetany and convulsions. Intravenous calcium should be given to the symptomatic patient provided hypocalcaemia does not result from hyperphosphataemia, in which case dialysis may be necessary. Intravenous calcium may be given slowly in a dose of 12 mmol/m^2 over a period of 3 hours, which would be expected to increase plasma calcium by 0.5–1.0 mmol/l. Serum magnesium levels should also be checked as hypomagnesaemia may lead to a refractory type of hypocalcaemia.

Hypercalciuria

Hypercalciuria will generally be present in patients with hypercalcaemia but may occur when plasma calcium is normal in patients with renal calculi, urinary concentrating defects or unexplained haematuria. Normal urine calcium is less than 0.15 mmol/kg/day or less than 700 mmol per mol creatinine but values greater than 0.12 mmol/kg should be viewed with suspicion. Hypercalciuria may be of renal, osseous or intestinal origin, or due to hyperparathyroidism. Differentiation of the cause is not always easy but may be helped according to Table 58.1. Most laboratories cannot measure a low blood PTH level but urinary phosphate excretion index (PEI which is high in hyperparathyroidism and low in hypoparathyroidism) may give valuable information concerning PTH status.

Phosphate depletion, in the patient on parenteral nutrition or on special diets, may also be an important cause of hypercalciuria. Most patients with renal calculi do not have significant hypercalciuria. However, urine calcium levels tend to be higher than in children who do not form stones. Approximately 50% of calculi in children are due to triple phosphate (struvite) crystals and result from infection, with or without obstruction. Rare metabolic causes of calculus formation, such as hyperoxaluria and cystinuria, need to be excluded in other patients with calculi.

this condition but dietary phosphate restriction and oral calcium binders are also often necessary.

Pseudohypoparathyroidism is extremely rare and implies an end-organ resistance to parathormone. This presents in a similar fashion to hypoparathyroidism, though mental deficiency and skeletal abnormalities, particularly of the metacarpals, may be associated features. Blood parathormone levels are high in this condition. Treatment is the same as for hypoparathyroidism.

Neonatal hypocalcaemia is common, and levels of plasma calcium down to 1.8 mmol/l may be considered normal in the neonatal period. This results from the considerable transfer of calcium from the mother to the fetus during pregnancy, so that at the time of birth the baby's parathyroid gland is relatively inactive. Such a condition may persist for several days and will be aggravated by high phosphorus feeding (as with many artificial formulas), by prematurity, or by conditions associated with anoxia or tissue catabolism.

Hypocalcaemia results in increased neuromuscular ex-

Table 58.1 Hypercalciuria: differentiation of cause

Cause of hypercalciuria	Plasma Ca++	PEI*	Intestinal Ca absorption	Urine Ca response to low Ca diet
Intestinal	High or N	Low	High	Decrease
Osseous	High or N	Low	Low	Remains high
Renal	Low or N	High	High	Remains high
Hyperparathyroidism	High	High	High	Slight decrease

* Phosphate excretion index

METABOLIC DISORDERS OF THE SKELETON

Rickets and osteomalacia

Rickets may be defined as impaired mineralization of the growing ends of bone with accumulation of cartilaginous matrix, whilst osteomalacia refers to an increased amount of unmineralized osteoid covering bone trabeculae. In practice the condition is called rickets in children, where marked deformities occur in the growing bone, and osteomalacia in adults. Causes are outlined in Example 58.3.

Example 58.3 Causes of rickets

Vitamin D deficiency
  Dietary deficiency
  Lack of sunlight
  Malabsorption in gastro-intestinal, hepatic or pancreatic
    disease.

Abnormal metabolism of vitamin D
  Chronic renal failure
  Vitamin-dependent rickets (1-hydroxylase deficiency)
  Anticonvulsant osteopathy

Phosphate depletion
  X-linked hypophosphataemia
  Fanconi syndrome

Renal tubular acidosis

Vitamin D deficiency. With adequate exposure to sunlight Vitamin D supplementation is unnecessary; however, with reduced sunlight and darkly pigmented skin the dietary intake is important. The recommended daily intake of vitamin D is 400 international units. Although breast milk is quite low in vitamin D content rickets is uncommon in breast fed infants in the first year of life, provided mother's nutrition is adequate. A small amount of late afternoon sunlight is sufficient to provide adequate vitamin D to a fair-skinned infant.

Recently, the incidence of vitamin D-deficient rickets has increased in many Western societies. In Australia this increase has been seen largely in migrants from southern Europe, the Middle East and Asia. Aboriginal people living in cities may also be affected. Important factors are poor housing conditions, lack of adequate infant welfare services for non-English speaking migrants, unusual feeding patterns and lack of sunlight. The last may be especially important in dark-skinned children living in a temperate climate.

Clinical features of rickets

The diagnosis is often suggested from a chest radiograph performed for an intercurrent chest infection, the physi-

cal signs being either too subtle or missed. The clinical features comprise some or all of the following – delayed closure of the anterior fontanelle, frontal and occipital bossing of the skull, thickening of costochondral junctions (rickety rosary), widening of the end of the long bones and, when the child walks, bowing and bending of the legs. Dentition may be delayed. Muscular weakness and ligamentous laxity are frequent. Vitamin D deficiency early in life may present with convulsions because of hypocalcaemia when none of the above features are apparent.

Radiology of the long bones shows a widening of the space between the metaphysis and epiphysis (Fig. 58.2). The bones are generally rarefied with widened trabeculae. Cupping and fraying of the metaphyseal ends of the long bones is characteristic and related to the accumulation of poorly mineralized cartilaginous matrix. Serum alkaline phosphatase is high, serum phosphate low and serum calcium normal or low. Iron deficiency anaemia is also commonly present but children appear otherwise well-nourished.

Treatment is with oral vitamin D – 1500–5000 units

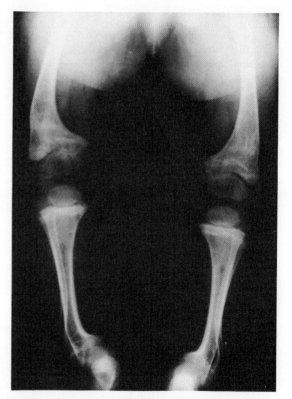

Fig. 58.2 Radiograph of the lower limbs of a child with severe nutritional rickets. Note the bowing of the long bones and the widening and fraying of the metaphyseal ends.

(1 microgram = 40 units) per day for 4–6 weeks by which time clinical and radiological healing is occurring and the dose can be reduced to 1000 units per day. Parents must be instructed to allow the child adequate exposure to sunlight and a diet of eggs, fish and fortified milk.

In X-linked hypophosphataemia, rickets tends to present later with bowing of the legs noticed after the onset of walking. This is an X-linked dominant condition so there is often a family history. The primary defect is renal phosphate wasting but vitamin D 1-hydroxylation may also be deficient. Treatment consists of dietary phosphate supplementation, with 1–2 g of extra phosphorus per day, and calcitriol, usually 0.25–1 μg daily. Frequent serum calcium estimations are necessary to avoid vitamin D overdosage.

A particular form of osteopathy may be encountered with the prolonged use of anticonvulsants, particularly barbiturate and phenytoin derivatives. It may be seen in severe form in association with cerebral palsy and mental retardation where poor diet, relative inactivity and minimal sun exposure may be added factors.

Renal osteodystrophy

This is a complex disorder which occurs when glomerular filtration falls below about 25% of normal. Of major importance in causation is the rise in plasma phosphate levels leading both to an inhibition of the vitamin D 1-hydroxylase enzyme and to a fall in plasma calcium and hence stimulation of parathormone secretion. A combination of rickets and secondary hyperparathyroidism ensues, resulting in gross skeletal deformities.

Treatment consists of dietary phosphate restriction combined with a phosphate binder. This is best given as calcium carbonate in divided doses. Calcitriol (0.25–1 μg per day) may be added once plasma phosphate levels are below 2 mmol/l, but serum calcium, phosphate and alkaline phosphatase levels must be checked frequently. Aluminium hydroxide may also be used but care must be taken as aluminium toxicity may lead to a particularly refractory form of rickets as well as progressive brain damage.

Osteoporosis

Osteoporosis is apparent radiologically only when approximately half the bone mineral content has been lost. It may result from nutritional deficiency or malabsorption of calcium, from bone disease or replacement of bone by malignant cells (as in leukaemia), from endocrine disorders (hyperthyroidism and Cushing's

disease), certain metabolic disorders (e.g. homocystinuria), and from prolonged disuse in neurological disorders or resulting from immobilization. Voluntary disuse, combined with local inflammatory disease, is probably a factor in its association with juvenile chronic arthritis. Of particular severity is a form of osteoporosis associated with deficiency of both calcium and phosphorus in the low birthweight infant. Sometimes osteogenesis imperfecta may present as osteoporosis in later childhood (see Ch. 7). Idiopathic juvenile osteoporosis is a rare form which tends to occur in middle childhood. This may present with backache or a gait disturbance following relatively mild trauma. Despite extensive vertebral crush fractures, this type tends to remit spontaneously with the onset of puberty.

Osteopetrosis

Osteopetrosis is a rare familial disorder of the skeleton in which there is a defect in bone and cartilage resorption and hence of bone remodelling. This leads to a dense but brittle type of bone which is easily fractured. Infants usually present early in life with a severe leukoerythroblastic anaemia, symptoms of compression of cranial nerves (particularly optic atrophy leading to blindness) and marked hepatosplenomegaly. Bones show a characteristically dense and poorly modelled appearance on radiograph. Some patients with this condition have recently shown dramatic improvement following bone marrow transplantation.

Disorders of magnesium homeostasis

Although magnesium is the fourth most abundant cation in the body and is of vital importance in many physiological processes, comparatively little is known about its control. Vitamin D appears to have some enhancing effect on its intestinal absorption, and both parathormone and aldosterone affect its renal tubular reabsorption. In many reactions magnesium competes with calcium, and magnesium has been referred to as 'nature's physiological calcium blocker'.

Hypermagnesaemia

This is rarely a problem but may occur in severe renal disease, particularly if extra magnesium salts have been given.

Hypomagnesaemia

Hypomagnesaemia may occur with the same disorders that lead to hypocalcaemia, and should be thought of in states of hypocalcaemia which do not respond readily to calcium administration. Hypomagnesaemia may result from acute or chronic intestinal disease, from states of chronic acidosis (e.g. diabetes), and is commonly seen with chronic diuretic administration where it may lead to muscle weakness and, in the presence of heart disease, refractory cardiac failure.

Rare isolated defects of intestinal absorption of magnesium and hereditary disorders of renal tubular reabsorption of magnesium have also been described.

FURTHER READING

Bell N H 1985 Vitamin D – endocrine system. Journal of Clinical Investigations 76: 1–6

Berridge M J 1987 Inositol phosphates and cellular homeostasis. In: Cohn D V, Martin T J, Meunier P J (eds) Calcium regulation and bone metabolism Vol 9: 8–15. Excerpta Medica, Amsterdam

Fourman P, Royer P 1968 Calcium metabolism and the bone, 2nd edn. Blackwell, Oxford

Goldring S T, Krane S M 1981 Metabolic disorders of the skeleton. Disease a Month 27(4): 1–103

Harrison H E 1987 Vitamin D and metabolism of calcium and phosphate. In: Rudolph A M (ed), Pediatrics, 18th edn. pp 177–184

McCredie D A 1987 The kidney and disorders of calcium metabolism. In: Murakami K, Kitagawa T, Yabuta K, Sakai T (eds) Recent advances in pediatric nephrology 455–460. Excerpta Medica, Amsterdam

Rasmussen H 1986 The calcium messenger system. New England Journal of Medicine 314: 1094–1101, 1164–1169

Problems of gastrointestinal tract and liver

59. Vomiting in infancy and childhood

M. J. Robinson

In infancy and childhood, vomiting is symptomatic of many disorders. As the causes of vomiting in a number of these are poorly understood, a classification relating to disturbed physiology is impossible to construct. A sound clinical approach to the subject is to consider vomiting in relation to age, when three broad groups emerge:

1. The neonatal period
2. Infancy and early childhood
3. Older children.

Considerable overlap occurs but many disorders presenting with vomiting occur only in one of the groups and may be excluded on the basis of age in the others, for example, hypertrophic pyloric stenosis does not occur after the age of 3 months.

VOMITING IN THE NEONATAL PERIOD

It is not rare for neonates to vomit small amounts of mucus and blood swallowed during labour. This vomiting is probably due to mild gastritis and usually clears spontaneously within 24 hours. If not, a gastric lavage with physiological saline will usually relieve it.

In the early weeks of life many normal newborn babies regurgitate after feeds and, provided that they thrive, reassurance only is necessary. This type of vomiting usually stops within a few weeks. The cause of this 'spitting up' or 'possetting' is not clear.

Neonatal vomiting is often symptomatic, so that a careful enquiry and physical examination is necessary before reassurance can be given. The clinical history must show the following points:

1. The normality, or otherwise, and the duration of the pregnancy.
2. The labour, its duration, the presentation and any complications, for example, antepartum haemorrhage, prolapse of the cord, etc.

3. Any fetal distress during labour and asphyxia at birth.

At physical examination particular attention is directed to the degree of maturity, the detection of any birth defect and the neurological status of the infant.

Cerebral anoxia

This is frequently followed by vomiting. Signs of asphyxia will usually be present at birth when resuscitation will be required. Following this, some infants remain lethargic and feed poorly, others may be abnormally wide awake, cry frequently or be excessively irritable. The cry may be high-pitched and intermittent twitching may occur. Some of these infants are hypertonic and there may be head retraction with the thumbs adducted across the palms with flexion of the fingers. The Moro reflex may be exaggerated, but in severe cerebral anoxia it may be lost. The fontanelle tension is not increased initially unless there has been a cerebral haemorrhage, but within 24 hours cerebral oedema occurs often and the fontanelle tension rises. Occasionally, cerebral anoxia is the result of inappropriate timing of sedatives and analgesics during labour. In cerebral anoxia the vomiting often occurs before feeding, but is accentuated by feeding. It may be forceful and at times even projectile.

Treatment

Treatment is symptomatic. Spinal puncture will establish the diagnosis if a cerebral haemorrhage is present but is of little value in treatment. Cerebral haemorrhage is best defined in the neonatal period by ultrasound which will also provide evidence of cerebral oedema. Sedation with diazepam (Valium) 0.1–0.3 mg/kg IV or phenobarbitone 2 mg/kg IM will often be necessary. Careful observations on pulse, temperature, state of consciousness and the degree of hydration are important. Aspiration of vomitus is a real danger. Fluids given orally should be small in amount and offered frequently, for example, a quarter-strength formula offered at least 2-hourly. An intravenous infusion may be necessary, but it must be remembered that on the first day of life only 60 ml/kg is required. This amount is increased gradually each day until the end of the first week when the normal daily requirement of 150 mg/kg are met. Blood glucose estimations are important as hypoglycaemia occurs frequently in cerebral disorders in the neonatal period – this may compound the cerebral disturbance and accentuate the vomiting.

Subdural haematoma

With current high standards of obstetrics these are now rare in the neonatal period. In about 50% of cases vomiting is the only symptom. In the remainder, vomiting is accompanied by developmental delay, convulsions, an expanding head and retinal haemorrhages. The diagnosis is established by ultrasound and CT scanning. A subdural haematoma in any period in childhood must alert the clinician to the possibility of child abuse.

Hypoglycaemia

Vomiting may be the only symptom in the neonatal period. Hypoglycaemia is commonly associated with 'small for dates' babies and infants of diabetic mothers. However, it may be associated with any stressful situation in the neonatal period, for example, low birthweight, neonatal meningitis, septicaemia, severe Rh immunization, etc. Symptomatic hypoglycaemia does not usually occur with a blood glucose in excess of 2 mmol/l.

Systemic infection

Vomiting is one of the many non-specific signs of infection in the neonate. Thus, unexplained vomiting should be an indication for cultures of blood, stomach contents, urine and CSF.

Renal disease

In the neonatal period renal disease may present because of urinary infection, renal insufficiency or a combination of both. Also, vomiting and failure to thrive are commonly present, and often there is an underlying renal abnormality. This may be suspected clinically in an infant with dry, wrinkled skin, coarse facial features and abnormally shaped or low-slung ears – the 'Potter facies'. This is diagnostic of bilateral renal agenesis. Low-slung and abnormally shaped ears may be associated with less severe congenital renal lesions. Absence of the anterior abdominal muscles, wrinkled abnormal skin and bilateral undescended testes are associated with a congenital renal lesion and constitute the 'prune belly' syndrome. Gross abdominal distension with, at times, an ascites may indicate congenital bladder neck obstruction in the male. Usually both kidneys and the bladder are palpable and the urine stream is very poor. The obstruction is due to posterior urethral valves. Investigation may involve renal ultrasound, radiography of the renal tract, renal function studies and even renal biopsy. Renal tubular lesions may, on rare occasions, present in the neonatal period because of vomiting (see Ch. 52).

Adrenal insufficiency

In the neonatal period this is almost invariably the result of congenital adrenal hyperplasia due to a deficiency of the enzyme 21 hydroxylase (see Ch. 56). In the neonatal period the presentation is with ambiguous genitalia in the female, and in the male unexplained vomiting, dehydration, and collapse early in the second week of life. Failure to recognize the genital anomaly in the female will often result in vomiting, dehydration, and collapse also in the second week of life. The diagnosis is suspected by finding very low levels of sodium and elevated levels of potassium in the serum and is established by appropriate hormonal studies (see Ch. 56).

Inborn metabolic errors

Although individually rare, there are a number of inborn errors involving separately, amino acid, carbohydrate and organic acid metabolism. Most are inherited recessively and a number can now be treated. Frequently, the presentation is with unexplained vomiting, lethargy, seizures at times, collapse, and coma (see Ch. 28).

Neonatal intestinal obstruction

In high intestinal obstruction vomiting is early; the site of the block being usually at the third part of the duodenum distal to the ampulla of Vater, when the vomitus is bile-stained. The obstruction may be intrinsic, due to the presence of a septum or extrinsic, the result of congenital bands. Other anomalies, for example Down syndrome, imperforate anus, may co-exist. In the absence of birth asphyxia these infants are usually alert,

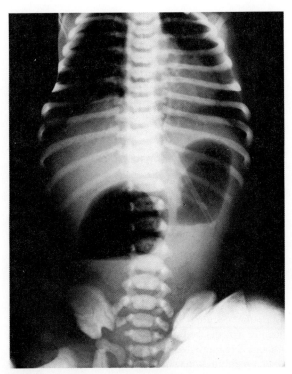

Fig. 59.1 Radiograph of the abdomen in a neonate, demonstrating the 'double bubble' sign. Note the absence of gas in the bowel distal to the second bubble. Diagnosis – duodenal obstruction.

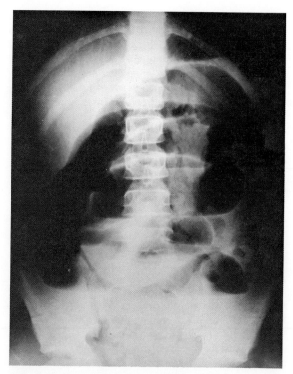

Fig. 59.2 Erect plain radiograph of the abdomen, demonstrating marked dilatation of loops of bowel and several fluid levels. Diagnosis – intestinal obstruction.

feed well, but vomit bile-stained material almost immediately. On physical examination a little upper abdominal distension is often apparent. The diagnosis is readily made by a plain upright radiograph of the abdomen, when the characteristic 'double bubble' shadow will be seen (Fig. 59.1). Little or no gas will be visible distal to the obstruction. Laparotomy is indicated after fluid and electrolyte correction.

Occasionally bile-stained vomiting may be seen in infants whose mothers have received medication during labour – particular antihypertensives used in treatment of pregnancy toxaemia. Also, it may be seen in acute gastroenteritis in infancy. The latter can usually be differentiated from the clinical history and a plain film of the abdomen when gas will be seen throughout the bowel.

Large bowel obstruction

In neonatal large bowel obstruction vomiting is frequent but tends to occur later and is always associated with gross abdominal distension. The vomitus may become faeculent if the obstruction is unrecognized. An erect film of the abdomen will show distended loops of bowel and fluid levels (Fig. 59.2). Similar radiological appearance may accompany acute gastroenteritis in infancy but the clinical history differentiates. More common causes of neonatal large bowel obstruction include ileal atresia, imperforate anus, meconium ileus and Hirschsprung's disease. In the latter disorder the obstruction is incomplete.

Hirschsprung's disease

Hirschsprung's disease (congenital megacolon) is the commonest of all neonatal obstructions and is the result of absence of ganglion cells in the bowel wall. This may extend a variable distance proximally from the anus. Peristalsis is abnormal in the aganglionic segment resulting in severe constipation and incomplete lower intestinal obstruction. The bowel proximal to the aganglionic segment becomes enormously dilated (megacolon). Obstruction is not complete in that small amounts of faecal material leak away. Putrefaction, with foul-smelling liquid faeces, occurs in unrecognized cases and, at times, an associated severe diarrhoea due to colitis. Most cases are recognized readily in the neonatal period because of failure to pass meconium, abdominal distension and vomiting. Symptoms are relieved temporarily by a rectal examination which usually produces large quantities of gas and faeces. In the milder case, symptoms comprise chronic and severe constipation with gross abdominal distension which may continue unrecognized into childhood. The diagnosis is confirmed by rectal biopsy which demonstrates complete absence of ganglion cells in the submucosa. On radiography distended loops of bowel and an abrupt change in calibre of the bowel at the junction of the normal and aganglionic segment are almost diagnostic. Treatment is surgical and involves excision of the aganglionic segment and subsequent anastomosis to the anal canal.

Oesophageal atresia

Oesophageal atresia will result in vomiting if the infant is fed. Feeding greatly compromises the infant so that the diagnosis should be made before feeds are offered. Any excessively mucousy infant at birth should be suspected of oesophageal atresia and an attempt made to pass a soft rubber catheter into the stomach (French 8 or 10) – failure is an indication for immediate referral.

VOMITING IN INFANCY

Vomiting is also a very common symptom in infancy and, again, a non-specific one. However, associated signs and symptoms are more likely to allow a definitive diagnosis to be made in this period without the need for investigation often so necessary in the neonatal period. Nonetheless, disease of any system may present in infancy with vomiting.

Infection

Perhaps the commonest reason for vomiting in infancy is in response to infection. Therefore, vomiting is a common presenting symptom of such diverse disorders as tonsillitis, otitis media, pneumonia, meningitis and urinary tract infection. A careful physical examination should exclude most of these, but early signs may be minimal in meningitis and pneumonia so that a spinal puncture and chest radiograph will be required if there is doubt.

An early diagnosis of urinary tract infection will not be made unless the non-specific signs are appreciated – vomiting is certainly one of them. In infancy dysuria, frequency of passing urine and loin pain cannot be relied upon for diagnosis, and the urine must always be examined. When the infection is controlled, imaging of the renal tract is indicated.

Lesions of the gastrointestinal tract

Those which produce vomiting are different from those in the neonatal period and by this time obstructive lesions have usually been recognized. However, duodenal obstruction associated with gut malrotation may present at any age with bilious vomiting. Failure to recognize malrotation of the gut may result in infarction and a massive bowel resection. This diagnosis is confirmed radiologically when a barium enema will indicate the caecum to be very mobile and a barium meal demonstrate an abnormal S-shaped curve of the intestine.

Gastro-oesophageal reflux

This is the commonest cause of vomiting in infancy. At times the vomiting commences soon after birth; frequently it is delayed a few weeks. After a feed, a small amount is regurgitated and from then until the next feed is due, regurgitation continues. At times there is forceful vomiting as well and it may even be projectile. Frank or altered blood or mucus may be present in the vomitus, which is never bile-stained. These infants usually thrive well and are rarely distressed by the vomiting. In some, the vomitus is sufficiently severe to restrict growth and in others milk is aspirated when the infant's major symptoms are cough and wheezing after feeds. Physical examination does not reveal any abnormality. The diagnosis is readily made from the history and can usually be confirmed by barium swallow when the barium is seen to reflux from the stomach into a dilated oesophagus (Fig. 59.3). Barium studies in oesophageal reflux are probably more useful to exclude other causes of vomiting in the gastrointestinal tract. Continuous oesophageal pH monitoring, which measures intra-oesophageal pH, appears to be a more sensitive method of detecting gastro-oesophageal reflux, but it is only available in specialized centres. Radioisotope studies are valuable in documenting the severity of gastro-oesophageal reflux and establishing the presence of aspiration in particular. The natural history of gastro-oesophageal reflux is for spontaneous recovery, usually before the first year of life. In a small proportion of these infants ulceration of the lower end of the oesophagus due to acid regurgitation occurs. This may result in repeated haematemeses and, rarely, the production of an oesophageal stricture. The symptoms of hiatus hernia are identical to those of gastro-

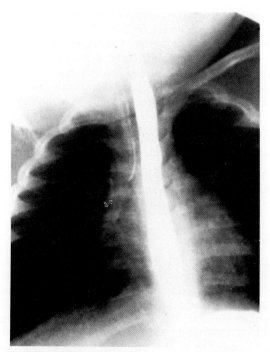

Fig. 59.3 Barium swallow. This has demonstrated gross gastro-oesophageal reflux during the screening. Note the fine line of barium adjacent to the oesophagus, demonstrating tracheal aspiration.

oesophageal reflux. Nursing the infant on a head-up sloping board, either in the prone or supine position, is helpful in relieving the vomiting. The addition of thickening agents to formulae, for example, cornflour, carob seed, and alginic acid preparations (Gaviscon) may also help but in general gastro-oesophageal reflux is characterized by exacerbations and remissions before spontaneous resolution. Severe disease with failure to thrive, oesophageal ulceration and recurrent or persistent aspiration may indicate surgical treatment. The operation of fundoplication is particularly successful in these situations.

Other lesions involving the oesophagus and producing vomiting in infancy are much less common and are recognized on barium studies of the oesophagus. The lesions include webbing of the oesophagus, achalasia and duplication. Acquired lesions of the oesophagus, for example, foreign body and corrosive ingestion, occur later in childhood.

Rumination

In this syndrome the infant consciously regurgitates and chews food which had already been swallowed. Some

infants initiate vomiting in this way by inserting their fingers into the mouth. Many of these infants are overactive and some are emotionally deprived.

Congenital hypertrophic pyloric stenosis

This is one of the most dramatic of the vomiting syndromes in infancy. Typically the onset is sudden between the second and sixth week. Males are affected five times more often than females and there is a definite familial incidence. Before the onset of vomiting, these infants have fed and thrived well. The vomiting is forceful from the onset and rapidly becomes projectile. Weight is lost rapidly and dehydration is an early feature. Despite the vomiting, which usually comes on immediately after feeding, these infants are hungry and will usually feed immediately after vomiting. The vomitus is not bile-stained but occasionally it contains altered blood. The diagnosis should be made clinically by feeling the firm pyloric tumour during feeding or immediately after vomiting. The tumour is typically hard, mobile and about the size of the terminal phalanx of the fifth finger. Peristaltic waves passing from the left costal margin to the right hypochondrium ('golf ball' waves) will usually be visible. Once the tumour is felt, further investigation is unnecessary. In congenital pyloric stenosis a barium meal will show delayed gastric emptying, a dilated stomach and a narrowed and attenuated pyloric canal – the 'string sign' (Fig. 59.4). A metabolic alkalosis is characteristic, which, together with the dehydration, must be corrected before surgery. There is little or no place for medical management of pyloric stenosis if surgery is available.

Pylorospasm

This is a well recognized cause of vomiting, particularly in the neonatal period. Occasionally pylorospasm may persist for some weeks and cause confusion in diagnosis with hypertrophic pyloric stenosis. However, no tumour is palpable even though peristaltic waves may be seen. A metabolic alkalosis is never present in this syndrome. The commonest associations with pylorospasm are cerebral birth injury in association with hyperkinetic and deprived infants.

Gastroenteritis

One of the commonest causes of vomiting in infancy is gastroenteritis. The association of vomiting with the typical fluid stools usually makes the diagnosis obvious, particularly if the stools also contain mucus or blood. However, vomiting and a few loose stools are seen in a

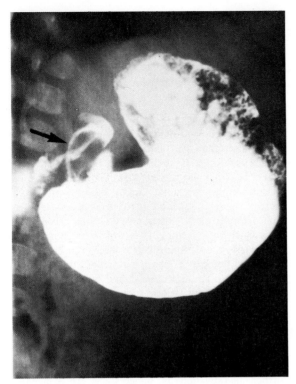

Fig. 59.4 Barium swallow. Note elongation of the pyloric canal (the string sign). Diagnosis – congenital hypertrophic pyloric stenosis.

variety of medical and surgical disorders in infancy; these include intussusception, acute appendicitis and pyelonephritis. Confusion with gastroenteritis is unlikely if a careful history is taken and a thorough physical examination performed. The diagnosis and management of gastroenteritis is covered in Chapter 60.

Malabsorption

In the majority of malabsorption syndromes vomiting is not a feature. At times, in the more severe cases of coeliac disease (gluten enteropathy), vomiting may be prominent. A gluten-free diet rapidly reverses the clinical features of this disorder.

Intestinal obstruction

As a cause of vomiting in infancy obstruction is most commonly due to intussusception or to an incarcerated or strangulated hernia. With intussusception, vomiting is usually present early. The typical history is of colicky abdominal pain, vomiting, pallor and the passage of

blood per rectum. It may be necessary to perform a rectal examination to detect the blood, but its absence does not exclude intussusception. A sausage-shaped mass is palpable abdominally or rectally in most cases. When symptoms have been present for less than 24 hours, reduction is almost always possible hydrostatically using barium or gas. Should there be doubts as to the viability of the gut, surgery is safer (see Ch. 62).

Incarcerated or strangulated hernias

These are almost invariably inguinal in infancy and childhood (Fig. 59.5) and will never be missed if a proper physical examination is carried out.

Poisons and drugs

Most major hospitals provide a drug screening service. In cases where the possibility exists that vomiting is due to poisoning, blood and urine should be sent off without delay. Drugs used for therapeutic purposes may also produce vomiting. The list of drugs is exceedingly large and no point would be served by listing them. Every effort should be made to identify the agent so that treat-

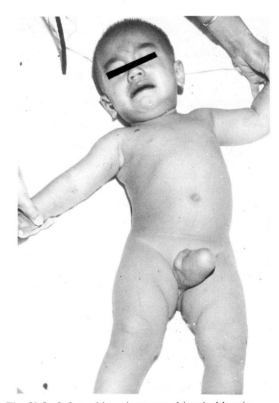

Fig. 59.5 Infant with an incarcerated inguinal hernia.

ment may be based on sound pharmacological principles. The more common ingestions in childhood include kerosene, aspirin, paracetamol, sedatives, tranquillisers, antidepressants, digitalis and aminophylline.

VOMITING IN OLDER CHILDREN

Usually, vomiting in older children presents few problems in diagnosis, because details of history are more specific. Vomiting in older children is still most commonly associated with infection. Viral or bacterial infection of the respiratory and gastrointestinal tracts is by far the most common. Less common, but clinically important, causes of vomiting in the older child, are described below.

In any child with unexplained vomiting the possibility of an intracranial neoplasm should always be considered. Vomiting with a cerebral neoplasm may or may not be accompanied by signs of increased intracranial pressure. In the absence of signs of increased intracranial pressure, the vomiting may be because of direct involvement of the vomiting centre which lies close to the dorsal nuclei of the vagus nerve in the medulla. This is seen in patients with midline cerebellar tumours, tumours involving the fourth ventricle or in tumours involving the pons or medulla. Initially, the vomiting tends to occur in the morning before breakfast and nausea may or may not be present. Remissions may occur for a few days but the vomiting invariably returns in a short time.

Other cerebral causes of vomiting in the older child include subdural haematoma, hydrocephalus, meningitis including tuberculous meningitis, encephalitis and cerebral abscess.

Vomiting may be due to lead poisoning; this diagnosis is confirmed by blood lead estimations. Radiology of skull or long bones and a blood film for red cell stippling are helpful in diagnosing lead poisoning.

Migraine

In the older child, the association of severe paroxysmal frontal headache with pallor and vomiting is very suggestive of migraine. Transient loss of vision, a transient hemiparesis, cerebellar ataxia or ophthalmoplegia are not infrequent in childhood migraine. In some children migraine is precipitated by minor trauma. In the younger child, attacks of pallor and vomiting may be the only symptoms. Treatment of the individual attack is difficult because of the vomiting. In frequently recurring migraine, pizotifen (Sandomigran) or a beta-adrenergic blocker, for example, propanolol may be helpful prophylactically.

Acute appendicitis and peritonitis

In acute appendicitis in childhood vomiting is the rule, but is usually preceded by pain. In the older child the physical signs usually confirm or exclude the diagnosis. However, in the younger child (1–3 years) vomiting with or without diarrhoea may be the only symptom. Physical examination in this age group may reveal little in the early stages. Thus, acute appendicitis needs to be considered in any young child with unexplained vomiting – it is only by repeated examinations and a high index of suspicion that the diagnosis will be made before perforation occurs (see Ch. 62).

Peritonitis is usually associated with vomiting. Abdominal pain or vomiting in a child with the nephrotic syndrome should alert the physician to the possibility of pneumococcal peritonitis. However, peritonitis most commonly results from perforation of an acutely inflamed appendix. Also, it may occur following mesenteric vascular occlusion.

Gut malrotation

Occasionally this condition presents in the older child – again with abdominal pain and bilious vomiting. If this disorder is unrecognized results can be tragic.

Metabolic disease

Vomiting in the older child, in association with metabolic disease, can still cause problems in diagnosis. While most inborn errors of metabolism present clinically in early life, this is not always the rule and many cases have masqueraded under the title 'cyclical vomiting'. A metabolic screen of urine is always worthwhile in a child with periodic episodes of vomiting.

Vomiting is not infrequent in acute poststreptococcal glomerulonephritis. Less commonly, it may indicate the onset of renal failure both in the child with a past history of renal disease or as the first clinical presentation. Urinary tract infection is also associated with vomiting in this age group but symptoms referable to the renal tract are more often present to suggest the diagnosis. Diabetic ketoacidosis must always be considered in the vomiting child and the appropriate blood and urine tests performed. In acute hepatitis the association of jaundice with vomiting makes the diagnosis clear but at times the onset of the jaundice may be delayed. Vomiting, gradual loss of consciousness in association with hepatomegaly, may suggest Reye's syndrome. Hypoglycaemia and elevated serum ammonium levels make this diagnosis more likely. Accidental poisoning must still be considered in the older child and attempted suicide is becoming more frequent.

Non-accidental poisoning

The diagnosis of attempted suicide is not always easy to make. Vomiting, respiratory and circulatory collapse in a previously well child should alert to the possibility of poisoning. As well as an increasing frequency, the age incidence of children attempting suicide is decreasing. A history of family discord and emotional problems in the child is not always volunteered at the onset of symptoms.

Psychological causes of vomiting

In any age group these must be considered. Psychogenic vomiting is often associated with attempts to force-feed a toddler or school child, after punishment, and as an attempt to avoid perceived threatening situations, for example, going to preschool or school. Almost any stressful situation may precipitate vomiting in a tense or anxious child. The absence of physical signs will be a feature. There should be a positive relationship between stress and vomiting to establish psychological factors as causative.

Cyclical vomiting

Cyclical vomiting is a syndrome of persistent periodic vomiting of childhood. The severity varies, but ketosis and a metabolic acidosis may develop rapidly and intravenous fluid therapy may be required. The aetiology is unknown and attacks usually cease quite dramatically. Children who have attacks of cyclical vomiting are often tense and anxious and may develop migraine or psychosomatic disease in later life. It is important to exclude recurrent intestinal volvulus and metabolic disease in these children before labelling them as cyclical vomiters.

FURTHER READING

Carre I J 1959 The natural history of the partial thoracic stomach (hiatus hernia) in children. Archives of Disease in Childhood 34: 344–353
Friesen S R, Pearse A G E 1963 Pathogenesis of congenital pyloric stenosis. Surgery 53: 604–608
Herbst J J 1981 Gastro-oesophageal reflux. Journal of Pediatrics 98: 859–870
Jones P G (ed) 1986 Clinical paediatric surgery, 3rd edn. Blackwell Scientific Publications, Oxford
Nixon H H 1964 Hirschsprung's disease. Archives of Disease in Childhood 39: 109–113
Thompson J A 1980 Diagnosis and treatment of headache in the pediatric patient. Current Problems in Paediatrics 10: 1–52

60. The child with diarrhoea

Graeme Barnes

ACUTE GASTROENTERITIS

Definition

An illness of acute onset, of less than 10 days' duration, associated with fever, diarrhoea and/or vomiting, where there is no other evident cause for the symptoms.

This definition implies that the diagnosis is often one of exclusion. The exclusions are very important as they include some of the most serious surgical emergencies which occur in children.

Although the severity and the mortality of acute gastroenteritis has been greatly reduced in recent years, the incidence of this disease is still very high. In Third World countries acute gastroenteritis constitutes a major health problem, causing enormous morbidity and mortality.

Aetiology

Rotavirus (Fig 60.1) is the most common cause of acute gastroenteritis in children under 5 years of age in developed countries, and is identified in 40–50% of cases where hospital admission is required. It probably also accounts for more episodes in infants in developing countries than any other single pathogen, and is associated with more severe disease than most other agents. The mucosal damage it causes, and hence the need for structural repair, has considerable nutritional implications for malnourished children. Asymptomatic reinfection several times each year maintains immunity throughout life, although mild disease can occur in older children and adults.

Many animals harbour rotavirus strains which have antigenic similarities to and differences from human

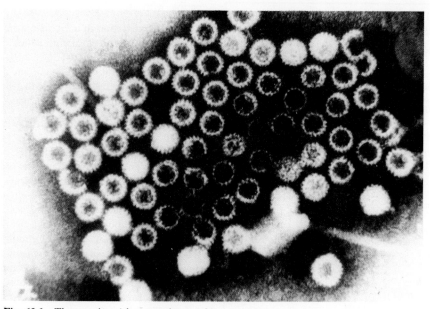

Fig. 60.1 The rotavirus (electron micrograph).

strains. Bovine and rhesus monkey strains have been tested as vaccines in humans. Enteric adenoviruses (types 40 and 41) cause 7–17% of cases requiring admission to hospital and several other virus candidate pathogens have been recognized.

Bacteria cause less episodes than viruses. *Campylobacter jejuni* may be responsible for 5–10% of cases in developed countries. *Salmonella* spp., *Shigella* spp., and various types of *Escherichia coli* each account for a small percentage. In developing countries, *E.coli* (enterotoxigenic, enteropathogenic and enteroinvasive) and *Shigella* are especially important – *Shigella* because it causes prolonged debilitating illness, and because antibiotic resistant strains are emerging.

Giardia lamblia rarely causes acute dehydrating diarrhoea, but another parasite, *Cryptosporidium*, is now known to cause 1–4% of cases of acute diarrhoea in infants admitted to hospital.

Clinical features

The presenting symptoms include poor feeding, vomiting and fever followed rapidly by diarrhoea. Vomiting and/or fever may not always be present. Stools are often watery, frequent (10–20 times per day) and of large volume in viral diarrhoea. Blood, mucus and frequent small motions associated with abdominal pain and tenesmus suggest a bacterial cause.

With increasing anorexia, vomiting and diarrhoea, the infant becomes lethargic, and signs of dehydration, with

---

Example 60.1 Differential diagnosis of acute diarrhoea and vomiting in infants and children

Enteric infection
   Rotavirus
   Other viruses
   Bacteria – *Salmonella* spp, *Shigella* spp, *E. coli*,
       Campylobacter jejuni
   Protozoa – *Giardia lamblia, Entamoeba histolytica
       Cryptosporidium*
   Food poisoning – staphylococcal toxin

Systemic infection
   Urinary tract infection
   Pneumonia
   Septicaemia

Surgical conditions
   Appendicitis
   Intussusception
   Partial bowel obstruction
   Hirschsprung's disease

Other
   Diabetes mellitus
   Antibiotic diarrhoea
   Haemolytic uraemic syndrome

---

accompanying metabolic acidosis, appear. It is of the greatest importance that these signs are recognized and interpreted correctly, as the management of diarrhoea basically involves the correction of dehydration and electrolyte depletion.

Differential diagnosis (see Example 60.1)

The diagnosis of gastroenteritis involves an appreciation of the history and assessment of the signs of dehydration. However, a few loose stools and vomiting may be the result of many other causes, for example respiratory tract infection, meningitis, urinary tract infection, etc. This has been called parenteral diarrhoea. Intussusception, acute appendicitis in the very young and, rarely, Hirschsprung's disease can mimic acute gastroenteritis. Therefore, it is vital that a proper and full physical examination is made, even though the history strongly suggests gastroenteritis. *It is sound practice to regard acute gastroenteritis as a diagnosis of exclusion.*

Dehydration

Water loss

The management of acute gastroenteritis hinges on the assessment and correction of fluid and electrolyte depletion. Fluid loss is assessed on the basis of percentage body weight loss. Physical signs of dehydration do not appear until there is a loss of 5% of body weight. Acute weight losses in excess of 14% are probably not compatible with life. Thus:

1. 5% dehydration in a 1-year-old infant weighing 10 kg involves a loss of 500 g, which is equivalent to 500 ml of water.
2. 10% dehydration in such an infant implies a weight loss of 1000 g, equivalent to 1 litre of water – an amount greater than the infant's blood volume.

Signs of dehydration in children with gastroenteritis are outlined in Example 60.2.

In early dehydration the infant is restless and cries frequently. The early physical signs of dehydration are listlessness, loss of skin turgor, dryness of the tongue, depression of the fontanelle and sunken eyes. These are signs of extracellular fluid loss. Intracellular losses occur concomitantly, but these cannot be determined from physical examination. With continuing fluid loss, contraction of the vascular compartment occurs with the development of a rapid, poor volume pulse, poor peripheral capillary return, cold blotchy extremities, and low blood pressure – signs of peripheral circulatory failure. With loss of base, consequent on diarrhoea, and

Example 60.2 Assessment of dehydration

Mild
   5% body weight loss
   Thirsty, alert, restless
   Otherwise normal

Moderate
   6–9% body weight loss
   Thirsty, restless, lethargic but irritable
   Rapid pulse, normal blood pressure
   Sunken eyes, sunken fontanelle★
   Dry mucous membranes, absent tears
   Pinched skin retracts slowly (1–2 secs)★
   Decreased urine output★

Severe
   10% or more body weight loss
   General appearance
   Infants: drowsy, limp, cold, sweaty cyanotic limbs,
      comatose
   Older children: apprehensive, cold, sweaty, cyanotic
      limbs
   Rapid feeble pulse, low blood pressure
   Sunken eyes and fontanelle★
   Very dry mucous membranes
   Pinched skin retracts very slowly (> 2secs)★
   No urine output★

★ Particularly useful in infants for assessment and
monitoring of dehydration.

poor tissue perfusion, metabolic acidosis rapidly ensues. This can be recognized clinically as the child develops deep sighing respirations; it is confirmed by acid-base studies. If this situation is not corrected rapidly death may occur.

Electrolyte loss

Electrolytes lost in acute gastroenteritis include sodium, potassium, chloride and bicarbonate. In most cases the dehydration is isotonic, water and electrolytes being lost in equal proportions. Thus, serum electrolyte values will be normal, as concentrations rather than total amounts are measured. Hypertonic dehydration implies a loss of fluid in excess of electrolyte. It occurs in 5–10% of cases admitted, and is more frequent in small infants. The increased surface to volume ratio and decreased renal concentrating capacity in young infants are factors. Irritability and underestimated dehydration are common in this situation. Rapid rehydration with hypotonic fluid should be avoided in hypertonic dehydration, or rapid shifts of water into cells may be followed by convulsions and brain damage. The message is to rehydrate slowly over 24–48 hours.

Hypotonic dehydration is rarely seen except in children with an ileostomy who have gastroenteritis. Their colonic sodium reabsorption capacity has been

lost. It is important to recognize this problem and to replace sodium vigorously, because death can occur quickly.

Treatment of gastroenteritis

No dehydration

Suitable fluids are listed in Table 60.1. Breast milk should be continued, but extra fluid will be required. The aim is to provide maintenance fluid and to keep up with ongoing losses. This usually means at least 5–6 ml/kg/hr. Reintroduction of food should begin within 24 hours, even if diarrhoea has not settled. Starvation beyond 24 hours may delay recovery.

Table 60.1 Suitable fluids for the non-dehydrated child

Solution	Dilution
Cordials (not low calorie)	1 in 6 with tap water
Carbonated beverages (not low calorie)	1 in 4 with warm water to remove bubbles
Unsweetened fruit juice	1 in 4 with tap water
Fruit juice drinks	1 in 4 with tap water
Glucose (Glucodin from chemist)	2 teaspoons in 240 ml boiled water

Each of these fluids has an osmolality of less than 200 mmol/kg water and sugar content below 200 mmol/l.

Mild to moderate dehydration

Oral rehydration will succeed in almost all children who are not shocked if appropriate fluids are given in an appropriate way. Elegant pathophysiological studies in cholera have led to formulation of oral rehydration fluids which have subsequently been shown to be suitable whatever the cause of the infectious diarrhoea episode. The critical items are the sodium and glucose concentrations which must be in the range recommended in Table 60.2 for maximum fluid absorption. Use of a nasogastric tube to achieve a steady infusion of fluid is appropriate if vomiting or fluid refusal is a major problem.

The volume of fluid required is calculated by adding estimated deficit to maintenance. Maintenance varies from 120 ml/kg/24 hours at 1–3 months of age to 100 ml/kg/24 hours (3–12 months) to 80 ml/kg/24 hours thereafter (see Example 60.3).

Severe dehydration (10% plus)

Circulatory insufficiency is present and intravenous therapy is required. The urgent requirement is to fill

Table 60.2　Oral rehydration preparations available in Australia

Solution	Na*	K*	Cl*	Citrate*	Glucose (%)
WHO recommended solution	90	20	80	10	2
Solution recommended for Australia	50–90	20	40–80	10	2
'Gastrolyte'	60	20	60	10	2
'Electrolade'	50	20	40	10	2
'Glucolyte'	45	20	35	15	2

* Concentrations expressed as mmol/l of made-up solution (except glucose %).

Example 60.3 An infant of 10 kg estimated at 7.5% dehydration has fluid requirements equal to:

$$\begin{aligned} \text{Maintenance } 100 \times 10 \text{ kg} &= 1000 \text{ ml} \\ \text{Deficit } 7.5\% \text{ of } 10 \text{ kg} &= 750 \text{ ml} \\ \text{Total} &= 1750 \text{ ml} \end{aligned}$$

Using oral rehydration the deficit can be replaced in 6 hours rather than 24 hours, so in the above example, the infant would be offered fluid as follows:

First 6 hours:

$$\begin{aligned} \text{Deficit} &= 750 \text{ ml} \\ \text{Maintenance } 6/24 \text{ of } 1000 &= 250 \text{ ml} \\ \text{Total} &= 1000 \text{ ml } (170 \text{ ml/hr}) \end{aligned}$$

Next 18 hours:
Maintenance 18/24 of 1000 = 750 ml (45 ml/hr)

Another simple method which gives about the right answer, is to calculate the fluid deficit, double it, and give that volume over 6–12 hours.

---

the vascular compartment quickly to restore circulation. This can be achieved by a bolus infusion of almost any isotonic fluid. 0.45% ('half normal') saline with added sodium bicarbonate, 75 mmol/l, is a satisfactory solution, given statim in a volume of 20–25 ml/kg. This puts the child into a position where management as for moderate dehydration is appropriate and this can be as intravenous or oral management – usually a combination of both.

See Chapter 51 for details of intravenous therapy in gastroenteritis.

Subsequent management of the severe case

Oral rehydration fluid (see Table 60.2) is offered and intravenous fluid is reduced to compensate. If intravenous canulas fall out or block after 24 hours they rarely need to be replaced. Introduction of formula and/or food can begin in the second 24 hours, usually beginning with half strength formula and/or starch based foods.

Clinical observations. Continued check on pulse, temperature and respirations must be made and careful fluid balance charts kept – this latter point cannot be stressed too strongly. The child should be weighed on admission and in severe cases after 6 hours and 24 hours. This is the best check on fluid replacement.

Breast-feeding after acute diarrhoea. In ideal circumstances, breast-feeding should be continued during a diarhoeal illness. In order to do this, extra fluid should be given to replace continuing losses. Even in the face of lactose intolerance, breast milk seems to be better tolerated than proprietary formulae containing lower lactose levels. Breast-feeding is better accepted by children during diarrhoea than artificially fed nutrients as it offers both comfort and fluids.

In less than ideal circumstances, when diarrhoea has been severe, a delay of 24 hours before recommencing breast-feeding may be required.

Drug therapy. There is no evidence that drug therapy with antidiarrhoeal agents is of benefit in childhood gastroenteritis. Drugs such as diphenoxylate with atropine (Lomotil) and loperamide (Imodium) are contraindicated as they may cause CNS depression and paralytic ileus. This particularly applies to Lomotil. Agents such as kaolin do not reduce fluid losses, although they may appear to promote a less fluid stool. Antibiotics have little or no place in treatment unless there is clinical suspicion of septicaemia. The use of erythromycin in *Campylobacter* infection, although theoretically valid is also usually of little practical value. It is important to remember that it is not the organisms themselves that are harmful, but the fluid loss they cause.

Complications of acute gastroenteritis

Febrile convulsions

They are not uncommon. Rotavirus infection is often associated with a rapid rise in temperature to 39–40°C.

Sugar intolerance

This is the most common complication. It occurs much more often in the younger infant. About 50% of infants under 6 months of age who require hospital admission, require a low lactose formula at the time of discharge, but in less than 10% of older infants is this a problem. It is recognized by the reappearance of diarrhoea when milk is reintroduced into the diet. The stools then become watery, acid, frothy and tend to excoriate the buttocks. If sugar intolerance is suspected the napkin should be lined with thin plastic material, or a rectal examination performed, and the fluid content collected and tested for reducing substances. It is pointless to test solid stool material.

Testing for sugar intolerance. Mix 5 drops of liquid stool with 10 drops of water and add a Clinitest tablet. A positive test indicates sugar intolerance. This test detects 'reducing' sugars such as lactose and glucose but does not detect sucrose. Specific glucose oxidase reagents such as Testape and Glucostix detect glucose only and will not detect lactose or sucrose.

The treatment of sugar intolerance is to remove the offending sugar (almost always lactose) from the diet. The most satisfactory preparations are Digestelact or Delact. These are commercial cow's milk based preparations in which the lactose has been enzymatically split by lactase to galactose and glucose. Other suitable and readily available preparations are Prosobee, Isomil, Nutramigen (see Ch. 13).

Diarrhoea due to lactose intolerance rapidly resolves on a lactose-free diet, which should be continued for approximately four weeks when most cases will have resolved. At that stage a normal milk can be gradually introduced and the effect observed. Should diarrhoea appear, a further four weeks of treatment is indicated, when the situation will normally have resolved.

A very small proportion of infants continue to have diarrhoea and sugar in the stools despite the exclusion of lactose and sucrose. Under these circumstances a carbohydrate free feed is given, with glucose and fructose (which have different cell transport mechanisms) added to tolerance.

Prevention of gastroenteritis

Whilst there can be no doubt that the prevalence of gastroenteritis relates to low living standards and inadequate hygiene, this does not totally apply in the case of rotavirus gastroenteritis. Progress towards a rotavirus vaccine is well advanced. It will be of immense value in developing countries, and will reduce admissions of children with gastroenteritis by 50% in developed countries. Better vaccines against typhoid, cholera and *E.coli* are also being developed.

CHRONIC DIARRHOEA

Chronic or persisting diarrhoea is a not infrequent problem in infancy. Causes are many, but only the more common will be discussed. Not infrequently, however, the cause of persisting diarrhoea is not found despite investigation.

Acute diarrhoea may progress to a chronic state, but more commonly chronic diarrhoea begins insidiously. A number of mechanisms are involved in the pathogenesis of chronic diarrhoea and the reader is referred elsewhere for discussion of these. The pathology may involve either the small bowel, the large bowel or both. When the pathology involves the small bowel, malabsorption is usually the major problem, although low-grade or intermittent diarrhoea may be associated.

The following are the more common causes of chronic or persistent diarrhoea in infancy and childhood:

1. Chronic non-specific diarrhoea
2. Postinfective diarrhoea
3. Milk allergy
4. Sucrase-isomaltase deficiency
5. Chronic inflammatory bowel disease
6. Enteric infection
7. Intestinal lymphoma.

Persistent diarrhoea is common in coeliac disease, giardiasis, cystic fibrosis and with persistent sugar intolerance. These are discussed elsewhere (Ch. 61).

Do not overlook constipation with overflow which often presents as spurious diarrhoea.

Chronic non-specific diarrhoea

This syndrome occurs most commonly in the toddler period – between 12 months and 4 years of age. It accounts for a large proportion of children with chronic diarrhoea although as knowledge of gut physiology and pathophysiology improves, the group becomes smaller. The history is one of frequent, poorly formed brown and slightly offensive stools. Food material is readily recognizable in the stools of these children, e.g. carrot, peas, beans, etc. The child, despite persisting diarrhoea, is constitutionally well, normally active, with growth unimpaired. Appetite is normal or increased and fluid intake is often increased. Physical examination in these children does not reveal any signs of wasting or of dietary deficiency. In addition, investigation is invariably negative. In the absence of an aetiology, management is not easy and it is not surprising that a large number of therapeutic agents have been tried without success. Diet assessment sometimes reveals a very high intake of fruit juices and cordials, or of sorbital which is often used as a sweetener. Reduction in intake of peas, corn and carrots (which are not chewed adequately by infants) reduces parental anxiety about poor digestion.

The parents of these children need a great deal of reassurance of the good outcome. Suggestions that toddler diarrhoea has a psychological cause have no basis in fact. The natural history of chronic non-specific diarrhoea is for the diarrhoea to resolve spontaneously at about the age of 3 years.

A similar type of diarrhoea occasionally follows dietary restriction, in particular a low-fat diet. When a normal fat intake (4 g/kg daily) is reintroduced, diarrhoea ceases. This is certainly not the cause of the majority of cases of non-specific diarrhoea of infancy, but the diarrhoea may be made worse if a low-fat diet is misguidedly recommended.

Postinfective diarrhoea

This not infrequently causes persisting diarrhoea in childhood. The diagnosis is established on clinical grounds from the following:

a. History of an acute attack of diarrhoea, preferably with documented evidence of ill-health and/or dehydration. The identification of a pathogen either viral or bacterial or parasitic is of added importance.
b. Poorly formed and frequent stools persisting after a period of two weeks when most episodes of acute diarrhoea have ceased.

Most cases of postinfective diarrhoea are associated with sugar intolerance. The finding of reducing substances in the stools or a positive breath hydrogen test confirms sugar intolerance and most will resolve when the offending sugar (usually lactose) is eliminated from the diet. Cow's milk protein may also need to be removed. A suitable formula which does not contain either cow's milk protein or disaccharide is Pregestimil. It should be emphasized that lactose intolerance is much more commonly associated with persistent diarrhoea than cow's milk protein intolerance.

Milk allergy

This is a difficult and controversial subject. Most paediatricians regard milk allergy as an uncommon cause of persisting diarrhoea, but few would dismiss it altogether. The diagnosis is essentially a clinical one and implies the development of diarrhoea while the infant is taking a cow's milk formula and its relief by elimination. Lactose intolerance must first be excluded. Some years ago Goldman and colleagues suggested that three separate trials were necessary to establish this diagnosis, but in genuine cases of cow's milk protein intolerance, this can be a dangerous procedure and even precipitate an anaphylactoid reaction. Skin tests and the currently available serological tests for allergy (RAST and IgE specific antibody) are usually unhelpful, expensive and may be misleading.

The diagnosis rests on meticulous history taking and observation, bearing in mind that reactions may be delayed for hours or a day or two. The pathology of milk allergy is not well understood, although a number of workers have documented evidence of mucosal damage following ingestion of cow's milk in a susceptible individual. In cow's milk protein intolerance, children may develop a diarrhoea similar to that associated with sugar intolerance. Occasionally, mucus and/or blood is present in the stools. Infants who are intolerant to cow's milk must be fed a cow's milk-protein-free formula. Most of these contain soya bean protein or protein hydrolysate. Unfortunately, infants who are intolerant to cow's milk may also become intolerant to soya bean, eggs, and wheat. The management of cow's milk protein intolerance obviously involves the exclusion of all dairy products and their substitution by alternate forms of protein, e.g. soya bean, wheat, etc. As a general rule, such children are able to tolerate cow's milk protein by about the age of two years. Great care needs to be taken in the reintroduction of cow's milk and, when attempted, it is wise to cover the possibility of an anaphylactoid reaction.

Sucrase-isomaltase deficiency

It is important to recognize this uncommon disorder because it responds well to treatment and because it is transmitted as an autosomal recessive trait. Occasionally, one obtains a history that diarrhoea follows ingestion of cane sugar, but this is far from the rule so that it is important to have a strong index of suspicion and pose the question, or undertake a trial of feeding sucrose and observing the effects. Many children with sucrase-isomaltase deficiency thrive well, but are subject to bouts of explosive diarrhoea when large sucrose loads are taken. The diagnosis is established finally by the demonstration of very low maltase and sucrase enzyme levels in a small bowel biopsy. The breath hydrogen test is a good indirect means of screening for sucrase-isomaltase deficiency. Management involves removal of the offending sugars. It should be noted that fruit juices are an important source of sucrose in children. Clearly this is a lifelong disorder.

Chronic inflammatory bowel disease in children

Ulcerative colitis

Approximately 5% of cases of chronic ulcerative colitis have their onset in childhood. Most occur in the latter part of childhood, but the disease has presented as early as the first year of life. As a rule, the presentation is with chronic diarrhoea and stools which contain fluid, mucus and blood. Abdominal pain and tenesmus are also common. The number of stools may vary from 1 or 2, to 20 or 30 in a day, seriously disrupting sleep. Patients with untreated active ulcerative colitis are generally unwell, rapidly lose weight, fail to grow and/or fail to progress normally into puberty. Occasionally, the disease is fulminating with gross abdominal distension, catastrophic diarrhoea, fever and collapse. The course of ulcerative colitis is one of remissions and exacerbations, even with treatment. The aetiology is unknown.

Pathology. Macroscopically the lesion is a granular proctocolitis with ready bleeding on contact. Microscopically the lesion is confined to the mucosa which is infiltrated with leucocytes and small round cells. Crypt abscesses may be present. Patches of mucosa of varying sizes are denuded producing shallow ulceration. Ulcerative colitis may involve part or the entire large bowel. In general the lesion tends to be more marked distally, so that if the rectum is only slightly involved it is unlikely that the remainder of the large bowel will be affected. The mucosa is affected uniformly without the patchy distribution or skip lesions seen in Crohn's disease.

Complications of ulcerative colitis include loss of haustration with reduction in calibre of the colon and consequent malfunction. Stenoses, perforation and internal fistulae may also occur. Extracolonic complications include hepatitis, cholangitis, skin lesions, e.g. pyoderma, arthritis, uveitis, erythema nodosum. Cancer risk is said to be higher in childhood onset disease, but this appears to be simply due to the duration of disease.

Diagnosis. This is established from colonoscopy and biopsy together with a barium study to define the extent of the disease (Fig. 60.2). Known infections must be excluded.

Treatment. This involves the administration of steroids in high doses to suppress activity, and long-term sulphasalazine. Correction of anaemia, a high protein, high caloric diet with additional vitamins and minerals are important. Failure to respond to medical treatment, inadequate growth and pubertal development indicate the need to consider surgery. Surgery will be necessary for the bowel complications mentioned above. Surgical treatment involves a total colectomy and is curative.

Crohn's disease (Fig. 60.3)

Crohn's disease is a chronic disorder of unknown aetiol-

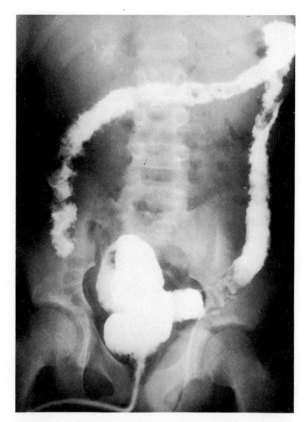

Fig. 60.2 Barium enema. Demonstrates diffuse continuous ulceration of the large bowel. Diagnosis – chronic ulcerative colitis.

ogy, characterized pathologically by involvement of all bowel wall layers in a chronic inflammatory process with non-caseating granulomas. Crohn's disease may involve any area of the gastrointestinal tract from mouth to anus, but usually it is the distal ileum and colon that are involved. Over recent years the incidence of Crohn's disease in children has increased dramatically. In Melbourne it has gone from less than 1 case per year in 1975 to 12–15 new cases per year in 1987, and it outnumbers ulcerative colitis 2:1. At times the distinction from ulcerative colitis can be very difficult and in 10–20% of cases the type of inflammatory bowel disease is not determined.

The clinical features. The presentation of Crohn's disease is extremely variable and a high index of suspicion is necessary if the diagnosis is to be made early. In one series, 50% of cases had been active for more than one year before the diagnosis was established. Suggestive modes of presentation include:

a. Abdominal pain with or without diarrhoea. The

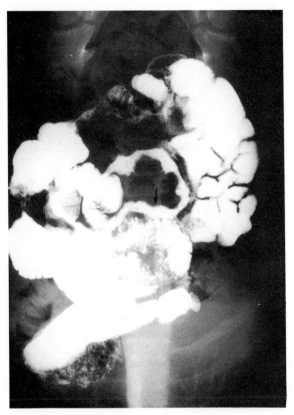

Fig. 60.3   Barium meal and follow-through demonstrating areas of irregular narrowing in the ileum. Diagnosis – Crohn's disease.

Investigations will usually reveal a significant elevation of the ESR and a mild anaemia. Occasionally hypoproteinaemia occurs.

Diagnosis. Confirmation of a suspected diagnosis is made from gastrointestinal endoscopy and biopsy. Both gastroduodenoscopy and colonoscopy are performed where IBD is suspected. Any involvement of oesophagus, stomach or duodenum makes Crohn's disease very likely whether or not typical granulomas are seen histologically. Macroscopically the appearances are often similar to those of ulcerative colitis and the distinction can only be made on histological grounds, but even this is not always easy. Radiologically the presence of small bowel disease and of 'skin lesions' are more important in making the distinction from chronic ulcerative colitis than narrowing of bowel and the so-called 'cobblestone' appearance (see Fig. 60.3). Complications of Crohn's disease include intestinal obstruction, fistulae and massive haemorrhage. Fortunately, these are not common in childhood.

Treatment. Treatment of the uncomplicated case is basically medical, but should be undertaken preferably by a paediatric gastroenterologist. A high protein, high caloric diet with vitamin and mineral supplements is essential but parenteral nutrition is sometimes necessary in the refractory case. Usually, steroids will produce a remission of the disease when long-term treatment with sulphasalazine is substituted. Exacerbations, which are frequent, require usually further steroid therapy. Recurrences are not uncommon after surgical removal of isolated areas of disease.

abdomen may be tender and there may be an ill-defined mass to palpate.
b. Diarrhoea with or without blood and mucus. Abdominal pain may also be present.
c. Anorexia, weight loss, lethargy and growth failure. In this group there may be few or no complaints referred to the abdomen.
d. As a PUO, again with few features referable to the gastrointestinal tract.
e. Abdominal features in association with perianal disease (fissure, fistula and abscess). This is particularly suggestive of Crohn's disease.
f. Extraintestinal manifestations, such as fever, arthritis, arthralgia and clubbing, may accompany the intestinal symptoms or may occur alone. Delay in pubertal development is frequent when the disease commences in this way. Occasionally stomatitis or erythema nodosum occurs.

Enteric infection

Occasionally chronic diarrhoea may be the result of an enteric infection which will include *Salmonella* sp, *Entamoeba histolytica*, *Giardia lamblia*, *Yersinia*, *Campylobacter*, and tuberculosis. In any case of persisting diarrhoea it is important to obtain aerobic and anaerobic stool cultures. Treatment clearly will depend upon the pathogen isolated, but specific therapy is often unavailable or unsuccessful and supportive measures will be required.

Intestinal lymphoma

Occasionally an intestinal lymphoma is responsible for chronic diarrhoea in infancy and, although rare, may need to be considered in the child with persisting diarrhoea for which no other cause is apparent.

FURTHER READING

Birman C W, Furnkawer C 1982 Food allergy. Pediatrics in Review 3(7): 213–220

Bishop R F 1984 Diarrhoea. Rotavirus in perspective – a personal view. Australian Paediatric Journal 20: 9–12

Cohen S A, Kristy M H, Eastman E J, Mathis R K, Walker W A 1979 Chronic non-specific diarrhoea. American Journal of Diseases in Children 133: 490–492

Diarrhoea in Children 1987 The Gut Foundation of Australia.

Ferguson A 1981 Chronic diarrhoeal disease in older children. In: Hull D (ed) Recent advances in paediatrics. Churchill Livingstone, Edinburgh

Fineberg L, Harper P A, Harrison H E et al 1982 Oral rehydration for diarrhoea. Journal of Pediatrics 101: 497–499

Goldman A S, Anderson D W Jr, Sellers W A 1963 Milk allergy: oral challenge with milk and isolated milk protein in allergic children. Pediatrics 32: 425–429

Harries J T 1987 Essentials of paediatric gastroenterology, 2nd edn. Churchill Livingstone, Edinburgh

Lloyd-Still J D 1979 Chronic diarrhoea of childhood and the misuse of elimination diets. Journal of Pediatrics 95: 10–13

Walker-Smith J A 1980 Toddler's diarrhoea. Archives of Disease in Childhood 55: 329–330

Walker-Smith J A, Hamilton J R, Walker W A 1983 Practical paediatric gastroenterology. Butterworths, Norwich

61. Malabsorption

Geoffrey Davidson

STRUCTURE OF THE INTESTINAL MUCOSA

Normally absorption occurs entirely in the small bowel where length and total surface area are particularly favourable. The surface area of the jejunum and ileum is greatly increased by the circular folds, villi and microvilli such that if it were stretched completely flat it would cover the surface of a tennis court. The process of absorption is remarkably efficient and can be completed in the proximal one-third of the small intestine.

Interference with intraluminal digestion will affect normal absorption and, thus, diseases affecting pancreatic function or bile flow will cause malabsorption. Similarly, not only is normal anatomy in terms of length and surface area of the small intestine important, but motility disturbances will interfere with propulsive movements and mixing of foods with gut secretions and can also lead to altered bacterial flora and hence malabsorption.

To have a better understanding of the mechanism of malabsorption, a knowledge of the normal processes of digestion and absorption of the dietary constituents (fat, protein, carbohydrate, vitamins, minerals and water) is essential.

Fat digestion and absorption

Dietary fats are water insoluble and are mainly ingested as triglycerides which are made up of three molecules of fatty acids (containing 16 to 18 carbon atoms, e.g. stearic, oleic acid) esterified to a glycerol backbone.

Fat digestion starts in the stomach, where lingual lipase (secreted from the glands of von Ebner at the base of the tongue) contributes to intragastric hydrolysis, which is particularly important in the first few months of life. The major function of the stomach is to regulate delivery of fat to the duodenum where triglycerides are hydrolysed by pancreatic lipase, colipase, esterase and phospholipase to yield two fatty acids and beta-monoglycerides (see Fig. 61.1).

Hydrolysis is aided by pancreatic secretion of bicarbonate which creates an optimal pH (near neutrality) and the detergent action of bile salts. Colipase is essential for adequate triglyceride hydrolysis.

The products of lipolysis are relatively insoluble and require bile salts for solubilization and dispersal in the aqueous environment of the small intestine. Bile acids, when present at a sufficient intraluminal concentration exist as small water-soluble aggregates called micelles which can solubilize fatty acids and monoglycerides by incorporating them into their molecular structure to form mixed micelles. These mixed micelles pass through the water layer at the mucosal surface and release lipid, which enters the intestinal absorptive cell by an, as yet, unknown process. The bile salt micelle is not absorbed and passes on to the terminal ileum where an extremely efficient reabsorptive process occurs, so that only a small amount of bile salt is lost in the faeces. The bile acids return to the liver by the portal vein, completing their enterohepatic circulation which occurs two to three times with each meal. The bile salt pool size in the full-term infant is half the adult level and in premature infants is about one-third adult level.

Within the mucosal cell monoglycerides and fatty acids are re-esterified to form triglyceride which is covered with a coat of phospholipid, cholesterol and protein to form chylomicrons. These leave the epithelial cell to reach the lymphatics and are distributed as chyle.

Medium chain triglycerides are lipids with fatty acids containing 6 to 12 carbon atoms. Their absorption is improved in the presence of pancreatic lipase and as they are moderately water-soluble micelles solubilization is not necessary. Medium chain fatty acids are not esterified but appear as unchanged free fatty acids in the portal venous blood. Because of these properties they can be used as dietary supplements for patients with defective fat absorption and fat digestion of varied aetiology.

In summary, the important factors for fat digestion and absorption include gastric emulsification, pancreatic

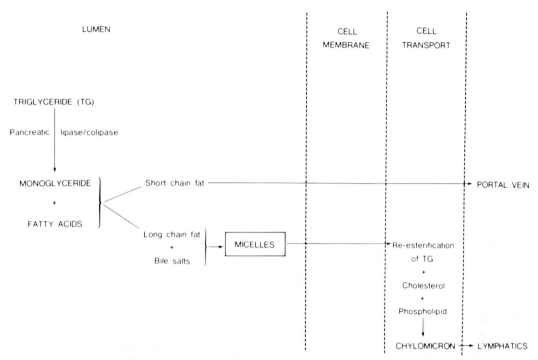

LUMEN   CELL   CELL
                                       MEMBRANE   TRANSPORT

TRIGLYCERIDE (TG)

Pancreatic | lipase/colipase

MONOGLYCERIDE   Short chain fat ———————————————————————→ PORTAL VEIN
      +
 FATTY ACIDS

              Long chain fat
                   +   → MICELLES   → Re-esterification
              Bile salts   of TG
                                                          +
                                                      Cholesterol
                                                          +
                                                      Phospholipid
                                                          ↓
                                            CHYLOMICRON ←→ LYMPHATICS

Fig. 61.1 Diagrammatic representation of fat digestion and absorption.

lipase and colipase, bile salts and a critical micellar concentration, and alkalization of the duodenum to optimize activity of the pancreatic enzymes.

Carbohydrate absorption and digestion

Carbohydrate constitutes about 10% of the calories of the infant. Dietary carbohydrates are primarily starch (mixture of polysaccharides, amylose and amylopectin), sucrose (table sugar) and lactose (milk sugar). Carbohydrates require hydrolysis to their component monosaccharides before absorption (see Fig. 61.2).

Starch

This is a polymer of amylose and amylopectin where amylose is a straight chain glucose polymer joined by 1–4 carbon linkages. Amylopectin is a branching glucose polymer with 1–4 linear chains joined at periodic branch points by 1–6 linkages which occur at intervals of about 25 glucose units. Starch digestion begins in the mouth by salivary amylase but the bulk of digestion occurs in the duodenum by pancreatic amylase which breaks the 1–4 linkages of both amylose and amylopectin. Starch digestion results in the production of a disaccharide (amylose), a trisaccharide (maltotriose) and a series of

branched oligosaccharides (alpha-limit dextrins). These are further hydrolysed by the brush border disaccharidases maltase and isomaltase to the monosaccharide glucose.

Disaccharides

The disaccharides sucrose and lactose are hydrolysed to their component monosaccharides by the respective disaccharidases sucrase and lactase to glucose and fructose and glucose and galactose, respectively. The monosaccharides glucose and galactose are absorbed by a sodium-dependent active transport mechanism whereas fructose absorption occurs by sodium-independent facilitated diffusion. This latter mechanism seems to have a limited capacity. The monosaccharides pass through the enterocyte into the portal circulation.

Protein digestion and absorption (see Fig. 61.3)

Protein provides 10–15% of total calories. Protein digestion is begun in the stomach by pepsin but the majority is digested in the small intestine by pancreatic proteolytic enzymes which are initially secreted as inactive precursors under the influence of cholecystokinin. Trypsinogen is activated to trypsin by the enzyme

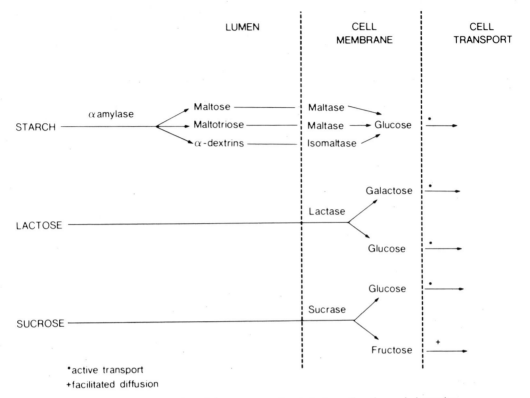

Fig. 61.2 Diagrammatic representation of the processes of carbohydrate digestion and absorption.

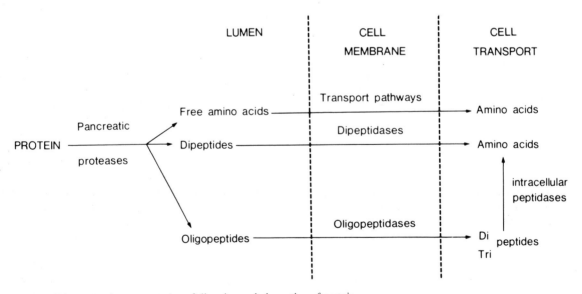

Fig. 61.3 Diagrammatic representation of digestion and absorption of protein.

enterokinase present in the brush border of the duodenum. Trypsin activates autocatalytically trypsinogen and the other zymogens chymotrypsinogen, proelastase and procarboxypeptidase. The products of proteolysis are a mixture of free amino acids and oligopeptides with 3–6 amino acid residues. The oligopeptides undergo further hydrolysis by brush border peptidases or intracellularly depending upon the type of peptide present. Amino acids as well as di- and tripeptides can be absorbed intact into the enterocytes where the di- and tripeptides can be digested by cytosolic peptidases. Amino acids are taken into and transported across the cell membrane by an active sodium-dependent process. The site in the small intestine at which digestion is complete varies with the type of meal but a greater length of intestine appears to be necessary for protein absorption than for carbohydrate. Thus protein digestion may not be complete in the upper ileum.

Vitamin absorption

Fat soluble vitamins (A, D, E and K)
Fat soluble vitamins are insoluble in aqueous solutions and are dependent on micellar solubilization which in turn is dependent on adequate bile production. Vitamins A and D require hydrolysis by pancreatic enzymes before absorption. Any disease associated with significant fat malabsorption usually leads to simultaneous malabsorption of fat soluble vitamins.

Water soluble vitamins

These do not require micellar solubilization for optimal absorption but several require specialized digestive and transport mechanisms, e.g. folic acid, vitamin B_{12}. However, the majority like vitamin C are absorbed by passive diffusion throughout the small intestine.

Folic acid

Folic acid is absorbed mainly from the duodenum and jejunum. Dietary folate from plant and animal sources are mainly in the form of pteroylpolyglutamates which are hydrolysed by a specific brush border peptidase (folic acid conjugase) to mono- and diglutamates before being absorbed.

Vitamin B_{12}

Vitamin B_{12} is present mainly in animal protein and is liberated in the stomach by gastric pepsin. The free vitamin binds in the stomach to a binding protein (R protein) which has a greater affinity for vitamin B_{12} than does intrinsic factor. R protein must be removed for absorption to occur and this happens in the upper small intestine under the influence of the pancreatic proteases allowing vitamin B_{12} to bind to intrinsic factor. The intrinsic factor-B_{12} complex passes through the small intestine and binds to specific receptors on the terminal ileal enterocytes where the vitamin B_{12} is absorbed.

Minerals

Iron

Absorption occurs in the duodenum and upper small bowel. Approximately 5–10% of dietary iron is absorbed, which corresponds with daily losses through gut, skin and urine. The process of iron absorption is complex and not fully understood but seems to be regulated at the level of the epithelial cell (see Ch. 42).

Calcium

Calcium absorption is maximal in the duodenum and proximal jejunum. The most important influence on calcium absorption is the vitamin D derivative, 1,25 dihydroxycholecalciferol. It enhances calcium absorption by increasing permeability of the intestinal cell membrane and induces production of a calcium-binding protein which carries the calcium across the cell to the baso-lateral membrane, where it is excreted as a result of the activity of CaATPase.

A wide variety of gastrointestinal diseases can affect calcium absorption, including the interference with vitamin D bio-availability by altering vitamin D absorption and the enterohepatic circulation, by disordered vitamin D metabolism because of liver or renal disease or by interrupting the normal absorptive process required for calcium absorption.

Zinc

20–30% of ingested zinc is absorbed. Zinc transport in the epithelial cell is via a zinc-binding ligand. Zinc deficiency occurs in the presence of fat malabsorption and is common in Crohn's disease and coeliac disease and will occur rapidly in children on parenteral nutrition without zinc supplements. Also there is an inherited deficiency of zinc absorption (acrodermatitis enteropathica). Zinc deficiency is manifested by scaly dry dermatitis (acrodermatitis), alopecia, diarrhoea, hypogeusia, delayed wound healing and failure to thrive.

Magnesium

About one-third of ingested magnesium (0.5 g per day) is absorbed in the small intestine, mainly in the proximal segments. Magnesium transport appears to be passive, occurring by simple diffusion. Magnesium deficiency most commonly occurs in conditions giving rise to malabsorption but there is also a genetically determined disorder of magnesium absorption (primary hypomagnesaemia) which appears to be a result of a defect in carrier-mediated transport. Magnesium deficiency can cause tetany and/or convulsions, chronic diarrhoea and muscle cramps.

Water and electrolyte absorption

The bulk of fluid and electrolyte absorption occurs in the proximal half of the small intestine. The major role of the duodenum is to rapidly equilibrate gastric contents with plasma, producing an iso-osmotic chyme, which remains so throughout the jejunum and ileum.

Water absorption is extremely efficient, with the bulk being absorbed in the jejunum and ileum and about 10% in the colon. Less than 2% of the many litres of fluid passing through the gut each day is excreted in faeces. Water is absorbed passively through mucosal pores and carries ions and small solutes with it (solvent drag). Electrolytes are also absorbed by active transport, a process stimulated by actively transported solutes such as glucose and amino acids. In the jejunum water absorption largely follows nutrient absorption, whereas in the ileum it occurs without nutrient absorption.

The jejunum avidly absorbs bicarbonate, whereas it is secreted into the ileal lumen. Chloride absorption is passive in the jejunum and active in the ileum. Potassium is absorbed passively from both jejunum and ileum.

The colon conserves water, sodium and chloride remaining in the lumen after the bulk of the products of digestion have been absorbed. Most of this occurs in the ascending colon. Although this absorption is small and is promoted by mineralocorticoids, it is important in the maintenance of fluid and electrolyte homeostasis, especially where small intestinal absorption is impaired such as in gastroenteritis.

For normal digestion and absorption the following are necessary (see Fig. 61.4):

- The gut must be of sufficient length, with undisturbed forward propulsive movement of content
- Unrestricted flow of normal quality bile and pancreatic secretions is required
- The small intestinal mucosal absorptive cells must carry out their normal digestive and absorptive processes.

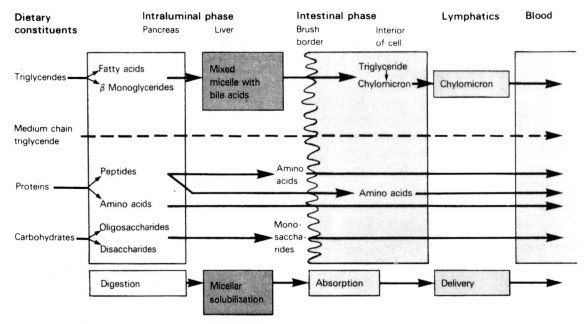

Fig. 61.4 Schematic representation of absorption of fat, carbohydrate and protein (adapted from Roy C C et al, Pediatric Clinical Gastroenterology, 2nd edn, C V Mosby, St Louis, 1975).

MALABSORPTION

Malabsorption is a syndrome, not a disease entity and is defined as any state in which there is a disturbance of digestion and/or net absorption of nutrient across the intestinal mucosa.

Aetiology

It is useful to consider the aetiology according to the intestinal pathophysiology responsible. The more common causes are outlined in Example 61.1. In developed countries the commonest causes of malabsorption relate to:

1. Mucosal injury secondary to gastroenteritis (post-enteritis syndrome with secondary disaccharide malabsorption)

Example 61.1 Aetiology of common causes of malabsorption in children based on the pathophysiological disturbance

Pathophysiological disturbance
Mucosal abnormality
Anatomical
  Post-enteritis syndrome ± carbohydrate malabsorption
  Giardiasis
  Cow's milk protein intolerance
  Coeliac disease (gluten-sensitive enteropathy)
  Immunodeficiency states
  Severe malnutrition
  Inflammatory bowel disease

Functional
  Primary disaccharidase deficiency, e.g. sucrase-isomaltase deficiency,
  Adult onset lactase deficiency
  Glucose-galactose malabsorption
  Congenital chloridorrhoea
  Enterokinase deficiency
  Acrodermatitis enteropathica (zinc deficiency)

Luminal abnormality
Exocrine pancreatic insufficiency
  Cystic fibrosis
  Pancreatic hypoplasia (Shwachmann-Diamond syndrome)
  Malnutrition
Bile salt insufficiency
  Bile duct obstruction (biliary atresia, choledochal cyst)
  Cholestatic liver disease
  Bacterial overgrowth
  Ileal resection

Anatomical abnormality
Short gut
  Surgical resection
Motility disturbance
  Stenosis
  Hirschsprung's disease

---

2. Cow's milk protein intolerance
3. Giardiasis
4. Coeliac disease
5. Interference with luminal digestion as in cystic fibrosis.

In developing countries and also in the Australian Aboriginal population the combination of poor hygiene, inadequate nutrition and recurrent gastrointestinal infections cause persistent mucosal injury, chronic diarrhoea and generalized malabsorption.

Clinical presentation

Malabsorption can present in any of the following ways although in practice the commonest feature would be chronic diarrhoea

Chronic diarrhoea

This is usually defined as diarrhoea of more than 14 days' duration. The frequency, fluidity and sequence of events surrounding the onset will provide important clues to the diagnosis, e.g. offensive, bulky stools since birth suggest cystic fibrosis, fluid-explosive stools since introduction of solids suggest sucrase-isomaltase deficiency, or fluid stools persisting for several weeks following a bout of acute enteritis suggest post-gastrointestinal syndrome with secondary disaccharidase deficiency. Stool colour is not usually a helpful clinical feature because of its variability. Similarly, a floating stool is not indicative of malabsorption but only of the amount of gas present in the stool.

Failure to thrive

Growth charts will indicate a marked reduction in weight and to a lesser extent, height (height/weight discrepancy). Slow weight gain since birth may be a feature of congenital conditions such as cystic fibrosis. Often, there is loss of subcutaneous fat and evidence of muscle wasting, best seen in the inner thighs, buttocks and arms. Failure to thrive can manifest simply as short stature, particularly in children with coeliac disease who may have no gastrointestinal symptoms.

Abdominal distension

Gaseous abdominal distension represents a combination of abnormal fermentation of food within the gut and poor muscle tone and is common in malabsorptive states. Abdominal examination may also reveal hepatomegaly, splenomegaly, an abdominal mass or tenderness which may also be relevant.

Pallor

Malabsorption can result in anaemia due to iron or folate deficiency. Deficient intake of folic acid, iron and vitamin B_{12} can cause pallor and failure to thrive.

Recurrent infections

The presence of chronic cough in association with growth failure should raise the suspicion of malabsorption and cystic fibrosis, which is one of the commonest causes of malabsorption in Caucasian children (1 in 2500 live births). Also finger clubbing and chest deformity are often present. However, a history of recurrent infections since birth or with onset during the first year of life occurs also in immunodeficiency states and pancreatic hypoplasia associated with neutropenia (Shwachman-Diamond syndrome).

Severe malnutrition

Most commonly this is seen in Aboriginal children, where there is a marked height/weight discrepancy although stunting may also be present, indicating a generalized calorie deficiency. If the deficiency has been related mainly to the inadequate protein intake or excessive protein loss, peripheral oedema with abdominal distension due to ascites may be present. Finger clubbing is often present with chronic liver, lung or bowel disease.

Previous bowel surgery

Malabsorption due to an anatomical abnormality or bacterial overgrowth should be considered if symptoms of vomiting, abdominal distension and chronic diarrhoea are present in a child who has had previous bowel surgery.

Behavioural changes

Children with coeliac disease can become anorexic, extremely irritable and manifest behavioural changes as a presenting feature. They can become very lethargic, as can children with severe malabsorption from any cause. In this context it is important to observe the mother-child relationship, as one of the commonest causes of failure to thrive is psychosocial deprivation without malabsorption.

Diagnosis

A detailed clinical history should provide the chronological sequence of events as well as a description of stool characteristics. Also an accurate dietary history is essential as inadequate dietary intake is a common cause of growth failure.

Physical examination may also provide clues to the diagnosis, such as surgical scars, or extra-intestinal manifestations of a malabsorptive disorder. The following features should be noted:

1. Weight, height and head circumference measurements and growth velocity
2. General appearance and evidence of recent weight loss
3. Muscle tone and muscle bulk
4. Abdominal distension or organomegaly
5. Pallor
6. Skin lesions and buttock excoriations
7. Finger clubbing (seen in chronic liver, lung or bowel disease)
8. Oedema (peripheral, ascites).

Investigations

The clinical history and physical examination should suggest the likely diagnosis and give direction to the subsequent investigations. The tests outlined below are of necessity simple and are extremely effective from a screening viewpoint.

Stool examination

If there is obvious steatorrhoea the stools will be large, pale, offensive and greasy, whereas with carbohydrate malabsorption they may be of fluid consistency and excoriate the buttocks. Stool microscopy may reveal fat globules (pancreatic insufficiency), fatty acid crystals (mucosal injury, biliary obstruction or deficiency) or cysts (*Giardia lamblia*). A Clinitest on the fluid portion of the stool may reveal presence of reducing substance (positive equals 0.75% and over), confirming the suspicion of carbohydrate malabsorption. The presence of red and/or white cells in the stool should suggest colonic pathology such as infective colitis or inflammatory bowel disease.

Breath hydrogen test

This test enables the diagnosis of incomplete carbohydrate digestion and absorption to be made in a sensitive non-invasive manner. The principle is that gaseous hydrogen (H_2) is released by fermentation of unabsorbed carbohydrate by intestinal bacterial flora. A portion of this H_2 is absorbed into the bloodstream and excreted by the lungs. Expired breath samples are collected at intervals and following a carbohydrate load and the H_2 measured by gas chromatography.

The breath hydrogen test is the most sensitive test for carbohydrate malabsorption. The commonest indication for its use is in lactose malabsorption but it can also be used to screen children with chronic diarrhoea for sucrose or fructose malabsorption. It is useful in screening for small intestinal bacterial overgrowth.

Full blood examination

Iron deficiency anaemia may be noted, either due to dietary insufficiency or malabsorption. A macrocytic anaemia may suggest folic acid or vitamin B_{12} deficiency. Acanthocytes in the blood smear suggest malabsorption related to abetalipoproteinaemia, a rare disorder of apoprotein B synthesis diagnosed by the absence of β-lipoprotein on serum lipoprotein analysis.

Sweat test

This is the only test that is diagnostic for cystic fibrosis, and at present the only acceptable method is pilocarpineiontophoresis. The presence of a sweat chloride in excess of 60 mmol/l is diagnostic provided a minimum of 100 mg of sweat has been collected.

Small bowel biopsy

In experienced hands, suction biopsy of the small intestine is a quick and safe procedure, even in neonates, and

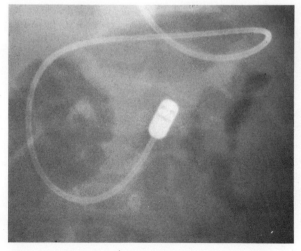

Fig. 61.5 The small bowel biopsy capsule in the 4th part of the duodenum at the level of the ligament of Treitz.

has proved to be a most valuable tool in the study of malabsorption (Fig. 61.5). This test is now performed much earlier in the evaluation of children with suspected malabsorption and growth failure because of its value in localizing and characterizing a digestive-absorptive defect. The procedure is performed under radiograph screening and the tissue obtained (lower duodenum or jejunum) is examined for its structure (by light and electronmicroscopy) and disaccharidase activities. Duodenal fluid obtained at the same time allows for intra-luminal enzyme assays, bile salt estimation, bacterial culture and microscopy of fluid for *Giardia lamblia* trophozoites. Small bowel biopsy and duodenal juice aspiration is the most reliable means of diagnosing giardiasis.

Other tests

There are many other tests proposed for the diagnosis of malabsorption in children but the above investigations will usually elicit a cause or give a guide to other more specific tests. Some of these are listed below.

Radiology. This is really only of value when an anatomical abnormality (e.g. malrotation, stenosis or blind loop) is suspected, or if there has been previous abdominal surgery.

Alpha-1 antitrypsin clearance. This is the preferred method of assessing protein-losing enteropathy in children and has replaced the radiolabelling techniques. Alpha-1 antitrypsin levels are measured in serum and a 24-hour stool collection and a clearance value calculated.

Fat balance studies. These are not diagnostic but rather confirm the presence or absence of fat malabsorption. It has only limited value in that it may be useful if all other investigations are normal to confirm a digestive-absorptive defect. In can be useful in monitoring enzyme replacement therapy in children with cystic fibrosis. It is also important to coincidentally measure fat intake so that a calculation of the percentage of fat absorption can be made. The test must be done over three days to eliminate dietary variation.

Pancreatic function tests. The most specific test involves duodenal intubation and collection of duodenal juice following stimulation with cholecystokinin and secretin. Pancreatic enzymes and bicarbonate secretion can be measured and quantified. A number of non-invasive (tubeless) screening tests are available but do not detect pancreatic dysfunction below the level of steatorrhoea and will not detect isolated enzyme defects.

Colonoscopy and colonic biopsies. These are indicated if inflammatory bowel disease is suspected as a cause of malabsorption and not confirmed by the above techniques.

COMMON DISORDERS CAUSING MALABSORPTION

Mucosal abnormality

Coeliac disease (gluten-sensitive enteropathy)

In this disorder the intestinal mucosa is damaged by gluten-containing foods (gluten is a glycoprotein found in wheat, rye and barley products). The nature of the toxicity of gluten is still unknown. The incidence in Australia is similar to that for cystic fibrosis. Coeliac disease is uncommon in blacks or Asians but can occur in 10% of first-degree relatives. The relationship between the incidence of the disease, breast-feeding, and the age of introduction of gluten into the diet is not known.

Coeliac disease classically presents between 9 and 18 months of age, when the previously thriving infant becomes anorexic, lethargic, irritable and demonstrates faltering growth, abdominal distension and offensive, frequent stools. Coeliac disease may present at any time of life and in other ways, which include:

1. Intermittent diarrhoea.
2. Short stature. Children with coeliac disease can present to an endocrinologist for investigation of short stature and have no gastrointestinal symptoms.
3. An obscure anaemia which may be hypochromic, microcytic or macrocytic.

At present there are no reliable screening tests for the diagnosis of coeliac disease, and if suspected a duodenal biopsy should be carried out. The diagnosis of coeliac disease is established in the following way:

1. A small bowel biopsy showing a completely flat mucosa carried out before there is any change in diet (Fig. 61.6).
2. A second biopsy (usually nine to twelve months later) showing the re-establishment of a normal mucosa following gluten withdrawal (Fig. 61.7).
3. A third biopsy three months after re-introduction of gluten, showing re-appearance of mucosal damage. This biopsy would be done earlier if symptoms developed. If this biopsy is normal a gluten-containing diet is maintained and a further biopsy carried out two years later or earlier if symptoms develop.

A small percentage of patients may not show relapse after two years of gluten challenge and may have had a temporary gluten intolerance. The treatment of coeliac diesase is the removal of gluten from the diet. The present evidence suggests that coeliac disease is a lifelong condition and thus it is extremely important to make an accurate diagnosis. There is no place for an empirical trial of a gluten-free diet.

Giardiasis

Infestation with *Giardia lamblia* is one of the commonest

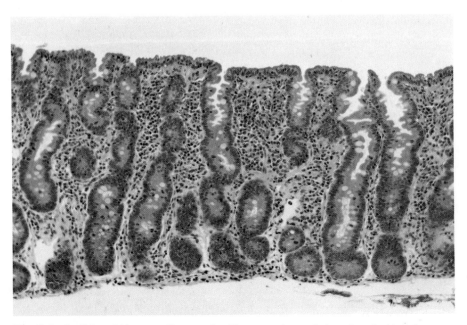

Fig. 61.6 Small bowel biopsy – villus atrophy. Note crypt hyperplasia and marked cellular infiltration into the lamina propria.

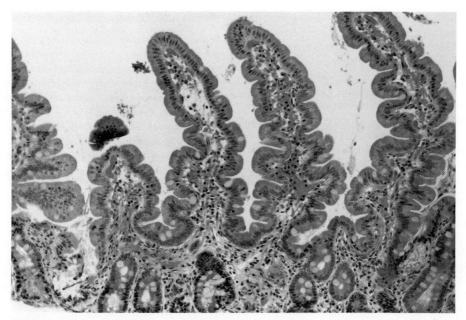

Fig. 61.7 Small bowel biopsy – normal appearances of mucosa.

causes of chronic diarrhoea with associated malabsorption, particularly of carbohydrate and fat. Clinically these children will have chronic, persistent or recurrent diarrhoea with very offensive stools, abdominal distension and weight loss. The clinical picture may mimic coeliac disease, although these children usually do not have temperament change and remain vigorous and active. Giardiasis can also mimic coeliac disease histologically, causing a flat mucosa.

The diagnosis can be made by stool microscopy, where typical cysts are seen. Microscopic examination of duodenal fluid however is the most reliable diagnostic test, showing the motile trophozoites (Fig. 61.8).

Treatment of Giardiasis is with metronidazole, tinidazole or related drugs. A metronidazole suspension (benzoyl-metronidazole) is palatable and effective in children. Recurrences are not infrequent as this parasite is quite infectious, being readily spread within families, day care centres and institutions. If a recurrence occurs in a child it is advisable to treat other family members.

Carbohydrate intolerance

The majority of cases of carbohydrate malabsorption/intolerance are secondary to mucosal injury which in children is most likely due to infectious diarrhoea, particularly rotavirus. Lactase deficiency is the commonest disorder and in fact is the commonest cause of

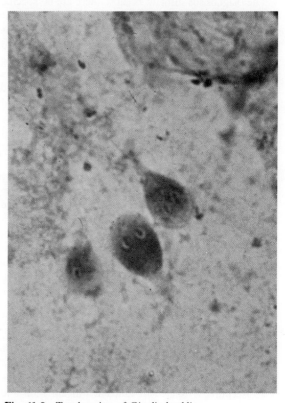

Fig. 61.8 Trophozoites of *Giardia lamblia*.

malabsorption in children. Almost any disorder causing mucosal injury with depletion of disaccharidases can cause carbohydrate malabsorption and diarrhoea. This includes inflammatory bowel disease, cow's milk protein intolerance, immunodeficiency states and bacterial overgrowth secondary to an anatomical abnormality. The diarrhoea that occurs is due to the osmotic effect created by fermentation of unabsorbed carbohydrate in the colon, producing fluid, acid, gaseous stools with associated peri-anal excoriation. Disorders of carbohydrate malabsorption have been covered in Chapter 60.

Dietary protein intolerance (cow's milk, soy, egg)

Cow's milk is responsible for 80% of cases of protein intolerance in children. The reaction is thought to be immunologically mediated and can result in a wide range of clinical features as well as significant intestinal mucosal damage, including a flat mucosa. Clinical features include acute anaphylaxis which is rare, gastrointestinal symptoms (diarrhoea, vomiting, acute colitis, occult blood loss, coeliac-like syndrome), skin disease (eczema, urticaria) and respiratory symptoms (wheeze).

The diagnosis is difficult because there are no specific diagnostic tests. If the diagnosis is suspected, more common non-immune causes of symptoms such as giardiasis, lactose intolerance, sucrase deficiency, and post-enteritis malabsorption should be excluded. The patient is then shown to improve on withdrawal of cow's milk from the diet with relapse on re-introduction and further remission on withdrawal. Skin testing and RAST tests are usually not helpful.

If the above criteria are met, dietary restriction must be carefully supervised by a dietitian. In children under two a substitute milk such as a protein hydrolysate (Pregestimil) is required. The challenge should be repeated every six to nine months as most children become tolerant by two years of age. If the original symptoms were severe or life threatening then the challenge procedure should be carried out in hospital. Also, it is important to acknowledge that breast feeding and antigen avoidance from birth will not prevent the development of atopic disease. The most important predictor of hypersensitivity is a family history of atopic disease.

Inflammatory bowel disease

Crohn's disease and ulcerative colitis are the clinical entities, Crohn's disease being more common in children. Malabsorption is related to mucosal inflammation and can affect all the dietary constituents. Treatment will depend on the cause.

Anatomical abnormalities and malabsorption

Malabsorption may be due to inadequate gut length, disordered motility, bacterial overgrowth or a combination of these. Lesions producing malabsorption include intestinal reduplication, congenital strictures and stenoses, malrotation and blind loops. Bacterial colonization causes malabsorption by bacterial enzyme destruction of the glycocalyx, microvilli and epithelium together with bile salt deconjugation. The diagnosis can be made by breath hydrogen analysis after a load of lactulose. Radiology of the gut is useful where an anatomical lesion is suspected.

Immune deficiency states

Chronic diarrhoea and malabsorption are important features of certain immunodeficiency states. Secondary immune deficiency can occur in malnutrition and intestinal lymphangiectasia. Lymphoid nodular hyperplasia is commonly associated with immunoglobulin deficiency, Giardia lamblia infestation, bacterial overgrowth, protein-losing enteropathy and malabsorption. Generally, the mechanism leading to malabsorption in immunodeficiency states is unknown but chronic infection with resultant mucosal injury seems most likely. Immunological reconstitution seems to be the only curative measure.

Disorders of protein absorption

Protein malabsorption as a primary disorder is very rare and it usually accompanies fat and carbohydrate malabsorption. Most disorders associated with protein deficiency are due to protein-losing states rather than malabsorption. Cystic fibrosis and congenital hypoplasia of the pancreas are two conditions where protein malabsorption occurs. However, enterokinase deficiency is the only example of a selective malabsorptive disorder of protein. This very rare condition is inherited in an autosomal recessive manner and presents in early life with hypoproteinaemia and oedema, failure to thrive and chronic diarrhoea. Pancreatic enzyme replacement therapy is effective.

Luminal abnormality

Malabsorption associated with exocrine pancreatic insufficiency

Cystic fibrosis (CF). This is the commonest recessively inherited disorder with an incidence of 1 in 2500 live births and a carrier frequency of 1 in 25. 1 in every 400 marriages is thus able to produce an affected child. The clinical features are described in Chapter 38.

Congenital hypoplasia of the pancreas (Shwach-man-Diamond syndrome). This autosomal recessively inherited disorder is about 100 times less common than CF. The major feature is a coincidence of clinical features associated with exocrine pancreatic insufficiency. These include chronic or cyclic neutropenia, skeletal abnormalities, growth retardation, recurrent infections, abnormal liver function, developmental delay and dental abnormalities. A sweat test will differentiate it from CF. Pancreatic enzyme supplements improve symptoms but not growth. The prognosis is much better than for CF, although in the past a significant mortality was associated with infection.

Malnutrition. Pancreatic insufficiency develops rapidly in malnutrition and is a primary cause of nutrient malabsorption. Function returns to normal with nutritional recovery.

Bile salt insufficiency

Malabsorption resulting from bile salt deficiency will be obvious in the presence of jaundice, when biliary atresia or hepatitis are most commonly causative. In non-icteric situations such as primary bile salt deficiency the diagnosis may be missed. The malabsorption is due to inadequate bile salt production with failure to achieve a critical micellar concentration and hence failure to carry the products of lipolysis to the mucosal surface. Stool microscopy may reveal fatty acid crystals.

SUMMARY

No present classification of malabsorption, whether based on clinical presentation or underlying pathophysiology is entirely satisfactory or complete. Many current reviews of the subject include all known disorders of small bowel function whether or not there is malabsorption and failure to thrive; these in fact are lists of disorders associated with chronic diarrhoea. Also it is important to realize that children with malabsorption may present with manifestations outside the gastrointestinal tract. In general, the simple clinical approach of demonstrating growth faltering followed by a few simple investigations will give a guide to the diagnosis. Only rarely will sophisticated tests be required. And it is important to realize that many children presenting with growth failure and suspected malabsorption will have social or emotional deprivation rather than any underlying mucosal pathology.

FURTHER READING

Hill D J, Ford R P K, Shelton M J, Hosking C S 1984 A study of 100 infants and young children with cow's milk allergy. Clinical Reviews in Allergy 2: 125–142

Lifshitz F 1982 (ed) Carbohydrate intolerance in infancy. Marcel Dekker, New York

Newcomer A D 1984 Screening tests for carbohydrate malabsorption. Journal of Pediatric Gastroenterology and Nutrition 3: 6–8

Sanderson I R 1986 Chronic inflammatory bowel disease. Clinics in Gastroenterology 15: 71–87

Walker-Smith J A 1986 Food sensitive enteropathies. Clinics in Gastroenterology 15: 55–69

Walker-Smith J A, Hamilton J R, Walker Y Y A 1983 (eds) Practical Pediatric Gastroenterology. Butterworths, London

62. The child with abdominal pain

M. J. Robinson

Acute abdominal pain is one of the commoner reasons for children being taken to the doctor. The causes of abdominal pain in childhood are many and diverse.

There can be fewer symptoms in children that cause more anxiety to parents than abdominal pain, the possibility of acute appendicitis often being present in their minds. In assessment, it is of major importance to differentiate those causes which demand surgery and, in particular, those which demand urgent surgery from those which have a medical basis. Abdominal pain in childhood does not always have a detectable organic basis; this concept is not easy to get over to parents and will certainly not be believed unless a very careful history and physical examination is undertaken before any discussions on the psychological causes of abdominal pain.

ABDOMINAL PAIN IN INFANCY

In very early infancy abdominal pain as a sole symptom is unusual and not easy to interpret. The more severe causes of abdominal pain are usually surgical emergencies and accompanied by other features, e.g. vomiting, constipation and abdominal distension. These disorders have been discussed in Chapter 59.

Colic

There is a group of infants who present in the first few weeks of life with attacks of screaming, drawing up of legs and refusing to be comforted. Despite these features, vomiting is absent, the bowels are almost normal and the infant thrives exceedingly well. Physical examination does not reveal any abnormality. This is the syndrome of infantile colic, the basis of which is poorly understood. There are those who would believe that it has to do with various aspects of feeding, e.g. amount, quality and technique. There are others who believe that it is a manifestation of cow's milk allergy and still others who believe that it is one manifestation of family distur-

bance. After a thorough assessment of the infant and the family dynamics treatment is supportive and the symptom almost invariably disappears by about the fourth month.

ACUTE ABDOMINAL PAIN IN OLDER CHILDREN

This should be considered against a background of the common surgical causes, as these must be excluded in the first instance. The major causes of acute abdominal pain which may require urgent surgical intervention in children are:

1. Intussusception
2. Acute appendicitis.

Intussusception

This is acute and fixed telescoping of a segment of bowel into the adjoining distal segment, resulting in intestinal obstruction. It should be suspected in an infant, usually aged between 5 months and 18 months of age, who suddenly develops screaming attacks with abdominal pain. During each bout the infant becomes pale and draws up the legs. The spasms tend to occur at intervals of about 10–15 minutes although they may occur with increased frequency. They tend to last 2–3 minutes. Vomiting is the rule and an early symptom. A few loose stools occur early but do not constitute true diarrhoea as the loose stools do not persist. This aspect should differentiate intussusception from acute gastroenteritis. Some infants with intussusception present with little more than pallor, abdominal pain appearing to be minimal. Should these symptoms be ignored, the infant rapidly develops signs of shock. The passage of blood or the 'red currant jelly' stool is by no means the rule and this latter is a late feature.

On examination, the infant with intussusception is usually pale, anxious and unwell. With care, a sausage-shaped mass may be felt usually in the right upper quadrant of the abdomen and particularly during a spasm of pain. However, a mass is not always palpable, particularly in ileo-ileal intussusception. The history is all important in making the diagnosis of intussusception but if there is doubt a barium enema must be performed. A plain erect radiograph of the abdomen will demonstrate bowel obstruction with abdominal distension and fluid levels. The barium enema will indicate the site of the intussusception.

Treatment

Hydrostatic reduction by barium enema under radiological control has been regarded as the treatment of choice where appropriate radiological facilities exist. Recently, hydrostatic reduction of acute intussusception with oxygen has been used in some centres (Fig. 62.1). It is claimed that hydrostatic reduction with oxygen is more efficient with an 80–90% success rate.

Indications for surgical intervention are

1. Infants less than 3 months and over the age of 2 years
2. Clinical signs of peritonitis
3. Obvious features of intestinal obstruction

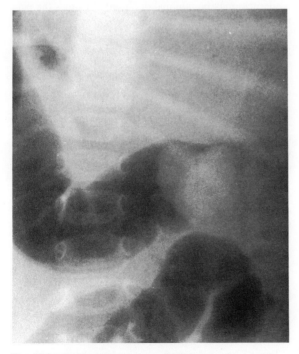

Fig. 62.1 Radiograph demonstration of apex of intussusception during reduction with oxygen.

4. Gross dehydration – this indicates severe intestinal obstruction
5. Failure of hydrostatic reduction.

The success of hydrostatic reduction is indicated by noting the barium flow into the ileum. There does not appear to be a greater incidence of recurrence of intussusception in those children treated by hydrostatic reduction compared with those treated surgically. At operation most cases are reduced without bowel resection, but, if after reduction there are areas of doubtful viability in the bowel wall, resection and end-to-end anastomosis is indicated.

Differential diagnosis of intussusception

The most important conditions to include are:

1. Gastroenteritis
2. Other causes of intestinal obstruction
3. Constipation
4. Haemolytic uraemic syndrome.

Gastroenteritis. In infancy, gastroenteritis is not infrequently associated with abdominal pain, vomiting, and the passage of blood and mucus in the stools. The diagnosis is usually obvious on clinical grounds by the passage of fluid and gaseous stools which persist. Occasionally a plain radiograph of the abdomen may show bowel distension and fluid levels in acute gastroenteritis; in cases where doubt exists a barium enema is indicated. The consequences of delay in diagnosis of intussusception far outweigh the risk of a barium enema in acute gastroenteritis.

Other causes of intestinal obstruction. In children who have not had previous abdominal surgery, intestinal obstruction may be the result of a volvulus, a band from a Meckel's diverticulum, duplication of the gut or, very rarely, an internal hernia. An irreducible inguinal hernia is the commonest cause of intestinal obstruction in young infants. The physical signs consist of pain, vomiting, abdominal distension and constipation. A careful examination of the groins will detect a firm tender mass – the incarcerated hernia.

Constipation. It is unusual for constipation to cause abdominal pain to a degree which might suggest a surgical emergency. However, there is no doubt that persisting constipation will result in abdominal discomfort and at times abdominal pain. A careful history, palpation of the abdomen after the bladder is empty and a gentle rectal examination should allow this diagnosis to be made without difficulty. A plain radiograph of the abdomen will demonstrate the extent of faecal retention (Fig. 62.2).

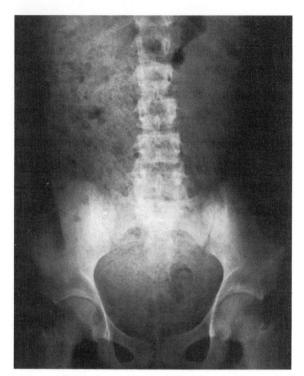

Fig. 62.2 Plain radiograph of abdomen demonstrating gross faecal overload.

The haemolytic uraemic syndrome. This disorder has already been discussed in Chapter 53. The onset is with diarrhoea followed by pallor and haematuria, but voiding may not have occurred at the time of presentation as oliguria is the rule. The pallor is due to anaemia; a blood film will identify the characteristic abnormal morphology of the red cells (red cell fragments). Thrombocytopenia will also be noted. The urine contains blood, casts and albumin, and the serum creatinine is grossly elevated in the haemolytic uraemic syndrome.

Acute appendicitis

This may occur at any age, although it is more common in children of school age and in adolescence. A problem of early recognition exists in the very young child (under 3 years) and in the mentally retarded child; the majority of these children present with peritonitis. Delay in diagnosis of acute appendicitis tends to relate to the variable symptomatology in childhood. For example, there may be few complaints of pain, vomiting may not be present and diarrhoea or dysuria may be predominant features.

The primary and most common symptom of acute appendicitis is localized abdominal pain. This tends to be intermittent and colicky initially and is usually situated in the epigastrium or peri-umbilical region. The pain soon shifts to the right lower quadrant. Constant pain is the result of peritoneal irritation. Vomiting occurs in at least 80% of children with appendicitis and diarrhoea in about 20%. The temperature is usually only slightly elevated, but in about 5% of cases it is in excess of 39°C.

Physical examination must be thorough, gentle and certainly not confined to the abdomen. The child's co-operation is essential and careful observation of a suspected case, with frequent abdominal examinations, may be necessary to make the diagnosis before perforation occurs. Attempts to elicit rebound tenderness do little more than destroy the child's confidence and confuse the doctor. Gentle palpation, while observing the child's face, will provide the most reliable evidence of abdominal tenderness and rigidity. The presence of an abdominal mass is a reliable sign, but this has to be differentiated from faeces in the pelvic colon. Rectal examination must always be performed, but with great gentleness if it is to be informative. Bowel sounds are usually reduced, but too much reliance should not be placed on this.

Difficulties in the diagnosis of acute apendicitis in childhood may be because the appendix is frequently located in an unusual position; if it is retrocaecal, tenderness may be minimal or absent. At times the pain may be constant from the outset, there may be no pain shift and, rarely, particularly in smaller children, little pain at all. Diarrhoea and urinary symptoms are at times sufficiently marked to obscure the clinical picture.

The presence of peritonitis is likely if the child is acutely ill with abdominal pain and fever and who, on examination, has generalized abdominal rigidity. Peritonitis in childhood is most commonly the result of acute appendicitis, but occasionally it may be primary, e.g. in the nephrotic syndrome and caused by *Streptococcus pneumoniae*.

It is this author's personal view that if abdominal pain in childhood is of sufficient duration (2 hours or more) and if local signs of guarding and tenderness are persistent, acute appendicitis cannot be excluded and laparotomy is indicated. That the cause of this may at times be the result of mesenteric lymphadenitis is irrelevant.

Laboratory studies in acute appendicitis are rarely helpful if the diagnosis cannot be made on clinical grounds. However, the urine should always be checked for sugar and albumen and examined microscopically if there are features suggesting renal disease. Radiology is of limited use in diagnosis, but a chest radiograph may be helpful in excluding a lower lobe pneumonia.

Differential diagnosis of acute appendicitis

This involves a large number of disorders but, with a careful history and thorough physical examination, differentiation is usually possible.

Mesenteric lymphadenitis. Perhaps this is the most difficult disorder to distinguish from acute appendicitis and at times the clinical distinction may be impossible. In general, localization of pain and tenderness is not as definite, the temperature is higher and rigidity is less of a feature in mesenteric lymphadenitis. Other conditions which may mimic acute appendicitis or an acute abdomen in childhood are mentioned below.

Henoch-Schönlein purpura. The abdominal pain associated with this disorder is often severe, colicky and be accompanied by vomiting. Usually the characteristic skin lesions are noted over the buttock and legs, but these may be few in number and consequently can be missed. Occasionally lesions in the gut precede the skin manifestations and the diagnosis may be made at laparotomy.

Sickle-cell anaemia. In the appropriate ethnic group sickle-cell anaemia is a prominent cause of acute abdominal pain and will need to be considered in a pale child with splenomegaly.

Meckel's diverticulitis. This is often cited in the differential diagnosis of acute appendicitis as the pain may be referred to the right iliac fossa. The symptoms may be identical so that differentiation may only be possible at laparotomy. A past or present history of melaena will suggest this diagnosis, but such a history is by no means the rule.

Cystic fibrosis. Children with cystic fibrosis frequently experience attacks of abdominal pain, the result of faecal impaction, a well known manifestation of this disease. Differentiation from acute appendicitis is occasionally difficult, but the symptoms will resolve following a bowel washout and recurrences will be infrequent if correct dietary measures are adopted.

Renal tract disorders. Acute abdominal pain may occur with renal colic, pyelonephritis and, at times, in acute glomerulonephritis. Pain and tenderness in renal disease is usually referred to the loin. The radiation of pain is different and abnormalities will be found on urinalysis.

The liver and biliary tract. Abdominal pain may be an early feature of acute hepatitis but the physical findings rarely indicate laparotomy and should indicate liver function studies. Cholecystitis is usually referred to the right hypochondrium. Gall bladder disease and gall stones are associated with some forms of chronic haemolytic anaemia, but more commonly occur for unknown cause.

Pancreatitis. Although this is a very rare disorder in childhood, it is important to diagnose. The clinical presentation is with severe epigastric pain referred posteriorly to the midline over the lower thoracic and upper lumbar spine. Nausea and vomiting are the rule and tenderness with guarding and abdominal rigidity prominent. These children often look ill and collapsed.

The aetiology of acute pancreatitis in childhood is usually obscure; there is rarely associated liver disease or gall stones as in the adult. Occasionally, viral infections may be causative, e.g. mumps. Abdominal trauma following a blunt injury is a well established cause. The diagnosis of acute pancreatitis is made on the clinical history and confirmed by estimations of the plasma amylase. In acute pancreatitis levels greatly exceed 500 iu/l. The management of acute pancreatitis involves correction of shock, intravenous fluid administration, nasogastric suction and analgesia. Surgery is rarely indicated.

Pneumonia. Abdominal pain and tenderness may be prominent features of pneumonia. Usually, however, the temperature will be high, the respiratory rate increased and some cough will be present. The diagnostic signs of pneumonia may be difficult to elicit clinically, so that a chest radiograph will be required.

Miscellaneous causes. Other systemic disorders associated with abdominal pain and which occasionally mimic appendicitis include diabetes mellitus, glandular fever, porphyria and some haemolytic anaemias.

Other causes of abdominal pain in childhood

Drugs

In any child complaining of acute abdominal pain, enquiry should be made into drug ingestion. Drugs commonly in use and which may produce abdominal pain include salicylates, non-steroidal anti-inflammatory drugs, corticosteroids, some antibiotics, imipramine, sodium valproate, phenytoin, iron preparations and some anticancer drugs.

Tortion of the testis

Torsion of the testis may occur at any time during childhood. These children present with pain and vomiting in association with swelling and extreme testicular tenderness. The pain commonly begins in the inguinal region just above the external inguinal ring. Differentiation from acute epididymo-orchitis is usually impossible on clinical grounds so that exploration will be required. Swelling of the testis with pain and tenderness may also be the result of mumps, Henoch-Schönlein purpura, a neoplasm or an incarcerated inguinal hernia.

Peptic ulceration

Abdominal pain due to peptic ulceration occasionally occurs in childhood. The abdominal pain of peptic ulceration is usually situated in the epigastrium, it is usually unrelated to meals, but frequently causes discomfort at night. Occasionally nausea and vomiting occur. The diagnosis will be made easier in the presence of haematemesis and melaena, which is a major mode of presentation of peptic ulceration in childhood. Occasionally the diagnosis is made following investigation of iron deficiency anaemia.

Acute gastritis and acute duodenitis produce abdominal pain usually associated with epigastric tenderness. Such children are usually considered to have peptic ulceration and the diagnosis is made on endoscopic examination of the upper gastrointestinal tract. Culture of biopsy specimens taken at this time frequently grow *Campylobacter pylori*. Treatment with ampicillin and a bismuth preparation (e.g. Denol) is usually successful, but relapses are common.

Reflux oesophagitis

Gastro-oesophageal reflux, a very common disorder in infancy, occasionally persists into later childhood when belching, acid eructations and intermittent vomiting persist. Substernal and epigastric pain will suggest reflux oesophagitis under these circumstances. Substernal and epigastric pain can be a very difficult symptom to assess so that in severe cases investigation will be indicated. Oesophageal pH monitoring is a technique which measures lower oesophageal pH via an electrode placed there and left in situ over a period of 24 hours. Reflux can thus be confirmed and a positive or negative relationship of pH to symptomatology established. Oesophageal endoscopy and biopsy is required to accurately establish the diagnosis. Management of reflux oesophagitis involves the administration of H_2 receptor antagonists and/or sucralfate and is usually successful. With intractable reflux oesophagitis the operation of fundoplication is indicated.

RECURRENT ABDOMINAL PAIN IN CHILDHOOD

The child with recurrent acute bouts of abdominal pain is a cause of great anxiety to parents and doctors alike. It is a very common paediatric problem. Many of these children are regarded as suffering from recurrent bouts of appendicitis and many will be operated on immediately after an attack. More frequently, however, surgery is performed as an interval procedure and based upon the number and severity of the attacks.

The syndrome consists of acute and frequently colicky abdominal pain localized to the umbilicus or just above it; radiation of the pain does not occur. Although the pains frequently double the child up and are associated with obvious pallor, they are usually over within an hour at most. Therefore it is unusual for the practitioner to see the child during the actual attack. Vomiting is unusual during these episodes, although nausea is frequent. The pain is also invariably diurnal, never waking the child through the night. Examination during or immediately after each episode occasionally reveals a little umbilical tenderness.

Doctors will be impressed by the anxiety exhibited by parents of these children who will vividly describe the severe pain the child experiences and dwell upon the gross pallor; the disparity between the parents description and the physical findings is very marked.

Once a few bouts have occurred, parents will usually demand investigations, but they are almost invariably negative. It is at this stage that a thorough enquiry into the personality of the child and into the home situation is indicated. This enquiry will usually reveal an anxious child, somewhat obsessive in personality and an individual who worries over the most trivial of things. Apley (1975) has compared these children with a group of controls and described them as highly strung, fussy, excitable, anxious, timid and apprehensive. They also tend to show undue fears, they suffer sleep disorders and over the years there may have been problems with eating. Other workers have noted overprotection by the very anxious parents of these children. In one particular study (Apley & Hale 1973) it was noted that one or both parents was intensely and almost obsessively occupied with the state of the child's health, personality and school progress. Thus the concept of anxiety and tension has come to be related causally with recurrent abdominal pain. Quite frequently an emotional disturbance will precede an episode of pain and on other occasions stress has preceded the pain and the pain has disappeared when the stress has been removed. The stress, however, is not always gross and perhaps most commonly is associated with minor tensions at home, difficulties with peer groups or minor school anxieties. However, episodes may occur for no apparent cause. A diagnosis of nonorganic recurrent abdominal pain can only be made after a very careful appraisal of the child in relation to the environment and a careful physical examination backed up by appropriate laboratory tests.

The following points are helpful in deciding whether investigation is indicated in these children:

Abdominal distension. The combination of abdominal pain and abdominal distension certainly indicates investigation, which will usually involve radiological studies of the gastrointestinal tract and specific investigation for malabsorption.

Vomiting. Abdominal pain and vomiting usually require investigation; the appearance of bile in the vomitus is very suggestive of intermittent small bowel obstruction.

Urine. This should be routinely examined for the presence of sugar, albumin, infection and porphyrins.

Fever. In the presence of fever with abdominal pain, investigation of the renal tract is particularly relevant.

Pallor. If this is associated with anaemia, conditions such as lead poisoning, sickle-cell and other haemolytic diseases must be considered and appropriately excluded.

The general status of the patient. Retardation of height and weight indicate a thorough search for the cause of the abdominal pain when such disorders as chronic inflammatory bowel disease, malabsorption syndromes and tuberculosis must be excluded.

Blood in the stools. This again may suggest chronic inflammatory bowel disease or a chronic dysentery.

Management

This is often difficult, but the mere uncovering of the personality of the child and of the family situation is often therapeutic. Of the greatest importance is for parents to realize that the problem has been taken seriously by the doctor and the necessary investigations performed. It is important that the doctor identifies the parents' perception of the abdominal pain. With this knowledge and the negative physical findings, reassurance can be much more positive. Once parents are convinced that there is no organic basis to the recurrent abdominal pain, advice in respect to removing unnecessary stress in the environment can be important. Constant criticism of the child by the parents should be stopped and unnecessary pressures avoided, e.g. to eat more, keep your room tidy, etc. These should be replaced by attitudes which encourage the child and improve self-esteem. Occasionally sedation and mild tranquillisers are helpful, but these should only be used against the background of an understanding of the family dynamics. Apley (1975) states that with such an approach, most cases respond. It is usual for this syndrome to disappear by the age of about 12 years, but in females it sometimes recurs about the time of the menarche.

The long-term outlook for children with recurrent abdominal pain is that many continue with personality disorders into adult life and present with digestive disturbances, bowel problems and neurotic behaviour.

REFERENCES

Apley J 1975 The child with abdominal pains. Blackwell Scientific Publications, London
Apley J, Hale B 1973 Children with recurrent abdominal pain and how they grow up. British Medical Journal 3: 7–9
Drum B et al 1988 Treatment of *campylobacter pylori* associated antral gastritis with bismuth subsalicylate and ampicillin. Journal of Paediatrics 113: 908–912

FURTHER READING

Barbero G J 1982 Recurrent abdominal pain in childhood. Pediatrics in Review 4(1): 29–34
Jones P G (ed) 1986 Clinical paediatric surgery, 3rd edn. Blackwell Scientific Publications, London

63. The problem of liver disease

Arnold Smith

Liver disease can most conveniently be considered in relation to age – infancy and later childhood. Overlap will be inevitable, but specific problems tend to occur in each group.

LIVER DISEASE IN INFANCY

In this age group the clinical presentation is usually jaundice. Neonatal jaundice has been discussed in Chapter 26 and in the first week of life is most commonly due to immaturity of bilirubin clearance by the liver (physiological jaundice and jaundice of prematurity). Haemolysis as the cause of the excessive bilirubin load should be sought if the onset of jaundice is unusually early (in the first 24 hours) or if unusually severe jaundice develops (a total serum bilirubin in excess of 200 μmol/l in term infants or 250 μmol/l in premature infants by day five of life). Causes of haemolysis in this period include maternal-infant ABO or Rh incompatibility, RBC enzyme defects such as G6PD deficiency and bacterial sepsis. The problem in this period is to control the level of unconjugated bilirubin to prevent kernicterus.

Jaundice persisting beyond the end of the second week of life always requires urgent investigation. Unconjugated jaundice may be due to serious causes such as hypothyroidism, congenital haemolytic anaemias (e.g. G6PD deficiency) or bacterial sepsis (especially urinary tract infections and umbilical infection). More often it is benign, a cause not found or being attributed to an undefined factor in breast milk.

If the jaundice is associated with a predominantly conjugated serum bilirubin and dark urine, liver damage or biliary obstruction are the likely causes. Usually there will be some hepatic enlargement and in about 50% of cases splenomegaly is present. Abnormally pale stools (clay coloured) suggest complete biliary obstruction or severe cholestasis associated with severe hepatocellular injury. Although the cause of this 'neonatal hepatitis syndrome' is unknown in the majority of cases, some patients have treatable conditions requiring urgent recognition and treatment if irreversible liver damage is to be avoided. Example 63.1 lists the more common causes.

Occasionally the neonatal hepatitis syndrome will present with the finding of hepatomegaly on routine physical examination or as a bleeding tendency in a baby not previously recognized to be jaundiced.

Example 63.1 Causes of hepatitis syndrome of infancy

Structural defects	Metabolic defects	Congenital infections
Biliary atresia	Galactosaemia	Rubella virus
Bile duct stenosis	α-1 antitrypsin deficiency	Cytomegalovirus
Choledochal cyst	Fructosaemia	Hepatitis B virus
Spontaneous bile duct perforation	Tyrosinaemia	Herpes simplex virus
Biliary hypoplasia	Niemann-Pick disease	Coxsackie B virus
a. intrahepatic	Gaucher's disease	Varicella zoster virus
b. extrahepatic		Listeria
Polycystic disease		Toxoplasmosis
		Acquired infection
		Septicaemias
		Congenital syphilis

Prolonged neonatal jaundice should always be considered a medical emergency demanding urgent referral to a paediatrician for extensive investigation.

Diagnosis

A careful history might identify:

1. Infectious illness in the mother during pregnancy
2. Addictive or other drug administration during pregnancy
3. Mother known to be a hepatitis B carrier
4. Known family history of heritable or metabolic disease or unexplained neonatal death of a sibling.

Physical examination

This examination may identify associated congenital abnormalities such as cataract, microcephaly, etc. suggesting intrauterine infection or cardiac or other abnormalities suggesting an identifiable syndrome.

Investigations

Rarely will history and physical examination alone lead to diagnosis.

Assessment of liver function

Conventional serum liver function tests – transaminases, proteins, alkaline phosphatase and gammaglutamyl transpeptidase – give an indication of severity of dysfunction but rarely help in identifying the cause of liver disease in this age group. Coagulation studies performed 24 hours after vitamin K1 2 mg IM are very useful in assessing the degree of liver damage.

Search for cause of liver disease

Exclusion of biliary obstruction

If, on personal examination, stool colour' is normal, a persistent complete biliary obstruction such as biliary atresia can be confidently excluded. Parents' reports of stool colour are, however, notoriously unreliable. If stools are pale the following three tests are necessary:

Abdominal ultrasound. This will enable diagnosis of a choledochal cyst or a congenital biliary stenosis. It cannot reliably diagnose or exclude biliary atresia or bile duct hypoplasia syndromes.

Radioisotope (HIDA) biliary scan. This may demonstrate patency of bile ducts by demonstrating flow of isotope into the gut. However, impaired hepatic isotope uptake from the circulation may make the test uninterpretable in some patients with hepatocellular disease and in some with liver damage secondary to obstruction.

Percutaneous liver biopsy. This can be safely performed in infants but histological interpretation requires the skills of a paediatric histopathologist.

Microbiological studies

Bacterial sepsis is a frequent cause of jaundice in early infancy. Swabs from the umbilicus, and urine and blood cultures are always indicated. *Escherichia coli* and Group B beta-haemolytic streptococcus are the organisms most frequently identified. Congenital syphilis may also present as a neonatal hepatitis; this treatable infection should be sought with serological tests on mother and infant. The most common viral agents causing neonatal hepatitis are rubella, cytomegalovirus, Coxsackie B, herpes simplex and hepatitis B. Often these are intrauterine in onset but herpes simplex type 2 and hepatitis B are usually acquired at the time of birth. Cytomegalovirus may be acquired either pre- or postnatally. Infection of the fetus with toxoplasma or *Listeria monocytogenes* may also cause neonatal hepatitis. Viral cultures and/or appropriate serology on mother and child will establish the diagnosis. Intrauterine infections are discussed in Chapter 27.

Metabolic studies

Galactosaemia can be excluded by estimation of galactose-1-phosphate uridyl transferase in red blood cells provided previous blood transfusion has not occurred. Alpha-1 antitrypsin deficiency should be sought by measuring serum levels. Diagnosis of alpha-1 antitrypsin deficiency requires confirmation by electrophoretic studies of the protein (Pi typing). Urine analysis for excess amino acids and fatty acid metabolites should also be routine. Diagnosis of some disorders (e.g. hereditary fructose intolerance) requires enzyme studies on liver biopsy material. Sweat electrolyte estimation is sometimes warranted as neonatal hepatitis is more common in cystic fibrosis.

Management of obstructive jaundice in the neonatal period

Differentiation of hepatocellular damage from biliary obstruction as the cause of obstructive jaundice is both difficult and urgent. Surgical procedures designed to relieve biliary obstruction in biliary atresia have the greatest prospect of success if performed early (four to six weeks of age) and are rarely successful in infants over the age of three months. Although no system of diagnosis is completely reliable, it is our experience that using the investigations above we can achieve a correct diagnosis and undertake surgery within a week of referral in 95% of cases. Satisfactory bile drainage leading to clearing of jaundice and prolonged (five and ten years) survival can be achieved in 50% of infants with biliary atresia. For those in whom bile drainage is not achieved, liver transplantation now offers an alternative to certain death from liver failure before the age of four years.

Alpha-1 antitrypsin deficiency

Alpha-1 antitrypsin is a protein with wide antiprotease activity made by hepatocytes. It constitutes about 90% of circulating alpha-1 globulins in the blood. Its function is to protect 'bystander' normal tissues from polymorph leukocyte elastase and other proteases liberated in response to tissue injury. Alpha-1 antitrypsin is controlled by a single autosomal gene but many genetic variants of this protein occur. Most have no importance as the site of variation does not alter the protease binding site. One variant, known as the Z variant, occurs commonly in people of northern European ancestry. The homozygous condition for this Z protein occurs in this group with a frequency of approximately 1 in 2500 births. Although the hepatocytes produce adequate amounts of the protein, there is a defect in the transport of the protein into the circulation. This results in the Z protein accumulating in liver cells and very low (less than 20% normal) levels of alpha-1 antitrypsin in the serum.

Approximately 10–20% of homozygous PiZ individuals develop liver disease in infancy and in about 5% hepatocyte destruction becomes chronic with eventual progression to cirrhosis and liver failure in childhood. Liver biopsy histology in early infancy may be indistinguishable from other forms of neonatal hepatitis but later biopsies may show globules of alpha-1 antitrypsin in periportal liver cells. In the patients with most severe involvement the clinical picture of severe cholestasis and periportal hepatocyte damage on biopsy can mimic biliary atresia. There is also an increased risk of chronic liver disease throughout life.

There is no established effective treatment available. Liver transplantation for children with decompensating liver function offers about a 70% prospect of continued survival. The transplanted liver produces alpha-1 antitrypsin of the donor's type and thus protects the recipient against subsequent emphysema.

The majority of alpha-1 antitrypsin deficient individuals develop premature onset emphysema. The progression to symptomatic pulmonary insufficiency is greatly accelerated by cigarette smoking and PiZ homozygotes may be respiratory cripples by their thirties if the smoking habit is acquired in childhood or adolescence.

Management of neonatal hepatitis

The cause of this syndrome is unknown in 75% of cases. Bacterial sepsis can be expected to respond to antibiotic therapy and some metabolic disorders will respond to dietary restrictions (e.g. galactosaemia, hereditary fructose intolerance).

Prognosis

Death from liver failure in infancy results in up to 20% of cases in some series. Those who survive this period, who have only mild cholestasis and in whom a cause is not found, have a low risk of subsequent progression to cirrhosis and/or liver failure.

Supportive management

Malabsorption of fat and fat soluble vitamins (vitamins A, D, K and E) accompanies cholestasis. Dietary manipulation (e.g. use of medium chain triglycerides to improve fat and hence calorie absorption) and vitamin supplementation may be required.

HEPATITIS IN OLDER CHILDREN

Viral infection is by far the commonest cause of acute liver disease in the older child. Some of the viruses responsible have been identified and characterized.

Hepatitis A (HAV)

Hepatitis A (HAV) is the most common virus and causes a relatively benign illness with total recovery being available. HAV is transmitted by the faecal-oral route and after an initial viraemia massive excretion of the virus in the stools occurs for some days before the onset of jaundice. By the time the jaundice has disappeared the patient is no longer infective. Anicteric hepatitis is common but jaundice is more common in older children and adults. Chronic carrier states do not occur. HAV infection cannot be invoked as an explanation for jaundice in infants or children under three to four years of age. The diagnosis is confirmed by demonstrating antibodies (initially IgM followed by IgG) to HAV in serum. Although no vaccine against HAV is yet available, household contacts of patients with acute HAV infection can be partially protected by administration of pooled gammaglobulin.

Hepatitis B (HBV)

Hepatitis B (HBV) tends to be more severe, but although it can occasionally result in fatal fulminant hepatic failure, most episodes of infection in childhood are asymptomatic and anicteric. Infection is generally contracted from body secretions e.g. saliva, blood, vaginal secretions, etc., but the faecal-oral route infection can occur. About 50% of people infected with HBV will become chronic carriers of the virus. Most will be asymptomatic but some will develop chronic progressive hepatitis and some of these will eventually develop primary hepatocellular carcinoma. This chronic carrier state is more common in certain areas of the world (South East Asia and Africa) where 'vertical' transmission from carrier mother to newborn infant via blood or vaginal secretions at birth is frequent. In general, the younger the age of contracting HBV the more likely is the carrier state to develop. In developed countries, although some children acquire HBV infection 'vertically' from their carrier mothers, the carrier state may be associated with sexual promiscuity or drug abuse.

HBV can be recognized by radioimmunoassay and its structure defined by electron microscopy. The HBV consists of a distinct outer coat surrounding an inner core. Both the coat and core bear distinctive antigens known as the hepatitis B surface antigen (HBsAg) and the hepatitis B core antigen (HBcAg), respectively. In addition to mature HBV particles, serum from subjects who are acutely or chronically infected with HBV contains huge numbers of small spheres and tubules composed entirely of HBsAg. These particles, which are empty and thus non-infectious, represent excessive antigen produced by infected liver cells, but which are never assembled into complete virus particles. The core also contains another antigen – hepatitis Be antigen (HBeAg). In an uncomplicated infection all three viral antigens can be detected in blood for varying periods and each stimulates a specific antibody response. Only antibodies directed against the surface antibody protect against reinfection.

Certain children are at risk to HBV infection. They include neonates of HBsAg positive mothers, when the risk is markedly increased if the mother is also positive for the Be antigen. Household contacts of HBsAg carriers are at risk also, but less so than sexual partners. Other persons at risk include those with hereditary or acquired blood disorders necessitating repeated transfusions, e.g. haemoglobinopathies, clotting factor disorders, aplastic anaemia and other rare hereditary states. Renal dialysis patients are at very high risk of HBV exposure, although this risk has been greatly diminished in recent years by increased awareness of the mechanisms of viral dissemination and by the institution of appropriate isolation procedures.

Vaccination against HBV

The first vaccine to be developed depended on concentration and purification of the excessive hepatitis B surface antigen (HBsAg) obtained by plasmapheresis of chronic HBV carriers. In order to prevent transmission of intact HBV and other blood born viruses a complex process of inactivation was needed. An effective, safe but expensive vaccine resulted. This first generation vaccine has been superseded by second generation vaccines using yeast cells genetically engineered to produce HBsAg.

Vaccination should be offered to anyone living in the same household as a person with acute or chronic HBV infection. Along with a dose of hyperimmune anti HBV gammaglobulin, HBV vaccination should be commenced within 24 hours of birth in all infants of HBV carrier women.

Vaccination can be expected to ultimately eliminate this disorder and greatly decrease the incidence of hepatocellular carcinoma.

Non A non B hepatitis

There appear to be at least three other hepatitis viruses which have not been fully identified and characterized. One has a short incubation period like HAV and infection during pregnancy carries a high maternal mortality. The other two have longer incubations and are more likely to result in chronic infection and/or carrier states. They are the cause of the majority of post-transfusion hepatitis and of fulminant hepatic failure.

Other, but rarer, causes of viral hepatitis are cytomegalovirus (especially in immune-suppressed patients) and Epstein-Barr virus.

CLINICAL FEATURES OF ACUTE VIRAL HEPATITIS

The clinical features of HAV and HBV are identical. It should be remembered, however, that many children with either viral infection may be totally asymptomatic. The prodromal symptoms are of variable duration and consist of tiredness, anorexia, nausea and vomiting. Fever is usually low grade, but headaches and joint pains, together with pain in the right upper quadrant of the abdomen, may be prominent. At times the main complaint is one of pruritis prior to development of jaundice, which of course is the diagnostic clinical feature. With the onset of jaundice the urine is usually dark and the stools pale. The liver is slightly enlarged and tender and the spleen is mildly enlarged in at least 10% of these children. Jaundice may persist for only a few days or for many weeks. With the onset of jaundice constitutional symptoms tend to lessen. Continued anorexia, vomiting and lethargy usually indicate severe hepatic dysfunction.

Investigations

Serum aspartate amine transferase (AST) and gamma glutamyl transpeptidase (gamma GT) are elevated. Serum bilirubin levels are elevated and at least half of this is conjugated. The serum albumin concentration is usually normal, but gross reductions may be an early clue to incipient liver failure. The aetiological diagnosis is established by the finding of hepatitis A antibody or hepatitis B antigen or antibody in the serum. Serum transaminases usually return to normal (particularly in hepatitis A) by 2–4 weeks.

The outlook in childhood is very good, with the majority losing their jaundice within 4–6 weeks and complete recovery occurring.

On rare occasions, however, the illness is a fulminating one with increasing jaundice, anorexia, vomiting, confusion, restlessness and even coma. Bruising of the skin and bleeding from the gastrointestinal tract may occur. In this situation a characteristic odour to the breath is noted, the palms of the hands and soles of the feet become reddened, a coarse flapping tremor of the limbs occurs and characteristic changes appear on the electroencephalogram. This is the clinical picture of fulminating liver failure, a disorder carrying a high mortality.

It is uncommon for viral hepatitis to become chronic in childhood.

Management

The management of acute hepatitis is non-specific. Bed rest has been recommended but there is little to suggest its value. Fluids will be encouraged and the child allowed to dictate the fluid and food intake. The value of corticosteroids in the treatment of acute viral hepatitis is not proven. They increase the mortality in acute hepatitis B.

In the event of liver failure, fluid and adequate glucose must be provided by the intravenous route to correct the acid-base and electrolyte disturbance. Any coagulation deficit should be corrected if possible. Protein is eliminated from the diet and the gut sterilized to prevent absorption of protein, ammonia and possibly other toxins elaborated by intestinal bacteria. Renal failure and cerebral oedema may accompany liver failure and will require specific measures. Corticosteroids are usually given in fulminating disease. The outlook in acute liver failure is very guarded.

Drug-induced acute liver damage

Overdose quantities of paracetamol taken by older children may produce acute and even severe liver damage. Anticonvulsants (especially sodium valproate), antituberculosis antibiotics and some anticancer drugs may also produce acute hepatic injury.

CHRONIC HEPATITIS IN CHILDHOOD

Chronic hepatitis should be suspected if:

1. There are signs of chronic liver disease (such as fingernail clubbing, splenomegaly, ascites or spider naevi) in a child presenting as acute hepatitis.

2. A child is reputed to have had two attacks of hepatitis.

3. If, following an acute hepatitis, jaundice is prolonged more than four to six weeks or liver function tests have not become normal within three months.

4. Vague symptoms of lethargy and anorexia are accompanied by an enlarged liver and/or abnormal liver function tests.

Features suggestive of hepatic decompensation should be sought. These include hypoalbuminaemia with oedema or ascites, clotting impairment with spontaneous bruising or nose bleeds, gynaecomastia, nail clubbing, growth failure and spider naevi. Signs of portal hypertension may also be present if cirrhosis has already resulted.

Causes of chronic hepatitis include autoimmune processes, chronic infection with hepatitis B or non A non B viruses, alpha-1 antitrypsin deficiency, Wilson's disease, cystic fibrosis, drugs and liver damage secondary to biliary obstruction or inflammatory bowel disease.

Autoimmune chronic active hepatitis

This may be a process localized to the liver or part of a more widespread autoimmune process such as disseminated lupus erythematosus. Liver dysfunction can be accompanied by skin rashes, arthritis, pleurisy, iritis,

Coombs' positive haemolytic anaemia etc. The diagnosis is supported by elevated AST levels, hyperglobulinaemia, antinuclear and antismooth muscle or antimitochondrial antibodies and a liver biopsy showing plasma cell accumulation in portal tracts and periportal liver cell loss. A response to corticosteroid therapy can be expected and if instituted early cirrhosis may be prevented. Complete clinical control in excess of two years must be achieved before withdrawal of steroid therapy can be contemplated. Relapse will occur following withdrawal of therapy in more than 50% of patients and low-dose corticosteroid therapy will then need to be life long.

Wilson's disease

This disease involves an inborn error in copper metabolism which results in accumulation of large quantities of copper in the liver and subsequently in other organs (especially brain, cornea and kidneys). It is inherited in an autosomal recessive fashion. About 50% of cases present in childhood (after the age of four) with either asymptomatic hepatomegaly, mild non-specific symptoms plus hepatomegaly or with features of severe acute-on-chronic liver damage with or without acute haemolytic anaemia. The last presentation has a rapidly progressive downhill course and an often fatal outcome.

Neurological features of the disease – clumsiness, slurred speech and behavioural disturbances – are rare in childhood. Copper deposits in the periphery of the corneas are pathognomonic of this disease but are not present in most children with Wilson's disease and when present require slit lamp examination by an experienced ophthalmologist for their recognition.

Definitive diagnosis requires the finding of an excessive disparity between total serum copper (usually normal) and ceruloplasmin levels (usually low) indicating an elevated non-ceruloplasmin copper level in the serum. Confirmation of marked elevation of liver tissue copper by chemical measurement on biopsy tissue or demonstration of typical in vivo abnormal handling of radioactive copper is required also.

Treatment by low copper diet, penicillamine and pyridoxine needs to be life long. Cessation of treatment can prove fatal within a few months.

Siblings must be screened as they have a one in four risk of having subclinical disease.

Drugs

Drugs capable of causing chronic liver disease include isoniazid, rifampicin, methyldopa and some anticancer drugs.

Alpha-1 antitrypsin deficiency

Some infants with this disorder appear to recover from their neonatal hepatitis only to present later in childhood with cirrhosis and failing liver function.

CIRRHOSIS IN CHILDHOOD

Cirrhosis is the end result of chronic hepatic injury when the rate of injury exceeds the rate of cellular repair and replacement. Collapse of the reticulin supporting framework of the liver plus fibrosis and regeneration leads to the development of regenerative nodules surrounded by bands of fibrous tissue. These nodules lack the normal efficient vascular arrangement, hence the cells are less efficient metabolically and more at risk of ischaemia. This abnormal vascular pattern decreases ease of flow through the liver and causes portal hypertension. Cirrhosis is irreversible but may be compatible with normal growth and activity for many years. The large reserve capacity of the liver (three-quarters of the normal healthy liver) means that features of liver failure only arise when the functional liver volume is reduced to much below normal. A small cirrhotic liver is therefore the prelude to failure.

Patients with cirrhosis die either from liver failure (often precipitated by bacterial sepsis) or from gastrointestinal bleeding (usually from gastro-oesophageal varices (Fig. 63.1). Until recently the only forms of therapy available for cirrhosis and 'end-stage' liver disease were supportive – improved nutrition, diuretics, transfusion etc. Liver transplantation now offers some prospect of good quality prolonged survival.

Liver transplantation

Twenty five years of animal experimentation and human trials culminated in orthotopic (same site in the body) liver transplantation becoming an accepted form of life-prolonging therapy for 'end-stage' liver disease in the mid-1980s. Children with severe liver disease likely to be fatal within 6–24 months should be considered for liver transplantation. Survival results in children tend to be about 10% better than in adults. Most units report 50–80% survival through the operative and acute rejection phase, and 5-year survival figures of 50–70%. Lack of donors and the need to match for ABO blood groups and approximate body size, mean up to 40% of children seeking transplantation will die of their liver disease before a donor organ becomes available. The quality of life of survivors is good. Most achieve normal growth rates and a return to good physical health allows them to enjoy normal childhood activities. Life-long im-

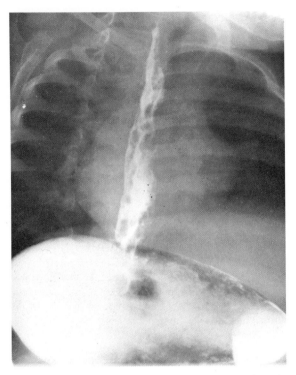

Fig. 63.1 Barium swallow demonstrating gross oesophageal varices in a child with cirrhosis.

munosuppression in order to retain the engrafted liver increases the long-term risk of development of malignancies, but experience with kidney transplantation indicates this is not an overwhelming risk.

Extrahepatic portal hypertension

Portal hypertension may arise from:

1. Impaired hepatic blood outflow e.g. hepatic venous thrombosis or constrictive pericarditis.

2. From increased hepatic vascular resistance e.g. cirrhosis.

3. Impaired hepatic portal inflow i.e. extrahepatic portal hypertension.

Although all forms of portal hypertension are uncommon in children, extrahepatic portal hypertension is proportionately more common than in adults. Whatever the cause of portal hypertension, some patients will develop portosystemic venous shunts in the submucosa of the gastro-oesophageal junction area – oesophageal varices (see Fig. 63.1). Some patients with varices will have episodes of severe, unexpected and sometimes potentially fatal bleeding. Thus haematemesis and melaena will sometimes be the initial presenting feature. In other cases the incidental finding of splenomegaly will lead to investigation. In some patients there is a

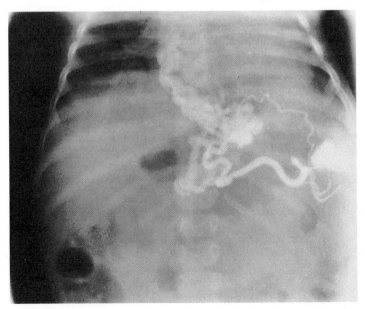

Fig. 63.2 Splenoportogram illustrating malformation of the portal vein with gross oesophageal varices.

premonitory small haematemesis followed hours later by a larger bleed impairing circulation and demanding transfusion. A third phase of bleeding may occur seven to ten days later. Painless bleeding associated with splenomegaly and visible subcutaneous venous shunts over the upper anterior abdomen help differentiate this cause of upper GI bleeding from peptic ulcer disease and ulcerated Meckel's diverticulum.

The cause of extrahepatic portal hypertension in childhood is not always known. The single large portal vein is replaced by a mass of tortuous smaller venous channels near the porta hepatis. In some children umbilical sepsis, dehydration or a temporary hypercoagulable state leads to portal vein thrombosis with subsequent imcomplete recanalization. In others it may represent a vascular malformation.

Diagnosis is established by splenoportography i.e. direct percutaneous needling of the splenic pulp to measure portal pressure and to inject radiographic contrast which outlines the portal vein and its associated 'shunt' vessels (often including gastro-oesophageal varices) (Fig. 63.2). Endoscopy or barium swallow will allow identification of varices in the oesophagus. Liver size and function is normal in extrahepatic portal hypertension.

Recurrence of variceal bleeding is common but, although each episode is frightening and potentially very dangerous, bleeding will usually cease spontaneously if managed conservatively by blood transfusion. Eventually spontaneous shunts develop at safer intra-abdominal sites. If blood loss is life threatening or bleeding frequency becomes intolerable, the varices may be obliterated by endoscopic injection sclerotherapy and/or an operative portosystemic shunt may be fashioned. Aspirin is a well-recognized precipitant of gastrointestinal bleeding episodes in these patients and parents need to be advised to avoid its use.

Hepatomegaly

The finding of an enlarged liver in a child demands full investigation. Of course it is essential to ensure that the liver is not pushed down by hyperinflated lungs. Should this be the case, there will be diminished or no liver dullness to percussion over the right side of the chest anteriorly. At times it is difficult to be certain of liver enlargement, particularly in a restless child. Abdominal ultrasound and/or technetium scanning will resolve the problem. It may also provide additional and valuable information regarding the structure of the liver, e.g. whether the enlargement is generalized or localized, solid or cystic, etc.

Example 63.2 Causes of hepatomegaly

Congenital
  Polycystic disease of liver
Infection
1. Septicaemias (particularly neonatal)
2. Hepatitis
  a. acute
  b. chronic
3. Parasitic
  a. malaria
  b. hydatids
  c. schistosomiasis
Neoplastic disease
1. Leukaemias
2. Lymphomas
3. Neuroblastomas
4. Primary and secondary hepatic tumours
Storage diseases
1. Carbohydrate
  a. fructose intolerance
  b. glycogen storage disorders
  c. galactosaemia
  d. diabetes mellitus
2. Protein
  urea cycle disorders
3. Lipid
  a. Gaucher's disease
  b. Niemann-Pick disease
  c. gangliosidoses
  d. mucopolysaccharidoses
  e. hyperlipoproteinaemias
Cardiovascular
1. Cardiac failure
2. Constrictive pericarditis
3. Inferior vena cava obstruction
Chronic haemolysis
1. Thalassaemia major
2. Sickle-cell disease

The causes of hepatomegaly are many and the more important are listed in Example 63.2. A careful history and thorough physical examination may allow the appropriate investigations required.

FURTHER READING

Biliary atresia – lessons from Japanese experience 1980 Lancet ii: 1283

Gust I 1983 Immunization against hepatitis B. Australian Family Physician 12(9): 657–660

Hussey H H 1981 The hepatitis B saga. Journal of the American Medical Association 245: 1317–1318

Mowat A P 1979 Recent advances in paediatric hepatology. Australian Paediatric Journal 15: 36–40

Mowat A P 1987 Liver disorders in childhood, 2nd edn. Butterworths, London

Shaw B W et al 1988 Liver transplantation therapy for children. Journal of Pediatric Gastroenterology and Nutrition 7: 157–166

Behaviour

64. Common behavioural disturbances

Robert Adler

Normal child development is a recurrent theme throughout this book. Most children develop in a predictable and orderly fashion emotionally and socially as well as physically and cognitively. Just as there is considerable variation in physical development, there is also variability in psychosocial development. Developmentally determined expressions of distress and variations in development are responsible for many common behavioural disturbances of infancy, childhood and adolescence. Thus, the infant is most likely to show his distress through feeding or sleeping difficulties while the toddler may have problems with learning which reflect specific learning difficulties or underlying emotional problems. The adolescent may express his or her distress by challenging parents' rules and values or engaging in provocative behaviour with peers. Many of these behaviours are normal if they are not excessive in intensity or frequency and provided they do not occur at an age which is developmentally inappropriate. Thus, the occasional temper tantrum in a 2-year-old is of no real significance, while prolonged tantrums occurring several times a day even at that age may be due to underlying emotional problems. Similarly, temper tantrums in an 8-year-old may well be indicative of underlying difficulties in the child, the family or at school. Whether a particular behaviour is perceived as a problem depends to a large extent on parental factors. Sometimes stress arising within the family may actually present as behavioural problems in a child.

One fundamental difference between child and adult psychiatry is in the presentation of problems. Adults usually come to a general practitioner or psychiatrist complaining of distress or discomfort which they experience. By contrast, children are usually brought because their behaviour is causing distress or concern to adults around them, most often parents or teachers. This means that some behaviours, such as withdrawal and depression, may go unnoticed unless they are particularly severe, leading to failure to thrive or attempted suicide.

In the past, great emphasis has been placed on the constitutional or environmental determinants (nature versus nurture) of particular problems. Nowadays, it is accepted that constitutional and environmental factors contribute to many problems.

CONSTITUTIONAL FACTORS

Genetic/chromosomal

Apart from some forms of intellectual handicap, e.g. phenylketonuria, fragile X syndrome and Down syndrome, there is little evidence to suggest that emotional and behavioural problems are determined by simple Mendelian inheritance or chromosomal abnormalities. There is considerable evidence from twin and adoption studies of a genetic contribution to many behavioural and emotional problems. These include temperamental differences and disorders as varied as enuresis, learning difficulties, hyperactivity and psychosis. Even in these disorders the impact of the problem on the child's development will be substantially influenced by environmental factors.

Handicapping conditions

Children with significant handicaps or chronic illness have at least a two-fold increase in the frequency of emotional disturbance. Intellectual handicap and disorders affecting the central nervous system may be associated with an even greater increase. Otherwise, there is little evidence of disease specific patterns.

Temperament

'Temperament' refers to a preponderant style in *how* an individual does things or how he or she responds to people and to situations, rather than to *what* the individual does, or to *why* he or she does it, or to the behavioural capacities or abilities that he or she manifests. This habitual pattern of responses is thought to be at least partly genetically determined. By the age of one year the infant's temperamental characteristics can be measured reliably using standardized temperament questionnaires. The pioneering work of Thomas et al (1968) suggested that infants could be classified on the following two dimensions 'easy – difficult' and 'slow to warm'. There is some evidence that 'difficult' infants are more likely to have subsequent behavioural and learning problems. However, the final outcome is mediated by environmental factors such as the parents' own temperament or personality and intercurrent events beyond the child's or the family's control.

ENVIRONMENTAL FACTORS

The developing child grows up in an environment in which the central figures during infancy are most often the parent(s). In our society it is still most commonly mothers who take the main caretaking role. This often lends particular significance to the mother-child relationship. As children grow older their world expands to include siblings, grandparents, other family members, other adults, school friends and many others. These relationships develop in the context of a socio-cultural milieu which has a profound effect on the values adopted by the family. Throughout development the child faces numerous stresses. Some of these, such as weaning, the birth of a sibling, starting school and puberty are normal and more or less predictable. These are often termed 'developmental' crises. Other stresses are much less predictable. These include death and serious illness in the family, parental conflict which may lead to separation and divorce, parental psychiatric illness, serious illness in the child which may lead to hospitalization and natural disasters. These are often termed 'accidental' crises. Children commonly respond to crises with emotional distress and/or behavioural disturbance. Regression is a particularly common response in children. When a child regresses in response to stress, skills which have been acquired most recently are usually lost first. Thus a 2-year-old child, hospitalized for the first time with asthma, may become incontinent of urine at night, may stop feeding himself and may have temper tantrums. These changes are usually rapidly reversible provided the stress is not too prolonged or intense and provided the parents can be supportive and understanding.

Some commonly occurring behavioural problems will now be discussed in developmental sequence.

DISORDERS OF INFANCY

Feeding disturbances

Problems with eating and feeding are common in the first three years. Estimates of their frequency range from 10–30%. In all cases a careful medical evaluation is essential before the problem is attributed to emotional causes. However, the diagnosis of an eating or feeding disorder should be made on positive grounds and not simply by exclusion of organic causes.

Problems can begin shortly after birth with refusal to suck. By three months the infant may actively resist feeding or begin to regurgitate food. Battles for control between infants and parents often centre around food intake during the second and third years of life. Anxious parents frequently see the child's rejection of food as a rejection of themselves. This may intensify their efforts to get the baby to eat which is counterproductive and may activate negativism and food refusal. At the other extreme, a neglected child may present in a malnourished state as a consequence of parental failure to provide an adequate, balanced diet. Feeding disorders are also more common in babies with underlying physical difficulties, especially if these involve the gastrointestinal system.

Management of these common problems should begin with a careful history and physical examination. If further investigations are warranted, these are best done early to avoid the cycle of repeated presentations with more investigations being done each time reinforcing the parents' conviction that there is something physically wrong. A diagnosis of milk allergy should only be made on positive grounds, not simply to give parents a spurious explanation for the infant's feeding difficulties. After a careful physical assessment the parents should be reassured if there is no evidence of physical abnormality. However, the reassurance should not simply dismiss the problem. Rather, it should lead to a careful discussion of the feeding situation which explores parental anxieties, identifies control battles and suggests alternative approaches. Puerperal depression should be considered as a possible aetiological factor. Tonics have no place in the treatment of feeding disorders although they may serve as a placebo. In severe cases, admission of mother and baby may be necessary. The purpose of admission is to help mother become more confident in her own ability to feed her baby.

In most instances, feeding difficulties resolve by three years. However, infants with feeding problems are more likely to have later emotional and behavioural problems.

Sleep disturbances

Parents fairly commonly complain that their children have problems sleeping. In infancy, these most often relate to difficulty falling asleep or waking through the night. In older children, nightmares, night terrors and sleepwalking may occur. In a study of 3-year-olds in

London, Richman et al (1975) found that 16% of children had difficulty settling and 14.5% woke at least three times a week. Many of these children still had difficulty sleeping when reviewed at eight years of age. Parents most often complain of disruption to their own sleep with resultant fatigue and irritability or interference with their own time together.

Assessment of a sleep problem must include a detailed history of the problem and should include a sleep diary. This may reveal that the child is sleeping for considerable periods which are not synchronous with the parents' pattern or that the child's sleep is being disturbed by overanxious parents 'checking on the baby'. This may be particularly common with parents who have had a previous cot death. In this case, the parents' anxiety is understandable but may not help the child establish a regular sleep-wake cycle.

Sleep patterns change throughout infancy. The normal newborn spends about 60% of sleep time in rapid eye movement (REM) sleep. This proportion may be even higher in premature infants. Usually each sleep cycle begins with a period of REM sleep and a regular diurnal rhythm is established by three months but only 70% of 3-month-old babies regularly sleep throughout the night. This rises to about 90% by nine months. A more adult pattern develops by one year with only 30% of sleep time in REM and the sleep cycle commencing with a non-REM period.

The cause of sleep disorders in early childhood is unclear. Some have suggested they are developmental/biological in origin, while others attribute them to psychological causes including separation anxiety or a response to marital conflict. In Richman's London study (1975), babies with sleep problems were more likely to have other behaviour problems, to have suffered accidents, to have mothers with psychiatric problems or to have a history of severe adverse perinatal events. Stressful events may lead to transient difficulties with sleeping. Sleep disorders are not uncommonly associated with difficulties with feeding.

Management begins with a careful assessment of the problem. Anxious parents may need reassurance and help to develop a routine which helps the baby settle. They may also need support to resist going to the baby as soon as crying begins. Parents need to be aware that infants also vary in their sleep requirements. A regular bedtime routine which involves settling things down rather than a highly stimulating interchange may be helpful. The child who has difficulty settling may benefit from being allowed to play quietly in bed. If a child is very anxious at bedtime or on waking through the night, the parents' presence may settle the child but the parent should be discouraged from too active an interaction. Gradual withdrawal over several nights may

then be possible. Occasionally, parents need support to allow the baby to cry until falling asleep. The sleep disorder may be a symptom of marital conflict which requires treatment in its own right.

Medication has little place in the treatment of sleep disturbances in early childhood. However, the judicious short-term use of a sedative-hypnotic may break the cycle of poor sleep, parental fatigue and irritability leading to increasing anxiety and poor sleep in the infant. The question is 'For whom to prescribe the sedative?'. Arguments can be mounted for sedating the child, the parents, or very rarely, both. Prescribing the parent a short-acting benzodiazepine for a few days may ease their fatigue. A similar goal may be achieved by asking the other parent, usually father, to take over responsibility for the child at night. The occasional use of a safe hypnotic such as chloral hydrate for the child is unlikely to be harmful unless used regularly or long term.

COMMON TODDLER PROBLEMS

Temper tantrums and breath-holding

The tantrum is the hallmark of toddlerhood or 'the terrible twos' as it has sometimes been termed. Tantrums which may be accompanied by breath-holding are very distressing for the parent, especially if they occur in public, but they rarely harm the child. Freud associated the negativism of 2-year-olds with the battle over bowel control. Whether this is true or not, the increasing mobility, curiosity and autonomy of the toddler coupled with a singular lack of awareness of danger and adult values frequently leads to conflict between parent and child. Tantrums may be inadvertently rewarded and supported by inconsistent and anxious parents who try to buy peace or avoid conflict. Depression in young women is commonly associated with being at home with several preschool children.

The assessment should, as usual, begin with a careful history. This serves several purposes. Firstly, it allows the parent to 'let off steam' or ventilate. Secondly, it identifies the frequency, severity and context of the tantrums. Thirdly, it can facilitate exploration of other family stresses which may be important aetiological factors. Finally, it prevents doctors giving premature advice based on insufficient information.

The management of tantrums depends on this history. Reassurance can be given that the occasional tantrum in a 2- to 4-year-old, while embarrassing for the parent, is commonplace and not harmful. Diverting the child's attention may help to abort a tantrum early in its course. However, it is virtually impossible to reason with a tantrumming toddler. In these circumstances, the parent is best advised to pretend to ignore the behaviour or to set a firm, non-punitive limit. The judicious use of 'time out' to give the child an opportunity to regain control may be helpful. This should not include locking the child in the bedroom which may be quite frightening. Medication, for the child at least, has no place in the management of tantrums.

Breath-holding also occurs most commonly in toddlers. There are two types: one is related to tantrums while the other is a simple faint. In the first, the distressed child usually cries several times and then stops breathing in full expiration. This is usually accompanied by cyanosis which, if prolonged, will lead to loss of consciousness and occasionally a brief grand mal fit. Epilepsy can usually be excluded on history alone as loss of consciousness and the fit precede cyanosis in the epileptic child. Breath-holding is self-limiting and will not harm the child apart from the risks of falling over. The simple faint usually follows a painful or frightening incident and is accompanied by vasovagal symptoms, including loss of consciousness, slow pulse and pallor.

CHILDHOOD PROBLEMS

Tics (stereotyped movement disorders – DSM 111R)

Tics are defined as 'the sudden, rapid and involuntary movements of circumscribed muscle groups which serve no apparent purpose'. These vary from minor, transient facial tics to the chronic debilitating tics of Tourette's disorder. The latter is a rare disorder with chronic tics which usually include vocal tics. These vary from grunts or sniffs to clear words. Coprolalia, or the involuntary utterance of obscenities, is said to be present in up to 60%. The lifetime prevalence of tics is 10–24% and boys are more frequently affected than girls. Facial muscles are most commonly involved followed by muscles of the upper limb and upper torso. Estimates of the frequency of tics in family members of a ticquer range from 10–30%. Some reports have suggested an increased frequency of psychiatric illness among the parents. However, the aetiological significance of this finding is unclear. Other symptoms of emotional disturbance, particularly non-aggressive symptoms, are more common among ticquers.

The aetiology of tics is largely unknown. A biochemical basis for Tourette's disorder has been postulated principally because of the favourable response to dopamine blocking agents such as haloperidol. Psychological explanations have described tics as a conditioned response to a frightening stimulus while others have explained them on a psychodynamic family interactional basis. None of these explanations should be considered proven at present. Most tics remit spontaneously but Tourette's disorder may persist well into adult life. Minor tics do not require treatment apart from reassuring the parent that they are likely to remit although psychotherapy and behaviour therapy have been recommended by some workers. There are few outcome studies and their results are varied. Haloperidol and other dopamine blocking drugs have been used successfully in the management of severe tics and Tourette's disorder. Their beneficial effect must be weighed up against the potential hazards, including tardive dyskinesia, of the long-term prescription of major tranquillisers.

Stuttering

This is synonymous with stammering and is characterized by interruption in the smooth flow of speech which may be accompanied by blinking or other tics. Many children go through a period of stuttering in their young pre-school years but approximately 80% will become fluent by adulthood. Stuttering is more common among boys and usually begins before the age of 6 years. It used to be thought that stuttering was a symptom of neurotic disorder but current evidence suggests that as a group, stutterers are no more disturbed than their more fluent peers. However, stuttering may cause secondary anxiety and social withdrawal. Twin studies suggest that there may be a genetic factor in the aetiology.

Many young stutterers improve spontaneously. However, speech therapy may be helpful for some children as young as two-and-a-half years. The type of therapy depends on the age of the child. Therapy is much briefer with young children.

Problems of bladder and bowel control

In the past, it was not uncommon for parents to commence toilet training their infants as early as nine months of age. Many claimed success but one might question who was trained, the infant, or the parent who was acutely attuned to the signs of impending micturition or defaecation. At present, parents are usually advised to wait until the child is 'ready'. This rarely occurs before the child is 18–24 months old. There is some evidence that children whose training starts before two years are less likely to be enuretic at 6–8 years. Most professionals advocate the use of reinforcement in the form of encouragement, praise or small rewards for success coupled with mild negative reinforcement, such as expressions of disappointment, for mishaps. More punitive approaches are unlikely to be helpful and may be associated with a more punitive approach to child rearing in general.

Developmentally, most children are continent of urine and faeces by 3–4 years of age with nocturnal urinary incontinence persisting most frequently beyond that age.

Enuresis

Nocturnal enuresis refers to 'the involuntary passage of urine during sleep in the absence of any identified physical abnormality in children aged above 4–5 years'. Enuresis is a common disorder affecting about 15% of 5-year-olds, falling to 1–2% of 14-year-olds. Sex ratio is equal in young children but males predominate among older children. A positive family history is common and twin studies suggest there may be a genetic component. Enuresis is more common among children with undiagnosed urinary tract infection and vice versa. Sleep studies show that wetting can occur at any stage of sleep and is not confined to deep sleep as was thought previously. Developmental delay in speech and motor development is more common among enuretics. Children who have previously been dry may develop secondary enuresis following stressful life events. There is an association between enuresis and psychiatric disorder but it is unclear whether this is causal, reactive or coincidental. Most studies report an increase in emotional wellbeing with successful treatment of enuresis.

Assessment of the enuretic child should include a urine examination to exclude urinary tract infection, diabetes insipidus or diabetes mellitus and measurement of serum creatinine to exclude chronic renal failure. A history of urinary dribbling or poor stream suggests the possibility of neurogenic bladder or anatomical urinary obstruction. In the vast majority these investigations will be negative.

There is little evidence to suggest that night lifting or fluid restriction in the evening are effective in clinical trials. But these measures, coupled with simple rewards, may help the child verging on continence to become dry at night. There is little justification for instituting more formal treatment measures for children under 5 years as one can expect 40% of wet 2-year-olds to become dry during the next year. Similarly, 20% of 3-year- olds, and 6% of 4-year-olds will become dry spontaneously. After this the spontaneous remission rate flattens out.

The two most effective treatments for more resistant bed wetters are tricyclic antidepressants or various alarm systems which wake the child. Tricyclic antidepressants have been shown to be effective in up to 85% of children. Imipramine is the most widely used in doses of 1–2.5 mg/kg as a single night time dose. Medication should be continued for a month after dryness is achieved. Dryness is often achieved quite quickly, making them useful for children who want to go away to a camp or to stay overnight. Alarm systems rely on a pad or sensor placed under the sheets which detects the passage of a small amount of urine and sets off an alarm to wake the child. Parents can be reassured that there is no chance of an electric shock but they must understand the importance of the alarm not the parent waking the child. Success rates of 50–100% have been reported using the pad and bell. Highest success rates are likely when the child is motivated, treatment is part of a collaborative venture between child, parents and doctor and there is no evidence of serious psychopathology in the child or family. Relapse rates of up to 40% have been reported with both drug and alarm treatment although relapse is said to be more likely after cessation of drug treatment.

Faecal soiling or encopresis

Most children who do not have any physical abnormality, develop normal bowel control by four years of age. Nevertheless, 1–2% of 5 to 12-year-olds continue to soil by day with boys outnumbering girls by about 2:1. These can be broadly divided into three groups. Firstly, there is a group of children who have adequate bowel control, but may transiently soil in response to a psychological stress. Secondly, there are those children who have never learned bowel control. A few have evidence of neurological damage, including cerebral palsy, spina bifida or intellectual handicap, while others may have enuresis, learning difficulties and problems with aggression. The latter are more likely to come from socially disadvantaged families with parents who are borderline or mildly intellectually handicapped.

The third group, and clinically the most important, consists of the children who present with soiling due to faecal retention with overflow of liquid faeces. Severe faecal retention may cause marked rectal and colonic dilatation (psychogenic megacolon) with faecal impaction. In some of these children there is a history of an episode of diarrhoea often followed by constipation and painful defaecation due to an anal fissure. If this occurs around the time of toilet training it may lead to a refusal to sit on the toilet and active withholding of faeces. In other cases, a psychological stress coinciding with toilet training appears to be the precipitant. Harshly coercive toilet training is also said to be more common among encopretics who retain faeces. Clearly, what subsequently evolves is a 'battle of the bowel' which the parents are unlikely to win unless a more co-operative spirit can develop. In other aspects of their lives, many encopretic children may be very good and even excessively compliant. These children seem to feel that they can only be autonomous in areas beyond the control of their parents.

History alone should be sufficient to exclude Hirschprung's disease from constipation due to psychological causes. In Hirschprung's disease, the constipation is present from birth which is rarely if ever the case in encopresis. If doubt persists, a suction biopsy of the rectum will demonstrate the presence of normal ganglia in encopresis. A plain radiograph of the abdomen is usually sufficient to demonstrate faecal retention and a barium enema is rarely warranted.

Many approaches to treatment have been tried and no single approach has been shown to be superior in the treatment of constipation with overflow. The principles underlying treatment include:

1. Defusing the control battle between parents and child so that the child is encouraged to use the toilet appropriately.

2. Emptying the bowel of impacted faeces, using microenemas and even disimpaction under anaesthesia if necessary.

3. The use of a high fibre diet and stool softeners to ensure the passage of soft, painless stools.

4. A behaviour modification programme based on positive reinforcement and desensitization of the fear of using the toilet.

5. Psychotherapy aimed at resolving underlying conflict and assisting the child with appropriate expression of aggression.

6. Parent or family therapy.

There are few systematic outcome studies but clinicians and parents may be reassured by the fact that faecal soiling is almost unknown among intellectually normal adults.

Attention deficit hyperactivity disorder (ADHD) (DSM 111R)

This rather cumbersome term is the most recent name given to a syndrome which has at times been called hyperactivity, minimal brain dysfunction and hyperkinetic syndrome (ICD-9). The criteria for the diagnosis of ADHD include age-inappropriate inattention coupled with impulsivity and hyperactivity commencing before seven years and extending over a period of more than six months in a child with no evidence of other major psychiatric disorder or severe mental retardation. The disorder is much more common in boys and is often associated with learning difficulty and other evidence of developmental delay as well as problems with defiance and aggression. Many of these problems also occur among children with conduct disorder. Although 'soft' neurological signs and non-specific abnormalities on EEG occur in up to 50%, there is no evidence of structural neurological abnormality.

Estimates of prevalence vary widely with much higher rates being reported among American children than in the United Kingdom or Australia. These differences are reflected in different rates of prescription of stimulant drugs. In making the diagnosis it is important to exclude those children whose behaviour and attention is well within age-appropriate limits but whose environment either home or school, is excessively intolerant of normal childhood curiosity and activity.

Drug treatment with stimulants, e.g. methylphenidate, has been shown to be effective in improving performance on tests of concentration and motor speed and reducing the severity of problem behaviours. However, their long-term value in terms of improved learning and social development remains unproved. The medication is usually given in morning or morning and lunchtime doses to avoid the sleep reduction associated with night time administration. Growth retardation in height and weight may occur but is reversible on cessation of the drug. Dosage is between 0.25–0.5 mg/kg/day. Drug free periods during school vacations reduce growth retardation and allow the indications for medication to be reviewed. Various behavioural therapies have been used to good effect, particularly in improving classroom behaviour and increasing time 'on task'. Family therapy has a role in addressing family issues which may be perpetuating the problem.

Separation anxiety disorder

Some anxiety about separation from key attachment figures usually appears in the second six months of life. For the next few years one expects some distress in young children who are separated from key figures, especially if they are in unfamiliar surroundings such as hospitals. Indeed, children who fail to show any anxiety on separation and who are non-discriminating in their relationships with adults may be showing signs of significant emotional deprivation and failure to form healthy attachments. One only has to observe children and parents on the first day at kindergarten and schools to see how common separation anxiety is in these new situations. It usually settles within days or at most a few weeks given understanding teachers and supportive parents who are not excessively anxious about letting their children go. In a few children the separation difficulty may be more prolonged and may foreshadow subsequent difficulties with separation.

The term Separation Anxiety Disorder (DSM 111R) encompasses many children who present with school refusal and some who present with recurrent abdominal pain. In the case of children who are not attending school it is important to differentiate school refusers from truants and those who are being kept at home by parents. Truancy is commonly associated with a range of antisocial behaviours and learning difficulties. The children often come from socially disadvantaged families. By contrast, school refusal is rarely associated with antisocial behaviour or learning difficulties. In fact, anxiety symptoms or recurrent abdominal pain which lead to absenteeism are more usual and the children are often average or above average students who are excessively compliant at home, provided there is no threat of separation. A small proportion may really be reluctant to go to school because of fears arising at school. However, the majority is anxious about separation from parents. This may be because of previous unhappy separation experiences or concerns about parental wellbeing. Parental threats of suicide or abandonment of the family, marital conflict or parental ill health may be important aetiological factors.

Assessment begins with a careful history including questions about problems in the family. Appropriate investigations should be carried out early. Prolonged, unnecessary investigations 'for fear of missing something' should be avoided as it reinforces an organic explanation for the problem.

The first goal of treatment is usually to get the child back to school because prolonged absence is associated with a worse prognosis. This often necessitates enlisting the aid of the parent who has not been involved, usually father. Behavioural strategies including relaxation and desensitization may be helpful. Some trials of tricyclic antidepressants as an adjunct to family and behavioural approaches have yielded encouraging results. The child

with severe underlying anxiety may benefit from individual psychotherapy provided this is combined with counselling or therapy for the parents. Liaison with the school is a vital part of treatment to support the child's re-entry and to minimize ostracism by peers.

Masturbation, thumbsucking, nailbiting and other non-problems

Children exhibit many behaviours which concern their parents and grandparents a great deal but have no clinical significance unless they predominate or continue beyond a developmentally appropriate stage. There is a great variety of child rearing books which offer parents advice on the management of these non-problems. Most sensibly reassure parents that the problem is very likely to go away provided that they do not pay too much attention to it. This is generally very safe advice as most are self-limiting.

REFERENCES

Richman N, Stevenson J, Graham P J 1975 Pre-school to school: a behavioural study. Academic Press, London
Thomas A, Chess S, Birch H G 1968 Temperament and behaviour disorders in children. University Press, New York

FURTHER READING

Connell H 1985 Essentials of child psychiatry, 2nd edn. Blackwell, Oxford
Green C 1987 Toddler taming. Doubleday, Sydney
Minde K, Minde R 1986 Infant psychiatry: an introductory textbook. Sage Publications, California
Rapoport J, Ismond D 1984 DSM-111 Training guide for diagnosis of childhood disorders. Brunner/Mazel, New York
Rutter M, Hersov L 1985 Child and adolescent psychiatry: modern approaches, 2nd edn. Blackwell, Oxford

65. Major psychiatric disorders in children and adolescents

Robert Adler

Children and adolescents may experience most of the psychiatric disorders which affect adults. Some disorders such as schizophrenia commonly begin during adolescence while others such as Huntington's chorea and dementia of the Alzheimer's or atherosclerotic type rarely, if ever, present before adult life.

In this chapter only a few of the major psychiatric disorders which affect children and adolescents will be described. These include autism and conduct disorders which usually present during childhood. Depression, suicide and eating disorders are of particular importance in adolescence even though they also commonly occur in adults. For consideration of other psychiatric disorders including schizophrenia, the reader is referred to the major psychiatric texts.

CLASSIFICATION

The classification of psychiatric disorders, particularly those presenting in infancy, childhood or adolescence can be somewhat confusing. It is made more difficult by a relative lack of information about the natural history, family patterns and developmental aspects of most disorders. Furthermore, children are rarely self-referred necessitating information from multiple sources, including parents, teachers and other professionals. The recent development of multiaxial classification systems is a significant advance in the description of complex psychiatric disorders. The axes cover primary psychiatric diagnosis; developmental state including intelligence; medical conditions; severity of psychosocial stressors; and the highest level of adaptive functioning in the previous year. As yet no axis to describe family functioning has been included.

Diagnoses should only be used to describe disorders and not to label a person as if the disorder is a life-long attribute of that person. Thus, it is more appropriate to describe someone as suffering from schizophrenia rather than calling them a schizophrenic which suggests that this is all they are. Indeed, the same principle could well be applied to chronic medical conditions such as asthma, diabetes or epilepsy.

Epidemiology

Studies of the prevalence of significant behavioural disturbance in children generally report rates of 6–15%. Before mid-adolescence, boys are referred more frequently than girls and prevalence rates are higher among urban children than among rural children. Children with physical illnesses, especially neurological disorders and intellectual handicap, have a non-specific increase in behavioural problems. Most studies have identified two main clusters of disorders, namely, emotional disturbance and conduct disturbance. These are sometimes termed internalizing and externalizing disorders, respectively. Emotional disturbances are characterized by fear, anxiety, misery and somatic complaints, while conduct disturbances are characterized by disobedience, disruptiveness, destructiveness and aggression often with delinquent behaviour. Organic brain syndromes and the psychoses constitute rare but important diagnostic groupings.

Autistic disorder

Autistic disorder or early infantile autism as it used to be known, is a rare disorder affecting 2–4 children in every 10 000 live births. It is approximately three times more common in boys. A further 20 children in every 10 000 may have some autistic features associated with severe mental retardation. Previously, autism was classified among the psychoses; however, recognition of its qualitative differences from schizophrenia led to its reclassification as a pervasive developmental disorder. Onset is usually before 36 months but a later onset type is recognized. Autism is characterized by four groups of symptoms.

1. Qualitative impairment in reciprocal social interac-

tion. The autistic child tends to relate to others as objects rather than people. They may not seek comfort when hurt nor engage in imitative or social play.

2. Qualitative impairment in verbal and non-verbal communication and in imaginative activity. Language development is severely impaired and when language is present words tend not to be used for communication. There is usually a lack of eye contact and a failure of non-verbal response to others.

3. Markedly restricted repertoire of activities and interests. Stereotyped behaviours and marked resistance to change are common.

4. Absence of delusions, hallucinations or schizophrenic thought disorder.

Approximately 75% of autistic children show some degree of general intellectual impairment. 20–30% develop epilepsy by late adolescence. Almost two-thirds continue to be severely disabled in adult life and are unable to live independently. 5–15% are able to work and lead some kind of social life in the community. Indicators of a good prognosis include performance IQ over 50–60 and the development of functional language by 5 years of age.

The aetiology of autism is unknown but there is no evidence to support earlier suggestions that autism is caused by cool, unresponsive parents. There is evidence of a genetic component with an increase in language disorder, learning disabilities and mental retardation as well as autism among siblings.

Special educational and behavioural approaches are the mainstays of treatment. Major tranquillisers may be useful in controlling disturbed behaviour but have no impact on the core pathology. Parents will usually need considerable support and may require counselling or therapy.

Somatoform disorders

States of emotional arousal are commonly accompanied by somatic symptoms. Generally these are part of an autonomic response and their psychological origin is both obvious and readily acknowledged. In a small proportion of child psychiatric clinic referrals children may present with a major alteration in physical functioning that suggests physical disorder but which is apparently an expression of a psychological conflict or need. Physical functions commonly affected include:

- altered motor functioning
- altered sensation
- altered perception, e.g. blindness, deafness
- psychogenic pain
- pseudoseizures.

Psychogenic disturbances in these functions are called hysterical conversion reactions. They only make up a small proportion of child and adolescent psychiatric referrals but paediatricians and paediatric orthopaedic surgeons report that they are not uncommon in their clinics.

The psychoanalytic explanation of hysteria is that the symptom is a way of avoiding an unconscious conflict (primary gain) often related to the oedipal stage of development. The symptom leads to an altered response by key figures in the person's life which may perpetuate the problem (secondary gain). Family therapists see the child's symptom as a powerful way of diverting attention from unacknowledged conflict between family members, particularly parents. In some cases of conversion illness a relative may have an illness affecting the same part of the body. In several follow-up studies of hysteria an organic illness related to the presenting symptom has been found in a number of cases. Misdiagnosis is most likely if an emotionally stressful event precedes the insidious onset of unusual symptoms with few definite physical signs.

Treatment. Mild cases of short duration will often respond well to reassurance that there is no serious underlying organic pathology and that the condition can be expected to improve spontaneously. The judicious use of physiotherapy may help the patient relinquish the symptom. Psychiatric referral may be necessary for more severe and persistent cases. Psychiatric treatment will usually involve a careful assessment of the child and the family followed by family or individual psychotherapy.

Conduct disorder, delinquency and drug abuse

Minor antisocial behaviours such as defiance, disobedience, occasional stealing or lying and minor acts of vandalism are common in childhood. These are of little clinical significance in families where there are clear, consistent behavioural expectations which are firmly but flexibly enforced with appropriate consequences for their infringement. However, the antisocial behaviour of a small minority of children is much more serious and persistent. These children exhibit behaviours which repeatedly violate major social norms and the rights of others. The behaviours commonly affected include:

- fighting
- disobedience
- destructiveness
- stealing
- running away
- lying

– truancy
– fire setting
– sexual coercion of others.

The DSM-111R criteria for conduct disorder include the presence of three or more of these behaviours over a period of at least six months. Regular smoking from an early age and the abuse of alcohol and non-prescribed drugs occur commonly among conduct disordered children. Delinquency is a legal rather than a clinical entity. The juvenile delinquent is a young person who has been found guilty of an offence that would be classified as a crime if committed by an adult.

There is a clear association between conduct disorder in childhood, adolescent delinquency and maladjustment in adult life. Robins (1966) followed up a group of conduct disordered children (mean age 13 years) five years after referral to a child guidance clinic and found that only 16% could be regarded as permanently 'recovered'. A thirty year follow-up of the same sample showed that more than 25% warranted a diagnosis of 'sociopath' or antisocial personality disorder.

Aetiology. The aetiology of conduct disorders is unclear. They are almost certainly symptomatic of many environmental and constitutional factors. Despite the lack of a specific aetiology a great deal is known about their occurrence. They occur more frequently in families where there are high levels of family violence, marital conflict and marital breakdown. Boys are more likely than girls to show evidence of conduct disorders in response to such family disharmony. Children who have been raised in institutions and those whose early development is marked by multiple changes of caretaker are also much more likely to exhibit serious antisocial behaviour.

Both girls and boys often have marked educational difficulties, with reading retardation severe enough to warrant a separate diagnosis of specific developmental disorder. Poor concentration and over-activity are commonly associated. Boys are more likely to have IQ levels slightly below average but this is not so for girls.

Management. The treatment of conduct disordered children is important because of its serious prognostic implications. However, treatment remains difficult at least in part because of the difficulty of involving the family. The advent of family therapy, more behaviourally oriented approaches and group psychotherapy in schools have provided some encouraging results.

Drug and alcohol abuse

There is considerable evidence that the rate of drug and alcohol abuse among children and adolescents has risen sharply in recent years. This is also true for the inhala-tion of volatile solvents (glue sniffing). The use of illicit drugs peaks in the 18–25 age group. Previous sex differences in usage are disappearing with increasing rates of use of all drugs, including alcohol, among girls.

Some experimentation with these substances is widespread in the community, but the majority of those who experiment with drugs and alcohol do not progress to dependence or addiction. However, this is no cause for complacency. The health and social consequences of drug and alcohol abuse are far reaching. Their misuse is often involved in physical violence, child maltreatment and motor vehicle accidents. Accidental or intentional overdosage is a common cause of morbidity and mortality. Emotionally, drug and alcohol abuse is commonly associated with depression and poor self-esteem. The use of illegal drugs contributes significantly to teenage crime. Intravenous drug use is associated with an increased risk of hepatitis B and AIDS.

Depression and suicide

Clinical features. The diagnosis of depression in childhood and adolescence is still controversial. It has long been recognized that children are often sad in response to loss. However, this is very different from the experience of depression as a symptom and a far cry from a diagnosable 'depressive disorder' requiring or warranting treatment. Unlike sadness, depression is characterized by feelings of unworthiness and self blame, a sense of helplessness that one cannot change the situation and a sense of hopelessness that things will not improve in the future. In adults the diagnosis of a depressive disorder usually depends on the presence of associated phenomena (sleep and appetite disturbance, psychomotor retardation, etc), social impairment and the duration of symptoms as well as the existence of depressed mood. Community surveys of children and adolescents have shown that depressed mood is much more common than was previously believed. Parents are often unaware of their child's depression. Although there is still disagreement about the necessary criteria for the diagnosis of a depressive disorder in childhood and adolescence, it is generally agreed that depression occurs more commonly with increasing age. Before adolescence, depression is more commonly diagnosed in boys but girls are more frequently affected after puberty. The reason for this sex ratio reversal around puberty is unknown. Depression is commonly associated with other childhood emotional and behavioural disorders. In particular, depression is common in adolescents with a history of attention deficit hyperactivity disorder in childhood, in children with conduct disorders and in those with eating disorders.

Aetiology. Clinical descriptions of depressed children

and adolescents have existed for many years but the systematic study of depression in children and adolescents only began in the last twenty years. Previously, Spitz (1965) described a phenomenon he termed 'anaclitic depression' in infants separated from their primary caretakers. Affected infants became withdrawn, apathetic and often failed to thrive. John Bowlby (1975) described a pattern of protest, despair and detachment occurring in preschool children separated from parents as a result of hospitalization or institutionalization. While it is recognized that these phenomena are a response to separation or loss, their relationship to depression in later life is unknown. Depression occurs more commonly among children of parents with a history of depressive disorder. It seems likely that this increased prevalence is genetic in origin but current studies do not allow environmental influences to be differentiated from genetic influences. The biological accompaniments of depression in adults, such as alterations in noradrenalin and serotonin levels, altered cortisol secretion and altered sleep physiology have not been found systematically in children.

Treatment. There is little evidence from double-blind controlled trials of a response to antidepressants which have been shown to be effective in adult depression. Indeed, in one controlled trial both placebo and drug groups had a 60% response rate. As one approaches adulthood the clinical picture becomes more like that in adults. These results suggest that at present the treatment of choice for depressed young people is psychological rather than pharmacological. However, there is no evidence that one psychological treatment has definite advantages over another.

Suicide and attempted suicide

Few children under the age of twelve years commit suicide but there are well-documented reports of children as young as seven or eight years who have killed themselves intentionally. Younger children are unlikely to have a clear concept of death, its irreversibility or a knowledge of how to kill themselves. The suicide rate climbs rapidly throughout adolescence with males having higher rates of completed suicide than females at all ages. Males are more likely to use more lethal means than females which may account for their higher rate of completed suicide. In recent years, there has been an alarming increase in the incidence of completed suicide among adolescents of both sexes throughout the Western world.

Suicidal thoughts are far more common than attempted suicide which, in turn, is far more common than completed suicide. Some adolescent suicide attempts are characterized by a high intent and lethalness

of method. These adolescents are usually more psychiatrically disturbed than those whose less dangerous attempts are an impulsive response to some interpersonal crisis. Many studies have highlighted the frequency of severe family breakdown among adolescents who attempt suicide. Jacobs (1971) suggests that there is a three stage process leading up to most adolescents' suicide attempts. These are a longstanding history of problems, followed by a period of escalation of conflict with family and friends, culminating in a chain reaction-dissolution of key relationships. The actual attempt most commonly follows a disagreement with parents or with a boy or girlfriend.

Management. Urgent assessment of the young person and their family is always indicated and dismissing a suicide attempt as 'just attention seeking' cannot be justified. The assessment should include a careful history of the attempt and its lethality. Examination of mood for evidence of depression is basic. In addition, there must be a complete evaluation of the family searching for precipitants and exploring the support available to the teenager within the family. If the attempt was potentially lethal and there is evidence of persisting depression, a lack of family support and little has changed as a consequence of the attempt, an urgent psychiatric assessment is always indicated.

Admission to hospital may be necessary for medical reasons. More commonly it is necessary to ensure that the child is safe until a more complete assessment can be conducted and treatment commenced. A seriously suicidal adolescent may need to be admitted involuntarily for their own protection. Sometimes protective action through the Children's Court is required to persuade parents of the seriousness of their child's suicidal attempt. Treatment of the suicidal adolescent is principally psychotherapeutic, preferably involving the family, although antidepressants have a role in the treatment of some.

Eating disorders

Anorexia nervosa. Anorexia nervosa (see Fig. 65.1) was first described in the seventeenth century. In recent years, there has been growing concern about a rapid increase in the incidence of the disorder and an increasing awareness of an associated disorder, bulimia nervosa. The name anorexia nervosa is actually a misnomer as patients rarely have a true loss of appetite. In fact most are intensely preoccupied with food and have a morbid fear of becoming fat.

Bulimia nervosa. Bulimia nervosa is associated with episodic binge eating. These binges result in intense guilt which often leads to self-induced vomiting and purgation. It is this abnormal eating pattern rather than

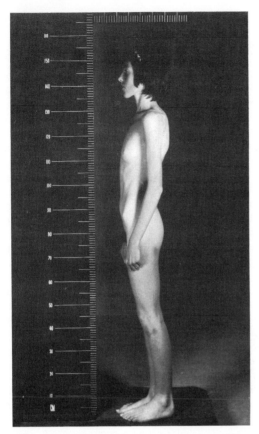

Fig. 65.1   An adolescent with anorexia nervosa.

pulse rate. High levels of activity are often maintained despite weight loss until the advanced stages of the illness. Depressive and obsessional symptoms are common. Occasionally anorexic symptoms may occur in a patient with schizophrenia.

Plasma luteinizing hormone and follicular stimulating hormone levels are often low and may remain low for several weeks after weight gain has been achieved. These hormonal changes are secondary to the weight loss. However, an anterior pituitary tumour may rarely present with a similar picture to anorexia nervosa.

Recently, community surveys have suggested that anorexic symptoms are far more widespread than was previously thought. The incidence is probably increasing with the emphasis on 'thin is attractive' among young women. Particular groups such as ballet students and gymnasts have a higher incidence than their peers. There is some evidence to suggest that anorexia is more common among girls from higher socioeconomic families. Many of those with mild anorexic symptoms remit spontaneously, especially if the behaviour is dealt with firmly, early in its course.

Aetiology. The aetiology of anorexia nervosa is unknown. Many theories have been put forward but none have stood the test of time. However, severe family dysfunction with overprotection of the child and a pattern of conflict avoidance is common. Whether this dysfunction is primary or secondary remains unclear. In many families the anorexic adolescent only feels able to be autonomous through food refusal. This leads to major battles with parents for control. Some teenagers become anorexic after a separation or threat of separation. Others seem to develop their symptoms as a means of remaining childlike and avoiding issues related to sexuality.

Treatment. Anorexia is best managed jointly by a paediatrician and a child psychiatrist. Children with severe weight loss may require hospitalization and intensive refeeding but many can be managed on an outpatient basis. Various psychotherapeutic approaches are the mainstay of treatment. Involvement of the family is essential with children and adolescents. Symptomatic use of medication for the relief of anxiety or depression may be helpful.

Prognosis. The outlook in anorexia nervosa is good although long-term follow-up reports have found a high frequency of disordered eating behaviour even among those who are no longer anorexic. Mortality rates of up to 10% through anorexia or suicide have been reported. Generally, the prognosis is better in younger patients who seek treatment early and who do not have evidence of bulimic symptoms.

weight loss which is the hallmark of bulimia. Bulimia more commonly occurs among older adolescents and young adults but there may be a past history of anorexia nervosa.

Clinical features. Anorexia nervosa is characteristically a disorder of adolescent females although it may continue into or even commence in adult life. Less commonly, it may present in premenarchal girls and occasionally in boys. The disorder is usually insidious in its onset with a failure to gain weight or a gradual loss of weight. This is achieved by calorie restriction but intensive exercise, self-induced vomiting and purgation are sometimes used to facilitate greater weight loss. Weight loss is associated with a marked disturbance in body image which results in the teenager feeling she is much fatter than she actually is. This feeling of 'fatness' may persist despite marked emaciation. Amenorrhoea or delayed menarche are usually present. In addition to the signs of weight loss the patients may have cool extremities, fine lanugo hair, low blood pressure and slow

FURTHER READING

Bowlby J 1975 Attachment and loss, vol. 2 Separation and anger. Penguin, London

Connell H M 1985 Essentials of child psychiatry, 2nd edn. Blackwell, Oxford

Jacobs J 1971 Adolescent suicide. Wiley, New York

Minde K, Minde R 1986 Infant psychiatry: an introductory textbook. Sage Publications, California

Rapoport J L, Ismond D R 1984 DSM-111 training guide for diagnosis of childhood disorders. Brunner/Mazel, New York

Robins L N 1966 Deviant children grown up. Williams & Wilkins, Baltimore

Rutter M, Hersov L 1985 Child and adolescent psychiatry: modern approaches, 2nd edn. Blackwell, Oxford

Spitz R A 1965 First year of life: psychoanalytic study of normal and deviant development of object relations. International University Press, new York

Steinhauer P D, Rae-Grant Q 1983 Psychological problems of the child in the family, 2nd edn. Basic Books, New York

66. Adolescence

John M. Court

Adolescence is the developmental process of physical, psychological and sexual maturation, starting with the first evidence of puberty and concluding with the emergence of the mature young adult. Adolescence proceeds through psychological stages which relate broadly to the physical stages of puberty as defined by Tanner (1962). Early puberty is characterized by preoccupation with a rapidly changing body and by an emergent ability for abstract thought. Mid-adolescence is characterized by conflict with parents as the adolescent asserts his need for independence, often expressed inappropriately. Sexual exploration is common and often uncomfortable. In later adolescence, the search for self-identity is largely achieved, the adolescent is capable of more mature relationships and is tackling the question of his or her role in society and in the workforce.

WHO (1989) defines the period of adolescence as the second decade of life from 10–19 years, and in Western society this represents about 18% of the population. Many health problems of childhood persist through adolescence, and some disorders of adult life (such as essential hypertension and alcohol abuse) may become manifest. Some problems, such as acne, anorexia nervosa, delayed puberty, the osteochondroses and the accidental consequences of risk-taking behaviour, are almost unique to adolescents.

Much of the significance of adolescence in medicine relates to the developmental process which underlies this period of life and influences health. The health needs of young people are often inadequately addressed, and this is particularly so for psychosocial problems, emotional stress, nutritional problems and those with chronic medical and physical disability.

HEALTH ISSUES

Adolescence is commonly regarded as a healthy time of life. At this age there is a lower prevalence of physical illness than at other ages. Most contact with a general practitioner is for physical illness. It has been suggested that many teenagers use their doctor in the same way they use a fast food outlet: when they are disturbed by physical illness they want relief at once, with little thought for the underlying medical implications and with an unwillingness to return for review once the immediate crisis or symptom is alleviated. This view is at variance with teenagers' own view of their health but is consistent with statistics indicating the reasons for attendance at a general practice.

The results of a survey of a group of 13- to 15-year-olds attending a primary care neighbourhood practice in a Melbourne suburb are listed in Table 66.1.

Table 66.1 Visits to doctors: 13- to 15-year-olds in a Melbourne suburb

Disorder	%
Upper respiratory tract infection	22
Injuries	11
Fever	6
Asthma	5
Warts	5
Other skin disorders	3

From Carmichael 1983

This list is very similar to surveys published in the United States and suggests the main reasons for seeing a doctor are upper respiratory tract and other infections, injuries and skin problems.

In contrast to this have been the results of studies on adolescents' own perception of their health. Parcel and others in 1977 reported that teenagers' major health concerns were school worries, drugs, sex, family problems and getting along with people. When asked what were the health problems for which they would most like help, they included acne, how far to go with sex, depression, overweight, getting along with parents and such other symptoms as nervousness and fatigue.

A series of consultations with some 3000 young people conducted in Victoria in 1987 showed that their

---

Example 66.1 Young people's perception of their main health issues

Fitness, wellbeing
Stress
Depression
Relationships
Boredom
AIDS, STD
Sexuality
Contraception
Healthy food
Alcohol, smoking
Menstruation
Overweight
Emotional problems
Health risks at work

---

major health concerns, and the issues on which they would most like information, also extended far beyond the common reasons for attending a general practitioner. Example 66.1 sets out their major concerns.

Mortality

Accidents account for over half of deaths throughout adolescence in Western society, and in the 10 to 14-year-old age group of the next most common causes are neoplasm and congenital anomalies. In the 10 to 19-year-old age group, suicide and homocide exceed other causes after accidents. Suicide rates during adolescence have increased steadily in Western society including Australia. The reported prevalence is 10 per 100 000 per year of 15- to 19-year-olds in 1980. Of 15-year-olds 7% have reported suicide thoughts, this is associated with almost 50% of adolescents experiencing feelings of depression at times.

For every successful suicide, there are about 100 suicide attempts or gestures. Boys are more likely to succeed at suicide attempts, and in Australia and the United States four males suicide for each female. Not all those who attempt suicide have a depressive disorder, but all should be taken seriously as an expression of distress.

AN APPROACH TO ADOLESCENTS

As adolescents are concerned about the wider emotional, developmental and social aspects of their health, it is perhaps surprising they seldom seek advice from their family doctor. Most teenagers prefer to discuss their problems with their friends and many claim that they never discuss health concerns with anyone.

Adolescents tend to underuse health services. The reasons for this are complex and relate to accessibility,

cost, confidentiality and intimidation. In a Victorian study published by the Youth Health Development Council (1988) it was said that many young people perceive doctors as lacking sensitivity, in not taking young people's problems seriously, in not listening, being judgemental and using medical terminology that young people did not understand.

Doctors may need to adopt appropriate strategies if they are to address themselves to the major health issues confronting youth. The main ingredients for such strategies are as follows:

1. Awareness of the physical, psychological and developmental process of adolescence.

2. Sensitivity to youth who may really be using a physical complaint to provide an opportunity to discuss more important personal problems with their doctor.

3. Provision of some time to see the adolescent alone without parents.

4. A willingness to listen to teenagers, giving them time to feel comfortable in speaking about themselves.

5. Avoidance of attitudes that a teenager may interpret as condescending, patronizing or overbearing.

6. Willingness to comment on findings during the examination, giving reassurance about normal variations in development.

7. Willingness to explain the illness and its treatment in understandable terms.

8. Respect for a young person's wish for confidentiality.

Examination of an adolescent

Examination of the adolescent affords an opportunity to raise health issues and allow screening for the early precursors of adult disease. Some young people, particularly in early adolescence, prefer to have a parent present during examination. For others, the examination provides an opportunity to discuss aspects of body development and function that he or she is embarrassed to raise in front of parents.

In addition to the standard paediatric approach to history and examination taking, Example 66.2 provides a checklist especially relevant to the adolescent.

Confidentiality and consent

It is usually in the best interests of adolescents, especially if they are still living at home, for parents to be fully informed of their health problem, and to give consent for treatment and participate in care. If an adolescent does not want this, their views should be respected. For serious conditions, however, it is wise to

---

Example 66.2 A checklist during interview and examination of an adolescent

Historical information
1. The teenager's own perception of his problem as opposed to that presented by a parent
2. Family function: the presence of conflict and disturbed family relationships may profoundly affect an adolescent's ability to cope with ill-health
3. Cross-cultural conflict in an ethnic family affecting a youth's social behaviour
4. School problems relating to learning and behaviour
5. Peer relationships
6. Menstrual difficulties: 40% of girls report problems associated with menstruation
7. Sexual activity: many adolescents welcome the opportunity to discuss contraception and the risks of sexually transmitted disease
8. Alcohol, smoking and drug use and abuse
9. The adolescent's strengths and skills: often overlooked when parents present a litany of faults

Examination
1. Stature: comparison of height with mid-parental height
2. Pubertal rating using Tanner's scale
3. Nutrition with formal evaluation of obesity
4. Orthopaedic problems including scoliosis
5. Skin: acne, tinea, warts, naevi
6. Genital development
7. Visual acuity: myopia may present during early adolescence
8. Blood pressure: essential hypertension may become manifest at this age
9. Dental caries and malocclusion.

---

discuss why they do not wish their parents to be informed. In many cases it may be appropriate to help them discuss their health problem with the parents.

If the adolescent insists on not involving parents, the doctor must act in the best interests of the child. In some cases, particularly if surgical treatment is proposed, it may be essential to involve parents if treatment is to be provided. If this is not really necessary doctors may need to consider the legal situation in respect to their own professional conduct.

There has been no consistent Australian State legislation to provide for underage patients who seek confidentiality from their parents. The concept of the 'mature minor', however, appears acceptable. It follows that any treatment or advice offered to the adolescent will be given in good faith and be defensible in law as in the best interests of the patient. A mature minor is one who appears to the doctor to be of sufficient maturity to give a reliable history, who is capable of understanding the nature of the medical complaint, who understands the nature and possible side effects and complications of treatment, and who is likely to follow treatment recommendations safely and reliably. This is usually readily applied to the adolescent 16 years or over, particularly if living away from home or working. It requires very careful consideration if the individual is 14 or 15 years of age and would apply only in very exceptional circumstances to a younger adolescent.

COMMON HEALTH PROBLEMS OF ADOLESCENCE

In a clinic established to provide a health service to adolescents, accepting both referrals from general practitioners, schools and youth agencies as well as self-referrals, the common problems encountered are set out in Table 66.2.

Adolescents with chronic illness and disability

The clinical manifestations of chronic illness may change during adolescence. Diabetes, for instance, tends to be more unstable and it is during this time that microvascular complications may become evident. It seems likely that this and other changes in metabolic disease are hormone-dependent. Epileptic seizures, previously controlled on medication during childhood, may recur during adolescence. This may be because of omission of medication, but the physician may fail to realize the need for increasing dosage with rapid growth. Other childhood illness, such as asthma, may improve through adolescence, but at this time the teenager may neglect consistent prophylactic therapy.

Of greater importance are the psychological changes during adolescence that influence the expression of chronic disease, and the social and emotional response to chronic disability. Children at this age frequently

Table 66.2 Attendance at an adolescent health service (130 consecutive consultations, excluding trauma and emergencies)

Disorder	Consultation (number)
Medical	
Obesity	23
Anorexia nervosa	10
Orthopaedic disorders	11
Respiratory tract infection	13
Acne	7
Menstrual problems	6
Vision problems	4
Hearing difficulties	2
Hypertension	2
Problems related to chronic disorders	3
Other medical disorders	16
Psychosocial problems	
Behavioural problems	11
Family dysfunction	8
School learning problems	7
Depression	4
Psychosis	1
Sexual assault	2

deny their disorder, fail to comply with treatment and reject advice and guidance.

Exasperating though this is for the physician responsible for the youth's care, it is usually entirely consistent with the developmental process of adolescence. Adolescents have to complete developmental tasks of adolescence if they are to achieve a mature and balanced adult life. These tasks are:

1. To establish independence from parents
2. To seek self-identity and self-esteem
3. To achieve adult sexuality
4. To define their social place in the community, and establish plans for a life career.

Often these tasks are in conflict with the satisfactory care of chronic illness. In the process of becoming independent of parents, children often go too far: they rebel against reasonable advice and they reject, at least temporarily, values and standards expected by their parents. They resent being reminded to take medication, or keep to a diet, or maintain personal hygiene.

In seeking new relationships with peers, it may be of over-riding importance to identify with them. Chronic illness or disability makes an adolescent feel different, and this feeling is reinforced when medication has to be taken, or when they have to conform to treatment demands. A teenager with epilepsy who had recently had a seizure said 'Every time I take my anticonvulsant pills I know that I'm an epileptic. If I don't take my tablets it means to me I don't have epilepsy. The risk of seizures is a risk I think is worth taking just to feel normal.'

A further task is the need to develop self-esteem and the feeling of self-worth. This is sometimes frustrated by chronic illness and disability. Teenagers with spina bifida or cerebral palsy, for instance, may react poorly during adolescence to a disability that they have coped with well during their earlier childhood. The task of deciding a career and finding a worthwhile position in society makes chronic disability a further burden. Many people judge their worth by the work they do or how large their income is. Inability to gain employment, or doubts on the future are further handicaps for the adolescent, who as a young child had felt secure within the supportive protection of his family.

The doctor caring for such adolescents may:

1. Help the adolescent sort out priorities for development and take responsibility for self-care. This may take time – perhaps years.

2. Support teenagers in their attempts to gain mastery over themselves and come to terms with their health problems.

3. Support the family, whose anxieties may increase over the adolescent years. The mother's role as care provider may be in part rejected, yet she may see her child's health neglected. The subsequent conflicts leave her frustrated and her child angry.

4. Take into account the changing physiological development of adolescents. There may be a need to re-evaluate drug dosage, nutritional advice, and the emergence of associated health problems, such as impaired visual acuity, sexual difficulties and acne.

5. Evaluate growth and sexual maturation as an index of the child's progress through puberty. Delayed puberty may be the consequence of inadequate treatment, and may further damage a child's developing self-esteem.

6. Enquire into school progress: this is an age when children under stress react badly to school. There may be difficulties imposed by school absence or by the handicap of the disease and its treatment. The school may be unaware of this or have insufficient facilities to provide remedial teaching or counselling.

Social issues

Many health problems of young people relate to social issues. Only 50% of Australian teenagers complete their schooling to year 12, the lowest percentages being from the lower socioeconomic groups and those living in the urban fringes. Of Australian 15- to 19-year-olds, 16% are unemployed. These are especially early school leavers, girls, the disabled and Aboriginal youth. Over 20% of children and young people are in families receiving Social Security supportive payment.

There are many government and voluntary agencies providing services for youth. These include family planning clinics, youth counselling services, drug abuse programmes, refuges and hostels. Referral to such agencies, that may have expertise and resources unavailable to the general practitioner, may be the most appropriate action for many of the psychosocial problems that confront the troubled adolescent in our society.

Sexuality

Many young people are concerned about their sexual feelings, about sex and personal relationships, and about variations in their own sexual development. Sexual activity may be both pleasurable and stressful or confusing. Many young people face moral issues when peer pressure or physiological urges are in conflict with family, cultural or religious mores. Teenagers may be torn between family attitudes towards sex, warnings about protective behaviour to avoid sexual abuse on the one hand and, on the other, the more open attitude of society towards sexual education, exploration and enjoyment.

There are increasing concerns about sexual violence, including incest, rape and harassment. Although most victims are girls, many boys have been sexually abused. Many teenaged youths, who may themselves have been the victims of sexual abuse, become the abusers and will also need help.

Unwanted pregnancy, and the difficulties facing the single teenaged mother and her child, are major issues in adolescence. Figures from the United States show that 50% of 15- to 19-year-old unmarried girls have had intercourse, and 70% of 17- to 21-year-old males. Adolescents tend not to use contraception, and those that do, do so unreliably. 11% of clients of Family Planning Association clinics in Victoria are under the age of 16 years.

Girls do not use contraception for a number of reasons, which include: lack of or misinformation, lack of access, unplanned sex, fear of loss of confidentiality, feelings of morality about contraception, feeling of invulnerability (I – or you – won't get pregnant) and lack of motivation to consider the consequences.

Many young girls seek contraceptive advice without the knowledge of their parents, and this may pose a concern for a general practitioner who is also the family doctor. Parents who discover their daughters are on the pill respond commonly with anger and a conviction that their child would not have been sexually active if contraception was not prescribed. Some are hurt that they were not confided in, and some are worried about side effects: good reasons why a doctor would usually suggest that a young adolescent should confide in her parents. It has been estimated that over 33 000 teenage girls in Australia become pregnant each year, 40% of these pregnancies result in abortion and 31% lead to birth outside marriage.

Menstrual problems

Menstrual problems are common in adolescent girls. In a survey of secondary schoolgirls in Victoria, 40% said they had concerns about menstrual periods. Worry about dysmenorrhoea and delayed menarche, irregularity and variable bleeding are common. Whereas simple advice, reassurance and appropriate use of analgesics will be sufficient care for most girls, some have disabling dysmenorrhoea and merit active medication with prostaglandin inhibitors. For some, especially those who are sexually active or potentially so, administration of the pill may be more appropriate.

Sexually transmitted disease (STD)

This has become increasingly common, especially amongst the young. In the United States, 75% of all cases of STD are amongst the 15- to 24-year-old age group. Of young people between the ages of 15–25, 10–15% will get a sexually transmitted disease. Conditions most likely to be encountered are *Chlamydia trachomatis*, often presenting as non-specific urethritis, Herpes simplex genitalis, genital and anal warts due to papillovirus, and *Neisseria gonorrhoeae* infections. The risk of pelvic inflammatory disease and subsequent sterility arising from STD has become increasingly recognized in teenage girls.

Adolescent risk-taking behaviour such as explorative sexual activity, unprotected sex, and sharing of IV drug needles, put teenagers at risk for HIV infection. US experience indicated that AIDS may become a significant issue for adolescent health in Western society.

Alcohol, smoking and drugs

Alcohol consumption has steadily increased amongst teenagers in Western society. In a survey amongst Victorian secondary school children, 46% of year 7 students, 80% of year 9 students and 92% of year 11 students had had alcohol. Males are more likely to drink heavily than females. Some 30% of females and 43% of males of year 11 had had five or more drinks consecutively at least once in the previous fortnight during the survey.

In the same survey, 48% of year 7 students, 70% of year 9 students and 78% of year 11 students had smoked. 30% of males and 38% of females in year 11 were smoking at present. A further Australian survey suggested that 43% of 16- to 19-year-old females smoke.

Marijuana smoking is much less common amongst younger adolescents in Australia. Of year 7 students 3.4% stated that they had used marijuana. This rose to 16% of year 9 students and 26.7% of year 11 students.

Recent reports indicate that volatile solvent abuse, including glue sniffing, has become common amongst younger adolescents, though most have stopped glue sniffing in their middle teens. Volatile solvent abuse can lead acutely to coma and cardiorespiratory depression, and there have been cases of suffocation from plastic bags used for the solvent. Chronic abuse can lead to damage to the nervous system, kidneys and liver.

Teenagers frequently use prescription and other drugs and medications. In Australia the survey indicated that 95% of teenagers have used analgesics, 25% tranquillisers and 18% of year 11 students have used sedatives. Teenagers have little difficulty in acquiring such drugs. They are often taken from parents, but are also obtained on prescription from a doctor. Drug overdosage may occur with young people experimenting with combinations of drugs. This is an important mode of attempted suicide, most commonly in girls. Many such overdosages represent a desperate gesture and plea for help rather than a true attempt to end life.

Most adolescents surveyed on their attitudes to alcohol and smoking do not acknowledge that they have a problem. However, some may seek help with an entrenched smoking habit or may be referred because of family or school concerns about drinking. Some may be referred by the Children's Court after conviction for an alcohol-related offence.

In helping young people to make decisions to change their drinking, smoking or drug-taking habit, it is useful to understand why young people take recreational drugs.

Many young adolescents and children start to drink or smoke as an experiment, and most have had their first cigarette or drink well before puberty.

Adolescents continue to smoke or drink alcohol for a number of reasons which may be important to them at the time. These include:

1. To help them relate socially to each other
2. As a means to help them identify with adulthood
3. An expression of rebellion
4. To enhance self-esteem
5. To compensate for frustration
6. To get pleasure and an altered state of mind.

It is obvious that it will be a very long time before the problem of smoking, drug and alcohol abuse in adolescence can be overcome.

REFERENCES

Carmichael A – Personal communication
Parcel G S, Narder P R, Meyer M P 1977 Adolescent health concerns, problems and patterns of utilisation in a urban population. Paediatrics 60: 157–164
Tanner J M 1962 Growth at adolescence. Blackwell Scientific Publications, Oxford
World Health Organization 1989 The health of youth. WHO, Geneva
Youth Health Development Council 1988 Health for youth. Health Department of Victoria, Melbourne

FURTHER READING

Bennett D L 1984 Adolescent health in Australia. An overview of needs and approaches to care. Australian Medical Association
Blum R W 1982 Adolescent health care. Academic Press, New York
Wilson J 1982 The teenager and you. Spectrum Publications, Melbourne

The skin

67. The neonate with a rash

George A. Varigos, Peter Fergin

ERYTHEMA

Several causes of neonatal erythema will be discussed but the most frequent ones include salmon patches and harlequin colour changes.

Salmon patches

Salmon patches (stork bites) are very common, being reported to occur in 35% of boys and 40% of girls. They comprise vascular ectasia without endothelial proliferation. They are commonly seen on the nape of the neck, as pink salmon-coloured flat lesions, and may also be seen on the upper eyelids, forehead and lip. The lesions fade in the first year of life, although those on the nape of the neck may persist.

Port wine stain (naevus flammeus)

Naevus flammeus affects less than 1% of the population, (Jacobs & Walton 1976, Pratt 1953), is usually seen at birth and can affect any site, but commonly the face. The lesions usually persist, and some can cover large areas. The colour of the naevus can vary, and depends on the size of vessel ectasia and the number of erythrocyte-filled vessels (Finley et al 1984). Associations with deeper structures and CNS changes have been reported.

Harlequin colour change

This is commonly observed over the first four days to three weeks of life in premature infants. Because of an immaturity of control of peripheral blood vessel tone, episodes of erythema of one (bottom) half of the body may occur, thus producing a sharp longitudinal demarcation, which is often obliterated by the flush caused by crying. The episodes last from only a few seconds to 20 minutes and there is a corresponding blanching of the upper half of the body.

In body folds

Other common causes of erythema in body folds are seborrhoeic dermatitis, flexural psoriasis and intertrigo from sweat irritation. Usually other signs of psoriasis or seborrhoeic dermatitis are present. Perianal erythema may develop from frequent loose bowel actions.

Candidiasis

Candidiasis of the nappy area involves the inguinal folds and results in erythematous eroded areas with an attached peripheral scale. Discrete satellite pustules are often present. Skin scrapings rapidly confirm the diagnosis. Nystatin, or one of the imidazole creams (clotrimazole, econazole or miconazole), produces a rapid improvement.

Cutis marmorata

The appearance of a mottled pattern due to vasodilation in a net or branching configuration is called cutis marmarata. The reaction may be a physiological response to cold, and continues to be seen in childhood. Occasionally, it may be associated with Down syndrome or other internal disorders. It should not be confused with a naevoid pattern, which is persistent.

Acrocyanosis

Acrocyanosis is a bilateral and symmetric bluish discoloration of hands and feet, which settles over several weeks. The features can be seen to be more pronounced in hyperviscosity states and hypothermia.

PUSTULES AND PAPULES

Toxic erythema (erythema toxicum)

This is a benign, self-limiting reaction consisting of erythema with pustules and papules over the face, trunk and limbs, sparing the palms and sides. It is relatively common: 30–70% of all neonates are affected. Onset is usually during the first two days of life, or up to two weeks. Recurring attacks, lasting several days each, are seen. The aetiology is unknown, but smears and histology show a sterile eosinophilic tissue response, which should be differentiated from incontinentia pigmenti and other infective causes of pustules. Toxic erythema requires no treatment and has no systemic associates.

Miliara neonatorum

This vesicular pustular papular grouped eruption is caused by blockage and subsequent rupture of eccrine ducts. Sweat in the dermis results in inflammation and a more marked lesion. The sites are usually the trunk, buttocks, napkin area and flexures. Secondary infection by bacteria may occur.

Milia

Milia are small epidermal inclusion cysts appearing as white pearly firm papules 1–2 mm in diameter. About 50% of newborns have milia on their faces, appearing after birth and usually fading after one month. No treatment is necessary. If widespread, genodermatoses should be considered.

Hypertrophied sebaceous glands

These small whitish papules on the nose and cheeks are common. Obstruction may produce a folliculitis, as in acne vulgaris. The lesions resolve after three to six months and no treatment is necessary unless more troublesome acne neonatorum develops.

In older infants, irritation caused by dribbling saliva, food contact and secondary infection by bacteria and sometimes *Candida* results in discrete folliculitis in the perioral region.

Transient neonatal pustular melanosis

This condition is marked by vesicular or pustular lesions present at birth and leaving a collarette of scale and pigmentation. It occurs on the face, limbs, trunk, palms and sides. No infective aetiology has been found.

Acropustulosis

Cyclical episodes of groups of sterile pustules lasting 10–14 weeks, and continuing with fewer lesions enduring at two or three years of age, is known as acropustulosis. No eosinophils are seen in the lesions.

SCALING IN NEONATES

Physiological desquamation shortly after birth is very common and of no consequence. A more severe, but equally benign, form occurs in post-mature neonates. 'Cradle cap' is very common, and is usually due to persistent dried vernix and desquamating epidermis inadequately removed after birth because of fear of traumatizing the fontanelle area. Seborrhoeic dermatitis also typically involves this area with a greasy, yellowish scale, but it rarely appears before the age of three to four weeks. Persistent dry, scaly skin may suggest one of the inherited disorders of keratinization (ichthyoses).

BULLOUS LESIONS

Bullous impetigo

The most common cause of blisters affecting neonates is bullous impetigo. Flaccid blisters with clear or cloudy fluid are present in the nappy area and elsewhere, and respond rapidly to appropriate antibiotics. The most common infection is a combination of *Staphylococcus aureus* and *Streptococcus* sp.

Mechanobullous disorders (epidermolysis bullosa)

Blistering at sites of trauma from birth may suggest the possibility of one of the inherited mechanobullous disorders.

PLAQUES

Neonatal lupus erythematosus

Erythematous plaques on the head may be seen in neonatal lupus erythematosus and may develop within one or two weeks of birth. The central portion may become depressed and there may be hair loss, scaling and telangiectasia. The histology and direct immunofluorescence is identical to adult cutaneous lupus erythematosus. Cardiac involvement (heart block) may occur. The mother may have lupus erythematosus or may develop it soon after the birth of the infant. Neonatal lupus erythematosus usually resolves in a few months.

REFERENCES

Finley J L, Arndt K A, Noe J, Rosen S 1984 Argon laser – port-wine stain interaction. Archives of Dermatology 120: 613–619

Jacobs A H, Walton R G 1976 The incidence of birthmarks in the neonate. Paediatrics 58: 218–222

Pratt A G 1953 Birthmarks in infants. AMA Archives of Dermatology and Syphilology 67: 302–305

68. The child with a rash

Peter Fergin

The diagnosis and management of skin disorders fundamentally relies on history taking skills and a thorough clinical examination. The history should include a chronology of development of lesions and associated symptoms – especially the presence or absence of itching and symptoms of internal disease. Enquiry for a past or family history is often useful, e.g. scabies. Specific questioning regarding drug intake or medication applied is essential.

The clinical examination must take place in good lighting and with the child fully undressed. Examination of the oral cavity, hair and nails is part of the routine examination of the skin. A general physical examination is always indicated.

Cutaneous lesions are classified often into primary and secondary lesions (see Example 68.1).

Often, various combinations of lesions are present in the one patient and may vary during the course of the illness. Accurate intermittent observation and description may be necessary to establish a diagnosis.

Investigation may be necessary. Skin biopsies are a convenient and useful technique for sampling cutaneous lesions to establish a diagnosis. Small lesions can be wholly removed by excision. Such specimens may also be submitted for special staining, direct immunofluorescence and electron microscopy.

Microscopic examination of skin scraping dissolved in 20% potassium hydroxide solution may confirm the presence of dermatophyte or *Monilia* infection. Culture of skin scrapings or nail clippings in Sabouraud's or other special media may be necessary to identify the organism involved. Examination of the scalp with a Wood's lamp (long-wave ultraviolet light) may detect green fluorescing hair infected by dermatophyte fungi and is a simple means of confirming the diagnosis of tinea capitis.

COMMON INFLAMMATORY DISORDERS

Atopic dermatitis (infantile eczema)

This is one of the most common skin disorders of children. It can be a very distressful condition for both the child and parents because of the persistent itching. The most common time of onset is at about three months of age. Itchy, erythematous, scaly patches on the cheeks usually present first; similar lesions may develop on the forehead and trunk but any part of the body may be involved. The lesions may be vesicular and subsequently weep (ooze plasma). Persistent crusting and scattered pustules may signal secondary infection (usually due to *Staphylococcus aureus*) and sleep disturbance may occur because of itching. Chronic lichenification of the popliteal and cubital fossae of older children is a characteristic feature (Fig. 68.1).

The cause of atopic dermatitis is uncertain. Frequently, a family history of atopic disorders can be elicited. Elevated immunoglobulin E levels are found in most patients, and decreased cell-mediated immunity may be present in some. Other abnormalities of phagocytes may be detected, but are variable in quality and quantity. Positive prick tests to multiple environmental allergens are frequently found, but hyposensitization does not

---

Example 68.1 Cutaneous lesions

Primary lesions include:

Macules – Small, flat changes of colour
Patches are large macules

Papules – Elevated, solid lesions less than 5 mm diameter
Nodules and tumours are larger

Plaques – Elevated, solid lesions which have a diameter far greater than their height

Vesicles – Small blisters

Bullae – Large blisters

Pustules – Opaque vesicles

Secondary changes include:

Weeping, crusting, scaling, ulceration, excoriation and lichenification from persistent rubbing. Ultimately atrophic, hypertrophic or keloidal scarring may result.

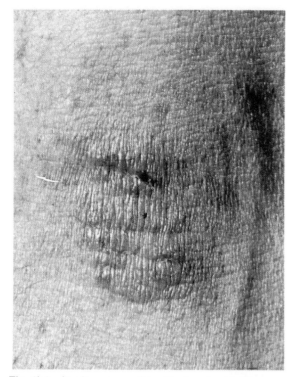

Fig. 68.1 Atopic eczema – lichenification of cubital fossa.

help in the management. The association of food intolerance with the pathogenesis of eczema is controversial as the majority of cases are managed successfully without any form of dietary manipulation. Non-specific aggravating factors include sweat, overheating and rough or woollen materials worn next to the skin. Spells of cold weather with low humidity can precipitate cracking of the skin. Atopic dermatitis is a chronic relapsing disorder for which no cure can be offered, although spontaneous improvement occurs in childhood. However, this improvement often takes months or years. Parents should be reassured that resolution will occur and no permanent scarring of the skin will develop. The most effective treatment involves the regular application of corticosteroid preparations; hydrocortisone 1% b.d. to q.i.d. is usually sufficient for infants with this disorder. For older children, the weaker fluorinated steroids suffice, e.g. Betamethasone 17 Valerate 0.02%; these should not be applied to the face and nappy areas. Occasionally half strength (0.5%) fluorinated steroid creams are used to small, persistent areas in older children. In general, creams are more soothing to acutely inflamed or weeping areas while ointments are more useful for dry and cracked lesions. Emollient creams and oils are frequently necessary, as generalized dry skin

(xeroderma) or even ichthyosis is a common association. Soap to the active areas should be avoided as should woollen clothing next to the bare skin and too much clothing. Nocturnal sedation is often very useful. Appropriate antibiotics are indicated for episodes of secondary infections and tar preparations for localized areas of lichenification on limbs. As this condition is a relapsing one, treatment should be maintained even when the skin is better. For maintenance treatment, the weakest steroid preparation necessary to control the lesions is indicated.

Special forms of atopic eczema

Eczema herpeticum. This occurs because of superinfection of active eczema by herpes simplex virus when discrete, umbilicated vesicles and pustules may develop rapidly. The patient may be febrile and toxic. Patients are usually admitted to hospital and barrier nursed. Antibiotics and antiviral chemotherapy (acyclovir) are usually indicated.

Juvenile plantar dermatosis. This form of atopic eczema is persistent erythema, scaling and cracking of the pressure bearing areas of the feet of primary school children. Sometimes itching may occur. Treatment involves the frequent application of emollient creams or low-potency steroid ointments. Cotton socks and leather-soled shoes and sandals are desirable. Treatment should be maintained until resolution occurs – usually by early puberty.

Pityriasis alba. Characterized by hypopigmented, slightly scaly patches on the cheeks of young children. They are usually manifested in summer when the non-affected skin tans. Hydrocortisone ointment or an emollient cream usually suffices; soap to these areas should be avoided.

Infantile seborrhoeic dermatitis

This condition, which is distinct from eczema, begins at about six weeks of age and is only mildly itchy. Erythematous patches covered with a greasy, yellow scale are present on the scalp, forehead and eyebrows. Scattered patches develop a little later on the trunk together with areas of erythema in the axillae and in the nappy area. Persistently weeping and infected patches behind the ears are common. The lesions may spread initially for a few weeks before resolving spontaneously after two or three months. Topical hydrocortisone is usually adequate.

Napkin dermatitis

This condition is regarded as an irritant dermatitis due

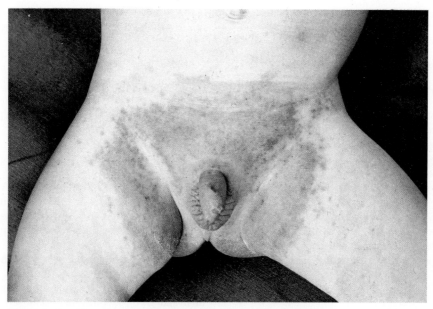

Fig. 68.2 Napkin dermatitis. Note the sparing of the inguinal folds.

to the action of several factors acting at the same time on a sensitive skin. These include urine, faeces, occlusion, friction (e.g. inner thighs) and pressure (e.g. over ischial tuberosities in children sitting in soiled nappies in car seats for prolonged periods). Secondary infection with bacteria and *Candida* is common, as is miliaria and occlusion folliculitis.

The erythema is evident on the convexities with sparing in the folds (Fig. 68.2), which is particularly noticeable in chubby infants. If the skin is allowed to dehydrate, a glazed appearance develops in 15–20 minutes, when scaling and cracking appears. Localized, thick-walled vesicles may appear on buttocks and pubis resulting in punched out ulcers which heal without scarring.

Meatal ulceration of circumcised males is a special variant of erosive napkin dermatitis. Occasionally bluish-red nodules develop in these areas (granuloma gluteale infantum). They are benign and resolve after several weeks (Fig. 68.3).

In treatment, frequent changing of nappies is essential. If the nappy is soiled, bathing is the most efficient and least irritating way of cleaning the area. Thick layers of zinc cream or paste as an inert barrier is often the only preparation needed. In addition, hydrocortisone 1% may be used if eczema, seborrhoeic dermatitis or psoriasis is also present. Anticandidal agents are used when indicated. Talc-based powders should be avoided as they can be abrasive, but cornstarch powder may be

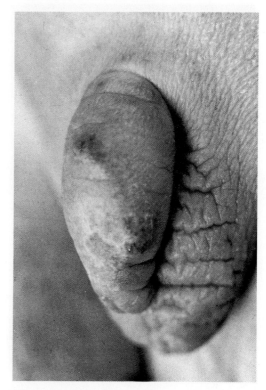

Fig. 68.3 Granuloma gluteale infantum – Blue-red nodules persisting for weeks.

useful. Treatment must be maintained until toilet training occurs.

Phytodermatitis

Contact dermatitis from plants is not rare. Ragweed pollen dermatitis and *Rhus* (poison ivy) dermatitis are extremely common problems in the US. Plants can induce skin disease via a number of mechanisms, e.g. prickles, foreign body granuloma, irritant hand dermatitis (tulips) and airborne contact dermatitis (Ragweed pollen). *Rhus* dermatitis develops from contact with any part of the *Rhus* plant. A linear vesicular or bullous eruption of the limbs is common. Vesiculation and oedema of the face is characteristic (Fig. 68.4). Fluorinated steroids topically, and at times oral steroids, may be required to obtain rapid improvement. The diagnosis can be confirmed by careful skin testing.

Phytophotodermatitis

This may occur from contact with plants containing psoralens, e.g. carrot tops, parsnip, parsley, and a num-

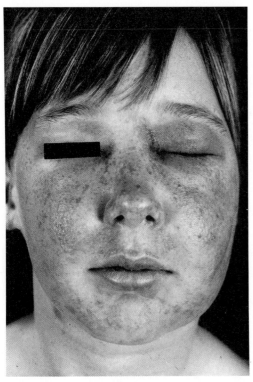

Fig. 68.4 Rhus dermatitis.

ber of weeds. A phototoxic erythema is precipitated if sun exposure occurs soon after contact with wet plants.

Psoriasis

Psoriasis can develop in any age group. In infants, involvement of the napkin area may occur and appears as sharply marginated erythema. Other typical lesions of psoriasis are usually present elsewhere.

Guttate psoriasis

This may develop suddenly in children and teenagers one to two weeks after streptococcal tonsillitis, when a shower of small, red scaly spots develops rapidly on the trunk. Many of these lesions resolve spontaneously in two to three months.

Plaques on the knees, elbows and in the scalp, are the common manifestations of psoriasis in teenagers (psoriasis vulgaris). Less common forms (flexural, pustular and erythrodermic) can occur with associated nail dystrophy and arthritis.

Tar and corticosteroid application are often successful in the treatment of psoriasis. Also, ultraviolet light and dithranol preparations may be used, and 0.5% crude coal tar (CCT) in zinc cream is useful for napkin psoriasis.

Urticaria

Urticaria may be defined as transient erythema, which usually lasts less than 24 hours. Itching and oedema are frequent accompaniments. Sometimes recurring localized oedema (angio-oedema) is the only manifestation. Most cases are acute, but some may persist for weeks or months.

The mechanisms involved in urticaria are:

1. Type 1 allergy – here tissue (mast cell) fixing IgE is produced in response to a number of allergens e.g. infection, drugs and food.

2. Type 111 allergy – when immune complex deposits in the skin vessels result in longer lasting painful urticarial lesions associated with arthralgia and fever, e.g. serum sickness, urticarial lesions in connective tissue disorders and in Henoch-Schönlein purpura.

3. Physical urticarias – less commonly urticaria is due to trauma (dermographism), exercise (cholinergic), sun, water, heat, pressure and cold. Cold urticaria may be associated with conditions producing cryoglobulins and cold agglutinins.

A careful history and examination is very important

to elicit the aetiology; indiscriminate investigations are rarely of practical benefit and the relevance of allergy tests is often difficult to interpret. Unfortunately, in many patients the cause is not obvious despite extensive investigation.

A diary of food intake in relation to attacks may be useful in diagnosis. Antihistamine therapy is the mainstay of treatment. Occasionally, total suppression of the lesions occurs, but more often some diminution of itch and erythema is achieved. Avoidance of foods containing salicylate, preservatives and tartrazine dyes has been demonstrated to be helpful in about 75% of cases. It should be noted that some antihistamine drugs contain tartrazine dyes and should be avoided; promethazine and cyproheptadine are satisfactory. Phosphodiesterase inhibitors may also help. Soothing applications, such as menthol 1% in calamine, are also quite useful. Oral steroids should be used only in special circumstances and for a short time, as this condition, even though long lasting, is benign.

Idiopathic immune complex urticaria appears to have a benign prognosis but renal involvement should be excluded. In all cases of angio-oedema the possibility of hereditary angio-oedema should be considered.

Granuloma annulare

This is a benign idiopathic inflammatory lesion of the dermis that may be present on hands, feet, elbows, and knees. The lesions begin as smooth, flesh-coloured papules that become annular, coalesce and appear serpiginous (Fig. 68.5). The central portion flattens and resolves. The lesions of granuloma annulare develop over many months and eventually resolve spontaneously without producing scarring; sometimes subcutaneous nodules may be present. Fluorinated steroids under occlusion, or intralesion steroid therapy may induce resolution.

PHOTOSENSITIVITY IN CHILDREN

This is not rare and children of all ages are subject to photosensitivity eruptions. A group of disorders known as polymorphous light eruptions may produce recurring erythematous, itchy vesicular papules on the cheeks, ears, side of neck and exposed limbs. The onset of the eruption may be delayed one or two days after sun exposure but the distribution of the lesions and history of exacerbation in the summer months is typical. Occasionally, lesions are transient and develop within a few minutes of sun exposure (solar urticaria) or are crusted and produce varioliform scarring. These eruptions are

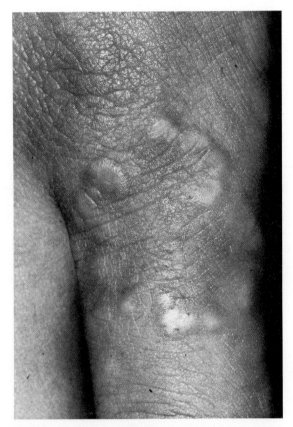

Fig. 68.5 Granuloma annulare.

chronic, but ultimately resolve. Action spectra are variable and include UVB and UVA wavelengths.

Other causes of photosensitivity in children include:

Drugs – these may be topical, e.g. sunscreens, or systemic, e.g. phenothiazines, antihistamines.

Lupus erythematosus – persistent, erythematous plaques of the face are classical, but solar urticaria and exaggerated sunburn (phototoxicity) may also occur.

Porphyria – these are rare but important disorders to exclude as systemic disorders may be associated, e.g. progressive liver disease in erythropoietic protoporphyria.

Rare inherited conditions that include albinism, PKU, Hartnup's syndrome and xeroderma pigmentosum.

Polymorphous light eruption is a diagnosis by exclusion and probably a skin biopsy and porphyrin estimations ought to be performed in all such patients. Avoidance of excessive sun exposure is essential through modifying life style, appropriate clothing and regular application of broad spectrum (UVA and UVB) sunscreens. Topical cortisone creams are often helpful. Antimalarials may be useful in lupus erythematosus and β-carotene in erythropoietic protoporphyria.

BACTERIAL INFECTIONS

Impetigo (school sores)

This is a superficial skin infection caused by *Streptococcus pyogenes* and/or *Staphylococcus aureus*. Honey-coloured crusts on an erythematous base develop in a few days and are often localized to one area of the body. Bullous lesions may be present in infants and sometimes in older children.

The lesions of impetigo respond to an appropriate antibiotic (flucloxacillin is probably the drug of choice) and the use of an antiseptic topically. Glomerulonephritis is an occasional complication of impetigo.

Boils (furunculosis)

Boils are due to staphylococcal infection of hair follicles. A topical antiseptic may be required in addition to a systemic antibiotic to rid the skin of surface bacteria which may cause reinfection when the oral antibiotic course ceases.

Staphylococcal scalded skin syndrome

A toxin produced by a particular *S. aureus* (phage type 71) causes this disorder in infants. It is characterized by the sudden onset of a generalized erythema and tenderness followed by dramatic shedding of sheets of epidermis, which begins in the perioral and nappy areas (Fig. 68.6). The infant is generally not unwell and the condition may spontaneously resolve in a week or two because the site of cleavage is superficial (subcorneal). Admission to hospital is usually necessary to monitor the fluid and electrolyte losses through the skin; cloxacillin should be administered.

Cellulitis

Cellulitis is a frequent bacterial infection of the skin of infants and children. The involved skin is red or reddish-blue, tender, slightly raised and indurated. Any area of the body may be affected, but it is very common over the face and the periorbital region. In past years the beta-haemolytic streptococcus was the major cause, but in the current era *S. aureus* and *Haemophilus influenzae* are the commonest pathogens. Children with

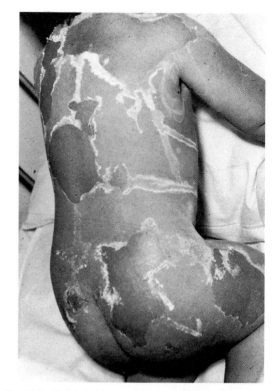

Fig. 68.6 Scalded skin syndrome.

cellulitis may be constitutionally ill; this is more common with cellulitis due to *H. influenzae* when the affected area may have a distinctly bluish colour. On other occasions children with cellulitis may have little constitutional upset. When the periorbital region is involved there may be sufficient swelling to prevent the child from opening the eyes. Eye movement is present in periorbital cellulitis in contradistinction to orbital cellulitis when the globe is fixed.

Diagnosis is made on the clinical picture and from blood culture. Needle aspiration and culture at the border of the lesion after instillation of a few drops of saline may provide the diagnosis, but this is usually not necessary.

Treatment is determined by the particular organism involved. Should the child be unwell, a combination of flucloxacillin and chloramphenicol will give reasonable cover until the organism is identified by culture. In children who are less toxic flucloxacillin given orally may be adequate. This is particularly appropriate in the older child. Periorbital and orbital cellulitis should be watched very carefully. Intracranial extension occasionally follows orbital cellulitis and in periorbital cellulitis the paranasal sinuses may be involved. Close co-operation with the ophthalmologist and/or ENT surgeon will be essential under these circumstances.

VIRAL INFECTIONS

Warts

Warts are benign tumours of the epidermis induced by inoculation of specific papova viruses. Several dozen serological types have been identified, some of which correspond to different clinical types. They may be classified as follows:

1. Common warts (verruca vulgaris). These are flesh-coloured papules with a rough top, found commonly on the fingers. However, they can be found anywhere on the body.
2. Periungual warts are notoriously resistant to treatment.
3. Plantar warts occur over pressure sites on the feet. They are usually tender and may not protrude above the skin surface level. Mosaic warts are a special form of plantar wart where multiple warts are so closely situated that they form largish verrucous plaques.
4. Plane warts are multiple, small, flat, slightly verrucous papules often on dorsum of hands and face. Scratching may result in autoinoculation to produce linear lesions.
5. Filiform (or digitate) warts are usually single and found on the face and scalp. They consist of a small cluster of spikes or fingerlike projections.
6. Genital warts (condylomata acuminata) are transmitted by sexual contact and are more commonly found in teenagers and young adults. Perianal warts in children may indicate sexual abuse. They present as cauliflower-like papules with a narrow stalk on the genitalia (especially under the foreskin) as well as in the perianal region.

Warts are typically benign infections that persist for months or years and finally resolve spontaneously. No systemic agents are effective so that each lesion has to be treated individually. Small numbers of warts may be eradicated by curettage, diathermy, or excision. Cryotherapy is a successful modality for many types of warts and some children tolerate this treatment well. Treatments at two- to four-weekly intervals are administered until all warts have resolved. Various keratolytics (e.g. salicylic acid), caustics (e.g. silver nitrate) and irritants (e.g. podophyllin) may be as successful as cryotherapy, if the treatment is long term. A solution of 3% formalin as foot soaks is useful for mosaic and multiple warts. Stubborn lesions may be treated with DNCB (dinitrochlorobenzene) as a form of immunotherapy.

Molluscum contagiosum

These are small, umbilicated pearly papules in groups. Sometimes itching and patchy eczema is associated. These lesions are caused by inoculation of a pox virus and may persist for months before spontaneous resolution occurs. Acute, pustular inflammation may occur just before resolution and result in scarring. Treatment is along the same lines as for warts. Cryotherapy is very effective.

Recurrent herpes simplex

Present as small, grouped vesicles on an erythematous base. An itching or burning sensation may precede the blisters which heal in one to two weeks. They are seen most frequently over the perioral and perinasal regions and on the genitalia. They typically recur in the same area at variable intervals. Genital herpes (HSV 2) can be distinguished serologically from other types (HSV 1). Herpes simplex are seen on the fingers (whitlow; Fig. 68.7) buttock and thighs. Eyelid lesions may be associated with dendritic corneal ulcers. Viricidal agents, administered topically or systemically, may reduce the severity of the eruptions but will not prevent future episodes, which tend to be precipitated by intercurrent infections, sun exposure, and menstruation. The

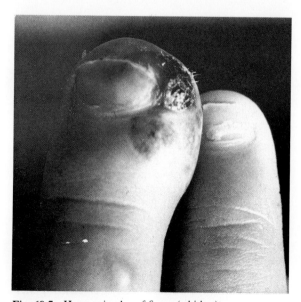

Fig. 68.7 Herpes simplex of finger (whitlow).

viricidal agents may be used as early as possible in an attack. Topically idoxuridine is useful and acyclovir is useful for severe infections especially in the immune suppressed.

Pityriasis rosea

This is a common eruption thought to be due to an infectious agent, as yet unidentified. Fawn-coloured, oval, scaly patches develop rapidly on the trunk and limbs. The longitudinal diameters of the oval patches are parallel to Langer's lines. An initial larger patch may be present some days before the multiple lesions erupt (herald spot). Usually a collarette of scale is present in some of the lesions; itching may be mild to moderate, but can be troublesome.

The condition lasts for about one to two months and resolves spontaneously. Usually steroids control the itching until spontaneous resolution occurs.

FUNGAL INFECTIONS

In Australian children, fungal infections of the skin (tinea) are usually due to *Microsporum canis* acquired from cats and dogs.

Tinea corporis

Tinea corporis begins as small, scaly itchy erythematous annular patches that become confluent and last a few weeks. Culture of skin scrapings confirms the diagnosis.

Tinea capitis

This is manifest as scaly patches with associated hair loss. Small broken-off infected hairs are normally present, which fluoresce a pale green colour when illuminated with a Wood's lamp (Fig. 68.8).

Treatment

For mild tinea corporis, topical antifungal therapy, such as imidazole creams or Whitfield's ointment, may suffice. However, oral griseofulvin for several weeks is necessary for more extensive skin infections and all scalp infections.

Kerion

This is an acute fungus inflammation in which tender, pustular plaques develop rapidly on the scalp or limbs; these lesions may be fluctuant. Kerion infection is often

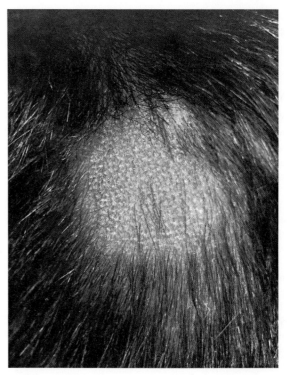

Fig. 68.8 Tinea capitis – a scaly patch with short hairs growing in it. These short hairs fluoresce a pale green when illuminated with a Wood's lamp.

due to *M. canis* but other fungi from animals or soil may be incriminated. Cultures are often negative and the lesions usually do not exhibit fluorescence. Prolonged administration of griseofulvin may be necessary for their resolution (Fig. 68.9).

PARASITIC INFESTATIONS

Scabies

This is a superficial infestation by a mite (*Sarcoptes scabiei*) transmitted by close personal contact. Itching first develops some three to four weeks after the infection is acquired. Non-specific erythematous papular lesions are often present on the trunk (Fig. 68.10) and vesicular lesion burrows in the finger webs, wrist and in the genitalia; involvement of the head and neck occurs only in infants. Secondary infection of lesions on the hands may occur and other family members may be affected. The diagnosis is confirmed by identifying the female mite in scrapings from burrows or vesicles (Fig. 68.11).

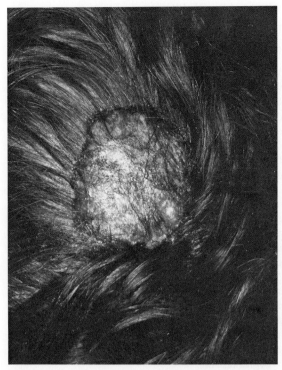

Fig. 68.9 Kerion – a boggy, tender crusted swelling of the scalp – an inflammatory form of ringworm.

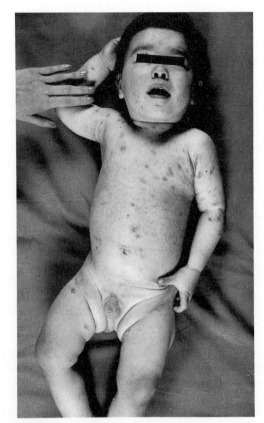

Fig. 68.10 Scabies.

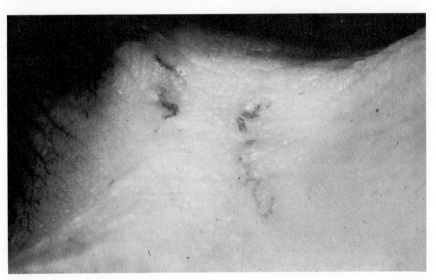

Fig. 68.11 Scabies burrows of interdigital spaces of the hands.

Benzyl benzoate (25% lotion), applied from the neck down, is usually curative. All itching contacts should be treated at the same time and bed clothes need to be laundered normally. A 10% crotamiton lotion (Eurax), applied twice daily, is an alternative treatment. Gammabenzenehexachloride 1% cream is also an efficient preparation, but this must not be used continuously as repeated application may result in significant absorption and CNS toxicity. Occasionally, itchy, red nodules may persist after successful treatment. These post-scabetic nodules do not indicate active infestation but may require topical or intralesional steroid therapy.

Lice

Lice infestation of the scalp and hair is a common problem in school children. Infestation occurs through close contact with infested fomites (e.g. combs, hats, etc).

Head lice infestation is due to *Phthirus capitis*. The cardinal symptom is itching of the occiput. Excoriation, eczematous patches and impetigo may also be present. Careful inspection of the hair usually reveals small, pearly nits (egg capsules) attached firmly to the shafts; lice are rarely seen. A single application of malathion 0.5% or gammabenzenehexachloride 1% is usually curative. A fine-toothed comb may be necessary to remove dead nits.

Infestation of eyelashes in children may occur and is often due to the pubic (crab) louse (*Phthirus pubis*). Persistent conjunctivitis is the presenting feature when eyelashes are infested and lice may be visible. Paraffin ointment to the eyelids is effective in treatment.

Insect bite allergy (papular urticaria)

In this condition, very itchy, erythematous papules with a small punctum, are usually present on limbs and face; these last one to two weeks. The lesions may be initially surrounded by an urticarial flare which resolves in one to two days. Excoriation and subsequent infection is common and small white scars may result. Clusters of three or four lesions suggest that fleas are the cause. New lesions may develop for months sometimes years.

Papular urticaria occurs because of hypersensitivity to an infected allergen(s). Dog and cat fleas are the most common cause, but many insects can produce similar eruptions. Thus, pets need to be treated and, if mosquitos are the cause, insect repellents and nets are useful. Sometimes fluorinated steroids may reduce itching and scratching and consequently minimize the scarring. Tolerance ultimately develops.

DISORDERS OF PIGMENTATION

Depigmentation

Vitiligo

Vitiligo may begin in children as sharply, circumscribed white macules of the limbs. Slow progression and confluence of the lesions result in patches and sheets of depigmented photosensitive skin. The cause of the loss of melanocytes from the skin is uncertain but this condition is thought to be an autoimmune disease and belonging to the thyrogastric cluster of autoimmune disorders.

Repigmentation may ocur with persistent exposure to ultraviolet light (solar and artificial). Sometimes photosensitizing medication (psoralens) is used topically and orally with UVA exposure. Treatment must be maintained for months when about two-thirds of patients achieve satisfactory results.

Vitiligo must be separated from temporary post-inflammatory hypopigmentation induced by eczema, psoriasis, or an infection such as impetigo and tinea corporis. Tinea versicolor may also present as white macules of the upper trunk in teenagers and young adults. Generalized hypopigmentation may occur in hypopituitarism.

Hyperpigmentation

Localized hyperpigmentation also often follows inflammatory disorders of the skin, especially in children who have generally pigmented skin because of their ethnic origin. Some drugs induce fixed pigmented patches that become worse each time the drug is administered. Such drugs include codeine, sulphonamides and tetracycline. These are termed fixed drugs eruptions. Generalized hyperpigmentation may also be induced by drugs, e.g. phenothiazine, minomycin and some cytotoxic agents. Generalized pigmentation may also be associated with systemic disorders such as scleroderma, dermatomyositis and Addison's disease.

DISORDERS OF THE PILOSEBACEOUS APPARATUS

Acne vulgaris

This is a very common disorder in teenagers. A detailed discussion of the pathogenesis and management is inappropriate here, but the effects of androgenic hormones on the sebaceous glands acting as end organs appear to be fundamental – eunuchs do not get acne! Sebaceous glands hypertrophy because of androgen stimulation during adolescence. Such glands are prone to obstruction by follicular keratotic plugs, resulting in the familiar comedone, papules, pustules, nodules, cysts, ulcers, and scarring of the face and upper torso.

In treatment, keratolytics (e.g. retinoic acid and salicylic acid) are useful for comedones, and broad-spectrum antibiotics suppress inflamed lesions. Benzoyl peroxide lotions are also helpful, partly as anti-inflammatory agents and partly as topical antiseptics. Intralesional steroids may hasten resolution of nodular and cystic lesions and minimize scarring. Isotretinoin is a retinoic acid derivative that is very effective for intractable acne but is used only in selected patients because of its teratogenic potential.

Acne neonatorum

This may develop at three to six months of age on the cheeks, the result of maternal hormones. This is usually mild and resolves after some months but scarring may occasionally occur. If it is accompanied by other signs of virilization, investigation is indicated.

DISEASES OF THE HAIR

Balding of the occiput of babies aged three to six months is very common. Friction on pillows causes fall of resting phase (telogen) hair. They regrow spontaneously after a few months. Slow growth of hair is common and of no significance, unless there are abnormalities of hair shafts, e.g. kinking, fragility or evidence of an underlying metabolic disorder, e.g. Menkes' disease.

Alopecia areata

This may develop at any age. Round bald patches may develop over one to two weeks. Short, tapering, broken-off hairs at the periphery (exclamation mark hairs) signify activity. There are usually no preceding symptoms. These lesions do resolve in the majority of cases in three to six months, but new lesions may develop at any time. More severe forms may cause cosmetic disability and even loss of all scalp hair (alopecia totalis) or even loss of total body hair (alopecia universalis). There may be associated nail changes (coarse pitting). The cause is uncertain but it appears to be an autoimmune disease.

The course of alopecia is extremely variable but most improve spontaneously. The application of a topical steroid may be a useful placebo and gain time, and small areas may respond to intralesional injection of steroids.

In certain circumstances a course of oral steroids may be justified. Various promising modalities are being developed and may be useful, e.g. PUVA treatment, DNCB treatment and topical minoxidil. Psychotherapy is very important and the acquisition of suitable wigs may help children recover self-esteem.

Trichotillomania

This presents as irregular single patches of hair loss. The hairs in the patches are of varying lengths and some are twisted. A history of playing or twirling of the hair is frequently obtained. This is regarded as a habit that eventually disappears. It does not signify severe underlying psychiatric disease.

Traction alopecia

This may develop where hair is constantly pulled tight, i.e. in parts for ponytails and pigtails. There may be some permanent hair loss.

NAIL DISORDERS

Paronychia

This results from thumb sucking; it is common and resolves on cessation of the habit. Chewing nails is also a common obsession. Repetitive pushing back of the cuticles on the thumb nails may result in a series of parallel depressions along the centre of the thumb nails.

Twenty-nail dystrophy

Characterized by rough linear ridges on many nails of the fingers and toes. The condition may last one or two years before resolution occurs. Sometimes, alopecia areata, lichen planus, or psoriasis induce this condition despite the lack of other cutaneous signs of these diseases. Persistent nail dystrophies, e.g. small or thick nail plate in addition to sparse hair and teeth abnormalities, suggest inherited ectodermal dysplasias.

MENDELIAN INHERITED CONDITIONS

Ichthyoses

These disorders are characterized by persistently dry, scaly skin. The most common is ichthyosis vulgaris with an incidence of 1:300. It has an autosomal dominant mode of inheritance and is a mild disorder. More severe forms have variable inheritance patterns and associated features, e.g. blistering and erythema with epidermolytic hyperkeratosis, which also has an autosomal dominant form of inheritance. The biochemical basis of some of these conditions is now known, e.g. steroid sulphatase deficiency in hyperkeratotic X-linked recessive ichthyosis. The development of an oral retinoic acid derivative (etretinate) for the treatment of these disorders is a significant advance on the persistent use of emollients.

Mechanobullous disorders

This is a group of conditions characterized by a life-long tendency to blistering following minor trauma. The deeper level of clefting, the worse the disease. Epidermolysis bullosa simplex is the mildest form and the blisters occur on hands and feet and heal without scarring. More severe forms result in scarring and nail dystrophy. The very severe recessive bullous disorders involve more extensive areas of blistering and erosion and there may be associated mucosal and nail dystrophy involvement. Death from sepsis and debilitation occurs frequently.

Xeroderma pigmentosum (autosomal recessive mode of inheritance)

A group of disorders characterized by a deficient repair of ultraviolet light damage to DNA. Sun-damaged skin from childhood is a feature, as are solar keratoses, squamous carcinomas and melanomas. Protection from ultraviolet light is paramount.

Prenatal diagnosis is possible via fibroblast culture.

Ectodermal dysplasias

Inherited disorders of adnexal structure, i.e. hair, nails, and teeth. In the anhidrotic type sweat glands may be rudimentary or missing. Hyperpyrexia (and fitting) may occur in early infancy.

Ehlers-Danlos syndrome

Abnormalities of collagen production result in bruised, wide scars, laxity of joints and hyperelasticity of the skin. Premature rupture of the membranes may be the first sign of this disorder. Herniae, dissecting aneurysms of the aorta and bleeding from the gastrointestinal tract occur at an early age.

Cutis laxa

Deficient elastic tissue causes progressive sagging of the skin folds, herniae and emphysema.

FURTHER READING

Hurwitz S 1981 Clinical pediatric dermatology: a textbook of skin disorders of childhood and adolescence. Saunders, Philadelphia
Levene G M, Calnan C A 1974 A colour atlas of dermatology. Wolfe Medical, London.
Rook A, Wilkinson D S, Ebling F J G 1979 (eds) Textbook of dermatology, 3rd edn. Blackwell Scientific, Oxford

69. Skin lesions in systemic disease

M. J. Robinson

Skin lesions are quite frequently associated with systemic disease in childhood. Sometimes the skin lesion constitutes the major physical sign and the systemic features are quite minor, while at other times the skin lesion, although of minor importance symptomatically, may be of great importance in establishing a diagnosis.

SKIN LESIONS INDICATING THE POSSIBILITY OF SYSTEMIC DISEASE

Skin bleeding

Apart from skin bleeding due to trauma which will usually be obvious, bleeding into the skin should always indicate haematological investigation, e.g. idiopathic thrombocytopenic purpura, leukaemia, haemophilia etc. It should be mentioned, however, that multiple bruises of differing ages and at unusual sites may indicate non-accidental injury.

Occasionally the distribution of the bleeding is helpful, e.g. in Henoch-Schönlein purpura the eruption is distributed over the legs and buttocks. Bleeding and clotting studies are normal here.

In some cases the general condition of the child and the acuteness of the presentation may suggest that the bleeding is part of a septicaemia. Meningococcaemia is the most life threatening of the septicaemias in childhood, but bleeding into the skin is occasionally seen in septicaemia due to *Haemophilus influenzae*, *Streptococcus pneumoniae*, Staphylococci and some Gram- negative organisms. Less extensive, but equally useful diagnostically, are the purpuric lesions of subacute bacterial endocarditis, typhus and typhoid fever.

Bleeding into the skin, as well as from other sites, is part of the syndrome of disseminated intravascular coagulation. Usually this indicates a serious underlying disorder, particularly an overwhelming infection, but the syndrome may occur in a number of other states associated with circulatory collapse. Bleeding here is the result of consumption of platelets and other coagulation factors.

Bleeding and bruising in association with bone pain and spongy gums may indicate scurvy. Radiographs of the wrists will establish the diagnosis. Large doses of vitamin C are curative within a week.

Easy bruising, the result of increased capillary fragility, is a feature of Cushing's syndrome. Cushing's syndrome may be the result of corticosteroids given for some underlying disease, e.g. leukaemia, the nephrotic syndrome, etc., or may be the result of hyperplasia or tumour of the adrenal cortex or anterior pituitary. This diagnosis should be obvious from the general appearance of the child.

Skin bruising in association with undue dermal fragility, abnormal skin elasticity and hyperextensibility of joints characterizes the Ehlers-Danlos syndrome.

Skin bruising is frequently associated with therapeutically administered drugs, e.g. salicylates and non-steroidal anti-inflammatory agents. A number of pharmaceutical preparations cause aplastic anaemia and the child presents with bleeding into the skin. These include chloramphenicol, antithyroid and antineoplastic drugs. The possibility of drug ingestion should always be considered in the child who presents with skin bleeding or bruising.

Pigmentation

Pigmentation may be increased or decreased, localized or generalized. Depigmentation is almost always localized. Generalized hyperpigmentation is seen in adrenal insufficiency, but, in addition, areas which are normally pigmented, e.g. nipples and genitalia, show even greater pigmentation.

Pigmentation is also a feature of the lipidoses – Gaucher's disease, Niemann-Pick – and Hand-Schüller-Christian disease. The cause of the pigmentation in these disorders is not clear, but examination of the skin reveals increased amounts of iron and melanin. Gaucher's disease is accompanied by gross splenomegaly; in Niemann-Pick disease, liver, spleen and the lymph nodes are enlarged and purpura is usualy present. Bone lesions and, at times, growth failure characterize Hand-Schüller-Christian disease. Appropriate tissue for histological examination is necessary to establish this diagnosis.

Hyperpigmentation and photosensitivity are important diagnostic features of porphyria. This rare metabolic error is unusual before adolescence. The diagnosis may be suspected in individuals with acute abdominal pain, personality change and, in some varieties of porphyria, the passing of burgundy red urine.

A dirty grey discoloration of the skin is sometimes seen in chronic renal failure.

Localized hyperpigmentation

Localized areas of hyperpigmentation is the first sign of von Recklinghausen's disease – neurofibromatosis. These lesions are described as 'cafe au lait' (coffee with milk) because of their colour. They vary in size and number but, to be of diagnostic value, at least four should be present. The lesions have a smooth border in contradistinction to the irregular border of other pigmented naevi which are not associated with systemic disease (Fig. 69.1). Large numbers of pigmented naevi in the axillae – axillary freckles – are another feature of

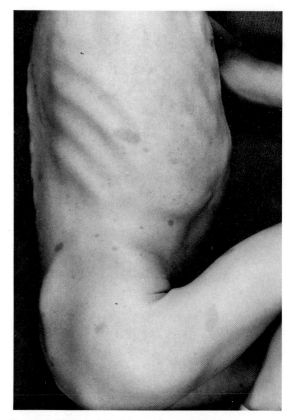

Fig. 69.1 Cafe au lait pigmentation and 'freckles' characteristic of neurofibromatosis in childhood.

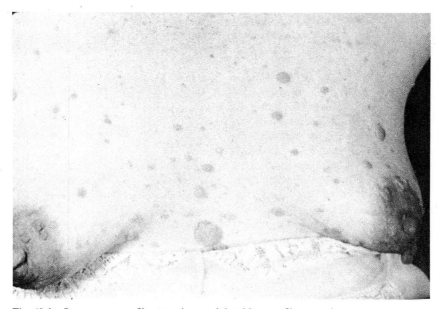

Fig. 69.2 Cutaneous neurofibromata in an adult with neurofibromatosis.

von Recklinghausen's disease. Neurofibromatosis is transmitted in a Mendelian dominant fashion and, as in all conditions of dominant inheritance, the phenotype is variously expressed. It is very important in a suspected case to examine both parents for signs of pigmentation as well as the other features of the disease. In most cases one parent will be affected but mutants are not infrequent. Neurofibromas which may involve peripheral, spinal and cranial nerves do not usually appear until after puberty; they vary in size from a pinhead to that of a grapefruit, as well as in number and in position (Fig. 69.2). Thus, a very variable clinical pattern results. Neurofibromas also involve the meninges (meningiomas) and occur within the brain and spinal cord as gliomas. Involvement of bone in neurofibromatosis results in swelling, deformity and easy fractures. Renovascular hypertension may occur due to involvement of renal vessels and, in later life, there is a strong association of phaeochromocytoma and neuroblastoma with von Recklinghausen's neurofibromatosis.

Tuberous sclerosis

Cafe au lait spots are also seen in tuberous sclerosis, which is also dominantly inherited. Adenoma sebaceum, epilepsy and progressive mental retardation comprise the fully expressed disorder. Tuberous sclerosis may present in infancy with infantile spasms and an EEG pattern of hypsarrhythmia. More usually the early manifestations of tuberous sclerosis involve the skin

(Fig. 69.3). The dermal lesions comprise areas of ash leaf hypopigmentation, angiomas and collagenous plaques (shagreen patches). Shagreen patches are distributed over the lower back, legs, and interscapular regions. Their colour varies from purplish red to a fleshy hue. Adenoma sebaceum usually appears later than the skin lesions described above. This term is a misnomer as they are neither adenomas nor do they affect the sebaceous glands; they are, in fact, fibroangiomatous naevi surrounding the hair follicles. Adenoma sebaceum vary in colour from fleshy to yellowish red and are typically distributed over the nasolabial folds and spread to involve the nose, cheeks, forehead and chin, but rarely extend below the neck (Fig. 69.4). The visceral lesions which characterize these disorders, such as cerebral tumours, phakoma, renal cysts and rhabdomyoma occur later. Mental retardation, which occurs in the full expression of the disorder, is progressive, but can usually be recognized by the age of about two years.

In any child with tuberous sclerosis it is very important to examine the parents carefully. Should skin lesions not be apparent in either parent, CT scanning may be indicated in them to exclude silent lesions of tuberous sclerosis within the brain. Only in this manner can appropriate genetic counselling be offered.

Albright's syndrome

In this disorder, which mainly affects girls, the cafe au lait pigmentation is associatd with bone lesions (fibrous

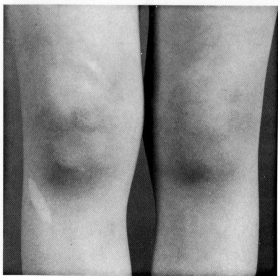

Fig. 69.3 Examples of depigmented patches of tuberous sclerosis.

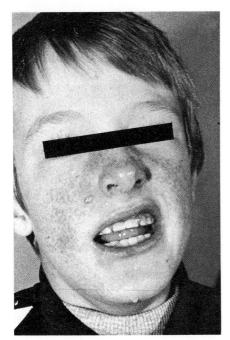

Fig. 69.4 Characteristic adenoma sebaceum of tuberous sclerosis. This young boy is developmentally delayed — note the excessive dribbling.

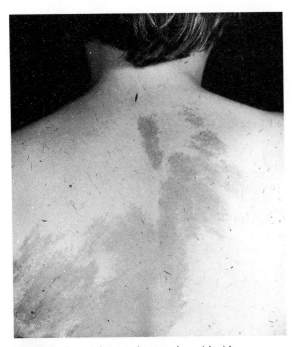

Fig. 69.5 Large pigmented naevus in a girl with Albright's syndrome.

dysplasia) and precocious puberty. The cause of this syndrome is unknown but the outlook is good (Fig. 69.5).

Incontinentia pigmenti

The pigmentation seen in incontinentia pigmenti consists of brown streaks, which have a whorled appearance but do not follow the distribution of peripheral nerves. The pigmentation is accompanied by mental deficiency, disturbed dentition and eye defects.

Focal dermal hypoplasia (Goltz's syndrome)

In focal dermal hypoplasia (Goltz's syndrome) pigmentation is associated with dermal atrophy and gross malnutrition.

Skin lesions of pellagra

These lesions consist of erythema involving and extending to be localized to the back of the hands, wrists, forearms, neck and fingers in the early stages. Later these lesions become pigmented and scaly (Casal's necklace).

Scleroderma

In scleroderma there is skin tightness with thickening; this is seen initially over the dorsum of the hands and over the fingers. Tightness of the skin of the face is responsible for the characteristic appearance of the patient with scleroderma. Other skin changes include hyperpigmentation and areas of depigmentation. Telangiectases are frequently seen on the face, lips, hands and upper chest and abnormal skin capillaries in the cutis adjacent to the finger nails.

Depigmentation

Depigmentation is less common and is usually localized. The hypopigmented patches of tuberous sclerosis have already been mentioned. Depigmentation is also seen in protein energy malnutrition which, if severe, may cause the hair to turn red. Localized depigmentation (vitiligo) is seen in chronic renal disease, but most frequently the cause of vitiligo is not apparent.

Generalized lack of skin pigment is characteristic of *albinism*. A number of variants have been described. The disorder is characterized by extremely fair skin, fine white silky hair and ocular problems. There is marked photophobia, consequent on the lack of iris pigment and a series of other ocular abnormalities. These children need to wear tinted spectacles when out of doors because of intense photophobia. They also have a great tendency to sunburn so that they must wear broad-brimmed hats and apply a protective cream to the skin which is uncovered. Partial forms of albinism with different modes of inheritance are also seen.

Angiomas (vascular naevi)

Vascular naevi are not commonly associated with systemic signs and produce their effects largely through ulceration, bleeding or by obstruction, if they are situated in the subglottic region. Most present because of cosmetic disturbance.

Encephalotrigeminal angiomatosis (Sturge-Weber syndrome)

This is characterized by a unilateral port wine-coloured naevus which follows the distribution of the fifth cranial nerve, most commonly the ophthalmic division. The lesion is present at birth, it is sharply demarcated in the midline and usually involves the mucous membranes and the sclera of the same side (Fig. 69.6). Intracranial

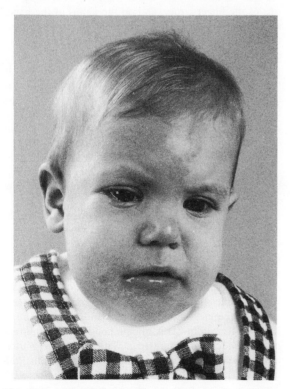

Fig. 69.6 Sturge-Weber syndrome. The lesion is confined to the right side of the face. (Reproduced with permission.)

extension to involve the brain is characteristic and a skull radiograph later in childhood may show fine sinuous double-contoured calcifications in the subcortical region parallel to the convolutions of the cerebral cortex; the EEG shows epileptic activity over the involved areas. In the fully developed Sturge-Weber syndrome, there is mental retardation, epilepsy and a contralateral hemiplegia. Involvement of the choroid may lead to glaucoma in childhood. Management of the epilepsy is difficult and the prognosis is poor. Transmission is in an autosomal dominant fashion.

Ataxia telangiectasia

The vascular lesions in this disorder commonly appear some time after the onset of ataxia. There is, of course, the association with severe and persisting infection and a variable immunological defect. The lesions most commonly involve the bulbar conjunctivae (Fig. 69.7), the lobes of the ears, eyelids, cheeks and the 'V' of the neck. In this disorder death is frequently the result of a lymphoreticular malignancy. Transmission is in an autosomal recessive fashion.

Less common symptoms associated with angiomas include *angiomatosis retinae-et-cerebelli* (von-Hippel-Landau haemangioma). This is characterized by haemangiomas of the retina and cerebellum together with tumours and cysts in various organs, and occasionally vascular naevi around the face.

Familial haemorrhagic telangiectasis (Rendu-Osler-Weber disease) is characterized by mucosal and skin telangiectases which occasionally occur early in life, but as a general rule do not present until adult life. Bleeding frequently occurs from these sites and may be considered as the cause of an iron deficiency anaemia in cases which are resistant to appropriate iron therapy. The anaemia is due to bleeding from the gastrointestinal tract and the diagnosis established by upper gastrointestinal tract endoscopy.

Erythema

Children presenting with fever and an erythematous rash will most frequently have one of the infectious exanthemas (measles, rubella, etc.) The type of rash, its distribution and the epidemiology will usually allow the diagnosis of one of the infectious diseases to be made without difficulty. The clinical features have been described in Chapter 29.

Erythema of various types accompanies a number of systemic disorders. The skin lesions of SLE have already been described. They have a characteristic butterfly distribution over both cheeks and the base of

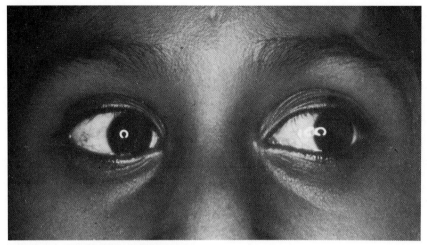

Fig. 69.7 Ocular telangiectases of ataxia telangiectasia.

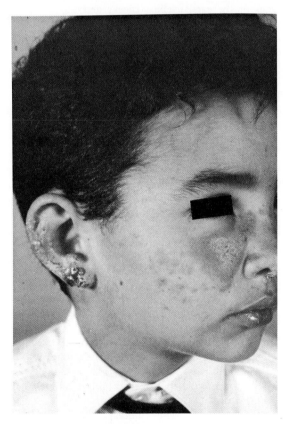

Fig. 69.8 Erythema and scaling particularly over the malar region, characteristic of systemic lupus erythematosus.

the nose (Fig. 69.8). Patchy lesions may also be seen to involve the ears, neck and less commonly the limbs. The initial lesions soon become confluent, scaly, ultimately ulcerate and finally scar. In SLE, erythematous macules are also commonly seen about the nail beds, along the tips of the fingers, toes, and on the palms of the hands and soles of the feet. The diagnosis of SLE is made from the clinical features described in Chapter 73 and the characteristic serology.

An erythematous maculopapular rash is often seen in the systemic form of juvenile chronic arthritis. This rash tends to have a salmon colour, it tends to come and go, being particularly evident at the time when the fever is at its height. The skin lesion of systemic juvenile chronic arthritis is occasionally urticarial in type.

The lesions of Henoch-Schönlein purpura, while usually purpuric, may be erythematous and urticarial but again the distribution typically involves the limbs and the buttocks.

An erythematous rash which is distributed over the extensor surfaces of the joints, particularly over the knuckles, elbows and knees, is characteristic of dermatomyositis. In addition, most children with this disorder show a violaceous facial rash and periorbital oedema. Later in the course of this disease, atrophy with scaling of the affected skin is noted and, in the quiescent stages, depigmentation. The outstanding clinical features of dermatomyositis in childhood are muscle pain, muscle tenderness and wasting. With progressive muscle atrophy, severe weakness, contractures and eventual calcification may produce severe disability. On the other hand, recovery may be almost complete. Skin and muscle biopsy initially show perivascular collections of inflammatory cells. Vascular occlusion by fibrin thrombi follows with secondary atrophy of structures supplied by these vessels (see Ch. 73).

Toxic shock syndrome

This refers to a syndrome characterized by high fever, vomiting and diarrhoea, with rapid progression into circulatory failure. These symptoms are accompanied by a generalized erythema which looks very much like sunburn. This erythematous rash ultimately peels, the peeling being particularly noticeable over the palms of the hands and the soles of the feet.

The toxic shock syndrome is most frequently a disorder of young females during the time of their menses, particularly in those who use vaginal tampons.

In the toxic shock syndrome vaginal cultures are frequently, but not always, positive for *Staphylococcus aureus*; occasionally this organism can also be grown from the nose, throat, blood, urine and/or stools.

Management. Individuals with the toxic shock syndrome are very ill and require urgent circulatory support with plasma expanders. Beta-lactamase-resistant antibiotics, e.g. flucloxacillin, will be prescribed after the various cultures are taken, but it is not certain if they play a significant role in treatment. With appropriate management most cases will recover.

Although it would seem that this syndrome relates to the menses, vaginal tampons and a pathogenic Staphylococcus, its incidence is not sufficient to recommend either routine vaginal cultures in all females or the abandonment of vaginal tampons.

Kawasaki disease

An erythematous rash is accompanied by oedema of palms and soles. Desquamation follows and is particularly marked over the tips of the fingers and toes. The aetiology of Kawasaki disease is unknown; it is certainly one form of vasculitis and many would regard it as identical to infantile polyarteritis nodosum (see Ch. 73).

Stevens-Johnson syndrome

Erythema multiforme exudativum, or Stevens-Johnson syndrome, is a hypersensitivity vasculitis, frequently to herpes simplex or *Mycoplasma pneumoniae* but also to a variety of drugs – usually sulphonamides, but penicillin, barbiturates and anticonvulsants may be causative. The skin lesion is originally blotchy and erythematous, beginning on the dorsum of the hands and the feet and trunk. Vesicles then develop within the erythematous

lesions; these frequently coalesce to form large bullae. The mucous membranes of the mouth, conjunctivae and urethra are involved. Fever, malaise and toxaemia are often present. The disorder is self-limiting, but occasionally may be life threatening, when steroids will be employed.

Skin nodules

These are present in a number of disorders including acute rheumatic fever, juvenile chronic arthritis, SLE and von Recklinghausen's neurofibromatosis. Diagnosis will be made without difficulty if the associated skin lesions, as already described, and the systemic features are appreciated.

Xanthomas are yellowish nodules usually with a faint erythematous base. Xanthoma plana are flat and usually located over the neck, shoulders and back. Xanthoma tuberosum are distributed over the elbows, knuckles, buttocks, knees, and heels, while xanthoma tendinosum are also associated with the tendo-Achilles, the fingers and the toes. Xanthelasma involves the eyelids. Xanthomas are associated with the hyperlipidaemias; the diagnosis of these is established by:

1. The finding of an elevated serum cholesterol.
2. Lipoprotein electrophoresis to determine blood levels of other lipids.
3. The exclusion of other disorders with xanthomas and secondary hypercholesterolaemia, e.g. hypothyroidism, biliary cirrhosis, diabetes mellitus, glycogen storage disease and the nephrotic syndrome.

Vesicles

Varicella

The commonest disorder associated with a vesicular rash is, of course, varicella, the clinical features of which have already been described (see Ch. 29). The majority of disorders presenting with vesicular or vesiculobullous eruptions are primarily disorders of the skin with minimal or no systemic features. A large number exist and will not be discussed in this section.

Dermatitis herpetiformis

This disorder is characterized by clusters of small, tense and intensely itchy papules and vesicles. In childhood the cause of dermatitis herpetiformis is unknown, but in adult life there is a frequent association with gluten-sensitive enteropathy. The diagnosis is best made from skin biopsy, as dermatitis herpetiformis may resemble a number of other primarily dermatological disorders.

Direct immunofluoresence labelling of a skin biopsy reveals a characteristic deposition of IgA at the tips of the dermal papillae.

Eczema

While eczema is almost always a primary allergic disorder, occasionally it may be part of a generalized disease. Eczema associated with recurrent infections suggest an immunological deficiency state, for example, Wiskott-Aldrich syndrome, combined immunodeficiency and occasionally sex-linked agammaglobulinaemia (see Ch. 22).

The association of perioral and perianal eczematous-like lesions with diarrhoea, hair loss and failure to thrive suggests the condition of acrodermatitis enteropathica in weaned infants. In this disorder body zinc stores are low. Administration of zinc rapidly improves the symptoms and signs.

NODULAR LESIONS

Haemangiomas

The most common nodular lesions are probably capillary haemangiomas, or strawberry naevi. Most are present or appear during the neonatal period as soft, bright red rapidly growing tumours; lesions may be single or multiple. There may be variable subcutaneous involvement in association, apparent as a soft, bluish subcutaneous swelling. Rapid growth over six to nine months may occur to produce severe cosmetic disability, obstruction of orifices, threatened viability of important organs (e.g. eye) and ulceration. Bleeding following trauma may occur and can be alarming to parents but is usually controlled simply by pressure. Inordinate bleeding and purpura may result from platelet consumption in some lesions (Kasabach-Merritt syndrome). Sometimes lesions also involve internal organs. Management is usually expectant, and spontaneous resolution ultimately occurs in most lesions. About 90% have resolved by ten years of age. Systemic steroids may help when the eye is threatened, where there is obstruction to breathing, feeding or defaecation, and in the Kasabach-Merritt syndrome.

ABNORMALITIES OF SUBCUTANEOUS FAT

Subcutaneous fat necrosis

This occurs in healthy neonates. Sharply circumscribed nodular areas may develop anywhere on the body. They may be tender and are a reddish-blue colour. Necrosis

of the overlying skin may occur. Most lesions spontaneously resolve in a few weeks.

Sclerema neonatorum

This is a most serious disorder involving subcutaneous fat. It usually occurs in very ill neonates (e.g. sepsis, congenital heart disease, etc.) or in premature infants. Rapid hardening of most of the subcutaneous fat occurs, and results in non-pitting induration and stiffness of the skin. Death occurs in about half of these neonates. With proper neonatal care this lesion should never occur.

DEVELOPMENTAL DEFECTS AND HAMARTOMAS

These occur in approximately 2% of all births. They frequently affect more than one component of the skin and subcutaneous tissues, but usually one specialized component predominates.

Aplasia cutis

Aplasia cutis may present as absent areas of epidermis (ulceration) on the scalp. Sometimes there are also skull defects and brain abnormalities. The lesions may be a portal of entry for bacterial meningitis. And they may be mistakenly thought to be due to birth trauma. Healing is the rule and the final result is an atrophic scar, i.e. it persists as a bald patch.

Sebaceous naevi

Sebaceous naevi may also present as hairless patches of the scalp at birth. In adolescence, due to the effects of androgens, they become raised and yellowish plaques. Various tumours may develop in these lesions in adult life; these include basal cell carcinomas and benign tumours of apocrine sweat glands and other adnexal structures. Extensive naevi can be associated with a variety of neurological and skeletal defects.

Epidermal naevi

These are warty, linear patches that become apparent after birth. They may be extensive and dermatomal in distribution and are occasionally associated with internal defects.

Congenital pigmented (hairy) naevi

These naevi are present at birth and may be very extensive. They may involve the meninges and eye pigment.

Melanomas may develop (even in childhood) but the risk is not accurately known.

Cafe au lait spots

Cafe au lait spots may be present at birth and, if numerous, strongly suggest the diagnosis of neurofibromatosis or Albright's syndrome. Single lesions are common and of no consequence.

Mongolian spots

These are large, bluish, macular, bruise-like areas on the lower back (especially in Asian infants). They resolve after one or two years. Melanocytes migrating from the neural crest are found in the dermis.

Ash leaf-shaped areas of depigmentation

These may be an indication of tuberous sclerosis. They are more easily seen under a Wood's lamp.

Other developmental naevi and disorders

Various other epidermal components can result in unusual developmental naevi, e.g. woolly hair naevus, eccrine naevus and naevus comedonicus. Localized developmental disturbances of the connective tissue of the dermis are known as connective tissue naevi, e.g. the shagreen patch of tuberous sclerosis.

Neurofibromas and capillary haemangiomas can be regarded as special types of developmental disorders of the dermis.

FURTHER READING

Barsky S H, Rosen S, Geer D E, Noe J M 1980 The nature and evolution of port wine stains: a computer-assisted study. Journal of Investigative Dermatology 74: 154–157

Cook C D, Rosen F S, Banker B Q 1963 Dermatomyositis and focal scleroderma. The Pediatric Clinics of North America 10(4): 979–1016

Epstein W, Kligman A M 1956 Pathogenesis of milia and benign tumours of skin. Journal of Investigative Dermatology 26: 1–11

Finley J L, Arndt K A, Noe J, Rosen S 1984 Argon laser – port-wine stain interaction. Archives of Dermatology 120: 613–619

Hodgman J E, Freedman R I, Levan N E 1971 Neonatal dermatology. The Paediatric Clinics of North America 18: 713–756

Hurley H J 1985 Diseases of the apocrine and eccrine glands. In: Moschella S L, Hurley H J (eds) Dermatology, 2nd edn. Vol 2. Saunders, Philadelphia, p 1323

Jacobs A H, Walton R G 1976 The incidence of birthmarks in the neonate. Paediatrics 58: 218–222

Jennings J L, Burrows W M 1983 Infantile acropustulosis. Journal of the American Academy of Dermatology 9: 733–738

Merlob P, Metzker A, Reisner S H 1972 Transient neonatal pustular melanosis. American Journal of Diseases of Children 136: 521–522

Pearson R W 1988 Clinicopathologic types of epidermolysis bullosa and their non-dermatological complications. Archives of Dermatology 124: 718–725

Perlstein M A, Perlstein M O 1967 Neurocutaneous syndromes. The Pediatric Clinics of North America 14(4): 933–948

Powell S T, Su W P 1984 Cutis marmorata telangiectatica congenita: report of nine cases and review of the literature. Cutis 34: 305–312

Pratt A G 1953 Birthmarks in infants. AMA Archives of Dermatology and Syphilology 67: 302–305

Rasmussen J E (ed) 1983 Pediatric dermatology. The Pediatric Clinics of North America 30: 3

Schachner L, Press S 1983 Vesicular, bullous and pustular disorders in infancy and childhood. The Paediatric Clinics of North America 30: 609–630

Smith M A, Manfield P A 1962 The natural history of salmon patches in the first year of life. British Journal of Dermatology 74: 31–33

Solomon L M, Esterly N B 1973 Transient cutaneous lesions. In: Schaeffer A J (ed) Neonatal dermatology. Saunders, Philadelphia, p 43

Stevenson R F, Morin J D 1975 Ocular findings in nevus flammeus. Canadian Journal of Ophthalmology 10: 136–139

Special senses

70. The eye

Geoffrey Harley

This chapter highlights problems which primarily affect the eye and visual apparatus. Many systemic conditions with ophthalmic manifestations are discussed in other chapters, e.g. those on genetics, neurology and metabolic diseases.

Can the child see? Is the eye turned? These two questions are intimately related. Poor vision in one eye is so often associated with a squint which may be large and obvious, or very small, only detected by careful and practised observation. If one eye turns and fixation is preferred by the other, then it must always be assumed that the vision in the turning eye is weaker.

ASSESSMENT OF VISION

By the age of seven years most children will confidently read the letters on the conventional Snellen chart and will manage a year earlier if the letters are replaced by numbers. Preferably the test is performed at the standard distance of six metres.

If a room of this size is not available the effective length of a three-metre room can be doubled by the use of a mirror. Remember that 6/60 denotes the visual acuity at 6 metres which would be expected of a normal person reading at 60 metres, whereas 6/6 denotes normal visual acuity. Visual acuity of less than 6/60 may be recorded as 3/60, 2/60, 1/60 as the chart is brought closer. Vision less than this is recorded as the ability to count fingers, perceive hand movements or just light (PL).

Younger children are given letter matching tests. The Sheridan Gardiner test is commonly used in the hospital situation and by the School Medical Service. In this the child is asked to match one of seven letters on a personally held card with a choice of similar letters presented by the examiner on a chart, or singly on cards. An alternative, more readily available in general practice, is the illiterate 'E' test where the subject matches the orientation of the 'E' presented in different directions using either the fingers or a cut-out 'E'. Many children have difficulty with left/right orientation, reducing the reliability of this test. Few children can manage these tests before the age of three years.

Although there are several tests designed for the documentation of visual acuity in younger children and those with physical and intellectual handicaps, they are not applicable in the normal clinical environment.

In younger children it is more practical to rely on objective assessment of social visual responses. Here, the parents' observations are of paramount importance.

Does the child appear to respond visually as other children of a comparable age?

A neonate will turn the head towards a lighted window and within the first few days, will follow a face, particularly the mother's and soon follow large objects and lights. By the age of 10 to 12 weeks there will be a response to a smile and within a short period the infant will attempt to reach for objects with increasing accuracy. The gaze will be steady and by the age of three months there should be firm binocular co-ordination.

A squint, nystagmus or poor visual responses inconsistent with the age of the infant are indications for referral and proper investigation.

Squint or strabismus

In the parlance of the ophthalmologist these are synonymous terms indicating misalignment of the visual axes of the eyes. Parents and other lay people will use the term squint or turned eye to describe this situation, but will also say that a child squints – meaning the eyes screw up. They will also describe the eyes as crossing when they are, in fact, diverging. Regardless of the confusion, parents are usually right in indicating some abnormality of eye movements. Detection of a squint is a very important part of a paediatric assessment.

Inspection. The alignment of the eyes may be obviously defective. The eyes may turn in – a convergent squint

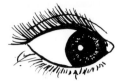 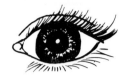

Fig. 70.1 Right convergent squint with eccentric light reflex.

or esotropia (Fig. 70.1). The eyes may turn out – a divergent squint or exotropia. The eyes may turn up or down – a vertical squint, hyper- or hypotropia which may be combined with horizontal deviation.

The squint may only be apparent in a particular direction of gaze and only detected when the child is observed using the full range of its eye movements. A broad nasal bridge and epicanthic folds very often give the appearance of a convergent squint when the visual axes are really quite parallel (Fig. 70.2).

Corneal reflections. Shine a torch at the child's eyes. If the reflection appears to come simultaneously from the centre of both corneae the eyes are probably parallel, though this test is not very reliable.

Cover test. This is the only reliable test for detecting squints, but requires practice, a co-operative patient and repeated observations. The patient must be encouraged to look at and fix on an interesting object, first at a distance across the room (or beyond if a divergent squint suspected) and then on close objects. The eyes are covered in turn and if the eye not being covered has to move to take up fixation it must be squinting. It will move outwards if the squint is convergent and so on. If the deviation recovers when both eyes are uncovered there is a latent squint (phoria). If recovery does not occur the squint is manifest (tropia) (Fig. 70.3).

Early detection and investigation of a squint or poor vision are essential to prevent or overcome amblyopia.

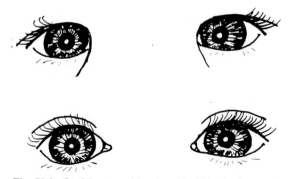

Fig. 70.2 Straight eyes with epicanthic folds. (top). Straight eyes without epicanthic folds (bottom).

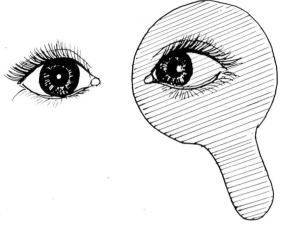

Fig. 70.3 Cover test – left eye turning in under cover.

Amblyopia

Any condition in which the image on the retina is not clear, steady and central during the first seven to ten years of life will lead to loss of normal functional and anatomical pathways between the retina and visual cortex, so that when the primary cause is corrected visual acuity is still poor. Treatment is aimed to eliminate the cause and institute some form of patching or fogging of the better eye to stimulate use of the amblyopic one. Amblyopia may be reversed in one or two weeks in the first year of life, but may take months at the age of seven years.

Refractive errors, with the error greater in one eye, can cause amblyopia.

Refractive errors (see Fig. 70.4)

Hypermetropia (long-sightedness). The eyeball is shorter than normal, but the young eye has the capacity to cope with this by increasing the power of its crystalline lens (accommodation). If one eye has a considerably higher error than its fellow the defocused image in the worse eye may lead to amblyopia. This may be detected on vision screening examinations or may precipitate the development of a convergent squint.

Myopia. Short-sightedness is rarely present at birth, but commonly develops between the age of 6 and 20 years and progresses to a variable degree during that period of development. The eyeball is longer than normal. While close objects may remain in clear focus, distant objects will remain out of focus unless an optical correction is worn.

Astigmatism (Fig. 70.5). Most of the refraction of light takes place at the interface between air and the corneal

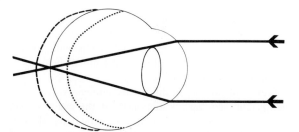

Fig. 70.4 Normal eye (solid line). Rays of light are in focus on the retina. Myopia (larger eye) focus is in front of the retina. Hypermetropia (smaller eye) focus is behind the retina.

surface. If the cornea is more curved in one meridian, tending to be shaped more like a lemon than an orange there will be a blurring of the retinal image. Small degrees of astigmatism may be detected universally and are insignificant. Large errors cause loss of acuity and if asymmetric may lead to amblyopia. This, again is detected by vision screening or routine examination and may occasionally result in a squint.

Refraction

Measurement of the refractive error is an essential part of the ophthalmic assessment of any patient at any age. In infants and young children reliance is placed on objective assessment which can be very accurate in experienced hands. The pupils are dilated and accommodation is relaxed using cycloplegic drops. Cyclopentolate 0.25% to 1% is a short-acting drug commonly used. It is not as effective as atropine sulphate 0.5% to 1% which requires several instillations before the examination and has a prolonged effect of up to ten days. Children may react to atropine with flushing and fever after the first instillation of the drops. If so, further administration should be discontinued. Refraction is assessed using the retinoscope (this is not an ophthal-

moscope). The movement of a streak of light projected from the instrument is observed on the red reflex of the fundus and lenses are put up in front of the eye to neutralize the movement. From this can be calculated the refractive state and the necessary corrective lenses can be prescribed. In older children and adults this process is refined by subjective confirmation of the results.

Other conditions causing visual deprivation

There are a number of disorders which occur early in childhood which, if not corrected, will cause amblyopia and possibly squints. Early detection and timely intervention will avoid these complications. They include problems mentioned below.

Eyelid problems

Ptosis or drooping of the upper eyelid may be sufficient to obscure vision. The commonest cause is congenital with varying degrees of under-development of the levator muscle of the upper eyelid. Other causes include the 'jaw winking' syndrome in which bizarre movements of the upper lid are coupled with mastication, due to misdirected innervation. Other disorders causing ptosis include Horner's syndrome, myaesthenia gravis, trauma and rarely congenital third nerve palsy. If the primary causes cannot be eliminated surgery is indicated to clear the visual axis. In general this is achieved by shortening the levator muscle or by procedures suspending the lid from the brow.

Corneal opacities

Many corneal opacities result from corneal ulceration and scarring. Keratoconus, some of the mucopolysaccharidoses, some other metabolic diseases and familial corneal dystrophies are also associated with corneal opacities.

Corneal foreign bodies

These should be removed as soon as possible. A drop of local anaesthetic, such as oxybuprocaine or amethocaine will relieve symptoms where a foreign body is suspected and will facilitate examination. If a foreign body cannot be easily removed and is imbedded the child should be referred quickly to an ophthalmologist. After removal of a foreign body an antibiotic ointment should be instilled and the patient reviewed daily until the cornea is healed and there are no symptoms.

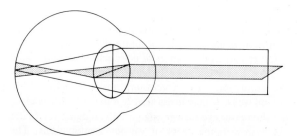

Fig. 70.5 Astigmatism. Rays of light in one meridian are in focus and out of focus in another. In this case the horizontal meridian (shaded) is out of focus.

Corneal abrasions

Superficial corneal abrasions can also be treated with antibiotic ointments and patched until healed. Deep and full thickness corneal lacerations require admission to hospital and specialist management.

Corneal ulceration

Corneal ulceration from purely infective causes is uncommon except for dendritic ulceration caused by herpes simplex. Recurrent attacks and involvement of the corneal stroma in young children can lead to varying degrees of scarring which can be a cause of amblyopia. If the typical dendritic figure is seen after staining the eye with fluorescein, acyclovir ointment instilled five times a day is now the treatment of choice pending specialist consultation. Steroids are strictly contraindicated.

Lens opacities

Any opacity in the lens may be termed a cataract. This may vary from a small developmental dot on the anterior pole of the lens which does not progress nor interfere with vision, to a totally opaque lens which precludes any useful vision whilst it remains. Some minor lens opacities may reduce vision slightly, don't progress and don't need surgical intervention. Others may progress and need removal of the lens. Significant cataracts degrade the retinal image and lead to amblyopia. This amblyopia is particularly severe if the cataract is unilateral. Thus early recognition and treatment provides the only hope of avoiding this amblyopia. Patients requiring treatment should have surgery as soon as possible. Infants with total cataracts are treated within the first weeks of life. The whole lens is removed and to compensate for the loss of the lens the infants are fitted with extended wear contact lenses a few days later. Intraocular lenses are generally contraindicated in children.

Significant cataracts present as a white pupil in infants (Fig. 70.6). All infants should be examined for any opacities in the ocular media using the direct ophthal-moscope. Whilst it is very difficult to obtain a detailed view of the infant's fundus with this instrument, the clarity of the media can be assessed by observing the red reflex from the fundus with the instrument held about 30 cm from the child's eye.

Causes of cataract in infants are numerous, but often no specific aetiology is identified. If the eye does not appear to be otherwise normal, particularly if it is microphthalmic, studies are indicated to eliminate an intra-uterine infective process. Maternal rubella in the first trimester of pregnancy still occurs causing congenital cataracts. A metabolic screen is also a mandatory part of the work-up. The one example of reversible cataract in infants is due to galactose-1 phosphate uridyl transferase deficiency. Cataracts are also common in Down syndrome (trisomy 21). Others are familial. Some are associated with other developmental defects in the eye.

Lesions behind the lens

Most conditions occurring in the posterior segment of the eye and causing visual loss are usually not amenable to prevention or treatment as causes of reversible amblyopia, though their recognition and management needs to be considered (see below).

Ocular misalignment (and the child is in the age group where amblyopia can occur)

Should one eye become misaligned (e.g. because of a weakness of an extra ocular muscle) the diplopia would naturally occur, is actively suppressed, and one eye develops amblyopia.

Squint management

The objectives of squint management are discussed below.

Good vision in both eyes

This is achieved by correcting refractive errors with appropriate visual aids after accurate refraction.

Other correctable causes of poor acuity are eliminated and the better eye is occluded to improve the vision in the amblyopic eye. 'Occlusion' may be achieved in several ways. It may mean simply a patch totally occluding the better eye for varying periods, fogging the better eye with atropine drops or various combinations. The sooner treatment is commenced the quicker the results. It is never too early, but it is often too late.

Don't ignore the observations of parents, infant welfare nurses or screening services.

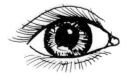 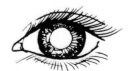

Fig. 70.6 White pupil.

Good alignment of the eyes

Spectacles alone may be all that is necessary. In hypermetropic children the stimulus to over-converge may be eliminated by provision of a full spectacle correction for the refractive error.

If there is a residual squint, surgery may be necessary to produce ocular alignment.

Overacting muscles may be weakened by several methods, usually by detaching the muscle from its original insertion on the globe and re-attaching it further back. Underacting muscles may be strengthened by resecting various amounts and repositioning them at or in front of their original insertions. Repeated procedures are often required. It is not necessary to remove the eye as some parents believe.

Restoration or attainment of binocular vision

There is a group of children who have squints from a very early age (2–3 months). It is probable that they have never had any binocular single vision i.e. the ability to fuse the images from each eye into a single image at the level of the cerebral cortex. If the eyes can be aligned before the age of 18–24 months, one-third of these children will develop some binocular association. Surgery is the essential part of their treatment.

There is a group of children who develop squints after the age of 18 months, but have probably had binocular single vision which has broken down. The sooner it is restored the better.

The management of childhood squints is ongoing and regular supervision is required at least for the first decade.

In summary. Poor visual acuity and squint are indications of amblyopia requiring immediate investigation and treatment.

OCULAR INFECTIONS

Neonatal

Gonococcal and chlamydial infections are uncommon but must be considered if a purulent discharge is found in the first few days of life. *Neisseria gonorrhoeae* conjunctivitis requires vigorous treatment with penicillin 120 mg/kg/day. In addition, sulphacetamide drops are used hourly to prevent corneal ulceration. The discharge is highly infectious.

The diagnosis of chlamydial infection is confirmed by serological tests on the conjunctival secretions. The infant is treated with oral erythromycin 50 mg/kg/day and local sulphacetamide eye drops. Treatment should be continued for two weeks. There may be associated chlamydial respiratory infection.

In both conditions the mother and father must also be treated.

Trachoma

Trachoma is a chlamydial conjunctivitis. It is rare in urban communities but prevalent in arid out-back areas and in the Aboriginal population. Recurrent and untreated disease leads to lid scarring and inturned lashes with corneal ulceration and visual loss. Tetracycline or sulphacetamide administered locally or trimethoprim orally is the recommended treatment. Control of the disease will come with improved living standards and hygiene.

Bacterial conjunctivitis

This is common in all children and causes red eyes with discharge. It is usually bilateral and cross infection within the family is frequent. Most cases respond rapidly to local antibiotics, particularly chloramphenicol 0.5% 2-hourly. Staphylococci and pneumococci are the usual pathogens, but it is unnecessary to culture the discharge unless the infection is resistant to treatment.

Viral conjunctivitis

A mild conjunctival inflammation with a follicular reaction in the conjunctiva of the lids may be the result of adenovirus infection. It is usually self-limiting and does not respond to specific treatment. Small epidemics of adenovirus conjunctivitis occur often with associated pharyngeal infections.

Herpes simplex, as a primary infection, causes a similar viral conjunctivitis. If vesicles are present around the lids the diagnosis will be made easier. Secondary infections will present as dendritic ulcers on the cornea (see above).

Allergic conjunctivitis

This may present in several forms. Mild irritation and watering may be present with other allergic manifestations, e.g. allergic rhinitis. Vernal conjunctivitis is a more persistent and chronic form usually without any identifiable allergen. Eversion of the upper lid will reveal a papillary reaction; large papillae, up to 3 mm in diameter may be seen in severe forms. These severe forms of atopy may have associated corneal plaques which can lead to corneal scarring. Vernal conjunctivitis usually disappears by the late teens. Treatment depends on its severity. Decongestant drops may be sufficient but sodium cromoglycate and steroid drops may be indicated for severe cases.

Lid infections

Blepharitis squamosa

This is a common condition in adolescence associated with scaling of the lid margin and mild chronic infection of the glands of the eyelid. The problem tends to be persistent and recurrent. The aim of treatment is to remove the scales either by saline bathing or by using baby shampoo on a cotton-tipped applicator. Local antibiotic drops or ointment and steroid drops may be necessary.

Acute infections of the lid

These may present as either a diffuse cellulitis which can be associated with infection in a gland related to a lash follicle (stye or hordeolum), or infection in one or more of the meibomian glands of the lid (meibomian cyst or chalazion). System antibiotics are only indicated if the infection is not localized. Otherwise antibiotic drops are sufficient. Styes usually discharge spontaneously and meibomian cysts tend to slowly resolve in children over a period of several weeks.

Allergic blepharitis

Itchy erythema and scaling of the skin of the lids may indicate a local allergy, the most frequent cause being local medication. The condition resolves with removal of the allergen.

Orbital cellulitis

This is a serious sight-threatening problem. Swelling of the eye lids and conjunctiva develop rapidly with proptosis and displacement of the globe and limitation of ocular movements. Infection of the paranasal sinuses is the most common cause and *Haemophilus influenzae* is the most frequent pathogen. Treatment involves hospitalization for intravenous antibiotic therapy and careful observation. Surgical drainage of the paranasal sinuses may be indicated so close co-operation with the ENT surgeon is essential.

Blocked tear duct

The nasolacrimal duct is formed from a solid core of tissue which hollows out and establishes a clear passage into the nose about the time of birth. In about 6% of infants this process is delayed so that the lacrimal sac, like any other blocked drain, becomes infected resulting in a persistent discharge from one or both eyes. In at least 50% of these infants spontaneous resolution of the problem occurs by the age of six months. During this period management is initially conservative with bathing, local antibiotics and massage over the lacrimal sac. Probing of the lacrimal passages should be done before the age of 12 months but may be indicated before 6 months if the discharge is profuse and irritating.

Uveitis

The iris, ciliary body and the choroid form the uveal tract which is the vascular coat of the eyeball. Its vascularity and cellular anatomy make it susceptible to blood-borne and local disorders, both infective and immunological.

Acute iritis

Acute iritis is a painful condition with a red eye, increased sensitivity to light and watering. The pupil may be small because of adhesions between the iris and the lens (posterior synechiae) and the vision is blurred. Iritis may also have an insidious onset and run a chronic course resulting in late complications such as cataract or glaucoma. In children, iritis often has a treatable cause. Investigation should exclude toxoplasmosis, syphilis and herpes simplex and any other generalized infective process. Acute iritis is frequently associated with chronic bowel disease and juvenile chronic arthritis. In the child with pauci-articular juvenile chronic arthritis who is antinuclear factor positive an insidious form of iritis frequently develops. This is asymptomatic in its early stages. Early diagnosis is made by regular examination of these children at risk with the slit lamp to detect cells in the normally clear aqueous humour.

Treatment of iritis involves pupil dilatation with atropine drops and steroids to suppress inflammation. Systemic steroids may be necessary if drops are not effective. The prognosis of iritis is good if treatment and follow-up are also good, but recurrence is likely.

Choroiditis

Choroiditis or posterior uveitis may involve the retina and vitreous in the inflammatory process. Blurred vision and floating opacities in the visual field are often the only symptoms. Pain is not a feature. Again, full investigation is mandatory. Choroiditis does not respond to steroids administered locally. Focal scars in the peripheral retina will not significantly affect vision but central scars (typical of intra-uterine toxoplasma infection) and diffuse scarring seen with some systemic diseases can lead to virtual blindness.

THE RETINA

Examination of the retina is extremely difficult with the direct ophthalmoscope in young children except under anaesthesia. The indirect ophthalmoscope, used by the ophthalmologist, provides an inverted virtual image of the retina in 'mid-air', but allows for examination of a much wider field of view, though with some decrease in magnification. Examination under anaesthesia is seldom necessary.

Non-inflammatory retinal diseases

These are mostly congenital or developmental; some are static and others progressive.

Failure in development of the eye in general can lead to microphthalmia, the extremes being a slightly undersized eye to a situation where only a tiny remnant can be found in the socket.

Defects caused by incomplete closure of the fetal fissure in the development of the optic cup causes defects in the uveal tract and retina – coloboma. If only the iris is involved there is just an irregular pear-shaped pupil; but colobomas may extend back to involve the posterior choroid and retina causing a visual field defect or loss of central vision. Colobomas may be associated with multiple congenital abnormalities. A coloboma of the choroid is seen as an area, extending inferiorly, where there appears to be virtually bare sclera.

The optic nerve may also show various developmental anomalies. One example is optic nerve hypoplasia where the optic disc is smaller than normal and edged by a double pigment ring in the choroid. Again, the manifestations and the effect on vision are variable. The association of optic nerve hypoplasia with absence of the septum pellucidum and pituitary abnormalities is de Morsier's syndrome.

Leber's amaurosis (blindness)

The fundus may appear normal in the early months, yet the child has no visual responses and develops nystagmus early. The diagnosis is established by the electroretinogram where no response is elicited. The differential diagnosis between a retinal cause of blindness and a cerebral cause can be difficult. A retinal problem will usually cause nystagmus, whilst the eyes may be quite steady if the cause is a cerebral one, for example porencephaly. Visually evoked potentials measured in-

directly off the occipital cortex are not yet a reliable aid in diagnosis or assessment of visual potential.

Pigmentary degeneration of the retina (retinitis pigmentosa)

Classical retinitis pigmentosa is a familial disease with variable inheritance. With progressive degeneration of the retinal pigment epithelium, there is formation of the 'bone spicule' pigmentation in the retina. There is also thinning of the retinal arterioles with increasing pallor of the optic disc. Symptoms in the early stages may be absent but increasing difficulty with night vision occurs with loss of peripheral visual fields. Central vision may be retained. Pigmentary degeneration of the retina may appear as part of a number of rare disease syndromes.

Full investigation with consultation with the medical geneticists is an essential part of the diagnostic work up. Electro-retinography can be diagnostic before signs or symptoms appear. Regrettably, there is no specific treatment.

Retinopathy of prematurity (retrolental fibroplasia)

This condition usually occurs in premature infants with a birthweight less than 1500 grams. Though there are many factors operating, the onset of this disease is related to the effect of oxygen on the developing retinal vasculature. Early stages of the disease may regress, but in more advanced progressive disease peripheral scarring of the retina occurs. Vitreous haemorrhage, retinal detachment and fibrous ingrowth with a retrolental membrane can finally result in blindness. Although there have been various treatments advocated including mega-doses of vitamin A, none has been proved effective.

Retinoblastoma

This is a rare tumour, with an incidence of 1:20 000 live births but is the commonest intraocular tumour in childhood. Untreated, the disease is fatal with spread along the optic nerve to the neuraxis or through blood-borne metastases. With early diagnosis and adequate treatment mortality should be less than 5%. Of all cases 60% are unilateral and sporadic and the remaining 40% are familial with an autosomal dominant inheritance. All bilateral cases are familial.

Retinoblastoma must be excluded in any child presenting with a white pupil (see Fig. 70.4). The differential diagnoses are cataract, parasitic endophthalmitis, Coat's disease and coloboma of the choroid. CT scans or plain radiographs of the orbit may delineate the tumour and reveal characteristic calcification. Detailed examination under anaesthetic is also necessary to confirm the diagnosis and to assess both eyes.

Most sporadic cases of retinoblastoma do not present until the tumour is large and useful vision is destroyed. The eye is removed with as much of the optic nerve as possible. Tumours are graded according to size and involvement of the internal eye. It is the routine at the Royal Children's Hospital in Melbourne to give children with grade five tumours prophylactic chemotherapy even if there is no evidence of metastatic spread.

Patients who have salvageable vision with small or bilateral tumours, may be treated by various conservative methods, including cryotherapy of the lesions and local radiotherapy.

Recent DNA studies have identified the exact locus of the retinoblastoma gene in some families, which will help with genetic counselling and management of children at risk. 13q chromosome deletion has been found in some families. These children also have other abnormalities.

OCULAR TRAUMA

Reference has already been made to some problems of minor ocular trauma. Others requiring special note are mentioned below.

Blunt trauma

This is caused by fists, missiles thrown by others or projected by machinery such as motor mowers. Hyphaema is haemorrhage into the anterior chamber of the eye from rupture of vessels at the root of the iris. This may result in an anterior chamber full of blood, a blood level obvious in the lower part of the anterior chamber or a minimal circulating hyphaema only detected on slit-lamp examination. It should be suspected from the nature of the injury. Usually a hyphaema will absorb within five days, but a re-bleed in 48–76 hours can occur with secondary glaucoma, blood staining of the cornea and profound visual loss unless intense specialist treatment is effective. Any hyphaema is, therefore, treated carefully, preferably with bed rest and sedation (avoiding aspirin) with instructions to report any pain within the first 72 hours which might indicate a secondary bleed.

Blunt trauma may also cause dislocation of the lens, rupture of the lens capsule with subsequent cataract formation, retinal detachment or haemorrhage into the vitreous. Assessment of visual acuity and an examination of the fundus are necessary.

Injuries to the orbit may also occur with fractures of the orbital wall (blow-outs). A limitation of ocular movements with double vision may be a clue to this. The problem may be associated with any 'black eye'.

Sharp trauma

Sharp trauma may perforate or lacerate the eyelids, the cornea or deeper structures of the eye and orbit in any combination and must be carefully sought in relation to any injury. It should always be suspected in any injury, as the history can be quite unhelpful and frankly misleading, particularly when a child's friend may have been responsible for the injury.

Prognosis for vision or even retention of the eye is dependent on early referral, competent surgical repair and follow-up.

Non-accidental trauma

This is seen in a few children who have been victims of physical assault. Vigorous shaking produces retinal and vitreous haemorrhages. These injuries have caused irreversible blindness, so examination of the fundus becomes an important part of the investigation.

Glaucoma

Congenital glaucoma is rare. Infants present with a cloudy cornea and enlarged eyes either at birth or within the first few months. The condition should be suspected in any infant with photophobia and a watering eye, and is usually bilateral. Treatment is surgical.

Learning problems, dyslexia and vision

A large number of children have been inflicted with spectacles containing useless lenses or incorporating mysterious tints. Others have been subjected to courses of eye exercises. There is no scientific basis for any of these regimes. Some children whose school performance is restricted by poor vision will be helped by correction of significant refractive errors. They are the exception rather than the rule.

FURTHER READING

Crawford J S, Morin J D 1983 The eye in childhood. Grune & Stratton, New York
Harley R D 1983 Paediatric ophthalmology, 2nd edn. W B Saunders, Philadelphia
Helveston E M 1984 Paediatric ophthalmology in practice, 2nd edn. C V Mosby, St Louis

71. Ear, nose and throat problems

Robert Webb

Disorders of the ear, nose and throat are common in children. They are partially related to immaturity of the immune mechanism but also to anatomical factors, such as the shape of the Eustachian tube and hypertrophy of lymphoid tissue; the adenoids may be sufficiently enlarged to cause obstruction. Interrelationships between the nasal and oral cavities, the pharynx, larynx, middle ears and paranasal sinuses are important. The relationship of these passages and cavities to the orbits, the cranial cavities and other structures in the head and neck must also be kept in mind.

THE NOSE

Congenital malformations

The commonest malformations of the nose are associated with the various types of cleft palate. These require surgical repair. The other important malformation of the nose is choanal atresia which, if bilateral, can present as a neonatal emergency. Neonates are obligate nose breathers so that an oral airway and surgical repair is required. Unilateral choanal atresia will present with a unilateral nasal discharge and it can be repaired surgically when required.

Acquired disorders

Acute viral rhinitis

The commonest disorder of the nose is acute viral rhinitis. This presents with nasal obstruction and a mucopurulent discharge. Associated symptoms include head fullness, malaise and sneezing. Physical signs include mucosal congestion and nasal discharge. Treatment is symptomatic with topical decongestants and analgesics.

Acute bacterial rhinitis

The symptoms are similar to viral rhinitis, but tend to be more severe and tend to follow on a viral rhinitis. An organism may be cultured – most frequently *Streptococcus pyogenes* or *Haemophilus influenzae*. Antibiotics are usually not indicated unless the child is toxic.

Acute sinusitis

The presenting features are acute rhinitis plus pain over the affected sinuses. The important physical sign is tenderness over the sinuses. The maxillary and ethmoid sinuses are present at birth, the sphenoid sinus develops at about the age of three years and the frontal sinuses at about the age of six years. The diagnosis can be confirmed radiologically when opacity or fluid levels may be demonstrated (Fig. 71.1). Treatment consists of decongestants, antibiotics and analgesics. Decongestants are best given topically in the form of nose drops. These should be given with the patient lying on the side with the head low and the face tilted slightly up and the

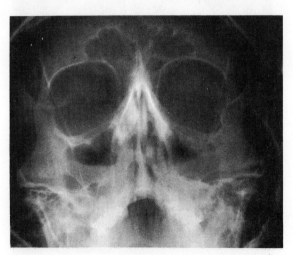

Fig. 71.1 Radiograph of paranasal sinuses demonstrating fluid levels in both maxillary antra.

drops put in the lower nostril. Systemic decongestants such as pseudoephedrine may be helpful.

If the condition persists an ENT specialist opinion should be sought as sinus washouts may be required.

Complications of sinusitis. The principle complication of ethmoidal sinusitis is orbital cellulitis. This varies in severity. In periorbital cellulitis the eyelids are swollen, the child has difficulty in opening the eyelids but eye movement is present. Progress to orbital cellulitis and a subperiosteal abscess causes proptosis and ophthalmoplegia. Intracranial extension of infection may result in cavernous sinus thrombosis.

A CT scan is indicated should there be any suspicion of intracranial or orbital extension (Fig. 71.2). Treatment involves decongestants as mentioned above and antibiotics given intravenously. The appropriate antibiotic is determined by the growth from a nasal swab, but until this is available, intravenous antibiotics covering Gram-positive and Gram-negative organisms are necessary. Should proptosis be present ENT specialist opinion should be obtained as a drainage procedure is usually required.

Intracranial spread occurs principally into the frontal lobe region from the frontal sinuses. It should be suspected with increasing headache, swelling over the frontal sinus, meningism or neurological features. A CT

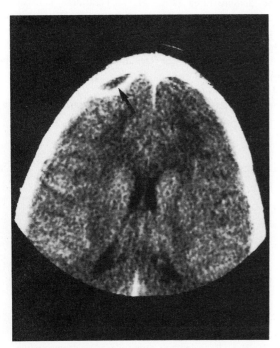

Fig. 71.2 CT scan of brain demonstrating an extradural abscess (arrow) over the left frontal lobe.

scan is required for confirmation. This complication is best prevented by referral of any persistent case of sinusitis for ENT specialist opinion.

Allergy

Children are affected by a wide range of inhaled and ingested allergens. The clinical features and management of acute allergic rhinitis are covered in Chapter 23.

Vasomotor rhinitis

This is nasal obstruction due to mucosal congestion. An anterior nasal discharge is not a feature and a posterior discharge is rare in children. It is caused by a sensitivity of the nose to mechanical, thermal and internal irritants. Examples include temperature change, fumes, smoke, emotional factors and medications such as some antihypertensives. The excessive use of decongestant nose drops can also cause this condition. Treatment involves the avoidance of the irritants, systemic decongestants such as pseudoephedrine and in persistent cases cautery of the nasal turbinates.

Many children will have features of infective, allergic and vasomotor rhinitis. Specialist referral is indicated in persistent cases.

Foreign body

The main symptom of an unobserved nasal foreign body is a unilateral purulent nasal discharge which may be blood stained. Rarely foreign bodies may be on both sides. The diagnosis is made by a good inspection of the nose with a suitable head light or head mirror after the discharge has been cleaned out. Removal may require general anaesthetic in a young or unco-operative child. Suitable hooks and forceps will be required and care must be taken to pull the foreign body out and not push it backwards.

Trauma

Obvious external deformity due to fractured nasal bones warrants operative reduction. Nasal obstruction following injury implies that either a septal haematoma or deviation of the nasal septum has occurred. The interior of the nose must be inspected carefully under these circumstances. A septal haematoma requires drainage.

Epistaxis

This is common in children and often occurs at night. The usual site is 'Little's area', which is on the nasal

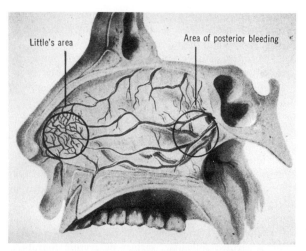

Fig. 71.3 The common sites for bleeding from the nose.

septum just inside the anterior nares (Fig. 71.3). The causes are listed below:

1. Infections – rhinitis, vestibulitis
2. Trauma, including nose picking and vigorous nose blowing
3. Over-heating – exercise, too many blankets, fever
4. Environmental factors – heat, low humidity
5. Mechanical factors – septum deviation and perforations, shallow blood vessels
6. Bleeding and clotting disorders
7. Anticoagulant drugs – particularly aspirin
8. Vascular disorders e.g. hereditary telangiectasia
9. Tumours e.g. angiofibroma, haemangioma
10. Foreign bodies
11. Chronic rhinitis – granulomas, atrophy.

Management. Management will depend on the cause which will be evident from the history, examination and investigations as appropriate. The first aid treatment of epistaxis is compression. Pushing just above the anterior nares with fingers and thumbs to compress the vessel in Little's area will usually stop the bleeding. A more posteriorly situated vessel can be occluded with moist cotton wool in the nasal cavity plus compression. Cold, such as an ice pack or a wet face washer, applied across the forehead is also useful.

If crusting is present in the nasal vestibule an antibiotic or antiseptic ointment such as neomycin or povidone-iodine can be usefully applied for about a week. This can be followed by the use of vaseline or a similar ointment to protect the area.

Nasal cautery. Apply local anaesthetic such as 5% cocaine or lignocaine and adrenaline. In most cases 10% xylocaine is satisfactory. Ensure that the local anaes-

thetic, particularly cocaine, is not swallowed. Apply for five to ten minutes and then cauterize with a silver nitrate stick. Larger vessels may require electric cautery, which in most children will require general anaesthesia. Nasal packing may also be needed.

THE PHARYNX

The pharyngeal mucosa contains numerous follicles of lymphoid tissue with 3 major aggregations of lymphoid tissue – the adenoids in the nasopharynx, the palatine tonsils in the oropharynx and the lingual tonsils in the hypopharynx. These aggregations are useful adjuncts to the immune system but are not essential. They are normally large in children and tend to shrink to adult proportions by the age of eight years.

Other important anatomical features are the Eustachian tubes which open into the lateral walls of the nasopharynx. The soft palate seals off the nasopharynx during swallowing, prevents nasal regurgitation of food and protects the Eustachian tubes which are opened by the pull of the tensor palatini muscle.

DISORDERS OF THE PHARYNX

Congenital

The main congenital abnormality is cleft palate. (Fig. 71.4)

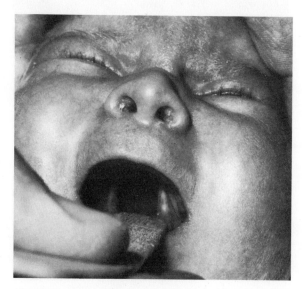

Fig. 71.4 A large cleft palate in a neonate. Note this infant does not have a cleft lip.

Acquired

Infection is common and usually the result of viral infection. The clinical features and management of pharyngitis is discussed in Chapter 35.

Adenoids

The main symptom of adenoidal enlargement is nasal obstruction which is usually of little concern to the child, but the parents are often worried by the mouth breathing and nocturnal snoring. However, some children are distressed by the continual mouth breathing. There may be other associated problems such as Eustachian tube obstruction, otitis media, nasal discharge, tonsillitis and dental disturbance.

The main sign of adenoidal enlargement is nasal obstruction in the absence of any narrowing of the

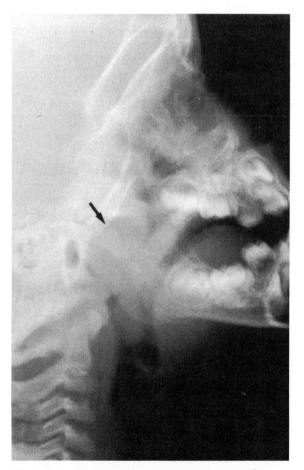

Fig. 71.5 Lateral radiograph of the neck demonstrating adenoidal tissue compressing the upper airway.

anterior nasal airways. This may be confirmed by a mirror examination of the postnasal space or a lateral soft tissue radiograph of the region (Fig. 71.5).

Treatment of uncomplicated nasal obstruction is by reassurance that the condition will probably spontaneously resolve. In other cases, adenoidectomy is indicated.

Tonsils

The tonsils are often involved in pharyngitis and will be enlarged and congested. In addition a specific infection can occur within the tonsils. This is usually due to debris in the tonsillar crypts which favours the proliferation of bacteria with the formation of pus and surrounding inflammation. This specific tonsillar infection is termed follicular, lucinar or cryptic tonsillitis. The clinical features and management of acute tonsillitis are discussed in Chapter 35.

The tonsils are frequently involved in infectious mononucleosis when the appearances are often characteristic, the tonsils being enlarged, congested and relatively smooth so that the crypts are obliterated. A whitish exudate frequently covers the tonsils in infectious mononucleosis. The diagnosis should be considered if there is no response to antibiotics and confirmed by the blood film and appropriate serology.

Complications of tonsillitis

The major complication of tonsillitis is quinsy. This is the spread of infection beyond the tonsils to the peritonsillar space. Initially it is a cellulitis and later an abscess. It presents as a progressive sore throat with increasing dysphagia, trismus and malaise. The diagnostic feature is the difficulty of opening the jaw and the displacement of the tonsil and uvula to the opposite side by a swelling lateral to the tonsils. A yellow discoloration on this swelling may indicate the site of pointing of the abscess. Treatment involves intravenous antibiotics, usually penicillin, and incision if it is pointing. A tonsillectomy should be considered to prevent recurrence.

Sleep apnoea

Hypertrophy of the tonsils and adenoids either as a complication of infection or due to their intrinsic size may cause marked obstruction to the airways. This is usually worse at night, when the child is recumbent as there may be some loss of pharyngeal muscular tone with sleep. The breathing becomes laboured with periods of total obstruction relieved by partial waking and change of position. In sleep apnoea blood gases reveal a low pO_2

which can be documented by oximetry. Electrocardiographic changes can also occur. The typical features of this syndrome are the nocturnal restlessness, inadequate sleep and consequent day time sleepiness. Sleep apnoea is an absolute indication for adenotonsillectomy. Enlarged tonsils may also cause dysphagia.

Tonsillar tumours

The commonest tumour of the tonsil in children is the lymphoma. it usually presents with unilateral tonsillar enlargement and is often associated with enlarged cervical lymph nodes. If suspected a biopsy by tonsillectomy is indicated.

THE LARYNX

The principle symptoms of laryngeal disease in children are hoarseness and stridor. Hoarseness is a roughness of the voice or cry. Stridor is a harsh high-pitched noise which in laryngeal disease is predominantly inspiratory. It is caused by turbulent airflow in a narrowed airway and is thus an indicator of partial respiratory obstruction. Increasing obstruction will lead to expiratory as well as inspiratory stridor. Of course there is no stridor with total obstruction. With increasing obstruction other symptoms such as restlessness, dyspnoea and ultimately cyanosis will develop. Stridor is thus an important symptom, the cause of which must be rapidly diagnosed and treated as an emergency.

Examination of the larynx

The larynx can be inspected by indirect or direct laryngoscopy. In indirect laryngoscopy a view of the larynx with a warmed mirror is obtained in a co-operative child. In direct laryngoscopy the larynx is directly viewed with a laryngoscope. In the neonate this may be performed without anaesthesia, but in older infants and children a general anaesthetic will be required.

DISORDERS OF THE LARYNX

Congenital

Laryngomalacia

This is the commonest congenital abnormality of the larynx and is characterized by stridor which commences soon after birth and is exacerbated with crying and exertion. There is no stridor with quiet breathing and no hoarseness. It is due to the laryngeal shape and the softness of the laryngeal cartilages. Laryngomalacia is a self-limiting condition requiring no treatment. However, it may exacerbate other conditions affecting the larynx. The diagnosis can usually be made from the history and in the mild case this is all that is needed. If the stridor is more severe, laryngoscopy is required to exclude other pathology.

Laryngeal webs

The degree of hoarseness and stridor depends on the size of the web. Treatment is by surgical division.

Cysts

Treatment is endoscopic removal.

Haemangiomas

Small ones can be observed. Larger ones may require tracheostomy and reduction in size by the laser technique.

Subglottic stenosis

Mild cases can be observed. Tighter ones may require either laser reduction, dilatation or open surgery.

Oesophageal atresia with tracheo-oesophageal fistula

The larynx may be involved in this malformation.

Acquired

Inflammatory conditions of the larynx are common and may be acute or chronic.

Acute viral laryngitis

The clinical features and management of this disorder are described in Chapter 35.

Acute epiglottitis or supraglottic laryngitis

The diagnosis and management of this life-threatening disorder is described in Chapter 35.

Vocal abuse

This is common in exuberant children who shout or sing excessively. In the acute form there is hoarseness after excessive voice use which improves with a rest. If the abuse is continued, the hoarseness will become chronic and vocal nodules will occur; these are swellings on the anterior part of the vocal cord. In the early stages vocal nodules are due to oedema. In established cases there can be a thickening of the epithelium and sub-epithelial fibrosis. The diagnosis is established by laryngoscopy. Treatment centres around vocal rest and in particular cessation of the shouting which is causing the problem. Once this is achieved speech therapy is of great benefit. If the hoarseness still persists surgical removal of the nodules is indicated.

Laryngeal tumours

The commonest childhood tumour is a papilloma. It is a wart-like condition and usually multiple. In severe cases all parts of the larynx, the trachea, and the bronchi may be involved. Treatment consists of surgical removal which may need to be repeated if regrowth occurs. In some cases numerous procedures are required to maintain a patent airway.

Recurrent laryngeal nerve paralysis

This may be congenital or acquired. In both cases it can be due to a poly- or mononeuritis. Other causes include CNS abnormalities, metabolic disorders, toxins, trauma, tumours, or the cause may be unknown. The voice has a breathy quality and the diagnosis is confirmed by laryngoscopy. The cause of this disorder should be determined and treated if possible. However, spontaneous improvement occurs in many cases but even if this does not the other side will compensate adequately. If recurrent nerve paralysis does not improve spontaneously a surgical procedure to improve the voice may be required.

THE EAR

The ear consists of external, middle and inner components. Examination of the external ear and the tympanic membrane is performed by otoscopy. This procedure plus any other form of instrumentation in the external canal must be performed with gentleness as the ear is an extremely sensitive structure.

Hearing loss

The effect of hearing loss in children, especially in the younger years, is particularly disabling because of its effects on speech development, learning capacity, and social interaction as well as the capacity to communicate. It is, therefore, very important that hearing loss should be detected as early as possible and effectively managed.

Common causes of hearing loss in children include:

1. Congenital factors
   a. Hereditary. In this situation there will usually be a positive family history
   b. Teratogenic agents, e.g. rubella, toxoplasma, syphilis, and thalidomide
   c. Hypoxia from birth trauma
   d. Prematurity
   e. Hyperbilirubinaemia from rhesus incompatibility
   f. External auditory canal atresia.

2. Acquired
   a. Wax inclusion
   b. All forms of otitis media
   c. Bacterial meningitis
   d. Viral labyrinthitis, e.g. mumps, measles, herpes zoster or influenza
   e. Trauma
   f. Ototoxic drugs – the aminoglycocides are the commonest
   g. Perilymph leak
   h. Metabolic disorders.

Presentation of hearing loss

This will depend on whether it is unilateral or bilateral, its severity and the age of onset. The more common presentations include:

1. Failure to respond to sound
2. Preference for or response only to loud sounds
3. Speech abnormality
4. Poor school progress
5. Behavioural disorders
6. Inability to detect sound direction – unilateral loss
7. Poor response in background noise
8. Visible malformation of ears, skull or facial structures.

A skilled audiological assessment is indicated if the child has the following:

1. One or more of the above symptoms or signs
2. A history of a condition which is likely to cause a hearing loss
3. Any doubts about hearing expressed by parents and teachers.

In addition some children, with a significant hearing loss will be missed if audiological testing was only carried out on the above grounds. Therefore, routine testing is important and should be carried out at infancy, kindergarten and primary school (Figs. 71.6 and 71.7).

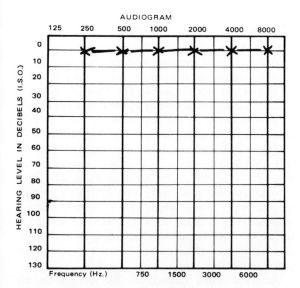

Fig. 71.6 Audiogram demonstrating normal hearing in the left ear. Audiogram of the right ear is not demonstrated in this figure.

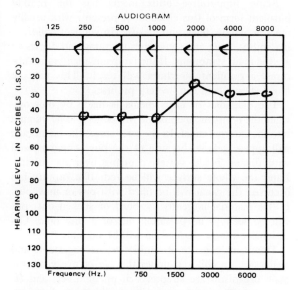

Fig. 71.7 Audiogram demonstrating right conductive hearing loss consistent with otitis media with effusion. Audiogram of the left ear is consistent with normal hearing.

Objective tests of hearing, such as measurement of the stapedial reflex and electric response audiometry can be carried out at any age. Subjective tests can be carried

out once the child has head control – from about 6 months of age.

Clinical testing of hearing also has a place. In the infant there is the auro-palpebral reflex which causes blinking in response to loud sounds. This is a crude test, but will probably exclude a severe bilateral hearing loss. A head turning towards sound can be assessed in older infants. The response to speech of varying loudness can be tested in co-operative children. Tuning fork tests can be of use, but are often unreliable. Otoscopic inspection of the ears is obviously very important.

The management of the hearing loss depends on its cause and severity. Some conditions such as otitis media with effusion or chronic otitis media can be managed medically or surgically. Other conditions, especially involving the inner ear, may warrant amplification with an appropriately fitted hearing aid or aids. In cases of moderate hearing loss the hearing aid alone will be adequate management. In many cases the use of the aid can be discretionery, in that it will only be required in certain circumstances where information must be accurately assimilated, such as in the classroom. More severe cases will require continuous use of the hearing aid. In children with a severe or profound loss, sounds will be distorted so that amplification alone will be adequate. Special rehabilitation programmes are most important and special education services will usually be required. Particular attention will be applied to the learning of skills such as lip reading and techniques of speech production. Sign language can be useful. A variety of other aids are available. In certain select cases where a hearing aid is of no benefit, a cochlear implant may be inserted.

SPECIFIC DISORDERS OF THE EAR

Congenital abnormalities

As the three parts of the ear develop separately, abnormalities of one part do not necessarily imply abnormalities of the others. However in certain syndromes multiple abnormalities may occur. Abnormalities of the external ear include malformations of the pinna and atresia of the external auditory canal. The pinna may require surgical reconstruction on cosmetic grounds. A unilateral canal atresia usually does not require surgery, but if bilateral surgical correction is necessary to provide adequate hearing. Before surgery the state of the middle and inner ears must be assessed radiologically and audiologically to ensure that reconstruction is feasible.

Acquired disorders

External

Wax is the product of glandular secretion plus exfoliated keratin and is normally in the ear and should continually appear on the surface where it should be wiped away and not pursued into the canal with a cotton bud. An excessive accumulation of wax may block the canal at any age. This may be removed by the use of softening drops, syringing, mechanical means or a combination of these.

Foreign bodies are frequently put into the external auditory canals of children. Treatment is judicious removal. A rough removal will often cause much more damage than the foreign body itself. A general anaesthetic is indicated in a young or unco-operative child.

Otitis externa

This is usually associated with swimming. The common form of otitis externa is an infectious dermatitis, the usual organisms involved being *Pseudomonas aeruginosa*, other Gram- negative bacteria and *Staphylococcus aureus*. Fungal superinfection may also occur. The diagnosis is made by inspection of the canal which is diffusely red and swollen. Any debris should be gently swabbed out and in persistent cases a bacteriological swab taken. Treatment consists of antibiotic-steroid drops, analgesics and strict avoidance of water and scratching. Anti-fungal agents may be necessary. Great care must be taken with otitis externa as it can become very intractable and difficult to treat. The pain can be very severe. ENT referral is required in any persistent case.

Myringitis bullosa

This is characterized by severe otalgia of sudden onset. Inspection of the canal will reveal clear or blood filled blisters on the canal skin and tympanic membranes. There is little or no hearing loss. A bloody aural discharge may occur and although very upsetting for the patient is associated with pain reduction. The differentiation from acute otitis media is made by noting the multiple swellings extending out on to the canal skin instead of a general bulge of the tympanic membrane. Treatment includes analgesia and an oral antibiotic. Topical warmth with warm drops or surface application of a poultice or hot water bottle is valuable in relieving discomfort.

The middle ear

The middle ear is an air-containing cavity, separated from the external canal by the tympanic membrane and ventilated by the Eustachian tube. Sound is transmitted through the middle ear by the ossicular chain to the inner ear. Normal function of the middle ear and the tympanic membrane requires the middle ear pressure to be that of the external canal. The Eustachian tube is normally closed and is opened by the tensor veli palatini as it contributes to the movement of the palate in separating the nasopharynx from the oropharynx.

If the Eustachian tube function is impaired, pressure within the middle ear decreases causing discomfort and hearing loss. If the middle ear pressure is sufficiently low and especially if allergy or infection irritate the middle ear lining, fluid, which can be serous, mucoid, mucopurulent or purulent, will develop in the middle ear cavity. This is currently termed otitis media with effusion (OME). The mucoid effusion is commonly called a glue ear.

Factors affecting Eustachian tube function include nasal and pharyngeal infection, allergy, adenoid hypertrophy and cleft palate. Children, as well as being especially susceptible to these factors have a less efficient tubal opening mechanism than adults. Therefore, OME is a predominantly childhood disease.

Acute suppurative otitis media has the frankly purulent form of this effusion. It presents with usually marked otalgia, fever and malaise. In younger children, irritability, fever and sometimes vomiting and diarrhoea are the main symptoms. If the tympanic membrane ruptures, a purulent otorrhoea will result. This may be blood stained and can be very profuse.

The diagnosis of otitis media is made by otoscopy when the tympanic membrane will be seen to be bulging into the external canal. In the early stages the membrane will appear yellow, because of the pus behind it, and with dilated blood vessels coursing over its surface. Later the whole surface will be red. If a rupture has occurred the canal will be filled with pus or mucopus. If this material is gently swabbed or sucked out, pus will be seen to be pulsating out of a tiny hole. Occasionally a large perforation will be present.

Treatment consists of antibiotics, decongestants and analgesics. In children under the age of five years the main organisms are streptococci, pneumococci and *H. influenzae*. The most appropriate antibiotic is, therefore, amoxycillin or co-trimoxazole. In older children *H. influenzae* is less common and penicillin or erythromycin are the agents of choice.

Decongestant therapy is particularly important. The most direct and effective way to reduce Eustachian tube congestion and oedema is to use a decongestant nose drop. Systemic decongestants such as pseudoephedrine are also useful. Analgesics, e.g. paracetamol, may be given by mouth. Warmed oil or medicated drops into the canal or topically applied warm compressors or hot water bottles are very useful for pain relief.

If a discharge is present, the antibiotic used can be adjusted according to the organism cultured. It is very important that an adequate course (10 days) of antibiotic is taken to eradicate the organism.

Complications of otitis media. The major complication is acute mastoiditis. This presents with pain, swelling and tenderness developing behind the ear, plus a general deterioration in the condition of the child. A more subtle version is masked mastoiditis where these symptoms are reduced or masked by inadequate antibiotic therapy. Complications of mastoiditis include chronic otitis media, facial nerve paralysis, acute labyrinthitis and intracranial spread. These may also occur directly from middle ear infection but are more commonly secondary to the mastoiditis. Early ENT specialist referral is indicated in any persistent or progressive case of acute suppurative otitis media.

Glue ear

The non-acutely infected type of OME presents with a mild to moderate hearing loss. Older children may complain of discomfort and younger children may be irritable at night. However, the child is usually unaware of the condition and the presentations include preference for loud TV and/or radio or poor school performance. Any speech disorder may be enhanced. Mild and unilateral cases may only be detected by routine audiological screening. The condition may be associated with acute episodes of infection.

The diagnosis is made by otoscopy with a pneumatic device attached. The movement of the drum is the best indication of the presence or absence of middle ear fluid. When there is thick mucus in the middle ear, drum movement will be restricted and very slow. If the middle ear is filled with air the movement of the drum will be wide and quick. When the middle ear is filled with air, but at a low pressure, the drum will not move outwards to any extent, but rapid inward movement will occur. In the presence of an air fluid mixture an in-between level of movement will occur. The tympanic membrane may have many appearances, but frequently it is dull, indrawn and immobile with a few dilated vessels on the surface. Other appearances include a yellowish tinge to the tympanic membrane, fluid levels and occasionally bubbles in fluid. A conductive hearing loss is present which can be detected clinically and audiologically. The diagnosis is confirmed with impedance audiometry (tympanometry).

Tympanometry

Measurement made here is the amount of sound absorption by the middle ear mechanism. Although it does not indicate the severity of serous otitis media, if the test produces a normal result it proves that there is an air-filled middle ear. The air canal is sealed and the air pressure in the canal is varied. This stretches the ear drum inwards and outwards and the effect of this movement on sound absorption provides the graph or pattern of tympanometry (see Figs 71.8, 71.9 and 71.10).

Treatment includes medical management of the contributing factors such as nasal allergy or infection. The decongestant regime as detailed under acute suppurative otitis media is given and is supplemented with the Valsala manoeuvre. Antibiotics may be useful in some cases, especially where there is some active inflammation as evidenced by dilated vessels. Many cases resolve within a week, and of course spontaneous resolution can occur.

Persisting or recurrent cases of OME of all types should be referred for ENT specialist opinion. Prolonged middle ear effusion can lead to tympanic membrane, middle ear mucosa and ossicular chain damage. This can result in a chronic otitis media, scarring or ossicular discontinuity which will require major ear reconstruction. But this can usually be prevented by the timely use of suction myringotomy and the insertion of middle ear ventilating or drainage tubes through the tympanic membrane.

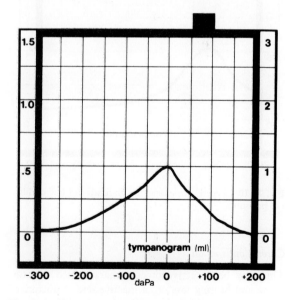

Fig. 71.8 Type A tympanogram (normal).

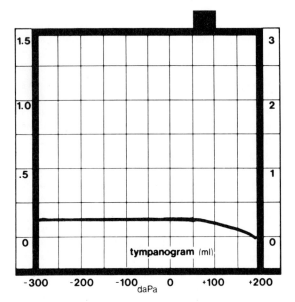

Fig. 71.9 Type B tympanogram (consistent with fluid accumulation in the middle ear).

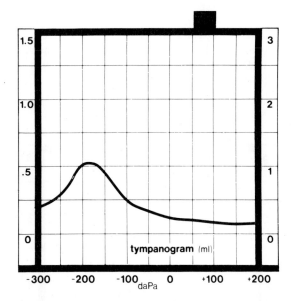

Fig. 71.10 Type C tympanogram. Indicative of low middle ear pressure.

Chronic otitis media

This may be an active process characterized by otorrhoea and hearing loss or an inactive one characterized by hearing loss alone.

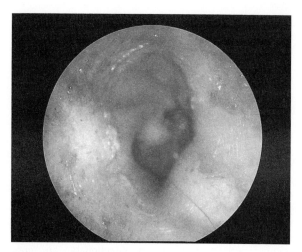

Fig. 71.11 A cholesteatoma.

The major sign of active chronic disease is a perforation of the tympanic membrane. The perforation may be central within the tympanic membrane or marginal at its edge. The central perforation will usually have a mucopurulent discharge which may be profuse. This is termed a safe perforation. The marginal perforation is often associated with an ingrowth of skin into the middle ear and mastoid air cells systems forming a cholesteatoma (see Fig 71.11). The cholesteatoma can be very erosive of bone in children with subsequent facial nerve paralysis, suppurative labyrinthitis or intracranial extension a real risk.

> Any child with a persistently discharging ear should be referred for specialist opinion.

Other forms of cholesteatoma can occur and may present only with a conductive hearing loss. For this reason all cases of conductive hearing loss should also be assessed by an ENT specialist.

Traumatic perforation

A perforation can result from a blow to the ear, explosions, impact with water, cotton buds or other devices used to clean the ear, including syringing the ear for wax. Most of these will spontaneously close and treatment is mainly to keep the ear dry unless the infection has occurred when antibiotics will be indicated. Specialist assessment is also required.

Facial nerve paralysis

This may be congenital or acquired.

Congenital causes. These include birth trauma, from which recovery is usually expected. Other developmental abnormalities may occur. These may be multiple or there may just be an isolated absence of the nerve or facial nucleus, e.g. Moebius syndrome.

Acquired causes. These include infection of which acute and chronic otitis media is the most important group. Thus it is essential to inspect the tympanic membrane in all cases of facial nerve paralysis. Other causes include skull base fractures, tumours and various types of neuritis and neuropathies. In a number no definite cause will be found. Idiopathic facial nerve paralysis is also called Bell's palsy. It is very important to remember that all facial paralyses are not Bell's palsy and that Bell's palsy is a diagnosis of exclusion. Specialist referral is indicated in all cases of facial paralysis whether it is incomplete or complete.

Vertigo

Vertigo is an illusion of motion which is usually rotary. An infected organ can involve the vestibulo-labyrinth or its associated central nervous pathways. It may be associated with unsteadiness, nausea or vomiting, hearing loss, tinnitus or other neurological symptoms and signs. The causes of vertigo are many and specialist referral is usually indicated.

Tinnitus

Tinnitus may occur in all abnormalities of the ear, but is uncommon in children. Occasionally it is the main presenting symptom of the abnormality. The investigation is that of the hearing loss; tinnitus normally improves with treatment of the hearing loss.

Most tinnitus is subjective in that it can only be heard by the patient. Occasionally an objective tinnitus will occur. This occurs in palatal myoclonus, tensor tympani spasms and also with vascular hums.

FURTHER READING

Bull T R 1974 A colour atlas of ENT diagnosis. Wolfe Medical Books, London

Cody C T R 1981 Diseases of the ear nose and throat. Year Book Medical Publishers, Chicago

Fox E H M 1980 Lecture notes on diseases of the ear nose and throat, 5th edn. Blackwell Scientific Publications, Oxford

Lucente F E, Sobol S M 1985 Essentials of laryngology, Raven Press, New York

Smith G D L 1978 Diagnostic ENT. Oxford Medical Publications, Oxford

72. The teeth

Roger K. Hall

Tooth formation commences in utero at the seventh week of fetal life for the primary teeth and at the fifteenth week of intrauterine life for the permanent teeth, beginning with the incisors and extending back to the molars. Calcification commences two months after the start of matrix formation. The structure of a normal tooth is shown in Figure 72.1.

THE MOUTH OF THE NEWBORN CHILD

The mouth of the normal newborn baby has well developed alveolar ridges with obvious bulges of tooth buds in both maxilla and mandible. The crest of the ridge anteriorly is initially a thin fibrous band with the maxillary labial frenulum crossing this and attaching into the incisive papilla. The palate is broad and flat and the alveolar ridges posteriorly are flattened (Fig. 72.2).

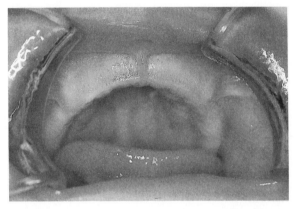

Fig. 72.2 Mouth of the normal newborn showing maxillary ridge with developing teeth, swellings and labial frenum attachment.

Natal and neonatal teeth

Teeth may be present at birth, or erupt in the neonatal period (1:3000 births) usually in the mandibular incisor region, but in infants with cleft lip and palate they occur high in the cleft, usually on the premaxilla.

. Published reports suggest that most natal teeth are normal primary teeth which have erupted prematurely, but clinical experience shows that many are 'supernumerary' teeth.

Natal teeth rarely interfere with breast-feeding because of nipple trauma, but where there is anxiety that a very mobile tooth may be dislodged and aspirated during feeding, careful removal soon after birth is indicated. Radiographs are not necessary before tooth removal as the decision to remove a natal tooth will be made solely on clinical grounds.

Congenital epulis

This is a benign pedunculated soft tissue tumour composed of sheets of granular cells. It is present at birth

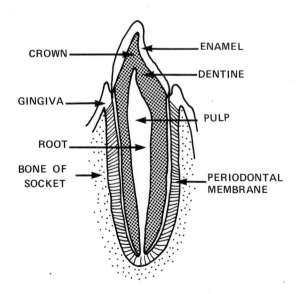

Fig. 72.1 The structure of the normal tooth.

CROWN — ENAMEL

— DENTINE

GINGIVA

— PULP

ROOT

BONE OF SOCKET

PERIODONTAL MEMBRANE

attached usually to the maxillary alveolar ridge. The lesion does not recur and management is by careful surgical excision.

Oral alveolar developmental (Bohn's) nodules

These are multiple creamy or grey nodules, consisting of mucous gland tissue, varying in size from 1 to 5 mm which occur predominantly on the outer surface of the alveolar ridges and are sometimes mistaken by parents for prematurely erupting teeth. They disappear by the third month.

Other similar nodules found along the palatal midline and composed of epithelial remnants are known as Epstein's pearls. Dental lamina cysts usually occur singly at the crest of the alveolar ridge. No treatment is indicated for any of these nodules or 'cysts'.

Eruption cyst and eruption haematoma

An eruption cyst is a blue or clear swelling overlying the crown of an erupting tooth, most commonly in the incisor region of the maxilla.

During tooth eruption, as vessels separate over the erupting tooth, blood may enter the loose tissue above the crown between oral and dental epithelium forming an 'eruption' cyst. If the bleed occurs more superficially the lesion is often then referred to as an eruption haematoma.

Eruption will be slightly delayed by such a cyst and discomfort can be eased by an occasional dose of paracetamol. Surgical intervention is contraindicated for an eruption cyst or haematoma.

This common lesion should not be confused with the very rare solid melanotic neuroectodermal tumour of infancy, the only other oral lesion which can appear bluish/grey.

Melanotic neuroectodermal tumour of infancy

This is a rare, multicentric, benign, but rapidly growing pigmented tumour associated with developing maxillary incisor, cuspid and first molar teeth in infants, and which occurs unilaterally. By three months of age the tumour is of sufficient size to produce facial asymmetry. Management is by thorough but conservative excision-curettage.

Frequent post-operative follow-up is necessary for twelve months.

TOOTH ERUPTION AND TEETHING

Tooth eruption following tooth development occurs at specific times and depends upon genetic factors and the health of the child. At six months of age eruption commences with the lower incisor teeth.

This normally occurs symmetrically with at most a few weeks separating left and right sides. Teething symptoms which are usually maximal some days before the tooth erupts include irritability, increased salivation and gingival erythema. Other symptoms such as transient mild diarrhoea, anal rashes and slight fever are frequent at the same time, but may be coincidental.

By twelve months of age all eight primary incisors are present. The first molars erupt at 15 months and the full primary dentition of 20 teeth is present by 2.5 years of age.

Delayed tooth eruption

At 6 years of age the primary lower incisors 'shed' following resorption of their roots by the erupting permanent central incisors. These erupted incisors are closely followed (often unnoticed) by the first permanent molars. The maxillary central incisors follow. For some time after eruption the anterior teeth may appear crowded or rotated because of the discrepancy between tooth and jaw size until maximum face and jaw width is reached at 9 years of age. The full permanent dentition (less the third molars) is normally established by 13 years of age.

There is a wide 'normal range' in eruption times of six to eight months, but eruption can be delayed much longer in chronic illness, Down syndrome, hypothyroidism and a number of rare conditions. A delay of eight to twelve months is not uncommon for the first primary tooth eruption. Failure of incisor teeth to erupt by twelve months of age may be an indication for early referral to a paediatric dentist.

ABNORMALITIES OF TOOTH DEVELOPMENT

For the infant the neonatal period is a time of metabolic stress when developmental defects of enamel matrix formation and calcification may occur. Hypoxia, and disturbance of calcium balance are the commonest 'insults' at this time which can be responsible for developmental enamel defects.

Developmental defects of enamel (DDE)

Disturbance of ameloblast metabolism will leave a permanent 'mark' on the erupted tooth enamel surface as a development defect as loss of tooth substance (hypoplasia) or opacity. By using published tables of normal tooth development such enamel defects can frequently be clearly related to prenatal, natal or postnatal events.

Such prenatal events (usually occurring between the fourth and seventh month of intrauterine life) are maternal rubella virus infection, maternal syphilis, and pregnancy toxaemia.

Natal events may be prematurity, hypoxia and hyperbilirubinaemia, and postnatally measles virus infection, gastrointestinal disease, hypoparathyroidism and administration of tetracycline.

In these situations defects will be found symmetrically and consistently distributed on areas of the tooth crown which were at that particular developmental stage at the time of insult (Fig. 72.3).

Genetic defects of enamel – amelogenesis imperfecta

Generalized defects of enamel affecting all teeth of both primary and permanent dentitions (amelogenesis imperfecta) may be inherited as autosomal dominant, autosomal recessive, or sex-linked trait. This may be either a single defect or associated with other disorders, e.g. pseudoparathyroidism, tuberous sclerosis and epidermolysis bullosa.

Clinical use of DDE in paediatric diagnosis

Knowledge of the aetiology of developmental defects of enamel is of importance not only to explain their apparent cause to parents, but is also of help diagnostically. Thus, should enamel defects be present, there must have been an infection or metabolic disturbance of significance, prenatally or neonatally (the exact developmental time depending upon the position of the defects on the primary teeth).

It is also well documented that 62% of very low birthweight, and 27% of low birthweight premature infants have developmental defects of primary tooth enamel (compared to 13% of normal birthweight full-term infants). A large number of aetiological agents capable of inducing developmental defects of tooth enamel has been identified.

Fluorosis

High serum levels of fluoride can produce an abnormality of the enamel known as fluorosis. This appears clinically as a white flecking or linear opacity of the enamel at its most minimal level and brown irregular opacity at its most severe. Minimal defects are sometimes difficult to distinguish from DDE arising from certain other causes.

Developmental defects of dentine (DDD)

Dentinogenesis imperfecta (opalescent teeth)

This occurs as an isolated genetically inherited disorder or as one feature in certain types of osteogenesis imperfecta (in other types of osteogenesis imperfecta the teeth appear normal). In affected teeth, changes in the structure of the dentine produce an opalescent appearance of the tooth crown.

Abnormalities of tooth crown form

In certain genetic disorders, the tooth crown form (and other ectodermal structures such as skin, hair, and nails) is disturbed in a consistent and characteristic way. The most common of these conditions is hypohidrotic ectodermal dysplasia where the anterior teeth have a

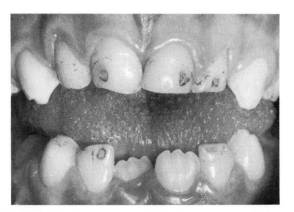
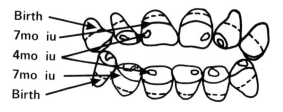

Birth
7mo iu
4mo iu
7mo iu
Birth

Fig. 72.3 Developmental defects of primary tooth enamel at 4 months iu, 7 months iu, and birth stages of tooth development, represented in photograph and diagram.

strange conical pointed form, and the molars an unusual shape. The teeth also occur in unusual positions. Crown form abnormalities also occur in other conditions with defects of ectodermal structures.

Other abnormalities of tooth development, in number, size and position of teeth may occur in conditions such as cleidocranial dysplasia, ectodermal dysplasia, hemifacial atrophy, hemifacial hypertrophy and in Russell Silver syndrome.

ORAL HABITS

Thumb sucking

Thumb sucking is a normal activity in utero, and most children continue this during infancy. Light thumb or other digit sucking does not disturb the dental arches, but vigorous or multiple digit sucking can produce an 'open bite'. Provided the thumb sucking ceases by the time the permanent incisors have erupted, there will be no residual deformity. Should thumb sucking continue this may distort the maxillary arch and incisor teeth to a point where orthodontic treatment will be necessary. Forcible control of thumb sucking is contraindicated.

When thumb sucking persists beyond the age of eight or nine years, it may be one sign of emotional disturbance.

Tongue thrust – abnormal swallowing

Tongue thrusting on swallowing can also produce an open bite. Correction of this oral habit requires the close co-operation of a speech pathologist and an orthodontist.

ABNORMAL FRENULA

Tongue tie (abnormal lingual frenum)

Parents and medical practitioners are often concerned about this problem. Interference with speech or swallowing occurs only in the most severe cases. Under these circumstances lingual frenectomy should be carefully carried out by an expert in this area.

Abnormal maxillary labial frenum

The upper labial frenum may be broad and large and separate the upper incisor teeth. Surgical frenectomy is not indicated unless the frenum is still attached to the incisive papilla by strong fibres which prevent physiological closure of the space between the incisors, and then not before the permanent cuspids have erupted at nine to ten years of age.

DENTAL CARIES

Dental caries is a declining disease in most developed countries of the world, due primarily to the use of fluoride and especially the use of fluoride toothpaste.

Dental caries results from the effect of acids produced by the action of bacterial enzymes on fermentable carbohydrates and sugars (mainly sucrose) on tooth enamel (Fig. 72.4).

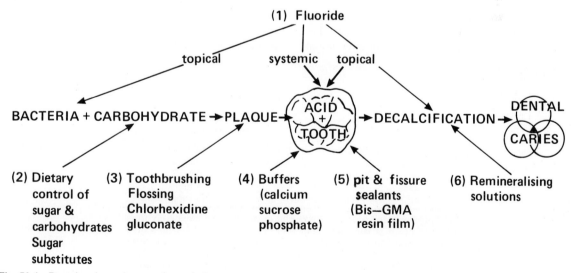

Fig. 72.4 Dental caries and preventive techniques.

Caries prevention*

The following preventive measures (see Fig. 72.4) have been developed to counteract the various phases of the caries process:

1. Fluorides act mainly topically, but when given systemically during tooth formation fluoride alters tooth morphology and crystal structure rendering the tooth enamel more resistant to acid dissolution. Fluorides also inhibit oral bacterial enzyme systems which convert sugar into acids in plaque. And they interfere with bacterial reproduction, inhibit storage of intracellular polysaccharides, reduce the tendency of enamel surface to absorb proteins and favour remineralization.

Fluoride supplement should be prescribed for all children in areas with less than the optimum 0.7–1 parts per million (ppm) fluoride in the water supply.

Table 72.1 gives the currently recommended dietary fluoride supplement dosage for different levels of naturally occurring fluoride in the water supply.

2. Dietary modification aimed at the reduction of refined carbohydrates and sucrose containing drinks

3. Plaque removal by correct toothbrushing, flossing, and the use of chlorhexidene gluconate mouth rinse or brush-on gel.

4. Buffering of acid formed using calcium sucrose phosphate.

5. Application of photocured Bis-GMA resin film to seal developmental pits and fissures

6. Remineralization of small areas of enamel decalcification.

Dental caries in infancy

Despite the incorporation of fluoride in developing and erupted tooth enamel, dental caries can still occur. This is seen with 'high frequency nursing bottle or breast-feeding' and the use of 'dummies' coated with sweeteners.

'Dummy' caries

This was the first of these conditions to be recognized and occurs because of the frequent use of a pacifier or dummy which has been dipped in a sweetening agent, most often honey. Severe destruction of all upper primary teeth, lower molars and canines can occur.

Nursing bottle caries (Fig. 72.5a)

This results from the undesirable infant feeding habit of leaving a nursing bottle containing milk, or fruit juice with a sleeping baby. The remaining bottle contents then continually bathes the teeth in contact with the teat, resulting in enamel decalcification and dental caries. The four maxillary incisors and first molars are the main teeth affected, because of the shape of the teat which spreads laterally in the mouth during sucking. Correct infant feeding practice is recommended with weaning from bottle to cup feeding after twelve months of age, 'mothering' during feeding, and removing the nursing bottle once the baby has fallen asleep.

'High frequency breast-feeding' caries (Fig. 72.5b)

Dental caries can occur when a mother encourages continual suckling (more than forty separate suckling periods are recorded during the day in such cases). These babies commonly sleep in the same bed as the mother and suckle at will during the night. The teeth involved in this type of caries attack are the maxillary incisors, which are almost continually in a decalcifying environment beneath a milk-moistened nipple. The palatal surfaces of these teeth break down, leaving a

Table 72.1 Recommended fluoride supplement dosage for different levels of naturally occurring fluoride in drinking water

Natural fluoride in drinking water	Age and daily supplement recommended		
	Birth–2 yrs	2–3 yrs	Over 3 yrs
< 0.3 ppm	0.25 mgF	0.5 mgF	1.0 mgF
0.3–0.7 ppm	No supplement	0.25 mgF	0.5 mgF
> 0.7 ppm	No supplement	No supplement	No supplement

For fully breast-fed babies: 0.25 mgF in orange juice or water daily from 3 months of age at latest for duration of breast-feeding. (2.2 mgm sodium fluoride is equal to 1 mg fluoride ion (F)) Note: 'Tank Water' may contain 0.14 ppm fluoride (0.94–0.38 ppm) (Galvanised Iron Tanks) or 0.58 ppm (0.10–2.30 ppm fluoride) (Concrete Tubs) (Hall & Storey, unpublished data).

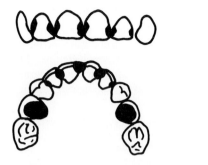 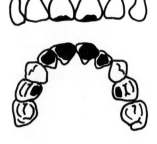 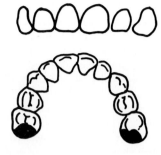

Fig. 72.5 **a** Nursing bottle caries. **b** High frequency breast-feeding caries. **c** Operculum caries.

ragged notch on the incisal edge. The smaller number of teeth affected is because of the smaller size of the human nipple in comparison to the bottle teat or dummy.

The family medical practitioner and paediatrician can do much to intercept, and help prevent this problem.

Management of such extensive dental caries at this young age requires intubation and general anaesthesia in an appropriate paediatric hospital setting.

'Operculum' caries (Fig. 72.5c)

In children who have had a period of chronic illness during the eruption of the second primary molar teeth, the natural gum flap (operculum) covering the distal half of these teeth may remain for an abnormally prolonged period of time before retracting. Under such circumstances the teeth may not complete normal eruption for up to six months, and the half erupted tooth is at risk of developing dental caries, beneath the soft tissue 'flap'.

DENTAL ABSCESS AND CELLULITIS

Dental abscess occurs following necrosis of the dental pulp from caries or trauma, and its subsequent infection by bacteria originating orally or systemically. A dental abscess may be acute or chronic. Acute flare up of a chronic abscess may follow trauma to the tooth or jaw.

In the primary dentition an abscess is usually superficial pointing beneath the oral mucoperiosteum (the 'gum boil'). Untreated these become chronic and a fistula forms discharging pus. Cyst formation may occur. Cellulitis occurs when infection spreads to the deeper

submandibular, infra-orbital or facial soft tissue planes. This is a more common sequence with abscess of permanent teeth, due to their longer and more deeply placed roots. Antibiotic therapy is urgent and delay can lead in the extreme case to mediastinitis or cavernous sinus thrombosis.

ORAL SOFT TISSUE INFECTIONS AND ULCERATION

Marginal gingivitis in children is due to irritation of the soft tissue attachment by plaque adherent to tooth surfaces.

Thrush (acute pseudomembranous candidiasis)

Thrush is the first oral infection most infants will experience and is the most common mucosal fungal infection in children.

Immunologically compromised children are at high risk of candidiasis. The chronic condition of mucocutaneous candidiasis involves nails as well as oral and other mucous membranes. Angular cheilosis is another chronic atrophic monilial infection. It is not uncommon in children, especially those with hypohidrotic ectodermal dysplasia.

Primary herpetic gingivostomatitis (see Ch. 29)

Vincent's infection (acute necrotizing ulcerative gingivitis)

This non-specific infection is almost never seen in children under the age of twelve years, except those suffering from extreme malnutrition and neglect, and is only seen in the adolescent if immuno-compromised or a poorly controlled diabetic.

---

* Immunization against dental caries is still at an experimental level.

Oral lesions in childhood leukaemia

It is often difficult to distinguish between oral complications of treatment (immunosuppression) and those of the malignant condition. Mucositis, drug-induced ulceration, oral gingival bleeding, neutropenic ulceration, candidiasis, viral (herpetic), bacterial and fungal infections all occur, but most can be prevented or minimized by strict oral hygiene using chlorhexidine gluconate and nystatin mouth washes.

Children who have received bone marrow transplants may show oral changes of graft-versus-host disease.

Oral features of HIV infection (AIDS)

In addition to the general clinical features of AIDS in children, persistent oral candidiasis and recurrent hepatic stomatitis are usually present.

Aphthous ulcers

These non-infective, extremely painful ulcers, most commonly occur on the labial and buccal mucosa, and tongue borders but are not seen in children before adolescence. A prodromal burning sensation precedes breakdown of a white papule to an ulcer with a crateriform base which slowly heals over eight to ten days. Aphthous ulcers are usually associated with stress, but the cause is unknown. Secondary infection can occur if the mouth is not kept clean.

OSTEOMYELITIS OF THE MAXILLA AND MANDIBLE

Osteomyelitis of the jaws in children is rare apart from neonatal maxillary osteomyelitis when the infection spreads rapidly involving developing tooth germs.

Osteomyelitis of the mandibular condyle occurs in the neonatal period or infancy, secondary to septicaemia (especially *Staphylococcus aureus*) producing rapid destruction of the growing cartilaginous condyloid process and leading to bony ankylosis or severe disruption of the temporomandibular joint, and severe growth disturbance of the mandible.

Osteomyelitis of the maxilla or mandible in later childhood occurs only rarely and usually in the immuno-compromised patient, from local or systemic infection. Infantile cortical hyperstosis (Caffey's disease) This inflammatory condition occurs before the fifth month of life, presenting with fever, hyperirritability and soft tissue swelling over the involved bones. The maxilla is never affected.

Proliferative periostitis (Garré's osteomyelitis)

In this condition the lower border of the mandible is affected unilaterally from either a dental cause or secondary to submandibular or cervical lymphadenitis. The layered (onion peel) radiographic appearance in periostitis may be confused with that of a malignant tumour.

ENLARGEMENT OF THE GINGIVAL TISSUES

Phenytoin hyperplasia of the gingivae

Enlargement of the gingival tissues occurs in epileptic children medicated with phenytoin for seizure control.

Much of the enlargement is inflammatory so that a high standard of oral hygiene and the use of chlorhexidine gluconate brush-on gel, will reduce the inflammation, and hence the enlargement. The enlargement slowly disappears on ceasing the drug.

Cyclosporin gingival hypertrophy

Cyclosporin administration in children who have had renal transplantation causes a distinctive interproximal enlargement of gingival tissues.

Gingival fibromatosis

This is an autosomal dominant inherited condition with dense firm general enlargement of the gingival tissue.

Mucopolysaccharidosis gingival enlargement

Extreme thickening of the gingival tissues is seen in the mucopolysaccharidoses.

TRAUMA TO THE TEETH AND ORAL SOFT TISSUES

One of every three children is likely to suffer an injury to a primary or permanent tooth. As with all trauma, boys suffer twice as often as girls, especially in the permanent dentition. The teeth most frequently injured are the more prominent maxillary central incisors. Dental injuries may involve actual fracture of the tooth crown and/or root, concussion, and partial or total displacement of a tooth from its socket.

Aetiology of injuries

In infants and very young children the usual cause is a fall while crawling or learning to walk – sometimes with an object in the mouth. Tongue and frenulum lacerations and displacement of teeth are the most common injuries. Dog bites are most frequent at this age and may cause severe injury.

From preschool and school ages, falls in playgrounds, and injuries from play equipment, especially swings, are most common; later falls from bicycles, sporting injuries and motor vehicle accidents as pedestrians, passengers or cyclists, become the most frequent cause of injury.

Injuries to the teeth may occur in children with epilepsy and cerebral palsy from 'head drop'.

Sublingual Riga-Fede ulceration

'Riga-Fede' ulceration is most common in mentally retarded and cerebral palsied children who continually rub the tongue backward and forward over the sharp edges of the lower incisor teeth. A small bonded splint covering the incisors allows the ulcer to heal.

Neuropathologic chewing trauma in comatose children

Self-trauma injury of tongue, lips and teeth occurs frequently in comatose children due to neuropathologic chewing activity.

A cast silver splint with a bite block on the molar teeth and cemented to the lower teeth prevents trauma and aids access for oral suction and nursing care.

Orofacial trauma in child maltreatment

Orofacial trauma is present in 50% of reported cases of child abuse. Bruising of lips and alveolar mucosa, avulsion of mucoperiosteum and teeth, alveolar bone fractures, finger and bite marks on face and neck are all frequent signs of child abuse. These result from slapping, punching, hand over mouth, forcible feeding with spoon or fork or forcible removal of a feeding bottle, dummy or toy from the mouth. Sexual abuse of children may also cause oral bruising. Oral signs should not be neglected when considering the possibility of child abuse.

Re-implantation of an avulsed permanent tooth

The most important dental injury is the partial or total avulsion of a permanent tooth from its socket. Re-implantation of the total avulsed permanent tooth should be accomplished within ten minutes and a flexible splint applied for six days. If immediate replacement is not possible, the tooth should be stored in milk until it can be re-implanted. This should be within two hours, to minimize the risk of loss of the tooth from root resorption.

Re-implantation of an avulsed tooth must be accompanied by tetanus prophylaxis and antibiotic therapy.

For further details on dental injuries, the reader is referred to *Traumatic injuries of the teeth* by Andreasen.

Fractures of the mandible and maxilla will not be considered here and the reader is referred to Chapter 13 on *Maxillofacial injuries* by Rowe & Williams

CLEFT LIP AND PALATE

Paediatric dentists, orthodontists and maxillofacial surgeons are essential members of the cleft palate 'team'. Management of the newborn baby with a cleft lip and/or palate may involve treatment with a small plate before lip repair to mould the palatal segments and control the otherwise unrestrained premaxillary growth. A high standard of oral hygiene is essential. Later treatment will include bone graft to the cleft in the alveolus to permit more normal tooth eruption and orthodontic correction of the teeth.

DENTAL CARE OF THE HANDICAPPED CHILD

Preventive dental care is of the utmost importance for the handicapped child, and parents or health care workers may need to learn special techniques and use special brushes to help clean the teeth. If co-operation or control of movement for treatment cannot be achieved, the use of pharmacological agents (such as diazepam), or general anaesthesia will be necessary.

ADOLESCENT TEMPOROMANDIBULAR JOINT PAIN/DYSFUNCTION

Pain in the temporomandibular joints occurs most commonly in adolescent girls and has an emotional basis. Pain, due to spasm of masticatory, neck and facial muscles leads to limitation and disturbance of jaw movement, with audible clicking and pain in the joints.

Management is by sensitive elicitation and counselling aimed at the underlying initiating problem, relief of pain with a potent analgesic such as Meosyndol, and most importantly by breaking the anxiety-muscle tension-pain cycle using a tranquilliser such as diazepam together with relaxation techniques. Dental malocclusions may also contribute to the problem. A lower bite plate is often used to correct overclosure and relieve pressure on the temporomandibular joint.

FURTHER READING

Andreasen J O 1981 Traumatic injuries of the teeth, 2nd edn. Munksgaard, Copenhagen

Magnusson B O, Koch G, Poulson S 1987 Paedodontics: a systematic approach. Munksgaard, Copenhagen

McDonald R E, Avery D R 1987 Dentistry for the child and adolescent, 5th edn. C V Mosby; St Louis

Mellberg J R, Ripa L W 1983 Fluoride in preventive dentistry. Quintessence Books, Chicago

Rowe N L, Williams J L 1985 Maxillofacial injuries Ch. 13: pp. 538–557. Churchill Livingstone, Edinburgh

Silverstone L M 1978 Preventive dentistry. Update Books, London

Disorders of connective tissue

73. Connective tissue disorders

M. J. Robinson, D. M. Roberton

This term is used to identify an inflammatory process, usually chronic, involving non-organ specific tissues or tissue components. These include blood vessels, synovial membranes, fascia, serosal membranes, muscle fibres and intra-cellular structures. Disorders of connective tissue in childhood are far less common than in adult life and often have a very different course and prognosis. Many of these disorders affect a number of organ systems so that a very complete history and physical examination is essential should a connective tissue disorder be suspected. Examples include the uveitis seen in some children with juvenile chronic arthritis and the recognition of involvement of the central nervous system in some children with systemic lupus erythematosus.

Pathology

Histological changes, which depend on the specific disorder, will include inflammatory cell infiltrates in blood vessels, proliferation of some tissues, e.g. synovium or glomerular cells, and degeneration in others, e.g. muscle fibres. Blood components may be involved with anaemia as a result of marrow suppression or haemolysis, thrombocytopenia and leukopenia.

Aetiology

A feature common to all connective tissue disorders is that their aetiology is unknown. In some, an autoimmune process may be demonstrated. The best example of this is the presence of antibody to cell nucleoprotein structures in systemic lupus erythematosus. Antinuclear antibody may be present also in the serum of some children with juvenile chronic arthritis. The association with particular genetically determined characteristics such as the HLA B27 leukocyte antigen and spondylitis syndromes suggests an abnormal host response in some children. Specific antigens may play a role, with antibody to cross-reacting antigens being important in the manifestations of rheumatic fever, or with the associa-

tion of some arteritis syndromes and hepatitis B. Recently, it has been suggested that a retroviral infection may be associated with the mucocutaneous lymph node syndrome (Kawasaki disease).

Incidence

There are few studies of the incidence of specific connective tissue disorders in childhood, but it is clear that their incidence is less common than that in adult life. Some have a tendency to be more frequent at specific ages or in particular racial groups. Thus, lupus erythematosus may be seen in the newborn and during infancy as a consequence of transplacental transfer of maternal autoantibody, but the disease is otherwise uncommon under the age of 8 years. Also, SLE is more common in Asian populations and children of Negro ancestry in North America than in Caucasian children. The more commonly recognized connective tissue disorders in childhood are listed in Example 73.1.

Example 73.1 Inflammatory connective tissue disorders of childhood

Juvenile chronic arthritis
Systemic lupus erythematosus
Juvenile dermatomyositis
Scleroderma
Mixed connective tissue disease and overlap syndromes
Systemic vasculitis syndromes
Mucocutaneous lymph node syndrome

JUVENILE CHRONIC ARTHRITIS (JCA)

This is the most common of the childhood connective tissue disorders. The disorder is also referred to as juvenile rheumatoid arthritis, but this term presupposes that the condition is similar to the adult disease. This is incorrect as juvenile chronic arthritis has a different presentation, course and prognosis. However, there is one form of juvenile arthritis that is similar to adult rheumatoid arthritis – the late onset polyarticular variety. This is seen commonly in females and is associated with a positive rheumatoid factor. It accounts for no more than 10% of all cases of JCA.

Diagnostic criteria of JCA

Universal agreement has not been reached on the diagnostic criteria for JCA, but most workers are agreed that arthritis in one or more joints should be present for at least 6–8 weeks, but preferably for 3 months (Example 73.2). JCA is readily subdivided into three groups each with different presentations, manifestations and prognoses. They are as follows:

1. Systemic onset disease
2. Pauciarticular (or oligoarticular) disease
3. Polyarticular disease.

Example 73.2 Criteria for the diagnosis of juvenile chronic arthritis

Arthritis in one or more joints, defined as:
    swelling or effusion
or two of:
    joint warmth
    pain on motion or joint tenderness
    limitation of motion
Duration of 6 weeks to 3 months
Age of onset less than 16 years
Absence of other rheumatic disease or other identifiable joint disorder

---

Systemic onset JCA

This is also known as Still's disease after the English paediatrician who first described it in 1896. Extra-articular manifestations are predominant and joint involvement may not occur for weeks or even months after the onset. Systemic onset disease may occur at any age in childhood. It affects both sexes equally and accounts for between 10 and 20% of cases of JCA. The presentation is with a high spiking fever. The temperature rises usually to over 39°C once or twice daily, being high in the latter part of the afternoon or early evening. Spikes of fever may be associated with the classical rash which consists of small, salmon-coloured erythematous macules. Usually, they are less than 5 mm in diameter and appear and fade rapidly. The rash is seen most often on the upper trunk, particularly around the axillae and nape of the neck, and on the proximal portions of the arms. It may be induced by a warm bath or by rubbing the skin gently (Koebner's phenomenon). When the child is febrile there is marked irritability, so that move-

ment appears painful even in the absence of overt arthritis. Generalized lymphadenopathy is frequent and hepatosplenomegaly maybe quite marked. Percarditis is not uncommon and is manifest by chest pain. Other serosal surfaces, such as the pleura, may also be inflamed.

Diagnosis

The diagnosis of systemic onset JCA may be very difficult in the early stages of the disease. Many infections may produce a similar clinical pattern so that infection must be excluded by appropriate blood, urine and CSF cultures. Other connective tissue disorders must be considered and a malignancy should be excluded. Thus, extensive laboratory investigation will usually be required and in many cases the diagnosis of systemic onset JCA will be one of exclusion. The diagnosis will become obvious with the onset of arthritis which, when it appears, tends to involve both the large and small joints. The cervical spine and temporo-mandibular joints are not infrequently involved in systemic onset JCA.

Clinical course

Systemic onset JCA runs a prolonged course with exacerbations of fever and fluctuating polyarthritis. This can be at least partially modified by therapy. Fortunately, many will recover with little or no disability, but a not insignificant number will progress to severe polyarthritis with growth failure and permanent incapacity due to joint deformity.

Pauciarticular arthritis

This is the most common variety of JCA and accounts for approximately half of all cases. The name of this form of arthritis derives from the term pauci, meaning few, and implies involvement of four or fewer joints. Pauciarticular JCA is more common in early childhood, being seen most often between the ages of 1 and 4 years. Girls are affected nearly twice as often as boys with the knee joints being by far the commonest joint involved (Fig. 73.1). Other joints commonly affected include the ankles, wrists, and elbows. Hip disease is rare in the early onset form of pauciarticular JCA.

A subdivision of pauciarticular arthritis (late onset group) commences between the ages of 8 and 10 years and is seen more often in boys, and large joints of the lower extremity are frequently involved. A number of these children go on to develop ankylosing spondylitis in late adolescence.

The diagnosis of pauciarticular juvenile arthritis is lar-

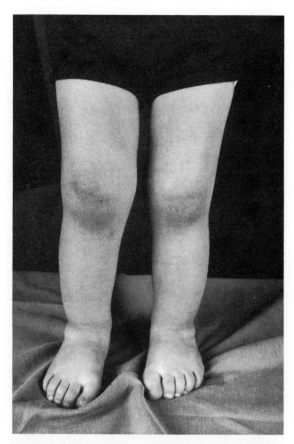

Fig. 73.1 Juvenile chronic arthritis: pauciarticular type involving the knee joint in a 3-year-old boy. There is swelling of the right knee due to an effusion in association with synovial proliferation. There is also increased growth of the right leg due to epiphyseal overgrowth secondary to the increased vascular supply in the area of chronic inflammation.

gely one of exclusion. Laboratory investigations reveal an elevated ESR, but an otherwise normal blood examination. The child is little disturbed systemically despite the moderate elevation of the ESR. Radiology of involved joints may show soft tissue swelling and even a joint effusion, but joint erosions are rare. Epiphyseal overgrowth and lengthening of the involved limb because of increased blood supply is frequent. Rheumatoid factor is rarely present in this form, but a number of children with early onset pauciarticular JCA have a positive serological test for ANA. This latter group is at particular risk of anterior uveitis.

Polyarticular arthritis

This subgroup is less common than the pauciarticular form, accounting for approximately 30% of all cases. Girls are affected almost twice as often as boys and although the presentation may be at any age in childhood, it is more common between the ages of 2 and 3 years. Most of these children have negative tests for rheumatoid factor.

There is a subgroup of polyarticular disease occurring in older girls. This subgroup has many features in common with adult rheumatoid arthritis, particularly involving symmetrically the small joints of the hands. This subgroup runs a course which is chronic and similar to the disease in adults; it is invariably associated with a positive rheumatoid factor. Rheumatoid nodules and extra-articular manifestations are seen in these children as in the adult (Fig. 73.2).

Young children with polyarticular disease have large joint involvement which is often symmetrical. Knees, elbows, wrists and ankles are most often affected (Fig. 73.3). The small joints of the hands and feet are oc-

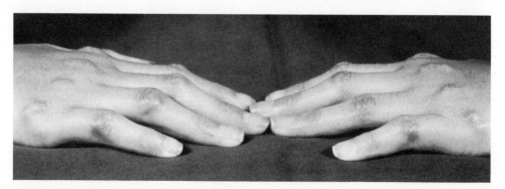

Fig. 73.2 Juvenile chronic arthritis: seropositive polyarticular type. Nodules are seen in the tendon sheaths over the dorsum of the metacarpophalangeal joints and some of the interphalangeal joints of the hands of this girl with rheumatoid factor positive arthritis.

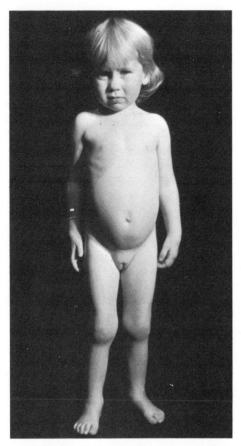

Fig. 73.3 Juvenile chronic arthritis: polyarticular type. This young girl has seronegative polyarticular arthritis. There is involvement of the ankles, knees, wrists, and fingers and swelling of the right shoulder. Both temporomandibular joints are involved as are her hips and cervical spine.

casionally affected later on and hip disease may occur. Despite the widespread nature of the arthritis the outlook for complete recovery in this group is very good. Systemic manifestations are minimal.

Eye disease in JCA

Inflammatory changes of the eye are a very important association with JCA being found in approximately 10% of all children. Those at particular risk are children with pauciarticular onset disease who are antinuclear antibody positive (20%). In this subgroup approximately 20% will have eye involvement. As the onset of eye complications is usually asymptomatic, regular slit-lamp examinations of the eyes by an experienced ophthalmologist is essential. Such examinations should be

undertaken at least three times yearly. The degree of inflammation does not relate to the severity of the arthritis so that it may be quite severe even in minor well controlled joint disease. Untreated eye disease may lead to severe impairment of vision due to cataracts or glaucoma. An acute iritis is sometimes seen in patients with pauciarticular disease of late onset and associated with ankylosing spondylitis.

Investigation of JCA

Children with systemic onset disease and polyarthritis of long standing will frequently have a mild microcytic and hypochromic anaemia. The ESR is usually elevated, but particularly so in systemic onset disease. Antinuclear antibody is most frequent in pauciarticular JCA of early onset. Rheumatoid factor (IgM antibody against IgG) is rarely seen except in late onset polyarticular disease. It is important to determine the reference range for the particular laboratory before making decisions on the basis of the rheumatoid factor. Immunoglobulin concentrations should be measured in JCA as some rare immunodeficiency disorders may present with a monoarticular or pauciarticular arthritis. The HLA B27 antigen is demonstrable on blood lymphocytes in approximately 8% of normal people, but is present in at least 90% of patients with ankylosing spondylitis.

Radiology

Radiological examination of involved joints may demonstrate overgrowth, erosions, progressive joint damage with subluxation and ultimately joint ankylosis. Radiology is also important in differentiating JCA from other disorders which may present as arthritis, for example, tumours of bone, unsuspected fractures and radio-opaque foreign bodies. However, in the majority of children with JCA little will be seen apart from some bone demineralization.

Arthroscopy is particularly indicated when mechanical derangement, foreign bodies or tumours are suspected. Synovial biopsies are taken routinely at the time of arthroscopy, but will only demonstrate a synovitis.

Management of JCA

The management of JCA is complex and is best achieved by a team involving a general paediatrician with appropriate consultation from paediatric rheumatologists, ophthalmologists and orthopaedic surgeons. The role of the physiotherapist is vital and the occupational therapist, schoolteacher and medical social worker will play roles similar to those in any other long-standing illness.

General principles of management only will be given here and the reader is referred elsewhere for details. Management basically involves suppression of the inflammatory process, relief of pain and preservation of joint function until permanent remission occurs. However, a small proportion of children with JCA will progress to chronic deforming arthritis. Management involves:

1. Pharmacological therapy
2. Rest, splinting and physiotherapy
3. Long-term measures

1. Pharmacological therapy

a. Anti-inflammatory drugs are the first line of treatment

They will relieve the pain and swelling and allow mobilization. Soluble aspirin is a very satisfactory means of achieving this, but dosages required (at least 100 mg/kg/day) are difficult to achieve in small children in whom a very careful watch for side effects is necessary. There is now much less acceptance of aspirin by the public since the association of infection, salicylate and Reye's syndrome appears to be more certain. Other side effects include hyperventilation, central nervous system excitation or depression, vomiting, gastrointestinal irritation and haemorrhage. Hepatotoxicity occurs occasionally and should this be suspected tests for liver function should be performed.

b. The non-steroidal anti-inflammatory drugs (NSAIDs)

These are probably less effective than aspirin in controlling fever, but the number of tablets required are less and consequently they are better accepted by children in general. Palatable NSAID syrups are required for very young children with JCA but so far only a limited number are available and are experimental. NSAIDs most commonly used are naproxen, piroxicam, ibuprofen, indomethacin and diclofenac sodium to name a few. Side effects include abdominal pain, vomiting, haematemesis, melaena and easy bruising. Recent reports of albuminuria and haematuria with their use are of concern.

c. Slow-acting antirheumatic drugs (SAARDs).

These second line drugs are useful additions to therapy when rapidly acting drugs (salicylate and NSAIDs) do not completely control symptoms. They have in common a significant delay period (up to 6 months) before their maximum effect is obtained. These drugs should never be used alone, and have side effects which are not inconsiderable. Therefore careful monitoring is mandatory. They should probably only be used under the

direction of a physician experienced in the management of JCA. Drugs in this category include D-penicillamine, hydroxychloroquine, gold salts, and sulphasalazine.

d. Corticosteroids

In severe systemic onset JCA it may be impossible to control fever and arthritis and obtain an adequate quality of life for the child without corticosteroids. As the ultimate outcome of JCA in the majority of children is good and the side effects of corticosteroids are not inconsiderable their use is usually contraindicated. They are not advised without expert supervision.

The use of intra-articular steroid is very useful in the management of the young child with monoarthritis. This applies particularly to the very young child where compliance with oral therapy is dubious and where there is an unwillingness to move an even slightly painful joint.

2. Rest, splinting and physiotherapy

In the acute stages of the illness, particularly in systemic and polyarticular JCA, rest is important. Even at these times all joints should be passively put through a full range of movement. Once disease activity decreases, active physiotherapy is encouraged under the direction of a physiotherapist expert in the management of JCA. Hydrotherapy is a valuable adjunct to treatment. This will involve warm baths and swimming or kicking in a heated pool.

Deformity before resolution must be avoided at all costs. Children will put their limbs in the position of comfort and this position is certainly not always optimal for ultimate good function. Therefore, involved joints may need to be splinted in the optimal position of rest, particularly during sleep.

3. Long-term measures

Although gross deformity is not common it does occur so that corrective orthopaedic surgery both to correct deformity during the active stage and to reconstruct joints permanently affected will be required. Unfortunately, a minority of children will require crutches or a wheelchair after the disease becomes inactive.

During the illness every attempt should be made to integrate the child into the community. Teachers should be made aware of the child's problems and when not able to attend school, correspondence courses should be arranged. Most states in Australia have Parents Support Groups to assist the families of children with JCA.

OTHER FORMS OF CHRONIC ARTHRITIS IN CHILDHOOD

Several forms of chronic arthritis occur in childhood other than JCA. The more important of these are listed

> **Example 73.3 Disorders presenting with chronic arthritis in childhood**
>
> Juvenile chronic arthritis
>   Systemic onset
>   Pauciarticular onset
>   Polyarticular onset
>   Rheumatoid factor negative
>   Rheumatoid factor positive
>
> Juvenile ankylosing spondylitis
>
> Arthritis associated with inflammatory bowel disease
>
> Reactive arthritis
>
> Arthritis associated with psoriasis
>
> Arthritis associated with other connective tissue disorders

in Example 73.3. They are differentiated clinically from JCA by their distinctive pattern of joint or connective tissues involvement, as in juvenile ankylosing spondylitis, or by the presence of co-existing involvement of other organ systems, as for example in inflammatory or infective bowel disease.

Juvenile ankylosing spondylitis

This disorder may have its onset in childhood in up to 10% of cases. It may present as arthritis of one or more joints distally in the lower limbs, often in association with pain and tenderness at the sites of insertion of the Achilles or patellar tendons and at the origin and insertion of the plantar fascia (enthesopathy). Sacroiliac and lumbosacral joint involvement may not become evident for some years (Fig. 73.4). These patients are usually male, have negative tests for rheumatoid factor and ANA, and have a high frequency (90%) of positivity for HLA B27. Other manifestations of ankylosing spondylitis seen in adults, such as aortitis, amyloidosis and pulmonary disease, are rare in childhood. Acute iritis may occur in childhood.

Inflammatory bowel disease and arthritis

Both Crohn's disease and ulcerative colitis may be complicated by arthritis. Usually only a few joints are affected, particularly those of the lower limbs. The arthritis is generally of only a few weeks' duration.

Reaction arthritides

Arthritis may occur after gastrointestinal infection with *Salmonella*, *Shigella*, *Yersinia*, and *Campylobacter* species. The arthritis is usually an oligoarthritis lasting

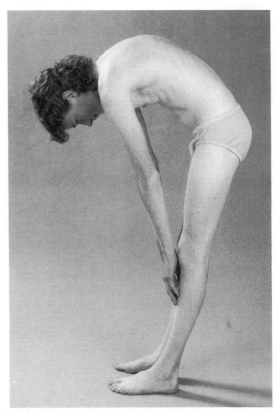

Fig. 73.4 Juvenile ankylosing spondylitis. There is marked loss of flexion of the spine and loss of normal curvature. This patient also had tenderness on palpation over the plantar fascia and over both sacroiliac joints.

only a few weeks. Treatment with NSAIDs is usually effective. Reiter's triad of conjunctivitis, urethritis and arthritis occurs in childhood, but is rare.

Psoriatic arthropathy

Arthritis may be seen in association with the skin lesions and nail pitting of psoriasis, although the skin lesions may not appear until much later. Usually only a few joints are involved, typically the distal interphalangeal joints. Sacroiliitis may also occur.

Other connective tissue disorders

Synovitis or arthritis may occur in systemic lupus erythematosus (SLE), dermatomyositis and mixed connective tissue disease. Other characteristics of these disorders are usually sufficiently obvious to make the diagnosis evident.

Other disorders with associated persisting arthritis

Haemophilia and malignancy may present with arthritis. Recurrent haemarthrosis in haemophiliac patients leads to joint destruction and dysfunction in adult life. Occasionally, leukaemia presents in childhood with hip or knee pain. Sarcoidosis presents rarely as a mono- or pauciarticular arthritis but chest changes are usually present on radiology.

Rheumatic fever and Henoch-Schönlein purpura

These disorders are described in Chapters 39 and 43, respectively.

Infections

Some viral infections may be associated with arthralgia or arthritis. These include Ross river virus, rubella, Epstein-Barr virus and hepatitis virus. Tuberculous joint disease is now rare in this country. Lyme disease is extremely rare in Australia and is the result of infection by the tick borne *Borrelia burgdorferi*, leading to a rash known as erythema chronicum migrans and a relapsing pauciarticular arthritis. It responds to treatment with penicillin. Joint swelling may occur in some allergic disorders, often in association with a pruritic rash.

A number of other conditions, many of which are described in other chapters, may present with joint pain or dysfunction in children (see Example 73.4).

Example 73.4 Miscellaneous conditions which may present as joint pain or dysfunction in childhood

Legg-Calve-Perthes disease
Slipped upper femoral epiphysis
Transient synovitis (e.g. irritable hip)
Foreign body synovitis (e.g. plant thorn synovitis)
Chondromalacia patellae
Unrecognized trauma (e.g. non-displaced fracture or 'toddler fracture')
Hypermobility syndromes
Reflex neurovascular dystrophy
Hysterical gait disorders

SYSTEMIC LUPUS ERYTHEMATOSUS

Systemic lupus erythematosus (SLE) is a chronic multisystem autoimmune disorder leading to inflammatory changes in blood vessels and connective tissues. The incidence of SLE in childhood differs in different populations, but is more common in girls, the female to male ratio being approximately 4:1. This is less marked

than the ratio of 9:1 seen in adult disease. SLE is rare under the age of 8 years, but the incidence increases throughout later childhood and adolescence to early adult life. It has a relapsing and remitting course with a high incidence of renal function impairment and a significant mortality.

Aetiology

The aetiology of SLE is unknown, but epidemiological studies have demonstrated racial, familial and immunological factors. For example, there is a high concordance rate for SLE in monozygotic twins. Certain drugs may precipitate the onset of SLE in childhood although drug-induced SLE in childhood is rarely chronic. Medications implicated are anticonvulsants (phenytoin, carbamazepine), sulphonamides, hydralazine and isoniazid.

Autoantibody formation is associated with many of the clinical features of SLE and antinuclear antibody is present in almost all patients. A high concentration of antibody against native or double-stranded DNA is associated with systemic disease activity, particularly in acute renal disease. The deposition of circulating immune complexes is associated with the vasculitic and renal manifestations of SLE.

Clinical features

The onset of SLE is usually insidious with vague symptoms of fever, tiredness, lethargy, loss of appetite and mouth ulceration. Weight loss is particularly prominent and in many alopecia occurs. By the time of presentation the characteristic rash is usually evident. It presents as a confluent, macular erythema with scaling and is typically distributed over the malar regions in a bat's wing configuration (Fig. 73.5). Localized patches occur occasionally on arms, thighs and the base of the neck. Some children may present with evidence of generalized vasculitis manifest by haemorrhagic lesions over the pulp of the digits of the hands and feet (Fig. 73.6). These may progress to ulceration.

In addition to these general symptoms, often the following number of body organ systems are involved:

1. Musculoskeletal – Joint pains and joint swellings are common, but usually disappear quickly with treatment and are rarely deforming.
2. Renal – Renal involvement is manifest clinically by the presence of microscopic haematuria and albuminuria. There may be generalized oedema and the renal disease, when severe, may rapidly progress to renal failure with or without hypertension. A number of dis-

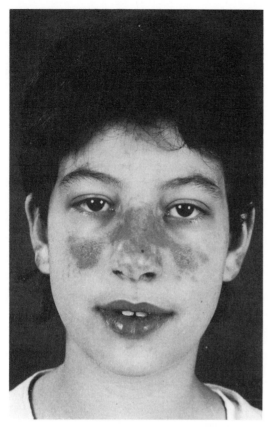

Fig. 73.5 Systemic lupus erythematosus: facial rash in a girl with active vasculitis. Note the vasculitic lesions on both ears.

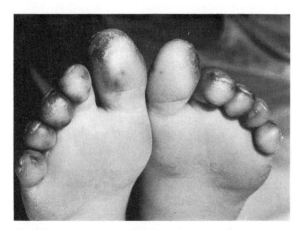

Fig. 73.6 Systemic lupus erythematosus: vasculitic lesions on the toes of a 9-year-old girl with active SLE. She also had a diffuse proliferative glomerulonephritis and anaemia in association with thrombocytopaenia.

tinct histological patterns of glomerulonephritis are seen in SLE (Ch. 53).

3. The central nervous system – Approximately one-third of children with SLE will manifest CNS abnormalities which, separately or in combination, may involve seizures, psychoses, headache, chorea and polyneuropathy. The features of CNS involvement are probably secondary to vascular abnormalities in the CNS although direct neuronal damage by antibodies may be important. Often, it is difficult to differentiate organic psychological manifestations which are the result of lupus from those associated with a serious protracted illness and with therapy which is disfiguring.

4. The respiratory, gastrointestinal cardiovascular and reticuloendothelial systems may also be involved singly or collectively.

5. Generalized lymphadenopathy is seen occasionally.

Diagnosis of SLE

This is made from the clinical features described and the many associated labortaory features. Antinuclear antibodies are present in high titre in the active stages and a diagnosis of SLE is untenable in their absence. Antibodies to many other cell and organ components may be found. Anaemia and leukopenia are frequent and thrombocytopenia occurs in approximately 10–15% of children. The ESR is invariably elevated and total haemolytic complement and in particular C3 and C4 are depressed when the disease is active.

Management

In the first instance a full assessment is required to define the extent of the disease. The philosophy of treatment is suppression of autoantibody formation and is achieved most reliably with corticosteroids. At times other immunosuppressants may be required. These include azathioprine, cyclophosphamide and more recently cyclosporin A. The treatment of SLE in childhood is difficult and prolonged and should only be undertaken by paediatricians expert in the field of connective tissue diseases. Ongoing assessment of disease activity is dependent upon the history, the wellbeing of the child, the physical examination, regular serology and tests of renal function. It must be emphasized that children on immunosuppressants are at significant risk from overwhelming infection, particularly viral infection. This is a common cause of death in SLE. Treatment is long term and spontaneous recovery uncommon. The more common causes of death are uncontrolled infection, involvement of the central nervous system or chronic renal failure.

Neonatal lupus syndrome

Some infants born to mothers with serological evidence of lupus will have transient manifestations of the disorder. The most common abnormality is lupus dermatitis which generally fades over several months. The most important complication of neonatal lupus syndrome is congenital heart block which persists through life and may require a cardiac pacemaker.

JUVENILE DERMATOMYOSITIS

The inflammatory changes of juvenile dermatomyositis involve striated muscle and skin, although there may also be minor involvement of other organ systems. Girls are affected approximately twice as commonly as boys and the peak incidence is from about 4–10 years of age. The disorder is recognized by a characteristic rash in association with proximal muscle weakness, muscle pain, tenderness or stiffness along with behavioural changes, malaise, lethargy or irritability. Behavioural changes often mask the muscle features at presentation. Muscle enzymes are elevated in most patients, but not all. There are abnormal electromyographical and muscle biopsy findings. The onset may be acute with severe or even life-threatening muscle weakness, subacute, or a slowly progressive muscle weakness becoming evident over many months.

Clinical features

Skin rash

The classical rash of juvenile dermatomyositis is a violaceous (heliotrope) discoloration over the eyelids which may extend over the bridge of the nose and on to the malar areas. Telangiectases are often seen over the eyelids. Erythema may be seen in a V-form over the upper trunk and elsewhere. Periorbital or limb oedema is sometimes prominent. Telangiectases and erythema of the nail folds are characteristic, and skin changes are often evident over the dorsum of the proximal interphalangeal joints and metacarpophalangeal joints of the hands. These areas of skin later become atrophic. Areas of dermal calcinosis may occur later in many children.

Muscle disease

There is general malaise, weakness and easy fatigability. The child experiences difficulty climbing stairs or onto chairs, arising from squatting or sitting, using the arms to climb or dress, or even with maintenance of head posture and respiration if the onset is acute or severe. There is often muscle tenderness.

Laboratory findings

Muscle enzymes such as creatinine kinase (CK) and aldolase are elevated in most children at diagnosis but some children may have normal enzymes. Electromyography of involved muscle shows the characteristics of a primary myopathy. Tissue obtained at muscle biopsy shows perivascular inflammation and focal muscle degeneration and necrosis. Less than half of children with juvenile dermatomyositis have ANA in serum.

Management

The mainstay of therapy has been high dose corticosteroid therapy (1–2 mg/kg/day of prednisolone). This has been responsible for a marked drop in mortality to well below 10%. In a few children with unremitting disease, further immunosuppressive therapy with azathioprine or cyclophosphamide may be helpful.

SCLERODERMA

Scleroderma is a rare connective tissue disorder which, in spite of its name, may have multisystem effects, leading to its description as progressive systemic sclerosis (PSS). One specific form of systemic disease is known as CREST, in which the features are calcinosis, Raynaud's phenomenon, oesophageal dysmotility, sclerodactyly and telangiectases.

Clinical features

Skin – The major feature is thickening and atrophy of skin in affected areas. This may be symmetrical and distal, localized as in linear scleroderma or morphoea, or generalized. There may be areas of abnormal pigmentation or depigmentation. Telangiectases over the face and nail folds may be present. Often calcinosis occurs later in areas of involved skin and periarticular contractures are common and may be severe.

Other features – Oesophageal dysmotility is frequent on barium swallow. Raynaud's phenomenon due to digital vasospasm is frequent. Bilateral basal pulmonary fibrosis occurs. Cardiac and renal dysfunction may develop.

Management

Therapy is supportive, with efforts to prevent digital vasospasm (warmth, nifedipine) and joint contractures. D-penicillamine is used often but its effect is variable. Some children have a spontaneous remission of the disorder but progressive disease may occur.

MIXED CONNECTIVE TISSUE DISEASE AND OVERLAP SYNDROMES

Several connective tissue disorders have features of more than one of the above entities. Mixed connective tissue disease (MCTD) may present with typical Raynaud's phenomenon as the major manifestation but arthritis, nodules and muscle tenderness and weakness may also occur. Antinuclear antibody directed against ribonucleoprotein helps to define the disorder serologically. The outlook appears to be very good in most, but renal or cardiac involvement may occur and some patients later develop features of SLE.

SYSTEMIC VASCULITIS SYNDROMES

Disorders which involve inflammatory changes of blood vessels as their primary manifestation are rare in childhood. Polyarteritis nodosa may be seen in infancy, with fever, a vasculitic rash, cardiac and renal involvement causing early death. Takayasu's arteritis and other forms of giant cell arteritis, Wegener's granulomatosis and Churg-Strauss syndrome have all been described in childhood.

MUCOCUTANEOUS LYMPH NODE SYNDROME (KAWASAKI DISEASE)

This disorder has well defined clinical manifestations due to inflammatory changes in blood vessels. It has been described worldwide but is more common in Japanese children. It is seen most often between the ages of 1 and 4 years. The diagnostic criteria are a fever with a temperature over 38.5°C, and four of the following five manifestations:

1. Bilateral non-purulent conjunctivitis.
2. Oral mucosal changes (erythema or dry cracked lips or strawberry tongue).
3. Cervical lymphadenopathy with one node 1.5 cm or larger in diameter.
4. Changes in the extremities (swelling of hands or feet, or erythema of palms or soles, or membrane-like peeling of the skin (Fig. 73.7).

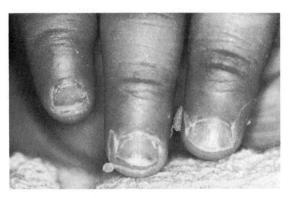

Fig. 73.7 Mucocutaneous lymph node syndrome (Kawasaki disease). Peeling of the hands or feet later in the course of this disorder may begin in a characteristic periungual distribution as seen in this 2-year-old boy who also had cervical lymphadenopathy, a rash, non-purulent conjunctivitis and intense erythema of the oral mucosa.

5. A generalized variable rash. The diagnosis is based on the clinical features and the absence of streptococcal infection or other disease process.

The importance of Kawasaki disease is that up to 20% of children may develop coronary artery abnormalities – usually proximal dilatation or aneurysm formation. Often these resolve with time, but severe coronary artery involvement may cause death. Treatment with intravenous immunoglobulin during the acute phase of the illness has been shown to decrease the risk of coronary artery aneurysm formation.

FURTHER READING

Ansell B M 1980 Rheumatic disorders in childhood. Butterworth, London

Cassidy J T 1982 Textbook of pediatric rheumatology. John Wiley and Sons, New York

Jacobs J G 1982 Pediatric rheumatology for the practitioner. Springer-Verlag, New York

Miller M L, Magilady D B, Warren R W 1986 Immunologic basis of lupus. The Pediatric Clinics of North America 33(5): 1191–1902

Pharmacology

74. Drug therapy in childhood and adolescence

Neil Buchanan

Paediatric pharmacology can be broadly subdivided into two major areas; that affecting intrauterine life and that involving extrauterine life. This chapter deals with drug therapy in extrauterine life, which can be divided into a number of distinct, albeit somewhat arbitrary, stages:

1. The early postnatal period – a phase of physiological immaturity during which there is rapid growth and there are alterations in drug metabolism and elimination.

2. Infancy – an extension of the first stage, but the type and severity of disorders being treated is different and requires a modified approach.

3. The toddler – mainly associated with recurrent minor infections, often leading to multiple short courses of therapy.

4. The young child – there is enhanced metabolism of a number of drugs, such as anticonvulsants and theophylline, in this age group, which make dosage more difficult than in adult practice.

5. Adolescence – whilst there does not seem to be any significant pharmacokinetic alterations at this stage of development, the problem of non-compliance may become a major issue.

GENERAL CONSIDERATIONS

Paediatric pharmacology developed from therapeutic practice in adults with children receiving 'scaled down' adult doses. Whilst this is clearly unsatisfactory, it should be remembered that this approach has been used for a long time with considerable clinical success. Much has been written about more precise dosage regimens and concepts such as the surfaced area method or the administration of drugs on a mg/kg bodyweight basis have become common practice. The evidence that these modes of dosage are actually scientifically very accurate is, in the main, lacking. Nevertheless, results are usually satisfactory. This is probably because many of the medications used in daily paediatric practice are relatively non-toxic and have a wide therapeutic margin. Thus,

the use of such drugs will be satisfactory – even with relative dosing inaccuracy, provided that the desired therapeutic end result is obtained with minimal side effects.

The situation with drugs with a narrow therapeutic margin, where there is but a small difference in dosage between efficacy and toxicity, is quite different. Thus for agents such as digoxin, aminoglycosides and cytotoxics much more specific dosage information is needed. This can be achieved by well-conducted pharmacokinetic studies which will allow the precise definition of dosage relative to variables such as age, renal and hepatic function and disease state to name but a few. Such studies are now being performed by a number of paediatric pharmacology units worldwide.

One of the bases of practical paediatric pharmacology, and, indeed, clinical pharmacology as a discipline, should be information on drug utilization. Obviously there is a very considerable difference between what is prescribed in a teaching hospital, a district hospital and a general practice. In this day and age, the majority of children are treated as outpatients. In addition, with the improvement in their general standard of health, most children have brief episodes of relatively mild acute illnesses. On the whole, these episodes require treatment, be it symptomatic or curative, with medications which have a fairly wide therapeutic margin. Obviously this is quite different in the sick child in hospital or the child with a chronic disease such as cystic fibrosis, epilepsy or severe asthma being treated as an outpatient. The differentiation between these two broad groups of patients is important, as it lends perspective to the appropriate development of paediatric pharmacology. It is easy for academic disciplines to get lost in the minutiae of a particular teaching hospital problem and lose sight of the realities of the community at large.

These comments do not represent a 'laissez faire' approach or minimize the importance of paediatric pharmacology. They support the contention that treatment of many minor illnesses, which represent a considerable amount of the day to day workload of general practitioners and paediatricians, can be dealt with by using tried and trusted medications, for which scientifically calculated dosage regimens do not exist. Nevertheless, experience has shown that the therapeutic end result is usually achieved. Thus, in the case of the child with pharyngitis, whose illness is probably viral in origin it is probably of little importance either in terms of therapeutic effect or side effects whether amoxycillin 125 mg tid or 250 mg tid is given. Although this rather simplistic approach may be disputed, it is essentially practical and recognizes the fact that for many of the commonly used medications, scientifically derived dosages do not exist. Nor, as these compounds have been available for some years, is there great incentive to obtain such data now.

DRUG ABSORPTION AND BIOAVAILABILITY

Drugs may be administered by a number of routes; orally, intravenously, percutaneously, intramuscularly and rectally.

Oral absorption

Physiologically it has been shown that newborns, especially the premature, have greatly reduced acid secretion with relative achlorhydria and that adult values are only achieved at about three years of age. In addition, gastric emptying, which has an effect on subsequent absorption, is prolonged and approaches adult values at about six months of life. The importance of delayed gastric emptying is probably not as great as believed previously. It is in the first few weeks of life that this is of clinical importance; however, sick newborns receive most of their medications parenterally. Because of the achlorhydria, absorption of the penicillins (ampicillin, amoxycillin, nafcillin and flucloxacilin) is enhanced.

On the other hand, for some other drugs absorption is reduced. Such agents include phenobarbitone, phenytoin, and rifampicin. With cephalexin, although the peak concentration is lower, the amount absorbed is similar to that in older children or adults. Orally administered carbamazepine suspension is well absorbed as are digoxin and diazepam. The lack of adequate absorption of some anticonvulsants during the first 2–3 weeks of life presents a practical problem and necessitates the continued parenteral administration of such medication to infants with seizures. Other than in the neonatal period, there are not really any significant differences in the gastrointestinal absorption of drugs between adults and children. Children with gastrointestinal problems, such as coeliac disease, may show abnormalities of drug

absorption and this should be borne in mind when treating them.

Of considerable practical importance is the question of drug absorption relative to meals. The present thinking is that all medications, with the exception of isoniazid, rifampicin, narrow spectrum penicillins and tetracyclines (except doxycycline and minocycline) should be taken with food. The importance of this is simplicity and to improve compliance: it should be the rule in paediatric practice.

Intravenous administration

This represents the 'gold standard' for bioavailability, for if all the drug is injected into the circulation, it represents 100% bioavailability. However, factors such as intravenous flow rate, the site of injection and the dosage volume, all affect the rate of drug delivery. It cannot be assumed that because a medication is injected into an intravenous line, it will be delivered evenly or adequately.

Percutaneous absorption

Percutaneous absorption of drugs is enhanced in infants, and to a lesser extent, in children, especially if the area of skin is burnt or excoriated. This has been documented with corticosteroids in infants with severe eczema and in babies in whom such medication is used for the management of nappy rash, especially in association with plastic pants. Topical steroids are rarely indicated for nappy rash and boric acid is both useless and potentially dangerous. The excessive use of topical aminoglycoside – polymyxin sprays on burned skin of young children has been associated with permanent hearing loss.

Intramuscular absorption

Rapid and complete absorption after intramuscular administration cannot be automatically assumed. From a practical point of view, it is known that certain drugs are poorly absorbed from an intramuscular site and should not be administered by this route. These drugs include phenytoin, digoxin, diazepam, and chlordiazepoxide.

Rectal absorption

Administration by the rectal route is generally less favoured in Anglo-Saxon countries than in Europe. The attractions of rectal administration are that it could be useful in patients who are vomiting, in infants and young children who are reluctant to take oral medication. Also rectal administration might avoid first pass metabolism to which a number of orally administered drugs are susceptible. In practice, the rectal route is not ideal because of considerable interindividual variations in rectal venous drainage. Probably the only drug to be recommended for rectal administration in children is diazepam for the home treatment of convulsions.

DRUG DISTRIBUTION

Numerous factors influence drug distribution including plasma protein-binding, circulatory factors, blood-brain barrier development and drug specificity for tissue receptor sites.

Body water

Newborn infants have a much higher extracellular fluid volume, especially the premature (50% of bodyweight) and full-term infant (45%), compared to older infants (25% at 1 year of age) or adults (20–25%). Total body water is also much greater in neonates, varying from 85% in the premature infant to about 75% in the full-term baby as opposed to about 60% in the adult. On the other hand, fat content is reduced, being about 3% in the premature infant, 12% in the full-term neonate, 30% at 1 year of age and about 18% in the average adult.

As drugs are distributed between extracellular water and depot fat according to their lipid water partition coefficient, these changes have considerable potential significance in the neonatal period in particular. In terms of drug dosage, especially with water soluble drugs, which are by far the most commonly used in paediatric practice, this implies that to get 'therapeutic' drug concentrations, larger doses on a mg/kg bodyweight basis need to be given to neonates to achieve levels similar to those seen in adults. This has to be balanced against diminished hepatic function and renal elimination.

Plasma protein-binding

Plasma protein-binding in the neonatal period and especially in the premature infant is decreased when compared to adult values. This implies that there is more circulating free (unbound) drug and as it is the free component which is pharmacologically active, this suggests the potential for an enhanced pharmacodynamic effect. The plasma protein concentrations in the newborn, especially plasma albumin, is lower than later in life, but, in addition, there are qualitative differences in the binding capacity of the proteins. Moreover, there may be competition between endogenous substances, especially by free fatty acids and bilirubin, and drugs for albumin binding sites. Whilst there are significant changes, both qualitatively and quantitatively, in neonatal plasma proteins the clinical significance of these changes is somewhat uncertain. From a practical point of view, the use of highly bound drugs such as cloxacillin, phenytoin and diazepam should be cautious in the presence of hyperbilirubinaemia.

In older children there are a number of disease states which may affect drug protein-binding. These include hepatic disease, the nephrotic syndrome, chronic renal failure, cardiac failure and malnutrition.

Blood-brain barrier

The two most important factors which determine the rate of transport of drugs across the blood-brain barrier are lipid solubility and the degree of ionization of the drug. Unionized drugs are much more lipid soluble than ionized drugs.

As meningitis is a relatively common problem in paediatric practice the following information on the passage of appropriate drugs to the CSF is given:

- Penicillin. Although the penetration of benzylpenicillin to the CSF is rather poor, the organisms for which it would be used – *Streptococcus pneumoniae*, streptococcus Group B and *Neisseria meningitidis* – are sensitive to low concentrations. Benzylpenicillin thus remains the drug of choice for these organisms.
- Ampicillin. This drug also penetrates the CSF poorly but, because of its activity against *Haemophilus influenzae*, it is extensively used in the treatment of meningitis. Its relatively poor penetration can be overcome, at least in part, by using high doses ranging from 200–400 mg/kg.
- Chloramphenicol. This drug achieves the highest CSF serum ratio of any antibiotic. CSF levels are about 40% of those in plasma, making it a particularly useful drug in the management of meningitis. The other advantage in children is that it can be used orally after 48 hours of intravenous or intramuscular therapy.
- Aminoglycosides. These drugs are the first line of therapy for systemic Gram-negative infections. However, passage to the CSF is poor and the levels achieved are inconsistent. The third generation cephalosporins are more appropriate in most cases.

– Cephalosporins. The early cephalosporins entered the CSF poorly, but the so-called third generation of cephalosporins, especially moxalactam and cefotaxime achieve CSF levels which are about 10–30% of serum levels. They are indicated mainly in the treatment of Gram-negative meningitis.

DRUG ELIMINATION

There are significant differences in the rate of elimination of drugs in neonates, infants and children and there is now sufficient information to allow a number of broad generalizations to be made. These are:

In the neonatal period, there is a physiological depression in the capacity of the liver to metabolize a large number of drugs. This leads to a potential increase in the serum drug concentration of the parent compound associated with a decrease in, or absence of, metabolites. Again, in general, the more premature the infant, the greater the degree of depression of hepatic metabolism.

The same principle applies to renal elimination of drugs. The more premature the infant the less the ability to eliminate the drug and thus the longer the half-life.

Hepatic metabolism

Recent work has shown that the elimination of many drugs in the newborn period is low compared to that in older children or adults. This is in part related to immaturity of hepatic drug metabolizing enzyme systems. In general, oxidation and glucuronidation are decreased in neonates, whilst demethylation and sulphation are much less affected. Interindividual differences in the rate of hepatic metabolism seen in adults are also seen in neonates.

The perinatal situation

In the newborn, the half-life of most drugs is prolonged. This is largely because of diminished renal function. However, immature hepatic drug metabolism also contributes to this phenomenon as exemplified by chloramphenicol. Glucuronidation is markedly deficient in most premature infants and some full-term babies. This reflects the low concentration of the enzymes glucuronyl transferase and uridine diphosphate glucuronic dehydrogenase. Thus, chloramphenicol given in the 'usual' doses based on weight might lead to high concentrations and accumulation of unchanged drug. It is this that led to the 'grey baby' syndrome. As a result

of these observations, numerous pharmacokinetic studies have been carried out with this drug in the neonatal period leading to more precise dosage based on factors such as weight and gestational age. Despite the achievement of more accurate dosage, there remain problems with the administration of chloramphenicol to newborn infants. It appears that the clearance of chloramphenicol correlates better with postnatal age than gestational age except in the first two days of life. In addition, the degree of illness, renal function and acidosis tend to elevate the serum concentration of chloramphenicol. Thus, despite quite precise dosage recommendations, if this drug is to be used in neonates blood level monitoring is of great importance.

The older child

Less attention has been paid to hepatic drug metabolism in the older child. The requirement of anticonvulsants on a mg/kg bodyweight basis, in the 1 to 8-year-old age group, is greater than in adults to achieve similar serum anticonvulsant levels. This is because the rate of metabolism of these drugs is more rapid in the younger age group, clearance is greater and thus half-life is shorter. All these factors dictate the need for a larger dose to achieve therapeutic blood levels. The same applies to theophylline. This rapid metabolism occurs almost certainly because during childhood, the liver is larger relative to bodyweight than in adult life. These proportions change to the usual adult pattern at puberty and it is at this time that drug dosage requirements lessen.

Renal excretion

Renal excretory capacity is immature at birth, more so in the premature infant and shows progressive maturation with postnatal age. Adult values for glomerular filtration rate are reached after about 3 to 6 months of age, whilst tubular function matures fully somewhat later than this.

As previously mentioned, there is now an accumulated experience as to drug disposition and the influence of altered renal function on drug elimination in neonates. Renal function is of particular importance to drug disposition in the neonatal period as most sick neonates receive antibiotics for suspected, or proven, infection and most of these agents are water soluble. The less mature the infant the lower is renal drug clearance and the longer is the half-life of the drug. These observations have led to the development of age and maturity related dosages for many of the drugs used in the neonatal period, especially antimicrobial agents (Table 74.1).

Table 74.1 Neonatal drug dosages: total daily dosage schedules of some drugs commonly used in the neonatal period. Dosage intervals are shown in brackets e.g. (q12h) = 12-hourly

Drug	Route	< 2000 g or 0–14 days	> 2000 g or 15–30 days
Aminoglycosides			
Amikacin	im/iv	15–25 mg/kg (q12h)	25 mg/kg (q12h)
Gentamicin	im/iv	5 mg/kg (q12h)	7.5 mg/kg (q12h)
Kanamycin	im	15–20 mg/kg (q12h)	20–30 mg/kg (q12h)
Tobramycin	im/iv	4 mg/kg (q12h)	6 mg/kg (q12h)
Cephalosporins			
Cephazolin	im/iv	20 mg/kg (q12h)	40 mg/kg (q12h)
Cephamandole	im/iv	25 mg/kg (q12h)	50 mg/kg (q12h)
Cefotaxime	iv	50 mg/kg (q12h)	75 mg/kg (q12h)
Cefoxitin	im/iv	—	90 mg/kg (q8h)
Cefuroxime	im/iv	30–60 mg/kg (q12h)	60 mg/kg (q12h)
Chloramphenicol	im/iv	10 mg/kg (q12h)	20 mg/kg (q12h)
Digoxin	oral/iv		
Premature infants 30 µg/kg load followed by 15 µg/kg/day (q24h)			
Full-term infants 25 µg/kg load followed by 10 µg/kg/day (q24h)			
Penicillins			
Benzylpenicillin	im/iv	50 000 u/kg (q12h)	75 000 u/kg (q8h)
Cloxacillin	oral/im/iv	50 mg/kg (q12h)	75 mg/kg (q8h)
Ampicillin	oral/im/iv	50 mg/kg (q12h)	75 mg/kg (q8h)
Amoxycillin	oral/im/iv	25 mg/kg (q12h)	30–40 mg/kg (q8h)
Carbenicillin	iv	300 mg/kg (q8h)	400 mg/kg (q6h)
Methicillin	im/iv	50 mg/kg (q12h)	100 mg/kg (q12h)
Phenobarbitone	im/iv	15–20 mg/kg as a loading dose, followed by 5 mg/kg/day (q12h) as maintenance. Reduce to 2.5 mg/kg/day if asphyxia present.	
Theophylline	oral/iv	6 mg/kg load followed by 4 mg/kg/day (q12h)	

ISSUES PARTICULAR TO DRUG THERAPY IN CHILDREN

Because of growth and maturation during childhood and adolescence, drug therapy in youngsters needs to be thought about somewhat differently to the situations in adults.

Early postnatal period

The administration of drugs

The oral administration of medication to neonates may result in aspiration and certain drugs are not well absorbed in the first few weeks of life. Intramuscular drug administration can be hazardous in infants as there is little muscle mass and the practice of using the buttocks as a site for intramuscular injections should be avoided because of the risk of damaging the sciatic nerve. The preferred site is the anterior or lateral aspect of the thigh although gangrene of the foot has occurred after injec-

tion in this area. Intravenous drug administration is not without hazard in the neonate, with problems of drug and fluid extravasation which may lead to local tissue necrosis.

Drug excretion in breast milk

Most drugs taken by the nursing mother will be excreted to some extent in her milk. However, for most drugs the amount ingested will be extremely small and will not be harmful. The decision to breast-feed while taking a medication needs to be made after weighing the benefits of breast-feeding against possible adverse effects in the infant.

For a few drugs, such as some of the anticonvulsants, relatively large amounts are transferred to the infant, with measurable plasma levels. However, clinical side effects in the infant are rare and, thus, the very presence of drug in the baby is not a contraindication to breast-feeding.

Despite a lack of accurate information, four groups of guidelines can be suggested, largely on a pragmatic basis:

1. Situations where breast-feeding is generally contraindicated (Example 74.1).

Example 74.1 Mothers taking these medications regularly should be recommended not to breast-feed. If the mother is adamant that she wished to breast-feed, an alternative medication should be sought if such is available

Carbimazole/methimazole
Chloramphenicol
Ergotamine
Gold preparations
Immunosuppressive/cytotoxic agents
Indomethacin
Phenindione

---

2. Situations where there is a small, but possible risk to the baby. Drugs in this category include alcohol, heroin, gold, indomethacin, chlorpromazine, lithium, cascara, senna and ergot. All these drugs need to be taken regularly to cause a problem.

3. Drugs which may suppress lactation (Example 74.2).

Example 74.2 A list of drugs which may suppress lactation. When these drugs are prescribed and breast feeding continues, infant growth should be carefully monitored by regular weighing

Bromocriptine*
Combined oestrogen/progesterone oral contraceptives
Dienoestrol*
Oestradiol*
Pyridoxine*
Stilboestrol*
Thiazide diuretics

* Used specifically to suppress lactation.

---

4. Drugs which represent a risk to the baby with G6PD deficiency (Example 74.3).

Thus with the exception of a limited number of drugs, it is generally appropriate to encourage mothers who are receiving medication to breast-feed. However, the infant should be closely observed for any side effects which should be reported.

Second to twelfth month of life

The physiological immaturity of the liver and kidneys

Example 74.3 Shows drugs which should be administered with caution to mothers whose infants have or may have G6PD deficiency. Babies are particularly sensitive to drug-induced haemolysis during the neonatal period

Aspirin	Naladixic acid
Chloramphenicol	Nitrofurantion
Chloroquine	Probenecid
Cotrimoxazole	Procaineamide
Dapsone	Quinine
Hydroxychloroquine	Sulphonamides
Isoniazid	

---

lessens during this period and after the first month of life, less detailed attention needs to be paid to drug dosages. Drugs are administered on a mg/kg bodyweight basis.

The main issues confronting those who prescribe for children in this age group include:

1. Getting the child to take medication. Many children are not keen to take medication and this can often be a major problem for parents. With the advent of syrups and suspensions this has become a little easier as many of the preparations taste quite pleasant. This very pleasantness can itself be a problem as children who receive multiple courses of liquid medications, which contain sweeteners, may develop significant tooth decay.

It is important to remember both from the point of view of compliance, and of actually getting the child to physically take the medicine, that very few drugs need to be given more than thrice daily. Most parents will develop their own ways of getting their children to take medication.

2. Normal childhood curiosity. Toddlers are in an exploratory phase of their lives and naturally very inquisitive. Therefore, it is important that medications and household products be safely stored in the home.

3. Recurrent infections. Young children, especially when they first go to school or preschool and are exposed to large numbers of other children, will get what seems to be more than their share of coughs, colds, sore throats and ear infections. In fact this is quite normal. During the first 6 years of life, the average child can expect to have approximately 17 minor colds, 7 severe colds, 3 ear infections, 6 other respiratory tract infections, 2 episodes of diarrhoea and 2 skin infections. Many of these infections will be viral in origin although this is difficult to prove at a clinical level. For this reason, young children are likely to receive recurrent courses of antibiotics, usually of a broad spectrum type.

Whether these are in fact necessary is a contentious matter.

4. Growth. Children grow throughout childhood and, therefore, those receiving medication for chronic disorders such as epilepsy, asthma, etc. will require to have their drug doses reviewed from time to time, perhaps with the help of blood level monitoring where this is appropriate.

Adolescence

Although the hormonal changes associated with puberty might be expected to produce alterations in drug disposition, there is no good clinical evidence that this is a major problem for the prescriber. Problems to bear in mind in the adolescent include:

1. Non-compliance. Adolescents may be very resistant to taking medication and whilst this may not be of great moment for acute self-limiting illness such as sore throats or tonsillitis, it can present difficulties in the management of chronic disorders particularly diabetes mellitus, asthma, epilepsy, juvenile chronic arthritis and cystic fibrosis.

2. Suicidal attempts. Self poisoning in this age group, unlike the inquisitive toddler, has a more sinister connotation and usually requires psychiatric intervention. Suicidal gestures and attempts are common in adolescence and this is a further reason for medication in the home to be securely stored.

3. Illicit drugs. The use of such agents begins to appear in adolescence and should always be borne in mind by the clinician.

DRUG PRESCRIBING PRINCIPLES IN PAEDIATRIC PRACTICE

Parents are becoming more demanding of information about their children's disorders and treatment. Doctors must respond to these demands by providing honest, factual information presented intelligibly. To achieve this, doctors must be honest with themselves. And it may be of value to consider the following five questions when writing a prescription:

1. What can reasonably be expected from drug therapy in the light of the natural course of the illness, i.e. is treatment necessary?
2. How long will treatment be needed?
3. Is the proposed drug effective?
4. Is it safe? Will it do more harm than good?
5. Is it economical? Is this the cheapest and most effective way of solving the patient's problem?

Is drug treatment really needed?

Drug treatment is not always required and whilst it is said that parents often demand treatment for their children, there is a growing trend in developed countries to avoid the use of medication if possible. This has gone hand in hand with a growing interest in natural remedies (naturopathy) and non-medical treatments such as acupuncture, iridology, etc. This trend allows the doctor more chance of not prescribing than was the case a decade ago.

There can be little doubt that antibiotics are overprescribed for sore throats, tonsillitis and ear infections, a large proportion of which are viral in origin. However, the argument between academics and practitioners which has gone on for years is of little value. We all know that the majority of upper respiratory tract infections in childhood are self-limiting in nature, but it is much more difficult for the academic to give the advice not to do so. The answers are dictated by common sense, the well child who has a cough and a sore throat may well not need any treatment at all. Diagnosis, explanation and reassurance may well suffice. On the other hand, the youngster with pus on his tonsils or who has a bulging red ear drum should sensibly receive antibiotics. In other words, the disease and the degree of illness should be taken into account. The same approach applies to the commonest symptom of all in childhood, fever. Whilst febrile convulsions are a matter of concern, fever per se is not a significant danger to the child and antipyretic drugs are by no means always necessary.

If treatment is needed, which drug is appropriate?

The choice of an antibacterial agent should be guided by a knowledge of the causative organism. In practical terms, especially in children, this is often not available or only becomes available after treatment has been commenced. Thus, it is important to be aware of the likely aetiological agents involved with particular conditions and to treat on the basis of this knowledge.

Certain antibiotics are less suitable for children than for adults. The risk of chloramphenicol toxicity is relatively high, especially in the neonatal period. This drug should not be used in children except in particular circumstances which include: certain neonatal infections (blood level monitoring is recommended), acute epiglottitis, *H. influenzae* meningitis and typhoid fever. Having said this, the reality of chloramphenicol is that it is a cheap and very effective antimicrobial agent with some unpleasant side effects. However, in certain situations, such as in developing countries, it may be one of the few affordable antibiotics. In Papua New Guinea for example, it is recommended as first line treatment for meningitis, osteomyelitis, septic arthritis, pyomyositis, severe pneumonia and typhoid.

Sulphonamides, including co-trimoxazole, should be avoided in the newborn because of the possibility of displacing bilirubin from its albumin binding site and the subsequent risk of kernicterus. Tetracyclines should not be used in childhood because of the risk of tooth staining and damage. Again, as for chloramphenicol, tetracyclines may be appropriate antibiotics in a developing country. Better a stained tooth than a dead child.

The use of aspirin in children is now less favoured than it used to be, firstly, because of toxicity in the young child and, secondly, because of its probable, but not proven, relationship to Reye's syndrome. Paracetamol (acetaminophen) has the advantages of being very safe and effective in young children as well as being available in liquid form.

Drug preparation and route of administration

Whenever possible the oral route should be used, although in the critically ill child, or the child with vomiting and significant diarrhoea, it may be more appropriate to administer the medication parenterally. There are very few indications for rectal drug administration in children, although the use of rectal diazepam in the management of febrile convulsions is reasonably well accepted and there are occasions where local rectal applications of glycerine suppositories are required in the management of constipation.

Liquid preparations are the most suitable for children under five years of age, followed by capsules which can be emptied and disguised in jam or honey. Tablets are often difficult to break and then crush. The decision as to which preparation to use is based upon a number of factors which include bioavailability, palatability, convenience, availability of various dosage forms, cost, stability and toxicity.

Inhaled medications are important in children and have revolutionized the management of asthma. Young children may not be able to use standard inhalers, but will benefit from the use of a nebulizer, where the medication is made available in fine spray form without the active participation of the child.

Drug dosage

There have been many formulae used to derive drug dosage in children. None of them are of any particular value. As mentioned, most drugs prescribed for children in the community have a wide therapeutic margin and thus absolutely accurate dosage may not be that important. For children with complex, or chronic disorders treated at a tertiary referral level, a much higher proportion of drugs with a narrow therapeutic margin is used and more specific dosage information is required. Such information is obtained by pharmacokinetic studies that allow the determination of dosage relative to age, weight, maturity and so on. The end result of such studies relate dosage to bodyweight, which is convenient as this is a variable which is almost always measured when children attend the doctor. There are some proponents of dosage based on body surface area. The advantages of this are scant and it also means that each child needs to be measured for length-height and then surface area calculated. Except for cytotoxic drugs, where there may be an advantage in using this system, it has no advantages over bodyweight. Recommended doses for commonly used drugs are shown in Table 74.2.

Duration of treatment

The duration of treatment is dictated by the nature of the illness. In general practice, clinicians will be involved mainly in short-term therapy, whilst tertiary referral paediatricians will be more involved in long-term therapy.

For certain conditions such as epilepsy, diabetes and cystic fibrosis, therapy will be prolonged and may be life-long. For other diseases such as tuberculosis, a defined course of therapy may be prescribed for 6, 9 or 12 months depending on the regimen being used. In most illnesses, however, the duration of therapy depends totally on the nature and duration of the illness.

Drug compliance and patient education

The failure of patients to take medication is well known. Non-compliance may take a number of forms; not filling the prescription, omission of doses, poor clinic attendance, discontinuation of therapy prematurely or in the case of children, difficulty in persuading the child to take the medication.

Antibiotic agents prescribed for the treatment of an acute infection are rarely taken for the number of days prescribed. Non-compliance occurs in 25–75% of paediatric patients receiving oral penicillin for an acute illness. In patients with a chronic illness, be they adults or children, it is known that compliance decreases the longer the duration of therapy. Studies of children receiving medication for asthma, juvenile chronic arthritis, diabetes, epilepsy, hyperactivity, immunosuppressants after renal transplantation or prednisone in the

Table 74.2 Recommended doses for infants and older children of some commonly used drugs. (Important neontal doses are shown in Table 74.1)

Drug	Dosage	Comments
Analgesics/antipyretics		
Aspirin	10–20 mg/kg/dose (q8h)	Antipyretic/analgesic dose.
	90–120 mg/kg/day (q8h)	Anti-inflammatory dose. Avoid use under the age of 1 year, potentially toxic.
Paracetamol (Acetaminophen)	5–10 mg/kg/dose (q8h)	Paracetamol has a wide therapeutic margin and is very safe in children. Double the suggested dose can be used.
Narcotic analgesics		
Morphine	0.1–0.2 mg/kg/dose SC (q3h)	
	0.1–0.2 mg/kg/dose IV (q3h)	
	0.035–mg/kg/h IV infusion	
Pethidine	1–2 mg/kg/dose IM (q3h)	
	0.25–0.5 mg/kg/dose IV (q1h)	
Antihelmintics		
Pyrantel embonate	10 mg/kg (single dose)	Threadworm, roundworm.
Thiobendazole	50 mg/kg/day (q12h)	2-day course for threadworm, ascaris, strongyloides; repeat in 1 week.
Vipyrium embonate	5 mg/kg (single dose)	Threadworm.

Antibacterial agents (see Table 74.1 for important neonatal doses. In principle, oral doses should be given for mild to moderate infections and parenteral doses for moderate to severe infections).

Amikacin	20–40 mg/kg/day (q12h) IM/IV	Monitor serum levels in renal failure.
Amoxycillin	20–50 mg/kg/day (q8h) PO/IM/IV	Better absorbed orally than ampicillin.
Ampicillin	50–100 mg/kg/day (q8h) PO/IM/IV	
Carbenicillin	400–500 mg/kg/day (q6h) IV	Modify dose in renal failure.
Cefotaxime	100–200 mg/kg/day (q8h) IM/IV	
Cephalothin	40–80 mg/kg/day (q6h) IM/IV	
Cephalexin	25–50 mg/kg/day (q8h) PO	
Cephazolin	25–50 mg/kg/day (q8h) IM/IV	
Cephadrine	25–50 mg/kg/day (q6h) PO/IM	
Cephamandole		
Cefoxitin	80–160 mg/kg/day (q8h)	
Cefuroxime	30–100 mg/kg/day (q8h)	
Chloramphenicol	PO/IM/IV 100 mg/kg/day (q8h) (1 year of age) 50 mg/kg/day (q8h) (1 month – 1 year of age).	

Chloramphenicol should only be used to treat *Haemophilus influenzae* meningitis, acute epiglotittis, typhoid fever or organisms resistant to other less toxic antibiotics.

Cloxacillin	50–100 mg/kg/day (q8h) PO/IM/IV	
Cotrimoxazole	(Suspension contains 40 mg trimethoprim and 200 mg sulphamethoxazole/5 ml). 5 ml/day (q12h) (6 months) 10 ml/day (q12h) (6 months–5 years) 20 ml/day (q12h) (5 years)	
Erythromycin	30–50 mg/kg/day PO	Avoid use with theophylline and carbamazepine, as it inhibits their metabolism and induces toxicity.
Gentamicin	2–6 mg/kg/day (q8h) IM/IV	Monitor serum levels in renal failure.
Kanamycin	20–40 mg/kg/day (q12h) IM	Monitor serum levels in renal failure.
Methicillin	100–200 mg/kg/day (q6h) IM	
Penicillin	50 000 u/kg/day (q6h) IM/IV	
Phenoxymethyl-penicillin	25–50 mg/kg/day (q8h) PO	
Sulphadiazine	150 mg/kg/day (q6h) PO/IV	Avoid in G6PD deficiency. Ensure adequate hydration to avoid crystalluria.
Ticarcillin	150–300 mg/kg/day (q6h) IV	Modify dose in renal failure.
Tobramycin	2–6 mg/kg/day (q8h) IM/IV	Monitor serum levels in renal failure.

Table 74.2   (cont'd)

Drug	Dosage	Comments
Antidepressants/antitipsychotics		
Chlorpromazine	2–4 mg/kg/day (q8h) IM/PO	
Haloperidol	0.05 mg/kg/day (q12h) PO	
Imipramine	Used in enuresis: 6 years and older, start with 25 mg at bedtime. May need to be increased to 50 mg. Over 12 years, can increase to 75 mg PO.	

Antidiarrhoeal agents: In most children, diarrhoeal illnesses are self-limiting and anti-diarrhoeal medications are not recommended.

Diphenoxylate hydrochloride	8 mg/day (q8h) (5–8 years) 10 mg/day (q6h) (8–12 years)	Best avoided in children due to atropine induced side effects.
Loperamide	Over 8 years of age; 2 mg to a maximum of 8 mg/day (q6h)	

Antiemetics: Antiemetics should **not** be used in the management of vomiting associated with gastroenteritis.

Prochlorperazine PO	10–15 kg: 2.5 mg q8h 15–20 kg: 2.5–5 mg q8h 20–25 kg: 5 mg q8h 23–35 kg: 5–7.5 mg q8h	Avoid under 10 kg. Extrapyramidal features common with overdosage.
Promethazine	1–2 mg/kg/day (q8h) PO/IM/IV	Extrapyramidal signs with overdosage.
Antifungal agents		
Amphotericin B	Test dose 0.1 mg/kg/day IV over 6 hours. Increase to 0.25 mg/kg/day and as tolerance allows, to 1 mg/kg/day	Used for life-threatening infections. Do not exceed 1.5 mg/kg/day.
Griseofulvin	10 mg/kg/day (q8h) PO	
Nystatin	1–2 million units/day (q8h)	
Antihistamines		
Chlorpheniramine	0.35 mg/kg/day (q8h) PO	
Dextrochlorpheniramine	0.15 mg/kg/day (q8h) PO	
Promethazine	0.25–0.5 mg/kg/day (q8h) IM/IV/PO	
Trimeprazine	3.75 mg/day maximum (2 years) (q8h) PO 7.5 mg/day maximum (3–12 years) (q8h) PO	
Antituberculous drugs		
Ethambutol	25 mg/kg/day for first 2 months and then 15 mg/kg/day thereafter single daily dose	Avoid in young children who cannot report the side effects of changes in red/green colour vision.
Isoniazid	Active Rx: 10–30 mg/kg/day (q24h) PO Prophylaxis: 10 mg/kg/day (q24h)	
Rifampicin	10–20 mg/kg/day (q24h) PO	Induces hepatic metabolism of oral anticoagulants. Potentially hepatotoxic when used with other antituberculous drugs.
Streptomycin	20 mg/kg/day IM (q24h)	
Antitussives		
Pholcodine	2 mg; (2–6 years) 2–4 mg PO (6–9 years) 4 mg/dose (q8h) (9–12 years)	
Dextromethorphan	1 mg/kg/day (q8h) PO	
Bronchodilators	PO	
Orciprenaline	2 mg/kg/day (q8h)	
Salbutamol	0.3 mg/kg/day (q8h)	
Terbutaline	0.15–0.2 mg/kg/day (q8h) 15–20 mg/kg/day (q8h)	
Theophylline	15–20 mg/kg/day (q12h)	Slow release preparation.
Cardiac glycosides		
Digoxin	Digitalizing dose 0.06–0.08 mg/kg PO; 0.04–0.06 mg/kg IV (1 month–2 years) Digitalizing dose 0.04–0.06 mg/kg PO; 0.02–0.04 mg/kg IV (over 2 years) Maintenance dose = one-fifth to one-third of the oral digitalizing dose/day Divide initial digitalizing dose into 3 administrations	

Table 74.2 (cont'd)

Drug	Dosage	Comments
Central stimulants		
Methylphenidate	5 mg morning and noon in hyperactivity. Can increase by 5–10 mg/week to a maximum 60 mg/day.	Avoid under 6 years of age.
Corticosteroids		
Cortisone acetate	This drug is used in complex and rare paediatric endocrine disorders. Dosage need to be closely related to plasma concentrations of renin activity and other hormones. Thus specific dosages cannot be given.	
Hydrocortisone	Status asthmaticus: 4 mg/kg/dose q3h IV	
Prednisone/Prednisolone	2 mg/kg/day (q12h) PO as an initial dose, with incremental reductions relative to progress.	
Haematinics		
Iron	Prophylaxis: 1–2 mg/kg/day (q24h) PO Treatment: 6 mg/kg/day (q24h) PO	
Laxatives		
Bisacodyl	0.3 mg/kg swallowed whole	Tablets should be swallowed whole and not crushed. Do not take with antacids or milk.
Senna	Powder: 40 mg/kg/dose PO Syrup: 0.15 ml/kg/dose	
Sedatives and hypnotics (see antihistamines)		
Chloral hydrate	Hypnotic dose: 50 mg/kg/day PO Sedative dose: 25 mg/kg/day (q8h) PO	
Diazepam	0.12–0.8 mg/kg/day (q8h) PO	
Trimeprazine	Hypnotic dose: 1.5–2 mg/kg/dose PO Sedative dose: 3–4 mg/kg/day (q8h) PO	
Vitamins		
Vitamin D_2	Prophylactic: 400–1000 u/day	
(Calciferol)	Therapeutic: 2000–4000 u/day	
Vitamin K	Haemorrhagic disease of the newborn	
	Prophylaxis: 1 mg IM/IV	Overdosage may induce kernicterus.
	Therapeutic: 5–10 mg IM/IV	
	Older children 5–10 mg IV/IM	

Abbreviations: SC = subcutaneous; IV = intravenous; PO = oral; IM = intramuscular; q6h = administer 6-hourly; q8h = administer 8-hourly; q12h = administer twice daily; q24h = administer once daily.

treatment of cancer have all shown non-compliance to be a reality. Adolescents are generally recognized as showing poorer compliance than younger children largely because children receive medication under parental supervision, whilst adolescents are no longer supervised to the same extent.

Does it matter if patients are non-compliant? Patients have the ultimate right to decide whether or not they are going to take the medication prescribed for them. However, failure to take medication does have both economic and therapeutic implications which extend beyond the non-compliance of the patient. Where treatment is unsuccessful because of unrecognized non-compliance, the patient, apart from suffering poor health, may be subjected to unnecessary diagnostic tests, the administration of alternative, and often inap-

propriate medications and, at times, repeated admissions to hospital. Early discontinuation of antibiotic therapy may lead to the emergence of resistant bacterial strains, whilst with some drugs, cessation of therapy may have life-threatening consequences. In addition, the accumulation of unused medications in a household may predispose to toddler poisoning. On the other hand, there is good evidence that overprescribing is a depressingly common phenomenon and, in this context, non-compliance makes good sense. 4–6% of adult admissions to hospital result from adverse drug reactions and 10–20% of patients experience an adverse drug reaction whilst in hospital. This may well predispose to non-compliance. Efforts to encourage compliance should be restricted to those patients in whom non-compliance is likely to have a deleterious effect.

The important factors which appear to influence compliance are:

1. The medication
2. Dosage frequency and the complexity of the therapeutic regimen
3. The illness
4. The prescriber
5. The therapeutic source
6. Prescriber-patient (parent) interaction.

These factors warrant discussion in some detail.

The medication

Of importance in paediatric practice is the dosage form. It is for this reason that liquid preparations are useful for most children up to about the age of five years. Parents should be reminded to shake bottles of suspension before the medication is given. Drug side effects are often cited as a cause of non-compliance, but this in fact is not a very common event, especially in children.

Dosage frequency and the therapeutic regimen

There are a number of studies which show that the frequency of dosage influences compliance both in adults and children. Whenever possible, dosage regimens should be tailored to the routine of the patient and his or her family. Meals are the most obvious times to take medication and there are indeed but six medications which need to be taken separately from food. Most medications can be taken three times a day, many twice a day, very rarely do they need to be given every six hours. Confusing dosage schedules, for example, one tablet twice daily, one capsule three times a day and a suspension at night should be avoided. The behavioural change expected from a patient to manage such a bizarre routine is unlikely to be achieved.

The illness

While nothing can be done to alter the nature of the illness, a great deal can be done to improve the patient's and parents' understanding of the illness and the need to take medication. Where the patient or the parents perceive the illness to be serious, compliance is likely to be better, while symptom free periods are associated with lapses in compliance.

In other words, patients will take medication when they are feeling ill and will cease to take it when they feel better.

The prescriber

The prescriber probably has the greatest influence in ensuring compliance. As stated by Green (1988) 'the physician's ability to have the child trust and like him, to be comfortable and friendly, to relate in a strong positive fashion and to identify with his or her attitude towards the child's health is a potent therapeutic force.' Seeing the same medical attendant on a regular basis also enhances compliance.

The therapeutic source

It is believed that inconvenient therapeutic sources lead to diminished compliance. Thus, if a patient waits several hours in a hospital outpatient clinic, is seen by the doctor, perhaps briefly, and then waits another hour for medication at the pharmacy, it can be imagined that their enthusiasm for the medication, let alone the entire health care system, may be slight.

Prescriber and patient/parent interaction

The doctor who is interested in the child and the family, who spends time discussing the illness and the medication and who is welcoming and remains interested at follow-up consultations, is much more likely to have compliant patients.

In summary, it has been proposed that non-compliance is a normal behaviour pattern in many situations with regard to taking medication. Efforts should be concentrated on those patients in whom compliance readily is important. Strategies to improve compliance in patients where it actually matters are discussed.

FURTHER READING

Boreus O O 1982 Principles of paediatric pharmacology. Churchill Livingstone, London
Briggs G G, Bodendorfer T W, Freeman R K, Yaffe S J 1983 Drugs in pregnancy and lactation. A reference guide to fetal and neonatal risk. Williams & Wilkins, Baltimore
Buchanan N, Baird Lambert J 1988 Prescribing medications for children. Williams & Wilkins, Sydney
Green C 1988 Toddler taming: a parents' guide to surviving the first four years. Doubleday, Sydney
MacLeod S M, Radde I C 1985 Textbook of pediatric clinical pharmacology. PSG Publishing, Littleton, Massachusettes

Index

Abdomen
  distension, 519, 530–1
  examination, 64
  pain, 526–31
    drug-associated, 529
    recurrent, 530–1, 549
Abetalipoproteinaemia, 521
ABO incompatability, 194, 336, 340, 532
Aboriginals, 71, 108, 129, 133–4, 245, 595
  age distribution of population, 133
  alcohol/substance abuse, 134
  available services, 134
  confinement statistics, 5
  education, 133
  employment, 133
  family life, 86
  health status, 133
  housing, 133
  infant mortality, 4, 133
  legal aid and, 133–4
  malabsorption syndromes, 519, 520
  malnutrition, 95, 133, 491
Absence (petit mal) seizures, 380–1
  status, 381
Absorption
  calcium, 517
  carbohydrate, 515
  electrolytes, 518
  fat, 514–5
  iron, 517
  magnesium, 518
  oral drug, 537, 634
  protein, 517
  vitamins, 517
  water, 518
  zinc, 517–8
Accessory auricles, 20
Acetazolamide, 409
Achalasia, 142, 501
Achondroplasia, 51, 408, 448, 456
Acid-base balance disturbance, 428–9
Acidosis, 428–9, 488
  chronic, 493
  diabetes mellitus, 481, 482
  heart failure and, 315
Acne neonatorum, 566, 577
Acne vulgaris, 556, 559, 576–7
Acquired immune deficiency syndrome

(AIDS) see HIV infection
Acrocyanosis, 565
Acrodermatitis enteropathica, 517, 586
Acromegaly, 451, 459
Acropustulosis, 566
ACTH therapy, 379, 380
Actinomycin-D, 368
Acyclovir, 203, 204, 221, 222, 224, 242,
    568, 574
Addison's disease, 161, 576
Addition mutations, 37
Adenoidectomy, 164
Adenoids, 601
  infection, 602
Adenosine deaminase (ADA) deficiency,
    160–1
Adenovirus
  conjunctivitis, 595
  gastroenteritis, 506
  respiratory infection, 262, 265, 267
    long-term complications, 279
Adolescent idiopathic scoliosis, 74–5
Adolescents, 556–61
  alcohol consumption, 560–1
  chronic disease/disability and, 558–9
  compliance, 639, 643
  confidentiality and, 12, 13, 557–8, 560
  developmental tasks, 559
  drug abuse, 561, 639
  drug therapy, 639
  examination, 557
  health concerns, 556–7
  health services utilization, 557
  menstrual problems, 560
  mortality, 557
  pregnancy, 149, 560
  sexuality, 560
  sexually transmitted disease and, 560
  smoking and, 561
  suicide/suicide attempts, 561, 639
  temporomandibular pain-dysfunction
    syndrome, 617
Adoption, 12, 57, 138–9
Adrenal disease, 140, 401
Adrenal insufficiency, 143, 333, 334, 476,
    489, 498, 579
  recurrent hypoglycaemia and, 486, 487
Adrenogenital syndrome (congenital

adrenal hyperplasia), 143, 442, 474,
    475, 479
  diagnosis, 477
  management, 477–8
  treatment in fetus, 479
Adrenoleukodystrophy, 392
Adriamycin, 366, 368, 369
Agammaglobulinaemia
  congenital, 364
  sex-linked, 158, 277, 586
Age, maternal, 55
  birth defects and, 20
  Down syndrome and, 125
  prenatal diagnosis and, 43
Agent orange, 25
Agyria, 385
Air embolus, 184
Airways obstruction, 64–5
Albinism, 582–3
Albright's syndrome, 581–2, 587
Alcohol abuse, 90, 93, 98, 128, 146, 552,
    560–1
  antisocial behaviour and, 132
  birth weight and, 24
  drinking patterns, 131–2
  employment and, 132
  family life and, 132–3
  health and, 132
  management, 133
  mortality and, 132
  physical complications, 132
  teratogenesis, 22, 24, 49
Aldosterone, 424, 492
Alkalosis, 428, 429, 488
  following vomiting, 426
Alleles, 29
Allergic blepharitis, 596
Allergic conjunctivitis, 165, 595
Allergic disease, 159, 335
  persistent cough and, 293
  see also Atopy
Allergic rhinitis
  perennial, 163–4
  seasonal (hay fever), 163, 164–5
Allopurinol, 365
Alopecia areata, 577
Alpha$_1$-antitrypsin clearance, 521

Alpha$_1$-antitrypsin deficiency, 195, 282, 533, 534
  liver disease and, 534, 536, 537
  pulmonary insufficiency and, 534
Alphafetoprotein screening, 41, 43
  neural tube defects and, 418
Alport's syndrome, 441
Ambiguous genitalia, 66, 474–9, 498
  androgen insensitivity, 477
  causes, 478
  congenital adrenal hyperplasia (CAH) and, 474, 477–8, 479
  counselling parents, 479
  diagnosis, 477, 478
  in female, 475
  information for child, 479
  in male, 475–6
  management, 476–9
  parents' psychological stress and, 474, 477
  prevention, 479
  sex of rearing and, 478–9
  testosterone biosynthesis abnormalities, 476
Amblyopia, 592, 593, 594, 595
Amelogenesis imperfecta, 612
Amethocaine, 593
Amikacin, 637, 641
Aminoglycoside-polymyxin sprays, 634
Aminoglycosides, 190, 207, 604, 633, 635, 637
Aminophylline, 175, 257, 287, 288, 503
Ammonium chloride preparations, 268
Amniocentesis, 43, 44, 48, 49
  neural tube defects and, 418
Amoxycillin, 190, 207, 317, 434, 606, 634, 637, 641
Amphotericin B, 642
Ampicillin, 224, 226, 234, 634, 635, 637, 641
Amputation, 117
Anaemia, 9, 181, 337–41, 522
  Aboriginal infants, 133
  blood film, 336–7
  blood loss and, 334, 336
  causes, 336–7
  classification, 337
  diagnosis, 335
  heart disease and, 317
  history, 336
  infection and, 336
  investigations, 336
  malabsorption and, 520
  management, 341
  neonatal, 334, 335, 336
  nutrition and, 336
  pallor and, 335, 531
  physical examination, 336
  preterm infant, 177
  red cell indices, 335
  renal disease and, 334
  transient erythroblastopenic, 339
Analgesics, 641
Anaphylactoid purpura, 351

Androgen insensitivity, 477
Anencephaly, 19, 56, 385, 413
Angioedema, 161, 168–9
Angiomas, 583
Angiomatosis retinae-et-cerebelli, 583
Angiotensin, 424
Animal danders, 166
Ankylosing spondylitis, 622, 624
Anogenital warts, 560, 573
Anorexia nervosa, 97, 553, 554, 556
Anthracyclines, 366, 367
Antibiotic therapy, 244, 246, 256, 257, 640, 643
  absorption, 615
  appropriateness, 638, 639–40
  asthma and, 287
  avulsed tooth and, 617
  candidiasis and, 153, 154
  cystic fibrosis and, 276
  dosages, 641
  ear infections and, 606, 607
  head injury, 257
  jaw infection, 234
  meningitis, 236, 237, 238, 256
  neonatal dosages, 637
  neonatal sepsis, 206–7
  osteomyelitis, 231–2
  prophylactic, 317, 318
  respiratory distress and, 190
  respiratory infection, 268, 272, 599, 600, 602
  urinary tract infection, 434
  vesicoureteric reflux and, 434, 435
Antibody
  deficiency with normal immunoglobulins, 159
  maternally derived, 155
  production, 154
Anticoagulants, 350
Anticonvulsants, 256, 376, 377, 379, 380, 381, 382, 383, 390, 391, 492, 536, 627, 633
  meningitis and, 238
  pharmacokinetics, 634, 636, 637
  seizure type and, 383
  serum level monitoring, 384
  side-effects, 384
  teratogenicity, 21, 24
Anti-D gammaglobulin, 194, 196
Antidiuretic hormone (ADH), 423, 424
Antihistamines, 165, 169, 265, 571, 642
  asthma and, 287
  non-sedating long-acting, 164
Antipyretics, 641
Antithrombin III deficiency, 353
Antithyroid drugs, 579
Anxiety, 335
Aortic coarctation, 64, 308, 312, 313, 314, 316, 320, 324–5
  pulses, 324–5
  treatment, 316, 325
Aortic incompetence, 307, 322
Aortic stenosis, 312, 316, 324, 325
  murmur, 307, 324

  pulses, 308
  treatment, 324
Aortopulmonary collateral arteries, 307
Aphthous ulcers, 616
Aplasia cutis, 586
Aplastic anaemia, 337–9, 350, 353, 364, 579
  clinical features, 339
  drug/chemical-associated, 338, 339
Apnoea monitors, 10
Apnoea, recurrent, 9, 10, 188
  preterm infant, 175
Appendicitis, acute, 502, 503, 506, 528–9
  diagnosis, 528
  differential diagnosis, 529
Aqueduct obstruction, 404, 406
Arachnoid cyst, 404
Arbovirus encephalitis, 240
Arch supports, 71, 72
Argininosuccinic acidaemia, 211
Arnold Chiari malformation, 404, 415
Arthritis, 233, 237, 239
  acute infantile, 232–3, 234
Arthrogryposis, 117
Artificial feeding see Bottle feeding
Artificial insemination by donor, 57
Aspergillus infection, 161
  osteomyelitis, 228
Aspiration pneumonia/pneumonitis, 187, 188, 274, 276
Aspirin, 168, 350, 503, 539, 625, 639, 640, 641
  platelet function studies and, 353
Asplenia, congenital, 337
Astemizole, 164
Asthma, 7, 117, 263, 267, 269, 275, 284–291, 293, 558, 639
  acute severe attack, 257, 287, 288, 289
  adolescents, 281–2
  allergen avoidance and, 286
  atopy and, 163, 165–166, 282, 284, 300
  bronchial hyper-responsiveness and, 284
  chronic, 141, 288–9
  clinical features, 285–6
  crisis plan, 289
  definition, 284
  drug therapy, 166, 286, 287–8, 289, 290–1, 640
  dry powder inhalation, 287, 288
  metered aerosols, 287, 288
    nebulizers, 287, 288
  episodic, 288–9
  failure-to-thrive and, 143
  'fat happy wheezer', 276
  fictitious, 282
  genetic aspects, 284
  growth failure and, 293
  hyposensitization and, 166, 286
  infants, 276, 279
  investigations, 166, 286
  mortality, 6
  natural history, 285
  pathophysiology, 284–5
  peak expiratory flow rate, 286, 294

persistent cough and, 300
preschool children, 279
prevalence, 285
pulmonary collapse and, 298
pulmonary function tests, 286, 293, 294
school-age children, 281–2
smoking and, 285, 289
sports and, 286–7, 289
triggers/inducers, 166, 284–5
Astigmatism, 593
Astrocytoma, 370, 371, 404
Ataxia telangiectasia, 161, 364, 391–2, 583
Ataxic cerebral palsy, 388, 389
Ataxic diplegia, 388
Atenolol, 443
Athetosis, 388, 389, 390
Atmospheric pollution, 263–264
Atonic diplegia, 385
Atopic dermatitis (infantile eczema), 163, 166–7, 567–8
   food allergens and, 166
   investigations, 167
   management, 167
Atopy, 163–9, 276, 282, 284, 300, 335
   definitions, 163
   dietary protein intolerance and, 524
   immunotherapy, 164–165, 166
   respiratory tract infections and, 263
   specific IgE and, 163
   symptoms, 163
Atrial septal defect, 316, 320, 323
   closure, 316, 323
   murmur, 308, 323
   ostium primum, 323
   ostium secundum, 323
   splitting of second sound, 308, 323
Atrioventricular septal defect (AV canal), 310, 323
   repair, 323
Atropine sulphate, 593
Attention deficit hyperactivity disorder (ADHD), 112, 548, 552
   drug treatment, 548
Attenuated microorganisms, 99, 100
Atwater factors, 90
Auditory problems see Hearing impairment
Auditory sequencing problems, 112, 115
Autism, 126, 391, 550–1
   intellectual impairment, 551
   symptoms, 550–1
   treatment, 551
Autoimmune chronic active hepatitis, 536–7
Autoimmune disease, 154–5, 159, 161, 353
   pyrexia of unknown origin and, 246, 247
Autoimmune haemolytic anaemia, 155, 336, 340
Autonomy, patients' 12–13, 15
Autosomal dominant inheritance, 29, 30
Autosomal recessive inheritance, 29, 30
Autosomal recessive microcephaly, 53
Avulsed tooth re-implantation, 617
Azathioprine, 441, 628, 629
Azidothymidine (AZT), 162

Babysitting groups, 89
Bag urine specimen, 433, 434
Barbiturates, 384, 492
Base substitution, 37
BCG vaccination, 99, 303
Becker muscular dystrophy, 43, 400
Beckwith-Wiedmann syndrome, 459
Behavioural disorders, 7–8, 543–9
   alcohol and, 132
   chronic illness and, 543
   environmental factors and, 129, 544
   failure-to-thrive and, 142
   genetic aspects, 543
   infancy, 544–5
   intellectual impairment and, 122, 124
   following meningitis, 239
   migrants, 136
   preterm infant, 178
   school-age children, 546–9
   temperament and, 543–4
   temporal lobe epilepsy and, 383
   toddlers, 545–6
Beikost, 93
Bell's palsy, 609
Beneficience, duty of, 12, 13
Benign focal epilepsy of childhood, 380, 382
Benign microscopic haematuria, 441
Benzathine penicillin, 202
Benzene exposure, 339, 364
Benzylpenicillin, 204, 232, 635, 637
Bereavement, 10
Berger's disease, 440
Bernard-Soulier syndrome, 351
Beta-2-sympathomimetics, 287, 288, 289, 290, 300, 301
Bicarbonate replacement therapy, 428
Bicillin allpurpose, 266
Bicuspid aortic valve, 308, 324
Bicycle accidents, 106
Bile salt insufficiency, 525
Biliary atresia, 195, 525
Biliary obstruction, 532
   diagnosis, 533
   management, 533–4
Biliary stenosis, congenital, 533
Bilirubin metabolism, 192–3
   drug therapy and, 635, 640
   inherited conjugation defects, 195
   jaundice and see Jaundice
Bilirubin encephalopathy/kernicterus, 193
   cerebral palsy and, 386, 388
   preterm infant, 176
Birth (perinatal) asphyxia, 118, 120, 181, 185, 186, 352, 376, 604, 612
   cerebral palsy and, 386, 388
   feeding difficulties following, 142
   preterm infant, 174
   small-for-gestational-age infant, 179, 180
   treatment, 257–8
   vomiting following, 497–8
Birth defects, 19–25, 187, 262, 557
   causes, 19
   cerebral palsy and, 385, 388

drug associations, 21, 22–5
failure to thrive and, 143
frequency, 20–1
functional, 20
   intellectual disability, 123
genetic counselling and, 55, 56
hydrocephalus and, 404
inborn errors of metabolism and, 208
neonatal deaths and, 5
parental age and, 20
parental reaction, 118
registers, 21, 23
respiratory infection and, 269, 270
screening, 21–2
small-for-gestational-age infants, 179
syndromes, 19–20
terminology, 19
Birthmarks, 67
Bisacodyl, 643
Bladder control, 546–7
Bleeding, abnormal
   anaemia and, 336
   associated disease, 350
   clinical history, 349–50
   coagulation disorders, 353–6
   diet and, 350, 352
   drug-induced, 350
   ecchymotic lesions, 350
   examination, 350
   family history and, 349, 353
   investigations, 350–1
   petechial lesions, 350
   platelet disorders, 349, 350, 351, 352–3
   vascular defects, 351–2
Bleeding time, 351
Bleomycin, 274, 369
Blepharitis, allergic, 596
Blepharitis squamosa, 596
Blindness see Visual impairment
Blood coagulation system, 353, 354
Blood film, 350–1
Blood gas measurement, 294
Blood group incompatability, 340
   maternofetal jaundice and, 194
Blood pressure measurement, infants, 64
Blood-brain barrier, 635–6
Body fluid distribution, 421
   drug distribution and, 635
Bohn's nodules, 611
Boils (furunculosis), 572
Bone age, 455
Bone disorders, metabolic, 491–3
Bone dysplasia, 47, 50
   counselling and, 51
   prenatal diagnosis, 44
Bone marrow transplant, 160, 161, 339, 362, 366, 492, 616
Bordetella pertussis infection see Pertussis
Bornholm disease, 225
Borrelia burgdorferi, 627
Bottle feeding, 87, 94, 422
   artificial milk formulas, 94
   dental caries and, 614
   underfeeding, 141

Botulism, 395, 398
Bow legs, 69, 70, 72
Bowel control, 546–7
Bowel obstruction, 424, 499
Brachmann-de Lange syndrome, 54
Brain injury, 181
  cerebral blood flow and, 254–5
  cerebral perfusion pressure and, 254
  coning and, 254, 255
  convulsions and, 256
  duration of treatment, 256
  fluid balance and, 255–6
  intellectual disability and, 117
  intracranial pressure and, 254, 255
  prevention, 128
Brain-stem glioma, 370, 371, 391
Breast feeding, 87, 93–4, 524
  acute gastroenteritis and, 507, 508
  bilirubin metabolism and, 193
  dental caries and, 614–5
  passively acquired immunity and, 94,
    155–6, 200, 262
  technique, 94
  underfeeding, 141
Breast milk, 422
  composition, 94, 200, 491
  drugs excreted into, 637–8
  production, 94
Breast milk jaundice, 195, 196
Breath-holding, 379, 545, 546
Breath hydrogen test, 520–1
Brodie's abscess, 231
Bromhexine, 301
Bromocriptine, 638
Bronchial adenoma, 282
Bronchial cyst, 297
Bronchial stenosis, 277
Bronchial stricture, 297
Bronchiectasis, 158, 279
  familial, 276–7
  growth failure and, 293
  management, 298
  persistent cough and, 294, 295, 297–8
Bronchiolitis, acute, 261, 269–70, 276,
    279
  age and, 263
  asthma and, 285, 286
  gestational age and, 263
  pathogens, 262, 282
  prognosis, 270
  sex, hospital admission and, 263, 269
  treatment, 269–70
Bronchitis, acute, 261, 267–8
  parental smoking and, 263
  pathogens, 262, 267, 282
  treatment, 268
  'wheezy'/'allergic', 279
Bronchodilators, 642
Bronchogenic cyst, 277
Bronchomalacia, 277
Bronchopulmonary dysplasia (BPD), 183,
    188–9, 276, 284
  aetiology, 188
  clinical features, 188

management, 189
  preterm infant, 177
  prognosis, 189
Brucellosis, 233, 234, 245
Bruton's agammaglobulinaemia, 158, 277,
    586
Bulimia nervosa, 97, 553–4
Bullous impetigo, 566
Burns, scalds, 7, 103, 104, 107, 147, 162,
    634

Caffey's disease, 616
Calciferol, 643
Calcitonin, 489
Calcitriol, 488
Calcium metabolism, 488–90
  absorption, 517
  hormonal control, 488–9
  plasma levels, 488–90
  urine levels, 490
Campylobacter infection, 233, 508, 512,
    626
Campylobacter jejunum, 506
Campylobacter pyloridis, 530
Candida albicans infection, 162, 184, 228,
    245, 318, 481, 489, 565, 569, 615
  following antibiotic therapy, 153, 154
  chronic mucocutaneous, 161
  immunodeficiency and, 157
Captopril, 443
Caput succedaneum, 67
Carbamazepine, 377, 380, 382, 383, 384,
    627, 634
Carbamyl phosphate synthetase deficiency,
    212
Carbenicillin, 637, 641
Carbimazole, 468, 638
Carbohydrate, dietary, 90, 93
  absorption, 515
  digestion, 515
  intolerance, 97, 523–4
Cardiac arrythmias, 318–9
Cardiac catheterization, 314, 320
Cardiac glycogenosis, 311
Cardiomegaly, 313–14
Cardiomyopathy, 312
Cardiovascular system examination, 64
Carnitine deficiency, 311, 401
Carnitine-palmityl transferase deficiency,
    398, 401
Carotenaemia, 333
Cat scratch disease, 245
Cataract, 120, 594
Catheter urine specimen, 433
Cefotaxime, 207, 238, 636, 637, 641
Cefoxitin, 637, 641
Ceftriaxone, 238
Cefuroxime, 637, 641
Cell division, 26–9
Cell mediated immunity, 154
Cellulitis, 572–3
Cephalexin, 634, 641
Cephalhaematoma, 67, 195, 334

Cephalosporins, 204, 206, 207, 232, 234,
    238, 635, 636, 637
Cephalothin, 641
Cephamandole, 637, 641
Cephazolin, 637, 641
Cephradine, 641
Cerebellar ataxia syndromes, 391
Cerebral abscess, 327, 503
Cerebral anoxia/ischaemia, 142, 254, 255,
    257
  vomiting and, 497–8
  see also Birth asphyxia
Cerebral blood flow, 254–5
Cerebral damage see Brain injury
Cerebral degenerations, 142, 390–3
  age of onset, 392
  evidence of regression, 391
  progressive disorders, 391–2
  treatability, 393
Cerebral gigantism, 408, 459
Cerebral oedema, 255, 256, 258, 428, 497
  head injury and, 256
  meningitis and, 238–9, 256
Cerebral palsy, 385–390, 547, 559, 617
  aetiology, 239, 385, 386, 388
  ataxic, 388, 389
  classification, 386
  clinical features, 386
  convulsions and, 385, 388, 389, 390
  deafness and, 119, 389
  definition, 385
  diplegia
    atonic, 388
    spastic, 387
  education and, 390
  employment and, 389, 390
  extrapyramidal forms, 388, 389
  feeding difficulty and, 389
  hemiplegia, 385, 387–8, 389
  incidence, 385
  intellectual deficit and, 117, 385, 386,
    388, 389
  malformations and, 385, 388
  mixed forms, 388, 389
  orthopaedic complications, 389
  preterm infant, 7, 386, 387, 388
  psychological complications, 389
  quadriparesis, 385, 387, 389
  spastic, 386–7
  speech difficulty and, 389
  treatment, 389–90
  visual impairment and, 389
Cerebral perfusion pressure, 254
Cerebral tumour, 363, 369–71, 381, 391,
    393, 503
  hydrocephalus and, 404–5, 406, 407
  investigations, 370–1
  posterior fossa, 370
  raised intracranial pressure and, 370
  treatment, 371
Cerebral vascular occlusions, 392
Cerebrospinal fluid (CSF)
  absorption, 403
  bacterial meningitis and, 237

circulation, 403
drug passage, 635–6
formation, 403
hydrocephalus and, 404, 407
drugs reducing production, 409
intermittent removal, 409
investigations, 246
Cerebroventricular haemorrhage, 183, 497
Chalazion, 596
Charcot-Marie-Tooth syndrome, 397
Chest deformity, 65, 293
Chest sounds, 64, 65
Chewing trauma, neuropathic, 617
Child abuse, 76, 103, 145–50, 177, 349, 498, 579, 598
alcohol and, 132
'at risk' children, 145, 146, 150
clinical presentation, 145–7
definition, 145
early identification/intervention, 145, 146
emotional, 145
examination, 146–7
family circumstances and, 129
history, 146
incidence, 145
investigations, 147–8
management, 149–50
neglect/non-organic failure-to-thrive, 141, 145, 147, 148, 149
orofacial trauma, 617
poisoning, 107–8
prevention, 150
spectrum of conditions, 145, 146
Child care groups, 89
Child disability allowance, 121, 127
Child sexual abuse, 145, 148, 560, 617
indicators of, 148–9
management, 149, 150
prevention, 150
Children's Court, 149–50
Children's homes, 138
Chlamydia trachomatis infection, 184, 293, 560
congenital, 204
conjunctivitis, 204, 595
prophylaxis, 204
Chloral hydrate, 643
Chlorambucil, 364
Chloramphenicol, 204, 226, 234, 238, 267, 338, 350, 572, 579, 595, 635, 636, 637, 638, 639, 641
phenytoin interaction, 238
Chlordane, 339
Chlordiazepoxide, 634
Chlorhexidine gluconate, 616
Chloroquine, 227, 245, 638
Chlorothiazide, 436, 443
Chlorpheniramine, 642
Chlorphenothane (DDT), 339
Chlorpromazine, 242, 642
Choanal atresia, 181, 187, 190, 599
Cholecystitis, 529
Choledocal cyst, 533

Cholera vaccine, 509
Chondrodystrophic myotonia, 401
Chondromalacia patellae, 76
Choreoathetosis, 388, 389
Chorionic villus sampling, 42, 43, 44
Choroid plexus papilloma, 405
Choroiditis, 596–7
Choroidoretinal degenerations, 120
Christmas disease (haemophilia B), 349, 351, 353–5
clinical features, 354
HIV infection and, 354
therapy, 355
Chromosomal abnormality, 19, 50, 53, 54
dysmorphic child, 47
failure-to-thrive and, 143
intellectual disability and, 124
leukaemia and, 364, 365
prenatal diagnosis, 43
amniocentesis, 42
chorionic villus sampling, 42
fetal blood sampling, 42
small-for-gestational-age infant, 179
Chromosome banding techniques, 19, 27, 57
Chromosome mapping, 40
Chromosome walking, 40
Chromosomes, 26
meiosis and, 27–8
mitosis and, 26–7
molecular organization, 33
functional aspects, 35–6
gene clusters/families, 35, 36
repetitive DNA, 33
unique sequence DNA, 33
sex, 26, 30
Chronic childhood spinal muscular atrophy, 394, 396–7
Chronic disease
learning difficulty following, 113
sick role and, 113
Chronic granulomatous disease, 161
Chronic lung disease in infancy, 188
classification, 188
Chronic lung disease of prematurity see Bronchopulmonary dysplasia
Chronic mucocutaneous candidiasis, 161
Chronic non-specific diarrhoea of infancy, 509–10
Chronic pulmonary insufficiency of prematurity (CPIP), 177
Churg-Strauss syndrome, 630
Cirrhosis, 537
Cis-platinum, 369
Citrullinaemia, 211
Cleft lip/palate, 20, 56, 67, 141, 599, 601, 610, 617
genetic counselling, 57
Cleidocranial dysplasia, 613
Clonazepam, 256
Clostridium botulinum, 398
Clotrimazole, 565
Cloxacillin, 572, 635, 637, 641
Coagulation defect, 186, 195

preterm infant, 176
Codeine, 268, 301, 576
Coeliac disease, 97, 343, 456, 458, 502, 517, 519, 520, 522, 634
growth failure, 140
Colds (coryza), 261, 265
management, 265
pathogens, 262, 265
Colic, infantile, 7, 526
Collagen disease, 398, 401
anaemia and, 340
diffuse lung disease, 273
genetic defects, 20
Collapse, 251–8
airway and, 251, 256, 257
brain injury and, 254–6
breathing/ventilation and, 251–2, 256, 257
intubation, 252
causes, 251, 256–8
circulation, 252, 254, 256, 257
fluid infusion into bone marrow, 252, 254
intravenous fluid, 252
drugs used in resuscitation, 252, 253
duration of treatment, 256
fluid balance and, 255–6
initial management, 251
intracranial pressure and, 254, 255
Coloboma, 597
Colonic biopsy, 521
Colonoscopy, 521
Colostrum, 94
Combined immunodeficiency, 159–61, 586
with enzyme defects, 160–1
Common variable immunodeficiency, 159
Community health centres, 87–8
Community health facilities, 87–9
primary health services, 87–8
social services, 88–9
Complement disorders, 161
Complement system, 154
Compliance, 638, 639, 640, 643–4
Conduct disorders, 550, 551–2
aetiology, 552
follow-up, 552
management, 552
Confidentiality, 13
adolescents and, 557–8, 560
Congenital adrenal hyperplasia see Adrenogenital syndrome
Congenital cardiac defects see Heart disease, congenital
Congestive heart disease, 183, 312
Conjunctivitis
allergic, 595
chlamydial, 204, 595
gonococcal, 204, 595
neonatal, 595
Connective tissue disease, 336, 621–30
aetiology, 621
incidence, 621
pathology, 621
pyrexia of unknown origin and, 246, 247

Consanguinity, parental, 55, 63, 208
Constipation, 547–8
Constrictive cardiomyopathy, 312
Convulsions, 7, 256, 375, 391, 392
  adolescents, 558
  anticonvulsants, 383–4
  breath-holding attacks and, 546
  cerebral palsy and, 385, 388, 389, 390
  febrile, 376–7, 508
  hypertensive, 440
  hypoglycaemia and, 484, 491
  infantile spasms, 377–9
  investigations, 383
  Lennox-Gastaut syndrome, 379–80
  management, 383–4
  meningitis and, 256
  myoclonic epilepsy, 379–80
  neonatal, 375–6
  preschool age group, 379–80
  reflex hypoxic seizures, 379
  school-age child, 380–3
  seizure type
    classification, 375
    drugs and, 383
Cornea
  abrasions, 594
  dystrophies, familial, 593
  foreign bodies, 593
  opacities, 593
  ulceration, 593, 594
Cornelia de Lange syndrome, 126
Cortical blindness, 120
Cortical hyperostosis, infantile, 616
Corticosteroid therapy, 162, 164, 165, 169,
    223, 247, 293, 299, 303, 318, 398,
    401, 529, 577, 586
  absorption, 634
  antenatal, 175
  asthma, 276, 288, 289, 291, 293
  atopic dermatitis, 568
  autoimmune chronic active hepatitis,
    537
  bleeding disorders, 351, 352, 353
  cerebral oedema and, 255
  congenital adrenal hyperplasia, 477
  convulsions, 379, 380
  dosages, 643
  encephalitis, 242
  growth failure and, 457
  head injury and, 257
  inflammatory bowel disease, 511, 512
  juvenile chronic arthritis, 625
  juvenile dermatomyositis, 629
  septic shock, 237
  skin disorders, 568, 569, 570, 571, 572
  systemic lupus erythematosus, 628
Cortisol, growth and, 451
Cortisone acetate, 643
Cost/benefit analysis, 14
Co-trimoxazole, 161, 226, 434, 435, 606,
    638, 640, 641
  side-effects, 435
Cough, persistent, 292–303
  blood gas measurement, 294

  causes, 303
  diagnosis, 293
  growth failure and, 293
  investigations, 293, 294
  management, 301
  psychogenic, 293, 300
  pulmonary function tests, 293–4
Cough reflex arc, 292
  disturbed, 301
Cough suppresants, 269, 301
Counselling, 51
  child abuse and, 150
  family, 138
  prenatal diagnosis and, 44
  preterm infant, 177
  see also Genetic counselling
Cow's milk hypersensitivity, 166, 167,
    168, 510, 519, 524, 526, 544
Coxsackie virus infection, 224, 225, 396,
    440, 480, 533
  meningitis, 240
  myocarditis, 311
  respiratory tract infection, 262, 265, 267
Cradle cap, 566
Cranial meningocele, 413
Cranial nerve assessment, 64, 65–6
Craniocleidodysostosis, 408
Craniofacial birth defects, 24
Craniopharyngioma, 125, 370, 391, 404,
    461–3
Cranium bifidum, 413
Crigler-Najjar syndrome, 195
Crohn's disease, 143, 233, 456, 511–2,
    517, 524, 626
Croup see Laryngotracheobronchitis
Cryptococcal meningitis, 393
Cryptosporidium infection, 162, 245, 246,
    506
Cushing's syndrome, 352, 492, 579
  growth failure and, 457
Cutis laxa, 352, 578
Cutis marmarata, 565
Cyanotic heart disease, 320, 326–9
Cyclical vomiting, 504
Cyclopentolate, 593
Cyclophosphamide, 367, 368, 369, 438,
    441, 628, 629
Cyclosporin, 438, 628
  gingival hypertrophy and, 616
Cyproheptadine, 571
Cysteamine, 436
Cystic fibrosis, 7, 19, 20, 87, 97, 117, 195,
    245, 279, 284, 295–7, 639, 640
  antenatal diagnosis, 42, 44, 295
  diagnosis, 297
  fat balance studies, 521
  fertility and, 297
  genetic counselling, 55, 57
  growth failure and, 140, 141
  hepatitis and, 195, 533
  incidence, 295
  lower airways obstruction, 296
  malabsorption, 519, 520, 524
  management, 276, 297

  neonatal screening, 21, 22, 295
  physiotherapy, 276, 297
  presentation, 62, 143, 293, 295, 529
  sweat test, 521
Cystic hygroma, 42, 190, 277
Cystinuria, 432, 436, 490
Cytochrome oxidase deficiency, 401
Cytomegalovirus (CMV) infection, 184,
    195, 223, 245, 246, 273, 376, 385,
    533, 535
  congenital, 202
  intra-uterine, 24, 119, 143
Cytosine arabinoside, 365, 366, 367
Cytoskeletal protein defects, 20
Cytotoxic chemotherapy, 162, 274, 299,
    300, 350, 365, 366, 367, 368, 369,
    529, 579, 598, 633, 638, 640

D_1, trisomy syndrome, 364
Dairy protein intolerance, dietary, 102, 524
Dandy-Walker syndrome, 404, 406
Dapsone, 638
Daunomycin, 366
Daunorubicin, 365
De Moisier's syndrome, 597
Deafness, 77, 78, 81, 118–9, 604–5, 607
  Aboriginal children, 133
  causes, 604
  cerebral palsy and, 119, 389
  education system and, 119
  hearing aids and, 605
  with intellectual disability, 117, 126
  learning difficulty and, 112, 113, 115
  management, 119
  following meningitis, 239
  otitis media and, 607, 608
  presentation, 604–5
  profound, 605
  risk factors, 119
  testing, 88, 604–5
  tympanometry, 607–8
  very low birth weight and, 7
Death, 10–11
  birth defects and, 21
  of child, 10–11
  hospital staff reactions, 10
  malignancy and, 363–4
  of parent, 10
  siblings' reactions, 10
Debendox, 25
Decongestants, 599, 600, 606, 607
Deformation, 19
Dehydration, 65
  acute gastroenteritis and, 506–7
  causes, 424
  clinical quantification, 424
  diabetes mellitus and, 481, 482
  hypernatraemia, 424–5
  hypotonic, 424
  intravenous fluids, 426
  intravenous treatment, 425–6, 507–8
  oral rehydration therapy, 507
  types, 424–5

Deletions, 37, 38, 45, 47
  cDNA probe detection, 39
Delinquency, 552
Dengue haemorrhagic fever, 351
Denis Brown splint, 70, 74
Dental abscess, 615
Dental age, 455
Dental caries, 613–5, 638
  aetiology, 613
  'dummy', 614
  high frequency breast feeding, 614–5
  nursing bottle, 614
  'operculum', 615
  prevention, 614
Dental health services, 88
Dentine, developmental defects (DDD),
  612
Dentinogenesis imperfecta, 51, 52, 612
Denver Developmental Screening Test, 77,
  124
Deontology, 14–15
Depigmentation, 582–3, 587
Depression, 391, 543, 550, 552–3
  adolescents, 556, 557
  aetiology, 552–3
  maternal, 8, 89, 129, 131, 135, 141, 545
  treatment, 553
Dermatitis herpetiformis, 585–6
Dermatomyositis, 273, 401, 576, 584–5,
  626
Desferrioxamine, 359
Desmopressin (DDAVP), 427
Desquamation, neonatal, 566
Developmental assessment, 66, 77–8, 87
  environmental stimuli and, 79, 81
  equipment, 81
  global delay and, 81, 82
  growth pattern, 79
  history, 78–9
  interpretation, 81–2
  language, 78
  milestones, 78, 79–80
  specific delay and, 81
  timing, 78
Developmental delay, 81, 82, 87, 122
  child abuse and, 147
  intellectual impairment, 123, 124, 126
  screening test, 77, 124
Developmental history, 63, 78–9
Developmental Record for Infants and
  Young Children (DRIYC), 77
Dexamethasone, 479
Dextrochlorpheniramine, 642
Dextromethorphan, 642
Di George anomalad, 161
Diabetes insipidus, 142–3, 424, 427, 436,
  547
Diabetes mellitus, 56, 97, 117, 142, 398,
    424, 428, 480–5, 529, 547, 639, 640
  adolescents, 484, 558
  aetiology, 480
  blood glucose measurement, 482
  clinical features, 481
  compliance and, 484

course, 481
  with cystic fibrosis, 297
  delayed puberty and, 484
  diagnosis, 481–2
  diet, 483
  exercise and, 483
  future therapeutic options, 485
  genetic aspects, 480
  growth and, 484
  hypoglycaemia management, 483–4
  indicators of glycaemic control, 483
  infection and, 481, 484
  initial treatment, 482
  insulin replacement therapy, 482, 483,
    485
  ketoacidosis, 481, 484, 498, 503
  management aims, 482
  maternal, 183, 196, 448, 458
    teratogenic effect, 45
  outpatient management, 483
  pathogenesis, 480–1
  prevalence/incidence, 480
  psychosocial stress and, 484
  type 2 (non-insulin-dependent), 480
  weight loss, 481
Diaphragmatic hernia, 186–7, 190
Diarrhoea, 334, 505–12
  anaemia and, 336
  chronic, 509–12, 519, 523
  failure-to-thrive and, 142
  immunodeficiency and, 157, 246
  malabsorption and, 519
  metabolic acidosis and, 428
  'toddler', 509–10
  vitamin A deficiency and, 95
Diazepam, 238, 242, 256, 377, 380, 497,
    617, 634, 635, 640, 643
Diazoxide, 439, 440, 487
Diclofenac sodium, 625
Dienoestrol, 638
Dietary guidelines, 93
Diethylstilboestrol, 20, 25
Diffuse lung disease, 273–4
Digestion
  disaccharide, 515
  fats, 514–5
  protein, 515–7
  starch, 515
Digitalis, 186, 189, 237, 503
Digoxin, 315, 319, 633, 634, 637, 642
Dihydrotestosterone, 475
Diphenoxylate, 642
  with atropine, 508
Diphtheria, 311
  immunization, 87, 99, 100, 102
Diplegia, 388
Disability, 117–21
  categories of, 117
  counselling and, 121
  diagnosis, 118, 121
  discrimination, 121
  doctor's role in care, 120–1
  early identification, 118, 121
  education and, 121

intellectual see Intellectual disability
  parental reaction, 118
  in previously normal child, 118
  special resources, 121
  team approach, 121
  WHO definition, 117
Discitis, 230
Disodium cromoglycate, 276, 287–8, 289,
  291
Disseminated intravascular coagulation,
  352, 353, 579
  meningococcaemia and, 236, 237
Divorce rate, 129
DNA
  chromosomal organization, 33
  functional aspects, 26, 35–6
  gene clusters, 35, 36
  highly repetitive sequences, 33
  moderately repetitive sequences, 33
  sequences involved in gene expression,
    34
  unique sequences, 33
DNA technology
  carrier detection, 400
  gene/protein product location, 40
  genetic disorder diagnosis, 38–9
  prenatal diagnosis and, 42, 43–4, 400
  sample collection for genetic
    counselling, 57
  Southern blot analysis, 39
DNCB, 577
Dobutamine, 252, 256
Dog bite, 108, 617
Domestic violence, alcohol and, 132
Dopamine, 315
Down syndrome see Trisomy 21
Doxycycline, 634
DPT (triple antigen) vaccine, 101, 102
Drowning/near-drowning, 103, 105,
    106–7, 257
  cerebral dysfunction following, 104, 107
  hypokalaemia following, 257
  resuscitation skills and, 106–7, 109
  safety education and, 109
  secular trends, 105
Drug abuse, 552, 561, 639
Drug therapy, 639–44
  administration route selection, 640
  blood-brain barrier and, 635–6
  body water and, 635
  breast milk, excretion in, 637–8
  compliance and, 638, 639, 640, 643–4
  distribution, 635–6
  dosage, 640, 641–3
    form, 644
    regimen, 644
  duration of treatment, 640
  elimination, 636
  hepatic metabolism, 636
  in infancy, 638–9
  intramuscular absorption, 634, 637
  intravenous administration, 634, 637
  neonates, 634, 635, 636, 637–8
  oral absorption, 634, 637

Drug therapy *continued*
  percutaneous absorption, 634
  plasma protein-binding, 635
  rectal absorption, 634–5
  renal excretion, 636
Duchenne muscular dystrophy, 56, 317,
    394, 399–400
  carrier detection, 400
  diagnosis, 399–400
  early symptoms, 399
  gene protein product characterization, 40
  genetic counselling, 57, 400
  intellectual disability, 126, 399, 400
  management, 400
  neonatal screening, 21
  prenatal diagnosis, 43, 400
'Dummy caries', 614
Duodenal obstruction, 500
Duodenitis, acute, 530
Duplications, genetic, 38
Dwarfism *see* Bone dysplasia
Dysgerminoma, 370
Dysmenorrhoea, 560
Dysmorphic syndromes, 19, 47–54, 113,
    114
  body proportions, 46
  diagnosis, 45, 47
  examination, 45–7
  facial features description, 46
  facial profile assessment, 46
  height, 46
  history, 45
  intellectual disability and, 126
  investigations, 47
  measurements, 45–6
  short stature and, 456
Dyspnoea, 313, 322
  food intake and, 141
  heart failure and, 314

Ear
  acquired disorders, 606–9
  congenital abnormalities, 605
  examination, 66, 604
    set/size, 46
  foreign bodies, 606
  wax, 606
Eating disorders, 97, 550, 552, 553–4
Echo virus infection, 158, 224, 225, 396,
    440
  meningitis, 240
  myocarditis, 311
  respiratory tract infection, 262, 265
Echocardiography, 314, 315, 318, 320
Econazole, 565
Ectodermal dysplasia, 578, 613
  hypohidrotic, 612–3
Eczema, 586, 634
  herpeticum, 224, 568
  infantile *see* Atopic dermatitis
Educational assessment, 115
Ehlers-Danlos syndrome, 20, 350, 352,
    578, 579

Eisenmenger's syndrome, 322
Electrocardiography, 309–11, 319, 320
  leads, 309
  neonate, 310
Electrolytes, 421
  absorption, 518
  balance, 423–4
  loss, 425
    acute gastroenteritis and, 507
    diabetes mellitus and, 481, 482
Elimination diets, 167, 169
Elliptocytosis, 20
Embryonic tumours, 363
Emergency child care services, 138
Emotional disturbance, 7–8
  alcoholism and, 132
  child abuse and, 147
  family break-up and, 129
  growth failure and, 456
  persistent cough and, 300
  recurrent abdominal pain and, 530, 531
  school problems and, 112, 115
Emotional needs, 85–6
Enalapril, 443
Enamel, developmental defects (DDE),
    611–2
Encephalitis, 142, 240–2, 376, 503
  arthropod vectors, 240
  clinical features, 240–1
  diagnosis, 242
  intra-uterine, 385
  pathogens, 240
  treatment, 242
  viral, 240–2
Encephalocele, 413
Encephalotrigeminal angiomatosis, 583
Encopresis, 547–8
Endocardial fibroelastosis, 311–2
Enhancers, 34
Entamoeba histolytica, 512
Enterokinase deficiency, 524
Enterovirus infection, 224–5, 240
Eosinophilic granuloma, 368
Enuresis, 543, 547
Ependymoma, 370, 371, 404
Epidermal naevi, 586
Epidermolysis bullosa, 566, 578, 612
Epiglottitis, acute, 261, 267, 639
  aetiology, 262, 267
Epilepsy, 97, 375, 583, 616, 617, 639, 640
  autism and, 551
  cerebral tumour and, 370
  drowning risk and, 106
  intellectual disability and, 117, 126, 127
  following meningitis, 239
  myelomeningocele and, 416
  myoclonic, 379–80
  post-traumatic, 108
  primary generalized, 380
  seizure classification, 375
  very low birth weight and, 7
  see also Convulsions
Epistaxes, 349, 600–1
  nasal cautery, 601

Epstein-Barr virus infection, 223, 224,
    245, 440, 535, 627
  myelitis, 241
Epstein's pearls, 611
Epulis, congenital, 610–11
Equal Opportunities (Discrimination
    Against Disabled Persons) Act
    (1982), 121
Ergotamine, 638
Erythema, 583–5
  neonatal, 565
Erythema chronicum migrans, 627
Erythema infectiosum ('slapped cheek'
    syndrome), 220
Erythromycin, 204, 269, 272, 273, 282,
    508, 595, 606, 641
Escherichia coli, 184, 195, 318, 411, 423,
    441, 506, 533
  detection in body fluids, 237
  neonatal sepsis, 205, 206, 207
  vaccine, 509
Ethambutol, 303, 642
Ethical aspects, 12–16
  autonomy of patients, 12–13
  beneficence, duty of, 12, 13
  decision-making for child and, 15
  deontology and, 14–15
  justice, duty of, 12, 14
  non-maleficence, concept of, 12, 13
  utilitarianism and, 14
Ethics committees, 15
Ethionamide, 303
Ethosuximide, 381, 384
Etretinate, 578
Eustacian tube, 601, 606
Ewing's sarcoma, 369
Examination, clinical, 13, 61, 63–7
  abdomen, 64
  adolescents, 557
  cardiovascular system, 64
  child abuse and, 146–7
  central nervous system, 67
  developmental assessment and, 66, 77
  ears, 46, 66, 604
  genitals, 66, 67
  head, 65
  hips, 66, 67
  infants, 63–6
  length/weight measurement, 66
  musculoskeletal system, 65
  neck, 65
  neonate, 67
  nervous system, 65–6
  older child, 66–7
  oral cavity, 66
  preliminary introduction, 61
  respiratory system, 64–5
  urine, 67
Exchange transfusion, 197–9, 210, 336,
    340
  complications, 199
Exomphalos, 41, 42, 43
Exons, 34
Expectorants, 301

External auditory canal atresia, 604, 605
External ear abnormalities, 66
Eye lid infection, 596

Fabry's disease, 392
Facial nerve palsy, 608–9
Facioscapulohumeral syndrome, 400–1
Factor XI (PTA) deficiency, 353
Failure-to-thrive, 140–4
  congenital abnormality and, 141
  cystic fibrosis and, 295
  diarrhoea and, 142
  dyspnoea and, 141
    with congenital heart disease, 313,
      322, 323
  endocrine causes, 143
  genetic causes, 143–4
  infection and, 143
  malabsorption and, 142, 519
  metabolic disorders and, 142, 143
  neglect/child abuse, 145, 147, 148, 149
  neurological lesions and, 141–2
  non-organic, 140–1
  organic causes, 141
  preterm infant, 276
  psychosocial deprivation and, 520, 543
  renal disease and, 142–3, 276
  severe combined immunodeficiency and,
    160
  underfeeding and, 141
  vomiting and, 142
Family allowance, 137
Family Assistance Payments, 137
Family day care, 89
Family environment, 85–9, 129–39
  child abuse and, 146, 149, 150
  child care services, 138–9
  community health facilities, 87–9
  counselling/information service, 138
  financial assistance, 137–8
  housing problems, 86
  marriage counselling, 139
  non-organic-failure-to-thrive and, 140–1
  nuclear, 86
  single parent, 86
  support units, 137
  with two working parents, 86
Family group homes, 138
Family planning, 139
Family support units, 137
Fanconi anaemia, 338, 364, 436
Fansidar, 227
Farmer's lung, 273
Fat, dietary, 90, 93
  absorption/digestion, 514–5
  balance studies, 521
Febrile convulsions, 376–7
  aetiology, 376
  afebrile convulsions following, 376, 377
  clinical features, 376
  treatment, 377
Feeding problems, 7, 8, 544, 545
Fetal alcohol syndrome, 19, 62, 132, 142

  aetiology, 49
  clinical features, 49
  failure-to-thrive and, 142
  prognosis, 49
Fetal biopsy, 42
Fetal blood sampling, 42, 44
Fetal varicella zoster syndrome, 203
Fetoscopy, 42
Fibrosing alveolitis, 273, 293
Fifth disease, 220
Flat feet, 69, 71, 72
  natural history, 71
  valgus deformity of heel and, 71
Floppy infant syndrome, 401–2
Flucloxacillin, 232, 234, 572, 585, 634
Fluoride supplements, 614
Fluorosis, 612
Focal dermal hypoplasia, 582
Focal segmental glomerulosclerosis, 438
Folic acid deficiency, 336, 520, 521
Fontanelles, 65, 67
Food colouring
  hypersensitivity reactions, 169
Food hypersensitivity reactions, 166,
    167–8
  allergens, 166
  atopic dermatitis, 167, 168, 568
  delayed, 167, 168
  immediate, 167
  spasmodic croup, 165
  symptoms, 168
  urticaria/angioedema, 168, 571
Food preservatives
  asthma and, 166
  hypersensitivity reactions, 169
Foot posture
  natural history, 71
  in newborn, 69–70
Footwear, 72
  modification, 72
Foreign body
  ear, 606
  ingested, 281
  inhaled, 279–81, 282, 293, 297, 298
  nasal, 600
Foster care, 138
Fracture, 76, 104
Fragile-X syndrome (Fra Xq27), 56, 124,
    125–6
  clinical features, 48
  genetic aspects, 48, 126
  prenatal diagnosis, 43, 48
  prognosis, 48
Frameshift mutations, 37–8
Frenula abnormality, 613
Friedreich's ataxia, 391
Fructose intolerance, hereditary, 142, 209,
    211, 486, 487, 533, 534
  diagnosis, 211
  treatment, 211
Frusemide, 186, 315, 427, 428, 438, 439,
    440, 443
Fucocidosis, 212
Fungal infection, 245, 246, 273, 318, 606

Funnel chest, 65
'Funny-looking kid' (FLK), 19
Furunculosis, 572

Gait abnormality, 395, 397
Galactosaemia, 142, 195, 209, 210, 211,
    486, 487, 533, 534
  diagnosis, 211
  neonatal screening, 21
  in pregnancy, 211
  treatment, 211
Galactose-1 phospate uridyl transferase
    deficiency, 594
Gall bladder disease, 529
Gallstones, 529
Gangliosidosis (GM$_1$ and GM$_3$), 212
Garre's osteomyelitis, 616
Gastritis, acute, 530
Gastroenteric cyst, 277–8
Gastroenteritis, acute, 225, 334, 501–2,
    505–9
  aetiology, 505–6
  breast feeding and, 507, 508
  clinical features, 506
  definition, 505
  dehydration, 424, 425, 426, 506–7
  differential diagnosis, 506, 527
  febrile convulsions and, 508
  metabolic acidosis and, 506, 507
  mucosal injury/malabsorption following,
    519
  prevention, 509
  sugar intolerance complicating, 508–9
  treatment, 507–8
    drugs, 508
    intravenous therapy, 507–8
    oral rehydration, 507
Gastrointestinal infection, 7, 153, 154
  Aboriginal children, 133
  immunodeficiency and, 159
Gastrointestinal lymphangiectasia, 162
Gastro-oesophageal reflux, 142, 500–1,
    530
  aspiration and, 9, 276, 298
Gaucher's disease, 213, 392, 579, 580
Gene therapy, 40
Generalized tonic-clonic seizures (grand
    mal epilepsy), 380, 381, 382, 416
Genes, 26
  allelic variants, 29
  autosomal dominant transmission, 29, 30
  autosomal recessive transmission, 29, 30
  cDNA probes, 39
  clusters, 35
  expression, 34–5
  families, 35, 36, 38
  linked/linkage analysis, 31–2, 35
  mapping, 31–2
  mutation, 19–20, 36–8, 45
  recombination, 28, 31
    errors, 38
  structural, 33–4
  unique copy, 36

Genes continued
    X-linked transmission, 29, 30–1
    see also DNA
Genetic code, 37
Genetic counselling, 20, 21, 55–8, 121,
        123, 128, 143, 208, 393, 394, 398,
        478, 598
    in absence of diagnosis, 56
    alternatives for families at risk, 57
    burden and, 57
    diagnostic precision and, 55–6, 118
    Duchenne muscular dystrophy, 399, 400
    emotional impact, 57
    haemoglobinopathies, 362
    indications, 55
    procedure, 57–8
    records for family, 58
    risk estimation, 56–7
        Down syndrome, 43
    timing, 58
Genetic disorders, 19, 20, 63, 118
    diagnostic, recombinant DNA
        technology and, 38–9
    gene/protein product location, 40
    screening newborns, 21
    Southern blot analysis, 39
    see also Inborn errors of metabolism
Genitals
    examination, 66, 67
    trauma, child sex abuse and, 149
Genotype, 30
Gentamicin, 190, 207, 234, 637, 641
Germ cell formation, 27, 28
Gestational age assessment, 173–4
    in neonate, 67
Giant cell arteritis, 630
Giant cell pneumonia, 217–8
Giardiasis, 159, 506, 512, 519, 520, 521,
        522–3, 524
Gilbert's syndrome, 195
Gingival enlargement, 616
Gingival fibromatosis, 616
Gingivitis, acute necrotizing ulcerative,
        615
Glanzmann's disease, 353
Glaucoma, congenital, 120, 598
Glioma, 404
Globin genes, 35
    deletions, 38
    β-globin gene family, 35
    hybrid globin chain production, 38
Glomerulonephritis, 437, 439–41, 529
    causes, 439
    definition, 439
    post-streptococcal, 223, 439–40
Glonazepam, 379
Glossitis, 49
Glucose-6-phosphate dehydrogenase
        (G6PD) deficiency, 195, 196, 336,
        340, 532
    breast feeding and, 638
Glue ear, 606, 607
    treatment, 607–8
Glue-sniffing, 393

Glutamate dehydrogenase deficiency, 213
Glutaric acidaemia type II, 208, 210
Glycogen storage disease, 316, 398, 401,
        486, 487
Glycogen synthase deficiency, 486
Goitre, 190, 470, 471, 472
    neonatal hypothyroidism and, 468
Gold, 339, 625, 638
Goltz's syndrome (focal dermal
        hypoplasia), 582
Gonadal dysgenesis, 476, 478
Goodpasture's disease, 273
Gout, 213
Gower's sign, 399, 400
Granuloma annulare, 571
Granuloma gluteale infantum, 569
Grasp reflex, 67
Graves' disease, 472
Grief reaction, 10
Griseofulvin, 574, 642
Growth, 140, 447–55
    clinical assessment, 87, 451–5
        bone age and, 455
        dental age and, 455
        percentile charts and, 66, 140, 451-4
    diabetes mellitus and, 484
    disorders, 455-465
    drug therapy and, 639
    genetic influences, 447–8
    hormonal control, 449–51
    intra-uterine influences, 448
    postnatal influences, 448–9
    protein-calorie malnutrition and, 97
    puberty and, 453, 454–5
Growth hormone, 448, 449–51
    control of secretion, 449–50
    deficiency, 143, 463
        recurrent hypoglycaemia and, 486,
            487
        short stature and, 457
    mechanism of action, 450–1
    recombinant DNA, synthesis and, 40,
        449
    replacement therapy, 143
Guillain-Barre syndrome, 395, 397
Guttate psoriasis, 570

H₂ receptor antagonists, 530
Haemangioma, 350, 586
    larynx, 603
Haematuria, 431
Haemoglobin Barts, 360
Haemoglobin E/ β thalassaemia, 360
Haemoglobin estimation, 350–1
Haemoglobin H disease, 360
Haemoglobin Lepore, 38
Haemoglobinopathy, 357–62
    gene manipulation and, 362
    genetic counselling, 362
    prenatal diagnosis, 42, 43, 44, 362
Haemolysis, jaundice and, 194
Haemolytic anaemia, 220, 335, 336,
        339–41, 529

confirmatory tests, 339–40
    neonatal, 340, 532
    with spleen enlargement, 340–1
Haemolytic uraemic syndrome, 340, 441,
        528
Haemophilia, 7, 87, 349, 350, 351, 353–5,
        579, 627
    antenatal diagnosis, 43, 44
    clinical features, 354
    HIV infection and, 354, 355
    home treatment, 355
    therapy, 354–5
Haemophilus influenzae, 158, 162, 217,
        318, 353, 572, 579, 596, 599, 606,
        635, 639
    acute epiglottitis, 262, 267
    antibody formation to polysaccharide
        antigen, 156
    bone/joint infection, 228, 234
    immunization, 263, 264
    meningitis, 235–6, 238
        detection in CSF, 237
        mortality, 239
        treatment of contacts, 239
    pneumonia, 269, 271, 272
    reactive arthritis, 233
Haemoptysis, 293
Haemorrhagic disease of newborn, 349,
        356, 386
Haemorrhagic telangiectasia, familial, 349,
        350, 352, 583
Hair disease, 577
Haloperidol, 546, 642
Hammer toe, 72
Hand, foot and mouth disease, 225
Hand preference, 388
Hand-Schüller-Christian disease, 367,579,
        580
Handicap, 7
    adoption and, 138
    birth defects and, 21
    community health centres and, 88
    dental care, 88, 617
    developmental screening and, 77
    ethical aspects, 12, 13
    self-help groups, 87
    special needs and, 86
    state-financed services, 87
    toddler groups and, 89
    WHO definition, 117
    see also Disability
Harlequin colour change, 565
Harrison's sulci, 65
Hartnup's syndrome, 571
Hashimoto's thyroiditis, 470, 471
Hay fever see Seasonal rhinitis
Head examination, infants, 65
Head injury, 103, 109
    collapse and, 256–7
    follow-up, 108
Hearing assessment, 65, 88, 114, 115, 119
    intellectual disability and, 124
    pure tone audiometry, 114
Hearing loss see Deafness

Heart block, 319
Heart disease, congenital, 20, 24, 25, 45,
    56, 117, 141, 181, 186, 245, 311–4,
    320–9
  acyanotic, 320–6
  antenatal diagnosis, 42, 44
  arterial desaturation and, 312–3
  bacterial endocarditis prophylaxis, 317
  cardiac catheterization, 320, 323, 324,
    327, 328
  chest radiography, 308–9, 314, 320, 322,
    323, 324, 325, 327, 328, 329
  cyanotic, 312–3, 320, 326–9
    growth and, 456
  diagnosis, 316, 320
  dyspnoea and, 313, 314
  echocardiography, 314, 315, 320, 322,
    323, 324, 327, 328, 329
  ejection sounds, 308
  electrocardiography, 308–11, 320, 322,
    323, 324, 325, 327, 328, 329
  examination, 313–4
  frequency, 320
  in infancy, 311–4
  murmurs, 307–8, 313, 320
  in older children, 316–7
  presenting features, 320
  pulses, 308, 314
  recurrent cerebral infarctions and, 392
  second heart sound, 308
  surgery, 315–6, 317
Heart failure, 64, 141, 189, 269, 314–5,
    322, 324, 325, 326, 334–5, 424,
    440, 635
  treatment, 315
Heart murmur, 307–8, 313, 320
Hemifacial atrophy, 613
Hemifacial hypertrophy, 613
Hemiplegia, 65, 385, 387–8, 389
Henoch-Schönlein purpura, 223, 440,
    529, 570, 579, 584
Heparin, 237
Hepatitis, 143, 503, 529, 627
  bile salt insufficiency and, 525
  chronic, 536–7
    arthritis and, 233
    drug-associated, 537
  neonatal, 282
    diganosis, 533
    investigations, 533
    management, 534
    prognosis, 534
  viral, 223, 534–5
    clinical features, 535–6
    investigations, 536
    management, 536
Hepatitis A, 534–5
Hepatitis B, 533, 535, 536, 552, 621
  antenatal screening and, 205
  antigens detectable in blood, 535
  chronic carrier state, 535
  congenital, 205
  transmission, 535
  vaccination, 205, 535

Hepatitis non A, non B, 535, 536
Hepatitis syndrome of infancy, 532
Hepatoblastoma, 369
Hepatocellular disease
  jaundice and, 195, 532
Hepatomegaly, 314, 322, 539
Hermaphroditism, true, 476
Hernia, incarcerated/strangulated, 502
  inguinal, 529
Herpangina, 225
Herpes simplex virus infection, 195, 224,
    376, 533, 568, 594
  conjunctivitis, 594, 595
  with eczema, 224
  encephalitis, 224, 240, 242
  genital, 560
  maternal, 203
  neonatal, 203, 224
  primary, 224
  recurrent, 224, 573–4
  teratogenicity, 24
Herpes zoster (shingles), 203, 221–2, 604
Heterozygote, 30
Hexosaminidase A deficiency, 213
Hiatus hernia, 500
Hip dislocation, congenital (CDH), 56, 66,
    67, 72–4, 233
  incidence, 72
  in neonate, 73
  in older infant, 73–4
  with scoliosis, 74
  time of diagnosis/treatment, 73
Hip examination, 66, 67
Hip, transient synovitis, 233
Hirschsprung's disease, 142, 499–500,
    506
Histiocytosis, 274
Histiocytosis-X, 367–8
Histone genes, 35
History
  clinical, 61–63
    child abuse and, 146
  developmental, 63, 78–9
  dietary, 90–1
HIV infection, 552, 560
  AIDS, 162, 246
    cumulative risk, 205
  congenital, 143, 205
  ethical aspects, 12
  haemophiliacs, 354, 355
  oral features, 616
Hodgkin's disease, 247, 274, 367
Holoprosencephaly, 54, 385
Homocystinuria, 392, 459, 492
  clinical features, 52
  neonatal screening, 21
  prenatal diagnosis, 53
  prognosis, 53
Homozygote, 30
Hopkins syndrome, 396
Hordeolum, 596
Horner's syndrome, 593
Hospitalization, 67–8
House dust mite allergen, 164, 166

Housing, 85, 86
Hunter syndrome, 49, 212
Huntingdon chorea, 14, 19, 55
  antenatal diagnosis, 40, 44
Hurler syndrome, 20, 49
Hyaline membrane disease, 175, 181, 183,
    185, 263, 274
  clinical features, 183
  complications, 183
  pathogenesis, 183
  prognosis, 183
Hydantoin, 21
Hydatid disease, 245
Hydralazine, 439, 443, 627
Hydramnios, maternal, 187
Hydranencephaly, 385, 408
Hydrocephalus, 388, 403–11, 503
  aetiology, 404–5
  aqueduct obstruction and, 404, 406
  associated malformations, 404, 406
  choroid plexus papilloma and, 405
  classification, 404
  'compensated', 406–9
  complications of treatment, 410–11
    infection, 411
    shunt obstruction, 410–11
  differential diagnosis, 408
  examination, 405–6
  history, 405
  intracranial mass lesion, 404–5
  investigations, 406–8
  meningeal adhesions and, 405
  natural history, 408–9
  with neural tube defect, 413, 415–6, 418
  postoperative care, 410
  progressive, 391
  shunts, 409, 410
  treatment results, 411
Hydrocortisone, 643
Hydronephrosis, 42
Hydrops fetalis syndrome, 360
Hydroxychloroquine, 625, 638
Hydroxyzine, 169
Hyperactivity, 112, 543, 640
  see also Attention deficit hyperactivity
    disorder
Hyperbilirubinaemia, 612
  preterm infant, 176
Hypercalcaemia, 142, 489
Hypercalciuria, 490
Hyperkalaemia, 401
  acute renal failure and, 427
Hypermagnesaemia, 492
Hypermetropia (longsightedness), 592,
    595
Hypernatraemic dehydration, 424–5, 426,
    427
Hyperoxaluria, 432, 490
Hyperparathyroidism, 432, 490
  renal osteodystrophy and, 492
Hyperphosphataemia, 490
Hyperpigmentation, 576, 579
  localized, 580–2
Hypertelorism, 46

Hypertension, 436, 442–3
  causes, 442
  examination, 442
  maternal, 196
  post-streptococcal glomerulonephritis
    and, 439–40
  treatment, 442–3
Hyperthyroidsim, 401, 471–2, 492
  clinical features, 471–2
  investigations, 472
  tall stature and, 459, 461
  treatment, 472
Hypertrophic cardiomyopathy, 312
Hyperventilation, 429
Hyphaema, 598
Hypocalcaemia, 488, 489–90, 491, 492,
    493
  convulsions and, 383
  neonatal, 376, 485, 486, 490
Hypoglycaemia, 9, 142, 185, 333, 378,
    485–7
  causes, 485
  clinical features, 484, 485–6
  convulsions and, 379, 383
  diabetes mellitus and, 483–4
  enzyme deficiencies and, 486, 487
  in infants, 487
  investigations, 486
  ketotic, 487
  neonatal, 379, 485, 486, 498
  in older children, 487
  preterm infant, 176
  recurrent, 486–7
    hyperinsulism and, 486
  small-for-gestational-age infant, 179, 180
  treatment, 486
Hypohidrotic ectodermal dysplasia, 612–3
Hypokalaemia, 401
Hypomagnesaemia, 376, 490, 492–3, 518
Hypoparathyroidism, 161, 612
Hypophosphataemia, X-linked, 492
Hypopituitarism, 486, 576
Hypoplastic left heart syndrome, 310, 316,
    325–6
Hypoplastic lungs, 186
Hypospadias, 66
Hypotelorism, 46
Hypothermia, 186
  preterm infant, 174
  small-for-gestational-age infant, 179
Hypothyroidism, 124, 125, 195, 335, 401,
    451, 468–70, 611
  acquired (transient), 468–9
  clinical features, 469
  jaundice and, 197, 532
  management, 469
  neonatal screening, 21, 128, 143, 468,
    469
  older child/adolescent, 456–7, 461, 470
  prognosis, 469–70
  short stature and, 456–7, 461
Hypotonia, 401–2
Hypoxic-ischaemic encephalopathy, 185,
    376

Hysterical conversion reactions, 551
Hysterical wheeze/stridor, 282

Ibuprofen, 625
I-cell disease, 212
Ichthyosis, 566, 577–8
Idiopathic juvenile osteoporosis, 492
Idiopathic pulmonary haemosiderosis, 273
Idiopathic thrombocytopenic purpura,
    352–3, 579
Idoxuridine, 574, 594
IgA disease (Berger's disease), 159, 440
Imipramine, 529, 547, 642
Immotile cilia syndrome, 299
Immune complex urticaria, 570, 571
Immunity, 153–5
  antibody production and, 154–5
  breast feeding and, 155–6, 200
  cell-mediated, 154
  developmental aspects, 155–6
  fetal, 155, 200
  non-specific mechanisms, 153–4
  passive (acquired), 155–6
  preterm infant, 177
  respiratory tract infection and, 263
Immunization, 63, 87, 99–102, 128
  combined vaccines, 100
  costs/benefit, 99
  definitions, 100
  egg allergy and, 102
  immunological basis, 99–100
  immunosuppression and, 102
  precautions/contraindications, 100, 101,
    102
  preterm infant, 102
  schedule, 101
  spacing of doses, 100
Immunocompromised patients see
    Immunodeficiency
Immunodeficiency, 273, 520
  AIDS and see HIV infection
  bone/joint infection, 288
  chicken pox and, 221
  chronic diarrhoea, 524
  complement disorders, 161
  diffuse lung disease, 274
  failure-to-thrive, 143
  familial bronchiectasis, 277
  herpes zoster and, 221
  infection causing, 162
  investigations, 157
  malnutrition and, 161–2
  measles and, 217, 219
  mucocutaneous candidiasis, 615
  phagocytic cell disorders, 161
  presentations, 157
  primary disorders, 157–61
    incidence, 158
  pyrexia of unknown origin, 245, 246
  recurrent cough and, 299–300
  secondary disorders, 161–2
  specific syndromes, 161
Immunoglobulin deficiency with increased

IgM, 158–9
Immunoglobulin therapy, 100, 158, 159,
    162, 352, 353
Immunoglobulins, 154
  breast milk and, 156
  developmental aspects, 155–6
Immunosuppressive therapy, 162, 166,
    217, 219, 628, 629, 638, 640
Impairment, definition, 117
Imperforate anus, 498
Impetigo, 572
In vitro fertilization with donor ovum, 57
Inappropriate ADH secretion, 424, 428
Inborn errors of metabolism, 20, 37, 97,
    208–13, 335, 376, 498
  in adulthood, 213
  in amino acid degradative pathway, 209,
    212
  cerebral degenerations, 392, 393
  diagnosis, 208, 210
  family history and, 208
  genetic counselling, 208
  heart disease and, 311
  hypoglycaemia and, 486
  intra-uterine protection, 209
  investigations, 210
  malformations and, 208
  myopathies and, 401
  neonatal presentation
    at birth, 209–10
    jaundice and, 195
    symptoms developing after birth,
      208–9
  in older child, 212–13
  prenatal diagnosis, 42, 44
  response to feeding change and, 209
  treatment principles, 210–11
  in urea cycle, 209, 210, 211
  vomiting and, 503
Incest, 148
Incontinentia pigmenti, 582
Inco-ordinate swallowing, 276
Indomethacin, 175, 189, 322, 436, 625,
    638
Infant feeding, 87, 93–4, 95
  transitional foods, 93, 95
  weaning, 95
Infant mortality, 4
  Aboriginal population, 133
  age at death, 5
  sex ratios and, 5
Infant welfare clinics, 87
Infantile idiopathic scoliosis, 74
Infantile spasms (West's syndrome), 377–9
  aetiology, 378
  cerebral palsy and, 389
  clinical features, 378
  EEG, 377, 378
  mental retardation and, 378, 379
  prognosis, 379
  treatment, 379
Infantile spinal muscular atrophy, 396
Infection, 3
  anaemia and, 336

arthralgia/arthritis and, 627
chronic diarrhoea and, 512
deaths and, 5, 21
diabetes mellitus and, 481, 482
diffuse lung disease and, 273
failure-to-thrive and, 143
febrile convulsions and, 376
frequency, age and, 156
immunodeficiency and, 157
intra-uterine, 179, 184, 200, 349
  fetal blood sampling, 42
morbidity and, 6–7
neonatal, 5, 200–7, 349, 376, 498
ocular, 120, 595–7
oral soft tissue, 615–16
pallor and, 333–4
preterm infant, 177
purpura and, 351–2
pyrexia of unknown origin and, 245–6
recurrent, malabsorption and, 520
resistance mechanisms, 153–4
respiratory distress and, 181
small-for-gestational-age infant, 179
sudden infant death syndrome (SIDS)
  and, 9
vomiting and, 500, 503
Infectious diseases, 217–27
Infectious mononucleosis, 223–4, 245,
  265, 266, 529, 602
  clinical features, 224
Infective endocarditis, 318, 322, 327
  clinical features, 318
  pathogenesis, 318
  prophylaxis, 317
  subacute, 245, 579
Inflammatory bowel disease, 531
  arthritis and, 626
  malabsorption and, 520, 521, 524
Inflammatory myopathy, 401
Influenza virus, 242, 273, 604
  respiratory tract infection, 262, 265, 266,
  267
  vaccine, 102
Information
  for parents, 15
  for patients, 13, 14
Informed consent, 12–13
Infundibular stenosis, 307, 322, 326
Insect bite allergy, 576
Insulin, 480
  growth and, 449
  recombinant DNA technology, synthesis
  and, 40
  replacement therapy, 482, 483, 485
Insulin-like growth factors see
  Somatomedins
Intellectual disability, 19, 20, 24, 25, 45,
  117, 122–8
  aetiology, 123, 124
  associated impairments, 126, 127
  cerebral palsy and, 385, 386, 388, 389
  children's services, normalization and,
  127
  chromosomal analysis and, 47

community response, 127
definition, 122
diagnosis, 123–4
differential diagnosis, 124–5
doctor's role in management, 127–8
Duchenne muscular dystrophy and, 399
dysmorphic syndromes and, 47, 48, 49,
  53, 54
education and, 126
effects on child, 126
ethical aspects, 12
family support, 127
genetic counselling, 55, 56, 57
hydrocephalus and, 405
inborn errors of metabolism and, 47
Lennox-Gastaut syndrome, 380
following meningitis, 239
parental reaction, 123, 126–7
with peripheral neuromuscular disease,
  395, 401
prevalence, 122–3
prevention, 128
residential care, 127
very low birthweight and, 7
Interferon, 40
Intertrigo, 565
Interview, 13
Intestinal obstruction, 142, 153, 502, 531
  differential diagnosis, 527
  neonatal, 498–9
  jaundice and, 195
In-toe gait, 69, 72
Intracranial pressure, raised, 65, 254, 255,
  256, 257, 391, 404, 405
  cerebral tumour and, 370
  differential diagnosis, 408
  hydrocephalus, 406
  treatment/blocked shunt, 410
Intramuscular drug absorption, 634, 637
Intra-uterine growth retardation see Small-
  for-gestational-age infant
Intravenous drug administration, 634, 637
Intravenous pyelogram (IVP), 435
Intravenous rehydration fluids, 426
Intraventricular haemorrhage, 405
  preterm infant, 176
Introns, 34, 35
  splicing defect, 37
Intubation, 252, 267
Intussusception, 502, 506, 526–528
  clinical features, 526–7
  differential diagnosis, 527–8
  treatment, 527
Invalid pension, 121, 138
Iodine deficiency, 467
Ipatropium bromide, 164, 287, 291
IQ test, 122
Iritis, acute, 596
Iron
  absorption, 342, 517
  chelation therapy, 359, 362
  deficiency, 520, 521
  in infant foods, 343
  preparations, 529, 643

requirements, 342–3
Iron deficiency anaemia, 335, 336, 337,
  342, 343–7, 358, 530
  aetiology, 343–4
  age-related iron requirements and, 343,
  344
  blood loss and, 343, 344, 345
  clinical features, 344–345
  dietary intake and, 343
  differential diagnosis, 346
  examination, 345
  investigations, 346
  malabsorption and, 343
  prevention, 347
  treatment, 346–7
Isoniazid, 303, 537, 627, 634, 638, 642
Isosorbide, 409
Isotretinoin, 24, 577
Isovaleric acidaemia, 212

Jaundice, neonatal, 67, 119, 192–9, 336,
  340, 522–3
  bilirubin encephalopathy and, 193
  breast milk, 532
  clinical approach, 195–6, 197
  conjugated, 195
  examination, 196
  exchange transfusion, 197, 199
  family history and, 195, 196
  general care, 196–7
  infant behaviour and, 196
  investigations, 196
  obstructive, 196, 333
  management, 533–4
  pharmacological treatment, 197
  phototherapy, 197
  physiological, 193–4, 196
  preterm infant, 176
  prevention, 196
  sepsis and, 206
  unconjugated, 194–5
  viral hepatitis and, 536
Jaw winking syndrome, 593
Joint infection
  acute
    infantile, 232–3, 234
    late, 233, 234
  chronic, 233, 234
  clinical features, 232–3
  microbiology, 228
  negative bacterial culture, 233
  pathology, 228–9
  subacute, 233, 234
  treatment, 233–4
Justice, duty of, 12, 14
Juvenile ankylosing spondylitis, 626
Juvenile chronic arthritis, 117, 233, 234,
  247, 492, 584, 585, 621–5, 639, 640
  aetiology, 621
  diagnostic criteria, 622
  education and, 625
  eye disease and, 621, 623, 634
  investigations, 624
  management, 624–5

Juvenile chronic arthritis *continued*
    pauciarticular, 622–3
    polyarticular, 622, 623–4
    radiology, 624
    social aspects, 625
    systemic onset (Still's disease), 622
Juvenile dermatomyositis, 629
Juvenile idiopathic scoliosis, 74
Juvenile nephronophthisis, 431
Juvenile plantar dermatosis, 568

Kanamycin, 637, 641
Kaposi's sarcoma, 246
Kasabach-Merritt syndrome, 586
Kawasaki disease, 233, 585, 621, 630
Kearn-Sayre syndrome, 401
Keratoconus, 593
Kerion, 574
Kernicterus *see* Bilirubin encephalopathy
Kerosene ingestion, 503
Ketogenic diet, 380
Ketoconazole, 161
Kidney duplication, 432
Klebsiella, 184, 206, 433
Klinefelter syndrome, 53, 364, 447, 459
Knock knees, 69, 70
Krabbe's disease, 392, 397
Kugelberg-Welander syndrome, 397
Kuru, 241
Kwashiorkor, 97

Lacerations, 104
Lactation, 94
Lactic acidosis, 208, 210, 212
Lactoferrin, 153
Lactose intolerance, 508, 509, 510, 523–4
Laryngitis, 603
Laryngomalacia, 190, 603
Laryngotracheobronchitis (croup), 261,
    266–7
    age and, 263
    hospital admission and, 263, 267
    pathogens, 262
    recurrent, 267, 285
    spasmodic, 165
    treatment, 266–7
Larynx
    cleft, 276
    cyst, 603
    examination, 603
    haemangioma, 190, 603
    infantile *see* Laryngomalacia
    obstruction, 190
    oedema, 190
    recurrent nerve palsy, 604
    tumour, 190, 604
    web, 190, 603
L-asparaginase, 365, 367
Lead poisoning, 142, 393, 408, 488, 531
Learning difficulties/school problems,
    111–16, 122, 543, 548, 549
    assessment, 114–15

associated problems, 111
attention deficit and, 112, 115
cerebral palsy and, 389
conduct disorder and, 552
constitutional factors and, 111, 112–13
developmental weakness and, 112
educational programmes, 115–16
environmental factors and, 111, 112, 113
family difficulties and, 129
genetic factors and, 113
health problems and, 113
hearing problems and, 112, 113, 115
incidence, 111
intellectual impairment and, 126
language problems and, 112
management, 115–16
following meningitis, 239
motor function and, 112
non-organic failure-to-thrive and, 145
following perinatal stress, 113
preterm infant, 178
repetition of grades and, 116
sequencing problems, auditory/visual,
    112, 115
shunt hydrocephalus and, 418
vision problems and, 113, 598
visual perceptual motor function
    problems, 112
Leber' amaurosis, 597
Leigh's disease, 392
Lennox-Gastaut syndrome, 379–80
    aetiology, 379
    clinical features, 379–80
    prognosis, 380
    treatment, 380
Leptospirosis, 245
Letterer-Siwe disease, 367
Leukaemia, 247, 274, 317, 336, 350, 353,
    363, 364–6, 492, 579. 627
    acute lymphoblastic, 8, 364, 365–6
    acute myeloid, 364, 366
    aetiology, 364
    clinical features, 364
    CNS prophylaxis, 365
    laboratory findings, 364–5
    management, 365–6
    oral lesions, 616
    prognosis, 365, 366
    relapse, 365, 366
Lice, 576
Linkage analysis, 32–2
Linked polymorphic markers, 32
Lipid storage disease, 20, 49, 379, 381, 579
Lipomeningocele, 413
Lissencephaly, 385
Listeria monocytogenes, 184, 205, 206, 207,
    533
Live birth
    definition, 3
    statistics, 4
Liver biopsy, percutaneous, 533
Liver disease, 350, 486, 532–9, 635
    cystic fibrosis and, 297
    diagnosis, 533

    drug-induced damage, 536
    infancy, 532–4
    liver function tests and, 533
    older children, 533–5
Liver failure, 97
    fulminating, 536
Liver transplant, 543, 537–8
Lobar emphysema, 185, 190, 277
London Dysmorphology Database, 47
Loperamide, 508, 642
Low birth weight, 5, 62, 119, 173, 498
    incidence, 173
    iron stores and, 342, 343
    osteoporosis, 492
    postnatal assessment of gestational age,
    174
L/S ratio ('shake test'), 181
Lucy-Driscoll syndrome, 195
Lung cyst, 190
Lyme diagnosis, 627
Lymphocytes, 154
    fetal, 155
    in neonate, 155
Lymphokines, 154
Lymphoma, 247, 274, 282, 353, 363,
    366–7, 512, 603
Lysosomal storage disease, 20, 47, 49, 210,
    212–13
Lysozyme, 153

Macrogyria, 385
Macronutrients, 90
Macrophages, 154
Macrostomia, 46
Magnesium
    deficiency, 518
    metabolism, 492–3
Malabsorption, 502, 519–25, 531
    abdominal distension and, 519
    aetiology, 519
    alpha-1 antitrypsin clearance, 521
    anatomical lesions and, 521, 524
    behavioural changes and, 520
    bile salt insufficiency and, 525
    breath hydrogen test, 520–1
    chronic diarrhoea and, 519, 520, 523,
    524
    colonoscopy/colonic biopsy, 521
    cystic fibrosis and, 295, 297
    diagnosis, 520
    failure-to-thrive and, 140, 519
    fat balance studies, 521
    full blood examination, 521
    medium chain fatty acid supplements,
    514
    mucosal abnormality and, 522–4
    pallor/anaemia and, 520
    pancreatic function tests, 521
    pancreatic insufficiency and, 534–5
    previous bowel surgery and, 520
    protein, 524
    radiology, 521
    recurrent infection and, 520

severe malnutrition and, 520, 524
small bowel biopsy and, 521, 522
stool examination, 520, 523, 525
sweat test and, 521
Malaria, 226–7, 245, 340, 353
anaemia and, 336
diagnosis, 226–7, 337
prophylaxis, 227
relapse, 227
treatment, 227
Malformation, congenital *see* Birth defects
Malignancy, 7, 8, 117, 363–71, 557, 627
common variable immunodeficiency
and, 159
death and, 363–4
diffuse lung disease and, 274
emotional problems and, 363
family support, 363, 366
palliative care, 363
pyrexia of unknown origin and, 247
Malignant hyperthermia, 398
Malnutrition, 21, 97, 270, 451, 582, 635
abnormal bleeding and, 350, 352
Aboriginal children, 133
anaemia and, 336
blindness and, 120
immunodeficiency and, 161–2
malabsorption and, 519, 520, 525
measles and, 217, 219
micronutrient deficiency, 95–6
neglect and, 544
short stature and, 456, 458
underfeeding, 141
Maloprim, 227
Malrotation, gut, 500, 503
Mannitol, 255
Mannosidosis, 212
Maple syrup urine disease, 21, 211, 212
Marfan syndrome, 20, 52, 56, 448, 459,
461, 463
Maroteaux-Lamy syndrome, 49
Marriage breakdown, 89
Marriage counselling, 139
Mastoiditis, 607
Masturbation, 549
Meadow's syndrome, 247, 393
Mean corpuscular haemoglobin (MCH),
335
Mean corpuscular volume (MCV), 335
Measles, 128, 160, 217–19, 265, 266, 267,
273, 274, 297, 352, 612
clinical features, 217
diagnosis, 219
ear infection complicating, 217, 219
encephalitis, 218, 219, 240
giant cell pneumonia and, 217–18
mortality, 99
myelitis, 241
subacute sclerosing panencephalitis and,
218–19, 241, 392
treatment, 219
vaccination, 87, 99, 100, 102, 219, 223,
583, 604
Mechanobullous disorders, 578

Meckel's syndrome, 19, 529
Meconium aspiration, 179, 185–6, 188
Meconium ileus, 195, 295
Meconium plug, 195
Meconium-stained amniotic fluid, 185
Mediastinal mass, 277, 281, 282, 293
Medium chain fatty acyl CoA
dehydrogenase deficiency, 212
Medullary cystic disease, 431, 441
Medulloblastoma, 370, 371, 404
Megalencephaly, 408
Megaureter, primary obstructive, 431
Meibomian cyst, 596
Meiosis, 27–8
non-dysjunction, 28
recombination errors, 38
Melanoma, 587
Melanotic neuroectodermal tumour of
infancy, 611
Meningeal adhesions, 405
Meningitis, 142, 158, 235–42, 246, 333,
376, 377, 428, 500, 503, 604, 639,
640
antibiotic treatment, 236, 237, 238, 256,
635, 636
cerebral oedema and, 238–9
complications, 238–9
contacts treatment, 239
convulsions and, 238, 256
diagnosis, 206, 237–8
fulminating onset, 236
hydrocephalus following, 405, 409
inappropriate ADH secretion and,
238–9
incidence, 235–6
long-term sequelae, 239
learning difficulties following, 113
lumbar puncture, 237, 238, 256
mortality, 239
neonatal, 206, 207, 235, 236, 498
neurological complications, 239
pathogens, 206, 240
presentation, 236
septic shock and, 256
subdural effusions and, 239
supportive therapy, 238, 256
vaccines, 236
viral/aseptic, 240–2
Meningocele, 416
Meningococcaemia, 236, 351, 579
chronic, 237
treatment, 236–7
Meningomyelocele, 67
Menke's disease, 577
Menstrual problems, 560
Mental retardation *see* Intellectual
disability
Mephenytoin, 338
6-Mercaptopurine, 365
Mesenteric lymphadenitis, 528, 529
Metabolic rate, 422
Metachromatic leukodystrophy, 392, 397
Metatarsus adductus, 72
Metered aerosols, 287, 288

Methaemoglobinaemia, 313
Methicilin, 637, 641
Methimazole, 638
Methotrexate, 365, 367
Methyl mercury, 19, 24
Methyldopa, 537
Methylmalonic acidaemia, 42, 211, 212,
486
Methylphenidate, 548, 643
Methylprednisolone, 257
Methylxanthine drugs, 300
Metoprolol, 433
Metronidazole, 523
Miconazole, 565
Microcephaly, 24, 25, 53–4, 124, 385
Micronutrients, 90
deficiency disease, 95–96
Microphthalmia, 24, 597
Micropolygyria, 385
Microsporum canis, 574
Microstomia, 46
Micturating cystourethrogram (MCU),
435
Midgut volvulus, 142
Midstream urine specimen, 433, 434
Migraine, 503
Migrants, 86, 88, 89, 129, 134–7, 245,
246, 491
community facilities, 136–7
education and, 135, 136
employment, 135, 136
family stress and, 135
language problems, 135, 136
numbers, 134–5
settlement problems, 135
sociocultural aspects, 135–6
TB screening, 303
Milestones, developmental, 78, 79–80
advanced, 81–2
developmental delay and, 81, 82, 124,
395, 400
Milia, 566
Miliara neonatorum, 566
Milk inhalation, 293, 298
Minerals, dietary, 90
Minocycline, 634
Minomycin, 576
Minoxidil, 577
Miscarriage, multiple, 55
Mitochondrial encephalomyopathy, 392
Mitochondrial function abnormality, 401
Mitosis, 26–7
Mitral incompetence, 307, 323
Mitral stenosis, 308
Mitral valve prolapse, 308
Mixed connective tissue disease, 626, 630
Moebius syndrome, 141, 609
Molluscum contagiosum, 573
Mongolian patch, 65, 587
Monoplegia, 388
Monosomy, 28
Mopp chemotherapy, 367
Moral values, 12–14
Morbidity statistics, 3, 6–7

Moro reflex, 67
Morphine, 186, 327, 641
Morquio syndrome, 212
Mortality, 3–4
　adolescents, 557
　causes in childhood, 6
　　trauma, 103, 104–5
　definitions, 3
　infants, 4, 5, 133
　neonatal, 4–5
　statistics, 4–6
Motor function problems, 112
Moulding, 67
Mouth in neonate, 610
Moxalactam, 636
Moyamoya disease, 392
mRNA processing
　capping of 5′ end, 35
　hnRNA processing, 34, 35
　polyA tail and, 34, 35
　promotors, 34
　spicing out of introns, 34, 35
　terminators, 34
Mucocutaneous lymph node syndrome see
　　Kawasaki disease
Mucolytic agents, 301
Mucopolysaccharidoses, 20, 49, 51, 125,
　　212, 213, 311, 317, 408, 593, 616
Mucosal secretions, 153
Mucus secretion, 153
Mullerian inhibitory substance (MIS), 475
Multifactorial inheritance, 56
Multiple endocrine adenomatosis, 473
Mumps, 222–3, 529, 604
　clinical features, 222
　complications, 222–3
　　meningoencephalitis, 222, 240
　　myelitis, 241
　diagnosis, 223
　treatment, 223
　vaccination, 87, 223
Muscular dystrophies, 19, 20, 55, 87, 117,
　　125, 301, 395, 399–401
Mutation, 36–8
　additions, 37
　base substitution, 37
　cDNA analysis, 39
　deletions, 37, 38, 45, 47
　frame shift, 37–8
　germ line, 36
　intron splicing and, 37
　meiotic recombination errors, 38
　nonsense, 37
　in promotors, 37
　restriction fragment length
　　polymorphism analysis, 39–40
　somatic cell, 36
Myasthenia gravis, 395, 398, 593
Mycobacterial infection, atypical, 162
Mycobacterium tuberculosis, 231, 301
Mycoplasma pneumoniae, 184, 262, 267,
　　271
　myocarditis, 311
　persisitent cough, 293, 295

pneumonia, 262, 271, 272
　respiratory tract infection, 265, 282
Myelitis, 240–1
Myelomeningocele, 404, 414
　adult life and, 418
　clinical features, 415–16
　conservative supportive care, 416
　education and, 418
　emotional/family support and, 416, 418
　hydrocephalus and, 415–16, 418
　limb deformity, 415, 417
　management, 416–18
　management team, 416
　mobility, 415, 417
　neurogenic bladder, 415, 416–17, 432
　neurogenic bowel, 415, 417
　pressure sores, 415, 417
　sexual function, 417
Myeloproliferative disorders, 364
Myocardial disease, primary, 316–17
Myocarditis, 311
Myoclonic epilepsy, 379–80
　status, 380
Myopathies, 395–6
　acute, 398–9
　chronic, 399–402
　congenital, 399
Myopia, 593
Myositis, acute viral, 401
Myotonia congenita, 401
Myotonic dystrophy, 43, 401
Myringitis bullosa, 606

N-acetyl-cysteine, 301
Nafcillin, 634
Nail biting, 549, 577
Nail disease, 577
Nalidixic acid, 435, 638
　intoxication, 408
　side-effects, 435
Napkin dermatitis, 568–70, 634
　treatment, 569–70
Naproxen, 625
Napthalene, 196
Nasal cautery, 601
Natal teeth, 610
Near-miss sudden infant death syndrome,
　　9–10, 257
Nebulizer therapy, 287, 288
Neck examination, 65
Necrotizing enterocolitis, 208
　preterm infant, 176
Needs of child, 85–6
　emotional, 85–6
　intellectual development and, 86
　physical, 85
　play and, 86
Neisseria gonorrhoeae, 204, 560, 595
Neisseria meningitidis, 635
　detection in CSF, 237
　meningitis, 235, 236, 239
　meningococcaemia, 236, 239
　　chronic, 237

treatment, 236–7
　treatment of contacts, 239
Neomercazole, 472
Neomycin, 601
Neonate
　clinical history, 62
　ECG, 310
　drug metabolism
　　absorption, 634
　　dosages, 636, 637
　　elimination, 636
　　plasma protein binding, 635
　examination, 67
　mortality, 3, 4–5, 173
　posture, 67, 69
　screening tests, 124, 295
Nephroblastoma, 363, 368
Nephrotic syndrome, 162, 334, 437–9,
　　528, 579, 635
　classification, 437
　complications, 438
　congenital, 438–9
　definition, 437
　focal segment glomerulosclerosis, 438
　incidence, 437
　management, 438
　minimal change, 437–8
　steroid resistant, 438
Nervous system disorders, diffuse, 392
Nervous system examination, 65–6, 67
Nesidioblastosis, 487
Neural tube defects, 20, 21, 25, 43, 56,
　　412–18
　aetiological aspects, 413
　classification, 413
　clinical features, 413–16
　definition, 412
　embryology, 412–13
　genetic counselling, 55
　incidence, 412
　prenatal diagnosis, 41, 42
　prevention, 418
　　screening, 41, 418
　　vitamin supplements and, 413, 418
　recurrence, 412, 416
Neurenteric cyst, 277–8
Neuroblastoma, 247, 363, 368–9
Neruodevelopmental assessment
　'hyperactive' child, 112
　school problems and, 114–15
Neurofibromatosis, 587
　intellectual disability and, 126
Neurogenic bladder, 432
Neuromuscular disease, 81, 394–402
　anterior horn cell, 395, 396–7
　classification, 395–6
　diagnosis, 394–5
　frequency, 394
　muscle, 395, 398–402
　neuromuscular junction, 395, 398
　peripheral nerve, 395, 397–8
　presentation, 394–5
Niemann-Pick disease, 213, 579, 580
Nifedipine, 439, 443, 629

Nitrofurantoin, 435, 638
  side-effects, 435
Nitrogen mustard, 367
Nodules, skin, 585
Non-Hodgkin lymphoma, 366–7
  classification, 366
Non-ketotic hyperglycinaemia, 209
Non-maleficence, 13
Nonsense mutation, 37
Non-specific urethritis, 560
Non-steroidal anti-inflammatory drugs
        (NSAIDs), 529, 579, 625, 626
Noonan syndrome, 50
Normalization, 127
Nose
  acquired disorders, 599–601
  congenital malformation, 599
  foreign body, 600
Nutrition, 90–98
  dietary history, 90–91
  disease aetiology and, 97–8
  disease management and, 97
  energy intake/expenditure, 90, 91, 92,
        422
  guidelines, 93
  infants see Infant feeding
  intake in healthy child, 91–93
  macro/micronutrients, 90
  neonatal jaundice and, 193, 195, 196,
        197
  preterm infant, 176
Nystatin, 565, 616, 642

Obesity, 96–7
  childhood onset, 96
  infancy onset, 96
  knock knees and, 70
  management, 96–7
  motor function delay and, 81
  respiratory tract infection and, 263
Ocular disease
  with juvenile chronic arthritis, 621, 623,
        624
  infection, 595–7
    neonatal, 595
Ocular misalignment, 594
Ocular trauma, 598
Oesophageal atresia, 187–8, 190, 297, 500,
        603
  clinical features, 187
  diagnosis, 187
  treatment, 187–8
Oesophageal duplication, 142, 277–8, 501
Oesophageal stricture, 142
Oesophageal varices, 537, 538, 539
Oesophageal web, 501
Oestradiol, 638
Oestrogen therapy, 459, 461
Oestrogens, growth and, 451
Oligohydramnios, 186, 430
Optic atrophy, 120
Optic nerve glioma, 370, 391
Optic nerve hypoplasia, 597

Oral alveolar developmental (Bohn's)
        nodules, 611
Oral cavity examination, 66
Oral cysts, neonate, 67
Oral soft tissue
  infection, 615–16
  trauma, 616–17
Orbital cellulitis, 572, 596, 600
Orbital wall fracture, 598
Orciprenaline, 642
Organ transplants, ethical aspects, 12
Organic acidoses, 212
Ornithine transcarbamylase deficiency,
        211, 212, 213
Orphans pension, 137
Ortolani's sign, 73
Osteochondroses, 75, 556
Osteogenesis imperfecta, 20, 51, 147, 408,
        492
  lethal neonatal (type II), 51–2
  severe deforming (type III), 52
  type I, 59
  type IV, 52
Osteomalacia, 491–2
Osteomyelitis, 158, 246, 640
  bone scan and, 231
  chronic, 231, 232
  clinical features, 229–31
  early acute, 229, 231–2
  late acute, 229, 232
  late treatment, 229
  microbiology, 228
  pathology, 228–9
  sites, 229–30
    maxilla/mandible, 616
  spine, 230
  subacute, 230–1, 232
    aggressive, 230
    non-aggressive, 230–1
  treatment, 231–2
Osteopetrosis, 408, 492
Osteoporosis, 492
Osteosarcoma, 369
Otitis externa, 66, 606
Otitis media, 6, 261, 500, 639
  Aboriginal children, 133
  atopy and, 165
  chronic, 608
  complications, 607, 609
  diagnosis, 606
  glue ear, 606, 607
    treatment, 607–8
  hearing loss and, 119, 604, 605
  immunodeficiency and, 158
  learning difficulty and, 112, 113
  pathogens, 262
  tympanometry, 607
Out-toeing, 69, 70–1, 72
Oxybuprocaine, 593
Oxygen therapy, 189, 269, 270
  toxicity, 183, 188, 276

Pacemaker insertion, 319
Pallor, 333–41
  acute blood loss and, 334
  allergy and, 335
  anaemia and see Anaemia
  anxiety-associated, 335
  congenital heart failure and, 334–5
  with fever, 333–4
  hypovolaemia and, 334
  infection and, 334
  leukaemia and, 364
  long-standing, 335
  metabolic disease and, 335
  renal disease and, 334, 335
  ß thalassaemia major and, 358
Pancreatic function tests, 521
Pancreatic hypoplasia
  congenital (Schwachman-Diamond
        syndrome), 520, 524, 525
  with neutropenia, 520
Pancreatitis, 529
Panhypopituitarism, 461, 463
Papular urticaria, 576
Papules, neonatal, 565–6
Paracetamol, 221, 223, 265, 266, 377, 503,
        536, 606, 640, 641
Parainfluenza, 262, 263, 265, 266, 267,
        270
Paramyotonia congenita, 401
Paraplegia, spastic, 387, 389
Parasitic infection, 133
  skin, 574–6
Parathormone, 488–9, 492
Paratyphoid fever, 245
Parent education, 85, 86, 87, 88, 150
Paronychia, 577
Paroxysmal atrial tachycardia, 318–9
Paroxysmal nocturnal haemoglobinuria,
        364
Partial thromboplastin time, 351
Parvovirus arthritis, 233
Patent ductus arteriosus, 64, 183, 188,
        189, 316, 320, 322
  bronchial compression and, 277
  echocardiography, 175
  medical treatment, 322
  murmur, 307, 313, 322
  preterm infant, 175
  pulses, 308
  surgery, 322
Pavlik harness, 73
Peak expiratory flow rate, 294
Pedestrian run-downs, 105
Pedigree, genetic, 30, 31, 32, 58, 349
Pellagra, 582
Pelviureteric junction obstruction, 431
Pendred's syndrome, 468
Penicillamine, 339, 392, 432, 537, 625,
        629
Penicillin, 190, 202, 206, 219, 223, 236,
        238, 266, 272, 317, 318, 359, 440,
        595, 602, 606, 634, 635, 637, 640,
        641
Peptic ulcer, 530

Percutaneous drug administration, 634
Perennial rhinitis, 163–4
Perinatal mortality, definition, 3
Periorbital cellulitis, 572
Peritoneal dialysis, 210, 211
Peritonitis, 503, 528
Periungual warts, 573
Periventricular haemorrhage
    preterm infant, 175–6
Periventricular leukomalacia, 176, 386
Peroneal muscular atrophy, 395, 397–8
Persistent fetal circulation, 181, 313
Persistent pulmonary hypertension, 185
Persistent truncus arteriosus, 326, 329
Persistent vernal keratoconjunctivitis, 165
Pertussis, 268, 293, 295, 297
    immunization, 87, 99, 100, 102, 264,
        268
        infantile spasms and, 378
Pethidine, 641
Petit mal (absence) seizures, 380–1
Phaeochromocytoma, 247, 333, 442
Phagocytic cells, 154
Pharyngeal inco-ordination, 141
Pharyngitis, 261, 265–6
    pathogens, 262
    treatment, 266
Pharynx, 601
    acquired disorders, 602–3
    congenital disorders, 601
Phenacetin, 360
Phenindione, 638
Phenobarbitone, 197, 256, 376, 377, 497,
        634, 637
Phenothiazine, 571, 576
Phenotype, 26, 29, 30
Phenozymethyl-penicillin, 641
Phenylbutazone, 338
Phenylketonuria, 7, 19, 20, 124, 211, 378,
        379, 571
    dietary treatment, 21, 143, 211, 393
    frequency, 21
    maternal, 19, 208, 211
    neonatal screening, 21, 128, 143, 211
    teratogenic effects, 25
Phenytoin, 238, 256, 376, 377, 380, 382,
        383, 384, 401, 492, 529, 627, 634,
        635
    chloramphenicol interaction, 238
    gingival hyperplasia and, 616
    teratogenicity, 24
Pholcodine, 268, 301, 642
Photosensitivity, 571–2
Phthirus capitis, 576
Phthirus pubis, 576
Physostigmine, 398
Phytodermatitis, 570
Phytophotodermatitis, 570
Pierre-Robin syndrome, 141, 190
Pigeon chest, 65
Pigeon fancier's disease, 273
Pigmented naevi, congenital, 586–7
Pinealoma, 404
Piroxicam, 625

Pituitary gigantism, 451, 459, 461, 463
Pityriasis alba, 568
Pityriasis rosea, 574
Pizotifen, 503
Plantar warts, 573
Plasmodium falciparum, 226, 227
Plasmodium ovale, 227
Plasmodium vivax, 227
Platelet dysfunction, 349, 350, 351, 352–3
Play, 86
Pleural effusion, neonatal, 190
Pneumocystis carinii, 157, 159, 162, 184,
        245, 246, 274
Pneumomediastinum, 184
Pneumonia, 261, 270–3, 333, 500, 529,
        640
    aetiology, 262, 270–2
    age and, 263
    atypical, 246
    bronchiectasis and, 297, 298
    gestational age and, 263
    intra-uterine, 184
    neonatal, 184, 188, 206
    parental smoking and, 263
    pulmonary collapse and, 298
    staphylococcal, 262, 269, 271–2
    streptococcal, 262, 269, 270, 271, 272
    treatment, 272–3
    viral, 262, 270, 271, 272
Pneumopericardium, 184
Pneumoperitoneum, 184
Pneumothorax, 181, 183, 184–5, 186
    tension, 190
Poisoning, 103, 104, 107–8, 502–3
    agents, 107
    intentional, 107–8, 504
    management, 257, 258
    prevention, 104, 107, 110
    second accidental ingestion, 108
Polio, 225, 301, 395, 396
    vaccination, 87, 99, 102
Pollen antigens, 164, 166
Poly-A tail, 34, 35
Polyarteritis nodosa, 273, 352, 585, 630
Polycystic kidney disease, 436
    adult type, 431
    infantile, 430–1
Polycythaemia, 181, 190, 313, 364
    neonatal jaundice and, 193, 194, 196
    small-for-gestational-age infant, 179
Polymorphonuclear phagocytes, 154
Polymorphous light eruptions, 571
Polymyositis, 401
Polyneuritis, 301
Pompe's disease, 311, 401
Porencephaly, 385, 406, 597
Porphyria, 213, 580, 529, 571, 572
Port wine stain (naevus flammeus), 565
Portal hypertension, 350, 353, 538–9
Possetting, 497
POSSUM database, 47
Posterior urethral valves, 431, 498
Postinfective diarrhoea, 510
Postinfective polyneuropathy, 395, 397

Post-neonatal mortality, 3, 4, 5–6
Post-streptococcal glomerulonephritis,
        334, 439–40, 442, 503
    clinical features, 439
    complications, 316, 440
    dialysis, 440
    hypertension management, 439–40
Postural proteinuria, 441
Posture
    foot, 69–70, 71, 72
    intra-uterine packaging defects, 69
    spine, 69
    toe, 71–2
    transient variations, 69
Potassium iodide preparations, 268
Potter syndrome, 186, 430, 498
Poverty, 86, 113, 129
    alcoholism and, 132
    financial assistance, 137
    malnutrition and, 97
    single parents, 130
Prader orchidometer, 454–5
Prader-Wili syndrome, 126
Prazosin, 439, 443
Prednisolone, 288, 289, 365, 367, 379,
        438, 441, 640, 643
Prednisone, 643
Pregnancy, teenage, 560
Prenatal diagnosis, 41–4, 48, 49, 51, 53, 57
    amniocentesis, 41–2, 43, 44
    Becker muscular dystrophy, 43
    bone dysplasia, 44
    chorionic villus sampling (CVS), 42, 43,
        44
    congenital nephrotic syndrome, 439
    counselling and, 41, 44
    cystic fibrosis, 295
    DNA analysis, 42, 43–4, 295
    fetal biopsy, 42
    fetal blood sampling, 42, 44
    fragile-X syndrome, 43
    haemoglobinopathies, 362
    indications, 43–4
    linkage analysis, 32
    maternal age and, 43
    neural tube defects, 418
    parental translocation and, 43
    previous trisomy and, 43
    RFLP analysis, 40
    serum alpha fetoprotein, 41, 43
    severe combined immunodeficiency, 160
    support for couples and, 41, 44
    ultrasound (sonar) screening, 41, 42, 44
    xeroderma pigmentosum, 578
Preschool education, 88–9
Preterm infant, 7, 8, 97, 118, 120, 173–8,
        181, 187, 270, 565, 604, 612
    aetiology, 173
    anaemia, 176–7
    associated factors, 174
    blood glucose monitoring, 176
    bronchopulmonary dysplasia, 177, 188
    calcium/phosphate deficiency, 177
    cardiovascular problems, 175

cerebral palsy and, 386, 387, 388
developmental assessment, 79
drug therapy, 634, 635, 636
gastrointestinal problems, 176
gestational age assessment, 173–4
hepatic problems, 176
hip joint laxity, 73
hypoglycaemia, 486
hypothermia, 174
immune system, 177
immunization, 101, 102
incidence, 173
infection, 177, 205, 206
iron deficiency anaemia, 336
jaundice, 192, 193, 194
late problems, 177
low birthweight and, 5
maternally transferred
    immunoglobulins, 155, 177
neonatal death and, 5
neurological problems, 175–6
oxygen therapy, 177
patent ductus arteriosus, 316, 322
perinatal asphyxia and, 174
periventricular leukomalacia, 386
prognosis, 177–8
psychosocial problems, 177
renal problems, 176
respiratory distress, 175, 181, 183
respiratory tract infection, 263
thyroid hormones and, 468, 469
vitamin K and, 176
Primaquine, 227, 360
Primary ciliary dyskinesia, 277
Primordial dwarfs, 143
Probenecid, 638
Procainamide, 401, 638
Procarbazine, 367
Prochlorperazine, 642
Prognathism, 46
Programme of Aids for Disabled People
    (PADP), 121
Proliferative periostitis, 616
Promethazine, 571, 642
Promotors, 34, 37
Propionic acidaemia, 212
Propranolol, 327, 472, 503
Propylthiouracil, 472
Prostaglandins, 325, 326
Protein C, 352, 353
Protein, dietary, 90
  absorption, 517
  digestion, 515–7
  primary malabsorption, 524
Protein losing enteropathy, 521
Protein S, 352, 353
Proteus, 206
Prothrombin time, 351
Prune belly syndrome, 432, 498
Pseudobulbar palsy, 141
Pseudophedrine, 265, 600, 606
Pseudohermaphroditism
  female, 375
  male, 476

Pseudohypoparathyroidism, 490, 612
Pseudomonas, 184, 318, 433, 606
  bone/joint infection, 228
  respiratory tract infection, 297
Psittacosis, 245
Psoriasis, 565, 570
  arthropathy, 626
Psychiatric disorders, 550–4
  classification, 550
  epidemiology, 550
  genetic counselling, 55
Psychogenic vomiting, 55
Psychological problems, 7
  post-traumatic, 108
Psychosis, 543
Psychosocial dwarfism, 456
Ptosis, 593
Puberty, 63, 454, 556
  delayed, 456, 559
  diabetes mellitus and, 484
  growth and, 453, 454–5
  precocious, 458
Pulmonary air leaks, 183, 184–5
Pulmonary atresia, 329
Pulmonary function tests, 293–4
Pulmonary haemorrhage, 186, 188
  small-for-gestational-age infant, 179
Pulmonary hypertension, 308, 322, 323
Pulmonary interstitial emphysema, 183,
    184, 188, 189
Pulmonary oedema, 188, 189, 274
Pulmonary stenosis, 316, 320, 323–4
  ejection click, 308, 324
  murmur, 307, 313, 324
  second heart sound, 308
  treatment, 324
Pulse, 64
Purine nucleoside phosphorylase
    deficiency, 161
Purpura fulminans, 352, 353
Pustular melanosis, transient neonatal, 566
Pustules, neonatal, 565–6
Pyelonephritis, 333, 502, 529
Pyloric stenosis, 56, 142, 195, 424, 428,
    501
  rehydration/electrolyte balance, 426–7
Pylorospasm, 142, 501
Pyomyositis, 640
Pyrantel embonate, 641
Pyrazinamide, 303
Pyrexia of unknown origin (PUO), 244–7
  autoimmune disease, 246, 247
  connective tissue disease, 246, 247
  history, 244–5
  infection, 245–6
  malignant disease, 247
  physical examination, 245
Pyridoxine, 376, 537, 638
Pyridoxine-dependency, 212, 376, 378, 393
Pyrimethamine, 203
Pyruvate carboxylase deficiency, 212
Pyruvate dehydrogenase deficiency, 208,
    212
Pyruvate kinase deficiency, 195, 340

Quinine, 227, 350, 401, 638
Quinsy, 602

Rabies, 99
Radiation
  genetic counselling following exposure,
    55
  teratogenic effects, 24
  therapy, 350, 367, 368, 369, 371
Radiography
  congenital dislocation of hip, 73
  trauma, 76
Ragweed pollen dermatitis, 570
Reaction arthritis, 626
Recombinant DNA technology, 38–40
  cDNA analysis, 39
  gene product synthesis, 40
  gene therapy, 40
  mutant gene/protein product location, 40
  restriction fragment length
    polymorphisms (RFLP), 39–40
Recommended Dietary Intakes (RDIs), 90,
    91
Records, genetic counselling and, 57, 58
Rectal drug absorption, 634–5
Rectal examination, 66
Rectal trauma, child sexual abuse and, 149
5-α Reductase deficiency, 477
Reflex hypoxic seizures, 379
Reflexes
  infants, 65
  primitive, 66, 67
Reflux nephropathy, 436, 441, 442
Reflux oesophagitis, 530
  cerebral palsy and, 389
Refractive error measurement, 593
Re-implantation of avulsed tooth, 617
Reiter's disease, 626
Renal agenesis, 430, 498
Renal anomaly, congenital, 245
Renal artery stenosis, 442
Renal calculi, 490
Renal colic, 529
Renal disease, 334, 335, 503
  acute failure, 424
    fluid/electrolyte correction, 427
  acidosis and, 269
  anaemia and, 36
  chronic, 97, 117, 333, 430, 431, 438,
    440, 441–2, 580, 582, 635
    growth and, 456, 458
    hypertension and, 316
    management, 441
    reflux nephropathy and, 434
  failure-to-thrive and, 142–3
  neonatal, 498
  tubular disorders, 142, 436, 498
Renal dysplasia, 430
Renal function
  preterm infant, 176
  water/electrolyte balance, 423–4
Renal isotope scan, 435
Renal osteodystrophy, 492

Renal transplant, 431, 438, 439, 441, 442
Renal tubular acidosis, 436
Rendu-Osler-Weber disease, 583
Renin, 424
Research
  ethical aspects, 12, 15–16
  NH&MRC principles, 16
Resource allocation, 13, 14
Respiratory disease
  chronic, 117, 133
  vitamin A deficiency and, 95
Respiratory distress, neonatal, 181–90, 182
  acid-base studies, 189–90
  antibiotics, 190
  causes, 181
  clinical features, 181
  fluid replacement and, 189
  investigations, 181
  oxygen therapy, 189
  physiotherapy, 190
  sepsis and, 206
  support for parents, 190
  supportive care, 189
Respiratory syncytial virus (RSV)
  infection, 262, 263, 265, 266, 267,
  269, 270, 276, 279
Respiratory system examination, 64–5
Respiratory tract infection, 6, 7, 261–4,
  265–74
  age and, 261, 262–3
  atmospheric pollution and, 263–4
  atopy and, 263
  classification, 261
  exposure and, 263
  failure-to-thrive and, 143
  gestational age and, 263
  heart failure and, 315
  immune function and, 263
  immunodeficiency and, 158, 159
  incidence, 261
  maternal care and, 262, 263, 264
  obesity and, 263
  parental smoking and, 262, 263, 264
  pathogens, 262–3
  persistent cough and, 295
  prevention, 264
  sex, hospital admissions and, 263
  social class and, 262, 263
Restriction enzymes, 38–9
Restriction fragment length polymorphism
  (RFLP) analysis, 39–40
  prenatal diagnosis, 43
Resuscitation see Collapse
Reticuloendothelial malignancy, 350
Reticulosis, 336
Retinal disease, 597–8
  non-inflammatory, 597
Retinal haemorrhage, child abuse and, 147
Retinitis pigmentosa, 597
Retinoblastoma, 371, 597–8
Retinopathy of prematurity (ROP) see
  Retrolental fibroplasia
Retrognathia, 46

Retrolental fibroplasia, 120, 177, 183, 189,
  389, 597
Retrovirus infection, 621
Rett's syndrome, 392
Reye's syndrome, 242, 408, 503, 625, 640
Rhabdomyolysis, 395, 398
Rhabdomyosarcoma, 369
Rhesus incompatability, 193, 194, 196,
  340, 498, 532, 604
  amniocentesis and, 42
Rheumatic fever, 223, 233, 266, 317–8,
  585, 621
  clinical features, 317–8
  genetic susceptibility, 317
  treatment, 318
Rheumatic heart disease, 316
Rheumatoid arthritis, 273
Rhinitis
  acute viral, 599
  allergic, 600
    seasonal (hay fever), 163, 164–5
  bacterial, 599
  vasomotor, 600
Rhinoviruses, 262, 265, 266, 267
Rhus (poison ivy) dermatitis, 570
Rickets, 65, 491–2
  anticonvulsants and, 492
  causes, 491
  clinical features, 491
  preterm infant, 177
  primary hypophosphataemia, 436
  renal, 492
  treatment, 491–2
  vitamin D deficiency, 491
  X-linked hypophosphataemia, 492
Rifampicin, 161, 239, 303, 634, 537, 642
Riga Fede ulceration, 617
Rights, minors', 12, 13, 85
Risk estimation, 56–7
RNA polymerase I, 34
Road trauma, 6, 103, 105–6
  bicycle accidents, 106
  pedestrian run-downs, 105
  secular trends, 105
  vehicle occupants, 106
    fatality prevention, 109
Roseola infantum, 220
Rose river virus, 627
Rotavirus gastroenteritis, 505–6, 508
  carbohydrate intolerance following, 523
  vaccine, 509
Rubella, 128, 195, 533, 583
  arthralgia and, 233, 627
  clinical features, 219
  complications, 291
  diagnosis, 219–20
  intra-uterine, 21, 24, 119, 143, 200–1,
  448, 594, 604, 612
  vaccination, 99, 100, 102, 201, 220, 223
Rumination, 501
Russell Silver syndrome, 408, 613

Sacral agenesis, 416
Safety legislation, 110
Salbutamol, 78, 257, 301, 642
Salicylates, 192, 318, 350, 529, 579
  poisoning, 269, 429
  Reye's syndrome and, 242
Salmon patches (stork bites), 565
Salmonella, 206, 506, 512, 626
  osteomyelitis, 228
Salmonella typhii, 225, 226
Salt, dietary, 93
San Filippo syndrome, 49, 212
Sarcoidosis, 273, 627
Sarcoma
  bone, 363, 369
  soft tissue, 363, 369
Sarcoptes scabiei, 574
Sauna baths, 25
Scabies, 574–6
Scarlet fever, 223, 352
Scheuermann's disease, 76
Schizencephaly, 385
Schizophrenia, 550, 554
School medical service, 88
School refusal, 549
Schwachman-Diamond syndrome, 520,
  524, 525
Schwartz-Jampel syndrome, 401
Sclerema neonatorum, 586
Scleroderma, 576, 582, 629
Scoliosis, 74–5, 389, 395
  intra-uterine packaging defect, 69
Scurvy, 95–6, 350, 352, 579
Seasonal conjunctivitis, acute, 165
Seasonal vernal keratoconjunctivitis, 165
Seasonal rhinitis (hayfever), 163, 164–5
Sebaceous gland hypertrophy, 566
Sebaceous naevi, 586
Seborrhoeic dermatitis, 565, 566, 568
Senna, 643
Separation
  anxiety, 68, 545, 548–9
    disorder, 549
  depression and, 553
Septate uterus, 19
Septic arthritis, 640
Septicaemia, 158, 351, 376
  meningitis following, 235
  neonatal, 205–7, 208, 209, 211, 498
    clinical features, 206
    diagnosis, 206
    jaundice and, 195, 197, 532, 533, 534
    osteomyelitis and, 228, 229
    pathogens, 205, 206
    source, 205
    treatment, 206–7
    pallor and, 333, 334
    skin bleeding and, 579
    subacute, 245
Sequestered lung, 297
Serratia infection, 161
Severe combined immunodeficiency,
  159–60
  antenatal diagnosis, 160

marrow transplant, 160
Sexual differentiation, 474–5
  aberrant in female, 475
  aberrant in male, 475–6
Sexually transmitted disease, 560
  child sexual abuse and, 149
Sheridan Gardiner test, 591
Shigella infection, 233, 506, 626
Shock, 333
  diabetes mellitus and, 481, 482
  fluid replacement, 427
  meningococcaemia and, 236, 237, 256
  neonate, 73
Short stature, 24, 45, 50–2, 143, 336,
    455–8, 522, 531
  case histories, 461–3
  causes, 455–7
  chronic disease and, 456, 458
  constitutional delayed puberty, 456
  definition, 455
  dysmorphic syndromes and, 456
  endocrine disorders and, 456–7
  examination and, 457–8
  genetic aspects, 455–6
  history and, 457
  immunodeficiency and, 157
  indications for investigation, 458
  low birth weight and, 456
  nutritional disorder and, 456, 458
  persistent cough and, 456, 458
  skeletal disorders and, 456
Sick euthyroid syndrome, 468, 469
Sickle cell disease, 220, 228, 236, 336,
    360–2, 529, 531
  anaemia, 361–2
    clinical features, 361
    crises, 361, 362
    pathophysiology, 361
  cDNA probe diagnosis, 39
  haemoglobin S, 37, 360–1
  trait, 361
Sickle thalassaemia, 362
Single base substitutions, 39
Single parent families, 86, 88, 89, 129,
    130–1
  children's problems, 131
  epidemiological aspects, 130
  Family Assistance Payments, 137
  financial problems, 130
  housing, 130–1
  social problems, 131
Single ventricle, 326
Sinuses, developmental aspects, 599
Sinusitis, acute, 599–600
  complications, 600
Skin disorders, 567
  Aboriginal children, 133
  acne, 576–7
  drug-associated, 579
    angiomas, 583
    pigmentation and, 579–82
  examination, 567
  infection, 7
    bacterial, 572–3

viral, 573–4
  inflammatory, 567–71
  inherited, 577–8
  parasitic, 574–6
  photosensitive, 571–3
  systemic disease, 579–87
    skin bleeding and, 579
Skull fracture, child abuse and, 146
'Slapped cheek' syndrome, 220
Sleep apnoea, 602–3
Sleep disturbance, 544–5
  medication and, 545
Slipped femoral epiphysis, 76
Slow-acting antirheumatic drugs
    (SAARDS), 625
Slow virus infection, 241–2
Small bowel biopsy, 521
  coeliac disease, 522
Small-for-gestational-age infant, 5, 6, 140,
    173, 178–80, 186, 193, 448, 498
  aetiology, 178–9
  complications, 179
  head enlargement and, 408
  incidence, 178
  iron deficiency anaemia, 336
  posthaemorrhagic hydrocephalus and,
    409
  postnatal growth failure and, 143
  prognosis, 179–80
  short stature and, 456
  spastic cerebral palsy and, 386
  trisomies and, 43
Smallpox vaccine, 99
Smoking, 25, 128, 561, 301
  low birthweight and, 62
  respiratory tract infections and, 262, 263,
    264
Snakebite, 108
Social class
  classification, 8
  respiratory tract infections and, 262, 263
Social history taking, 63
Socialization needs, 85, 86
Sodium cromoglycate, 164, 165
Sodium metabisulphite-precipitated
    asthma, 166
Sodium valproate, 21, 377, 379, 380, 381,
    384, 529, 536
Solar urticaria, 571
Solid tumours, 368–9
Solvent abuse, 552, 561
Somatic cell mutations, 38
Somatoform disorders, 551
Somatomedins (insulin-like growth
    factors), 448, 449, 450–1
Sotos syndrome, 126, 459
Southern Blot analysis, 39
Spas, 25
Spastic cerebral palsy, 386–7
  aetiology, 386
  clinical features, 386–7
Spastic diplegia, 183, 387
Spastic quadriparesis, 183, 385, 387, 389
Special benefit, 138

Spherocytosis, hereditary, 20, 195, 220,
    336, 340-1
Spina bifida, 7, 12, 41, 43, 56, 65, 67, 117,
    414–6, 432, 547, 559
  meningocele, 414, 416
  myelomeningocele see
    Myelomeningocele, 414, 415–6
  oculta, 413
Spinal cord lesion, 64, 65
Spinal cord tumour, 391, 393
Spinal injury, sports and, 108
Spinal muscular atrophy, 396–7
  chronic, 394, 396–7
  infantile, 396
Spinal posture, 69
Spiramycin, 203
Spirometry, 294
Spironolactone, 438
Splenectomy, 162, 353
Splenomegaly, 350
Sports injury, 108
Squint (strabismus), 591–2, 593
  corneal reflections, 592
  cover test, 592
  definition, 591
  inspection, 591–2
  management, 594–5
Staphylococcal infection, 184, 411, 440,
    481, 579, 595
Staphylococcal scalded skin syndrome, 572
Staphylococcus albus, 228, 318
Staphylococcus aureus, 158, 161, 205, 217,
    318, 411, 566, 567, 572, 585, 606,
    616
  bone/joint infection, 228, 231, 232, 234
  pneumonia, 262, 269, 271–2, 297
Status epilepticus, 376, 380
  absence, 381
Steatorrhoea, 142
Steinert's disease (myotonic dystrophy),
    43, 401
Sternomastoid tumour, 75
Steven-Johnson syndrome, 435, 436, 585
Stilboestrol, 638
Stillbirth, 3, 55, 58
Still's disease, 622
Stokes-Adams attacks, 319
STORCH infection, 196
  jaundice and, 195
Strabismus see Squint
Streptococcal infection, 245, 411, 566,
    570, 606
  diffuse lung disease, 273
  rheumatic fever and, 317, 318
Streptococcus group B, 184, 195, 228, 229,
    232, 533, 572, 635
  antenatal screening, 206
  bone/joint, 228, 232
  meningitis, 235
    detection in CSF, 237
  neonatal sepsis, 205, 206, 207
  scarlet fever and, 223
  tonsillitis/pharyngitis, 262, 265, 266

Streptococcus pneumoniae (Pneumococcus), 158, 162, 217, 353, 440, 528, 579, 595, 606, 635
  antibody formation to polysaccharide antigen, 156
  meningitis, 235, 236, 238
    contacts and, 239
    detection in CSF, 237
    mortality, 239
    pneumonia, 262, 269, 271, 272
    vaccine, 99, 162, 236, 359
Streptococcus pyogenes, 572, 599
Streptococcus viridans, 318
Streptomycin, 642
Stress reactions, 129
Stridor, 603
Sturge-Weber syndrome, 378, 583
Stuttering, 546
Stye, 596
Sub-acute sclerosing panencephalitis, 218–9, 241, 392
Subaortic stenosis, 307, 324
Subcutaneous fat necrosis, 586
Subdural haematoma, 386, 408, 498, 503
  child abuse and, 147
Subglottic haemangioma, 277
Subglottic stenosis, 190, 603
Sucking reflex, 67
Sucralfate, 530
Sucrase-isomaltase deficiency, 510, 519
Sudden infant death syndrome (SIDS)
  aetiology, 9
  age and, 9
  incidence, 5–6, 8
  monitoring and, 9
  near misses, 9–10
  parent support, 9
  risk factors, 9
Sugar intolerance, 508, 509, 510
Suicide/attempted suicide, 503, 504, 543, 553, 557, 561, 639
  management, 553
Sulphacetamide, 595
Sulphadiazine, 641
Sulphadoxine, 203
Sulphasalazine, 511, 512, 625
Sulphonamides, 192, 196, 338, 576, 627, 638, 640
Support groups, handicap and, 121
Supporting parents benefit, 138
Suppurative lung disease, 279
Suprapubic aspiration of urine, 433, 434
Surfactant, 181, 183
Sweat test, 521
Sydenham's chorea, 317
Syndactyly, 20
  toes, 72
Syndromes
  aetiology, 19, 20, 45
  computerized databases, 47
  diagnosis, 47
  see also Dysmorphic syndromes
Synovitis
  thorn, 233, 234

tubercular, 233, 234
Syphilis, 195, 201–2, 438, 533, 604, 612
  antenatal screening, 201
  clinical features, 201
  diagnosis, 201
  teratogenicity, 24
  treatment, 201–2
Systemic lupus erythematosus, 155, 161, 273, 319, 350, 353, 536, 571, 572, 626, 627–8
  aetiology, 621, 627
  clinical features, 627–8
    CNS, 628
    musculoskeletal, 627
    renal, 441, 627–628
    skin, 583–4, 585
  diagnosis, 628
  incidence, 621, 627
  management, 628
  neonatal syndrome, 566, 629

Takayasu's arteritis, 630
Talipes calcaneovalgus, 69
Talipes equinovarus (club foot), 56, 69, 74
Tall stature, 52–3, 458–9, 461
  associated syndromes, 459
  case histories, 463–5
  cerebral gigantism and, 459
  definition, 458
  examination, 459
  genetic aspects, 458
  history and, 459
  indications for examination, 459, 461
  large size in newborn and, 458–9
  oestrogen therapy and, 459, 461
  precocious puberty and, 458, 461
Tay Sachs' disease, 20, 213, 378, 392
Tear duct blockage, 596
Teeth, 610–7
  developmental aspects, 610
    abnormalities, 611–3
  eruption, 611
  natal/neonatal, 67, 610
  re-implantation, 617
  structural aspects, 610
  trauma, 616–7
Teething, 7, 611
Temper tantrums, 545–6
Temporal lobe epilepsy, 382–3
  behaviour problems and, 383
Temporomandibular joint pain/dysfunction, 617
Teratogenesis, 21, 22–5, 45
  agents, 23–5
  animal studies, 22
  detection methods, 22–3
  dose and, 22
  genetic aspects, 22, 55
  male parent and, 22
  mechanisms, 22
  timing and, 22
Teratoma, 278, 369

Terbutaline, 642
Terfenadine, 164
Terminators, 34
Testicular feminization, 477
Testicular torsion, 529
Testosterone
  biosynthesis defects, 476
  growth and, 451
  sexual differentiation and, 474, 475
Tetanus immunization, 87, 99, 100, 102, 617
Tetracyclines, 204, 576, 595, 612, 634, 640
  intoxication, 408
Tetralogy of Fallot, 308, 313, 320, 326–7
  clinical features, 326–7
  course, 327
  differential diagnosis, 327
  investigations, 327
  repair, 316, 327
Thalassaemia, 335, 336, 337, 353, 357
  alpha, 360
    cDNA probe diagnosis, 39
    molecular basis, 38
    silent form, 360
    trait, 360
  antenatal diagnosis, 40, 43
  beta major, 7, 333, 358–60, 340, 346
    chelation therapy, 359
    clinical features, 317, 358–9
    diagnosis, 359
    management, 359
    molecular basis, 37
    pathophysiology, 358
    prognosis, 359
  beta minor (ß thalassaemia trait), 341, 346, 358
  definition, 37, 38, 357–8
  haemoglobin H, 340, 341
  intermedia, 359
  RFLP analysis, 40
Thalidomide, 21, 22, 24, 604
Theophyllines, 175, 287, 289, 290, 626, 627, 633, 642
Thiazide diuretics, 638
Thiobendazole, 641
Thiopentone, 256, 377
Third and fourth arch syndrome, 161
Thirst, 423
Thomas heels, 72
Thomsen's disease, 401
Thrombocytopenia, 349, 351, 352
  secondary, 353
Thrombocytopenic purpura, 350
Thumb sucking, 549, 577, 613
Thyroid, 467
  cancer 473
  congenital absence, 468
  control of secretion, 467
  ectopic, 468, 470
  enzyme defect, 468, 470
  developmental aspects, 467
  function tests, 468, 469
  nodules, 473

Thyroid-binding globulin (TBG) deficiency, 468, 469
Thyroiditis, chronic lymphocytic (Hashimoto's), 470, 471
Thyroid-stimulating hormone (TSH), 467, 468, 469
Thyrotropin-regulating hormone, 467
Thyroxine (T₄), 467, 469
  growth and, 448, 449, 451
  iodine metabolism and, 467
  serum binding protein, 467
  serum levels, 468
  synthesis, 467
Thyroxine (T₄), replacement therapy, 469, 470, 471
Ticarcillin, 190, 641
Tics, 546
Tinea capitis, 754
Tinea corporis, 754
Tinea versicolour, 576
Tinidazole, 523
Tinnitus, 609
TM-26, 369
Tobramycin, 190, 637, 641
Toddler diarrhoea, 509–10
Toddler groups, 89
Toe walking, 395, 397
Tongue thrust, 613
Tongue tie, 613
Tonsillitis, 261, 265–6, 602, 639, 500
  complications, 602
  pathogens, 262
  treatment, 266
Tonsils, 601
  tumour, 603
Toroplasma, 223
Torticollis, sternomastoid, 75
Torula, 246, 405
Tourette's disorder, 546
Toxic erythema, 565–6
Toxic shock syndrome, 585
Toxoplasmosis, 24, 143, 195, 202–3, 245, 376, 385, 533, 604
  clinical features, 202–3
  incidence, 202
  treatment, 203
Tracheal stenosis, 277
Tracheomalacia, 277, 297
Tracheo-oesophageal fistula, 187, 276, 297, 603
  treatment, 187–8
Trachoma, 595
  Aboriginal children, 133
Traction alopecia, 577
Transcription, genetic, 26, 34
Transferrin, 342
Transient erythroblastopenic anaemia of childhood, 339
Transient familial neonatal hyperbilirubinaemia, 195
Transient hypogammaglobulinaemia of infancy, 159
Transient tachypnoea of newborn (TTN), 181

Transitional foods, 93, 95
Translation, genetic, 26
Translocation, 47
  chromosome staining techniques and, 57
  genetic counselling and, 55, 56–7
  prenatal testing, 43
  trisomy 21 and, 48
Transposition of the great arteries, 313, 314, 320, 326, 327, 328
  clinical features, 328
  heart block following correction, 319
  investigations, 328
  treatment, 316, 318
Trauma, 7, 76, 103–10
  causes, 103, 108
  child mortality and, 6, 103, 104–5, 557
  deafness and, 604
  follow-up, 108
  morbidity, 103–4
  nasal, 600
  ocular, 598
  prevention, 108–10
    design improvement, 104, 109–10
    education, 104, 107, 109
    safety legislation, 104, 110
  secular trends, 104–5
  teeth/oral soft tissue, 616–7
Treponema pallidum, 201
Trichotillomania, 577
Tricuspid atresia, 328
Tricyclic antidepressants, 547, 549
Tri-iodothyronine (T₃), 467, 468, 469
Trimeprazine, 642, 643
Trimethadione, 338
Trimethoprim, 595
Triplegia, 388
Trisomies, 19, 28–9, 456
  meiotic non-dysjunction and, 28
  parental age and, 20
  prenatal diagnosis, 43
Trisomy 13, 49, 54, 143
Trisomy 18, 48–9, 143
Trisomy 21 (Down syndrome), 12, 15, 19, 29, 45, 47–8, 123, 125, 143, 364, 402, 456, 498, 565, 594, 611
  associated malformations, 43
  clinical features, 47–8
  counselling on risk, 43
  epidemiological risk figures, 43
  genetic aspects, 48, 125
  incidence, 47, 125
  intellectual disability, 125
  maternal age and, 20, 125
  prenatal diagnosis, 41, 43, 48
  prognosis, 48, 125
Tuberculosis, 143, 219, 245, 246, 273, 293, 295, 301–3, 393, 512, 531, 627
  BCG immunization and, 303
  bronchial compression by hilar lymph nodes, 281, 282, 295
  cerebral, 405
  diagnosis, 302
  infection, 301
  meningitis, 246, 303, 503

  primary complex, 302
  social factors and, 302, 303
  spread, 302
  synovitis, 233, 234
  treatment, 302–3, 640
  tuberculin test and, 302
Tuberose sclerosis, 57, 126, 378, 581, 587, 612
Turner syndrome, 50, 143–4, 447, 451, 456, 476
Twenty-nail dystrophy, 577
Twin-to-twin transfusion, 344
Tympanic membrane perforation
  otitis media and, 606, 608
  traumatic, 608
Tympanometry, 607
Typhoid, 225–6, 245, 579, 639, 640
  chronic carriage, 225, 226
  clinical features, 225–6
  diagnosis, 226
  relapse, 226
  treatment, 226
  vaccine, 509
Typhus, 245, 579

Ulcerative colitis, 143, 233, 510–11, 524, 626
Ultrasound
  biliary obstruction and, 533
  birth defect detection, 41, 42, 43, 44, 51
  hydrocephalus and, 406–7
  urinary obstruction and, 431
  vesicoureteric reflux and, 435
Unemployment benefit, 138
Upper airways obstruction, 190–91
Upper motor neurone lesion, 65
Uraemia, 352
Urea cycle defects, 209, 210, 211–12
  diagnosis, 212
  presentation, 211–12
Ureaplasma arthritis, 158
Uridyl diphosphate glucuronyl transferase (UDPGT), 193
Uridyl diphosphate glucuronyl transferase (UDPGT) deficiency, 195
Urinary tract calculi, 432
Urinary tract infection, 245, 334, 431, 432–4, 500, 503, 547
  clinical presentation, 432
  diagnosis, 433
  epidemiology, 433
  failure-to-thrive and, 142
  treatment, 434
  urine sample collection, 433–4
  vesicoureteric reflux and, 434, 435
  vomiting and, 142
Urinary tract malformation, 430–2
Urinary tract obstruction, 153, 431–2, 436
Urine collection methods, 433–4
Urine metabolic screen, 47
Urine tests, 67
  antigens, 237, 271
Urticaria, 168–9, 570–1

Utilitarianism, 14
Uveitis, 596–7

Vaccines, 99, 100
Vaginal adenocarcinoma, 20
Vaginal discharge, child sexual abuse and, 149
Varicella (chickenpox), 160, 203, 220–1, 242, 273, 352, 585
  clinical features, 220–1
  congenital, 203–4
    prophylaxis, 204
  encephalitis complicating, 221, 240
  herpes zoster and, 221
  myelitis complicating, 241
  pneumonia, 221
  vaccination, 221
Vascular ring, 190, 191, 277
VATER association, 49–50
Vein of Galen aneurysm, 405
Venereal Disease Research Laboratory (VDRL) test, 201, 202
Venezuela equine encephalitis, 24
Venous hum, 307, 308
Ventricular arrhythmias, 319
Ventricular septal defect, 313, 316, 320, 321–2, 324, 326, 327
  bronchial compression and, 277
  closure, 316, 322
  murmur, 307, 313, 321, 322
Vernal keratoconjunctivitis, 165
Vertigo, 609
Very low birth weight baby, 118, 124, 612
  ethical aspects, 12, 13
  feeding difficulties, 142
  impairment and, 7, 178
  neonatal death and, 173
Vesicles, skin, 585–6
Vesicoureteric reflux, 245, 432, 434–6
  infection and, 434, 435
  investigations, 435
  management, 435–6
Vidarabine, 594
Vincent's infection, 615
Vincristine, 365, 368, 369, 428
Vipyrium embonate, 641
Virilization, 475
Visceral larva migrans, 245
Visual assessment, 114, 591
  at school, 88
  intellectual disability and, 124
  refractive error measurement, 593
Visual impairment, 77, 119–20, 392, 597
  aetiology, 120
  cerebral palsy, 389
  definition, 120
  diagnosis, 120
  education system and, 120
  following meningitis, 239
  intellectual disability and, 117, 126
  invalid pension, 138
  learning difficulty and, 113
  management, 120

with multiple impairment, 120
nervous system tumour and, 391
prevalence, 120
very low birth weight and, 7
Visual perceptual motor function problems, 112
Visual sequencing problems, 112
Vitamin A
  deficiency, 95
  intoxication, 408
Vitamin B_{12} deficiency, 336, 520, 521
Vitamin B group deficiency, 95
Vitamin C deficiency, 95–6
Vitamin D
  calcium metabolism and, 488–9, 517
  deficiency, 491
Vitamin K, 176, 643
Vitamins, 90
  absorption, 517
  deficiency, 393
Vitiligo, 576, 582
Vocal cord
  abuse, 603–4
  paralysis, 190
Vomiting, 334, 497–504
  failure-to-thrive and, 142
  infants, 7, 500–3
  neonate, 7, 497–500
  older children, 503–4
Von Hippel-Landau haemangioma, 583
Von Recklinghausen's neurofibromatosis, 580–1, 585
Von Willebrand's disease, 349, 350, 351, 353, 355–6
  diagnosis, 355
  treatment, 355–6

Walking reflex, 67
Warfarin, 22, 24
Warts, 573
Water
  absorption, 518
  balance, 421–2, 423
    abnormality, 424
    control of, 423–4
  daily maintenance requirement, 422
  distribution, 421
Weaning, 95
Wegener's granulomatosis, 273, 630
Werding-Hoffman spinal muscular atrophy, 142, 396, 402
West's syndrome see Infantile spasms
Wheezing, 275–82
  airflow in large airway and, 275
  airways malformation and, 277
  causes, 275–6
  infants, 276–9
    assessment, 279
  large airways obstruction, 277–8, 279–81, 282
  mediastinal cyst/tumour, 277–8
  preschool children, 279–81
  school-age children, 281–2

small airways obstruction, 276–7, 279, 281–2
vascular malformations and, 277
see also Asthma
Widow's benefits, 137
Widow's pension, 130, 137
Wilson-Mikity syndrome, 177, 189
Wilson's disease, 392, 393, 536, 537
Wiskott-Aldrich syndrome, 161, 350, 364, 586
Wolff-Parkinson-White syndrome, 319

X chromosome, 30
Xanthomas, 585
Xeroderma pigmentosum, 571, 578
  antenatal diagnosis, 578
Xerophthalmia, 95
X-linked agammaglobulinaemia, 158
X-linked hydrocephalus, 44
X-linked hypophosphataemia, 492
X-linked inheritance, 29, 30–1
XO see Turner syndrome
XXX syndrome, 459
47XXY see Klinefelter syndrome
XYY syndrome, 459

Y chromosome, 30
Yellow fever, 99
  vaccine, 102
Yersinia infection, 233, 512, 626

Zellweger syndrome, 47, 210
Zinc deficiency, 162, 517, 586
Zoster immunoglobulin (ZIG), 204, 221